Infectious Disease Surveillance

This book is dedicated with appreciation to all frontline public health
practitioners who carry out public health surveillance as the
first critical step in protecting communities from infectious diseases.

Infectious Disease Surveillance

First Edition

Nkuchia M. M'ikanatha
Division of Infectious Disease Epidemiology
Pennsylvania Department of Health
Harrisburg, Pennsylvania
USA

Ruth Lynfield
Minnesota Department of Health
St. Paul, Minnesota
USA

Chris A. Van Beneden
National Center for Immunization and Respiratory Diseases
Centers for Disease Control and Prevention
Atlanta, Georgia
USA

Henriette de Valk
Infectious Diseases Department
Institut de Veille Sanitaire (InVS)
Saint Maurice
France

Foreword by Anne Schuchat and Jean-Claude Desenclos

Blackwell
Publishing

© 2007 by Blackwell Publishing

Blackwell Publishing, Inc., 350 Main Street, Malden, Massachusetts 02148-5020, USA
Blackwell Publishing Ltd, 9600 Garsington Road, Oxford OX4 2DQ, UK
Blackwell Publishing Asia Pty Ltd, 550 Swanston Street, Carlton, Victoria 3053, Australia

First published 2007

1   2007

Library of Congress Cataloging-in-Publication Data

Infectious disease surveillance / [edited by] Nkuchia M. M'ikanatha . . .
[et al.]; foreword by Anne Schuchat and Jean-Claude Desenclos. – 1st ed.
        p. ; cm.
    Includes bibliographical references.
    ISBN 978-1-4051-4266-3 (alk. paper)
     1. Communicable diseases.   2. Epidemiology.   3. World health.
I. M'ikanatha Nkuchia M.
    [DNLM: 1. Communicable Disease Control.   2. Disease Outbreaks.   3. Public Health.
4. World Health. WA 110 I43 2007]

    RA643.I6537 2007
    614.5–dc22

                                                                        2007006425

ISBN-13: 978-1-4051-4266-3

A catalogue record for this title is available from the British Library

Set in Sabon 9.5/11.5pt by aptara Inc., New Delhi, India
Printed and bound in Singapore by Fabulous Printers Pte Ltd

Commissioning Editor: Maria Khan
Development Editor: Rebecca Huxley
Editorial Assistant: Jenny Seward
Production Controller: Debbie Wyer

For further information on Blackwell Publishing, visit our website:
http://www.blackwellpublishing.com

Contents

Section II: Use of Electronic and Web-Based Means in Infectious Disease Surveillance

Colour plates are found facing page 26 and page 266

Contributors

Abdel-Nasser Mohammed Abdel Ghaffar
Epidemiology and Surveillance Unit
Preventive Sector
Ministry of Health and Population
Cairo
Egypt

Katherine Ahrens
STD Prevention and Control Services Section
San Francisco Department of Public Health
San Francisco, California
USA

Andrea Ammon
European Centre for Disease Prevention
    and Control (ECDC)
Stockholm
Sweden

Roberta Andraghetti
Department of Epidemic and Pandemic Alert and
    Response
Communicable Diseases Cluster
World Health Organization
Geneva
Switzerland

Frederick J. Angulo
Enteric Diseases Epidemiology Branch
Centers for Disease Control and Prevention
Atlanta, Georgia
USA

Koye Balogun
Immunisation Department
HPA Centre for Infections
London
UK

Robert A. Bednarczyk
Department of Epidemiology and Biostatistics
School of Public Health
University at Albany
Rensselaer, New York
USA

John Besser
Minnesota Department of Health
St. Paul, Minnesota
USA

Guthrie S. Birkhead
Center for Community Health, and AIDS Institute
New York State Department of Health
Albany, New York
USA

Arnold Bosman
Epidemiology and Surveillance Unit
Centre for Infectious Disease Control
National Institute for Public Health
    and the Environment (RIVM)
Bilthoven
The Netherlands

Lynnette Brammer
Influenza Division
Centers for Disease Control and Prevention
Atlanta, Georgia
USA

James W. Buehler
Department of Epidemiology
Center for Public Health Preparedness and Research
Rollins School of Public Health
Emory University
Atlanta, Georgia
USA

Robert T. Chen
Epidemiology Branch
Division of HIV/AIDS Prevention
Centers for Disease Control and Prevention
Atlanta, Georgia
USA

Tom M. Chiller
Division of Foodborne, Bacterial
    and Mycotic Diseases
Centers for Disease Control and Prevention
Atlanta, Georgia
USA

Hermann Claus
Department of Infectious Disease Epidemiology
Robert Koch Institute
Berlin
Germany

Bruno Coignard
Infectious Diseases Department
Institut de Veille Sanitaire (InVS)
Saint Maurice, France

Nancy Cox
Influenza Division
Centers for Disease Control and Prevention
Atlanta, Georgia
USA

Richard N. Danila
Minnesota Department of Health
St. Paul, Minnesota
USA

Jean-Claude Desenclos
Infectious Diseases Department
Institut de Veille Sanitaire (InVS)
Saint Maurice
France

Henriette de Valk
Infectious Diseases Department
Institut de Veille Sanitaire (InVS)
Saint Maurice, France

Renny Fagan
State Services Section
Colorado Department of Law
Denver, Colorado
USA

Amy L. Fairchild
Department of Sociomedical Sciences
Center for the History and Ethics of Public
    Health
Columbia University Mailman School of
    Public Health
New York, New York
USA

Dennis Falzon
EuroTB, Department of Infectious Diseases
Institut de Veille Sanitaire (InVS)
Saint Maurice
France

Marc Fischer
Arboviral Diseases Branch
Division of Vector-Borne Infectious Diseases
Centers for Disease Control and Prevention
Fort Collins, Colorado
USA

Aaron T. Fleischauer
Bioterrorism Preparedness and Response Program
Centers for Disease Control and Prevention
Atlanta, Georgia
USA

Andrew Friede
Constella Group, LLC
Atlanta, Georgia
USA

Petra Gastmeier
Division of Hospital Epidemiology
    and Infection Control
Institute of Medical Microbiology
    and Hospital Epidemiology
Hannover Medical School
Hannover
Germany

Kathryn Gay
Division of Foodborne, Bacterial
  and Mycotic Diseases
Centers for Disease Control and Prevention
Atlanta, Georgia
USA

M. Kathleen Glynn
Division of HIV/AIDS Prevention
Centers for Disease Control and Prevention
Atlanta, Georgia
USA

Fernando González-Martín
International Health Regulations Coordination
  Programme
Epidemic and Pandemic Alert and Response
World Health Organization
Geneva
Switzerland

Richard A. Goodman
Public Health Law Program
Centers for Disease Control and Prevention
Atlanta, Georgia
USA

Samuel L. Groseclose
Division of STD Prevention
Centers for Disease Control and Prevention
Altanta, Georgia
USA

James L. Hadler
Infectious Diseases Section
Connecticut Department of Public Health
Hartford, Connecticut
USA

Rana A. Hajjeh
The Hib Initiative
Johns Hopkins Bloomberg School of Public Health
Baltimore, Maryland; and
The National Center for Immunization
  and Respiratory Diseases
Centers for Disease Control and Prevention
Atlanta, Georgia
USA

Douglas H. Hamilton
Office of Workforce and Career Development
Centers for Disease Control and Prevention
Atlanta, Georgia
USA

Max Hardiman
International Health Regulations Coordination
  Programme
Epidemic and Pandemic Alert and Response
World Health Organization
Geneva
Switzerland

Kathleen Harriman
Minnesota Department of Health
St. Paul, Minnesota
USA

D.A. Henderson
Center for Biosecurity
University of Pittsburgh
Balthimore, Maryland
USA

Joseph M. Hilbe
School of Social and Family Dynamics
Arizona State University
Tempe, Arizona
USA

Richard E. Hoffman
Department of Preventative Medicine and Biometrics
University of Colorado School of Medicine
Denver, Colorado
USA

John H. Holmes
Center for Clinical Epidemiology and Biostatistics
University of Pennsylvania School of Medicine
Philadelphia, Pennsylvania
USA

Teresa Horan
Division of Healthcare Quality Promotion
Centers for the Disease Control and Prevention
Atlanta, Georgia
USA

Richard E. Hoskins
Center for Public Health Informatics
University of Washington
Seattle, Washington
USA

Elmira Ibraim
Marius Nasta Pneumology Institute
Bucharest
Romania

Andrea Infuso
(Deceased)
EuroTB
Institut de Veille Sanitaire (InVS)
Saint Maurice
France

John Iskander
Office of the Chief Science Officer
Centers for Disease Control and Prevention
Altanta, Georgia
USA

Gerald F. Jones
National Center for Public Health Informatics
Division of Integrated Surveillance Systems
    and Services
Centers for Disease Control and Prevention
Atlanta, Georgia
USA

Marian Moser Jones
Department of Sociomedical Sciences
Center for the History and Ethics of Public Health
Columbia University Mailman School of
    Public Health
New York, New York
USA

Kathleen G. Julian
Division of Infectious Diseases
Penn State Milton S. Hershey Medical Center
Hershey, Pennsylvania
USA

Jeffrey D. Klausner
STD Prevention and Control Services Section
San Francisco Department of Public Health
San Francisco, California
USA

R. Monina Klevens
Healthcare Outcomes Branch
Division of Healthcare Quality Promotion
Centers for Disease Control and Prevention
Atlanta, Georgia
USA

Denise Koo
Office of Workforce and Career Development
Centers for Disease Control and Prevention
Atlanta, Georgia
USA

Gérard Krause
Department for Infectious Disease Epidemiology
Robert Koch Institute
Berlin
Germany

Lisa M. Lee
Office of the Chief Science Officer
Centers for Disease Control and Prevention
Atlanta, Georgia
USA

Richard Lemay
Global Public Health Intelligence Network
    (GPHIN)
Center for Emergency Preparedness and Response
Public Health Agency of Canada
Ottawa, Ontario
Canada

Mira J. Leslie
Washington Department of Health
Communicable Disease Epidemiology
Shoreline, Washington
USA

Ruth Lynfield
Minnesota Department of Health
St. Paul, Minnesota
USA

Frank Mahoney
Eastern Mediterranean Regional Office
World Health Organization
Cairo
Egypt

Abla Mawudeku
Global Public Health Intelligence Network (GPHIN)
Center for Emergency Preparedness and Response
Public Health Agency of Canada
Ottawa, Ontario
Canada

Toby McAdams
Minnesota Department of Health
St. Paul, Minnesota
USA

Louise-Anne McNutt
Department of Epidemiology and Biostatistics
School of Public Health
University at Albany
Rensselaer, New York
USA

Jennifer H. McQuiston
Division of Global Migration and Quarantine
Centers for Disease Control and Prevention
Atlanta, Georgia
USA

Nkuchia M. M'ikanatha
Division of Infectious Disease Epidemiology
Pennsylvania Department of Health
Harrisburg, Pennsylvania
USA

Elizabeth Miller
Health Protection Agency (HPA)
Centre for Infections
Epidemiology and Surveillance
London
UK

Eve D. Mokotoff
HIV/STD and Bloodborne Infections Surveillance
    Section
Michigan Department of Community Health
Detroit, Michigan
USA

Chester G. Moore
Arthropod-borne and Infectious Diseases Laboratory
Department of Microbiology, Immunology
    and Pathology
Colorado State University
Fort Collins, Colorado
USA

Matthew R. Moore
National Center for Immunization
    and Respiratory Diseases
Centers for Disease Control and Prevention
Atlanta, Georgia
USA

Alain Moren
Epidemiology Department
Epiconcept
Paris
France

Melissa A. Morrison
Division of Healthcare Quality Promotion
Centers for Disease Control and Prevention
Atlanta, Georgia
USA

Dale L. Morse
Office of Science and Public Health
New York State Department of Health
Empire State Plaza
Albany, New York
USA

Farzad Mostashari
New York City Department of Health
    and Mental Hygiene
New York, New York
USA

Hanna Nohynek
National Public Health Institute (KTL)
Department of Vaccines, Clinical Unit
Helsinki
Finland

Kurt B. Nolte
New Mexico Office of the Medical Investigator
University of New Mexico
Albuquerque, New Mexico
USA

Sonja J. Olsen
Division of Emerging Infections and Surveillance
    Services
Centers for Disease Control and Prevention
Atlanta, Georgia
USA

Umesh D. Parashar
National Center for Immunization and
    Respiratory Diseases
Centers for Disease Control and Prevention
Atlanta, Georgia
USA

Julie A. Pavlin
Uniformed Services University of the Health Sciences
Bethesda, Maryland
USA

Mindy J. Perilla
Center for American Indian Health
Department of International Health
Johns Hopkins Bloomberg School of Public Health
Baltimore, Maryland
USA

Lyle R. Petersen
Division of Vector-Borne Infectious Diseases
Centers for Disease Control and Prevention
Fort Collins, Colorado
USA

Richard Platt
Department of Ambulatory Care and Prevention
Harvard Medical School and Harvard
    Pilgrim Healthcare
Boston, Massachusetts
USA

Bruce J. Plotkin
International Health Regulations Coordination
    Programme
Epidemic and Pandemic Alert and Response
World Health Organization
Geneva
Switzerland

Alicia Postema
Influenza Division
Centers for Disease Control and Prevention
Atlanta, Georgia
USA

Catherine Quigley
Health Protection Agency North West
DBH House
Boundary Street
Liverpool
UK

Mary Ramsay
Immunisation Department
HPA Centre for Infections
London
UK

Sarah Reagan
Unexplained Death Project
Centers for Disease Control and Prevention
Atlanta, Georgia
USA

Guénaël Rodier
International Health Regulations Coordination
    Programme
Epidemic and Pandemic Alert and Response
World Health Organization
Geneva
Switzerland

Dale D. Rohn
Division of Communicable Disease
    Surveillance
Maryland Department of Health
    and Mental Hygiene
Baltimore, Maryland
USA

George W. Rutherford
Institute for Global Health
University of California
San Francisco, California
USA

Michael C. Samuel
STD Control Branch
Division of Communicable Disease Control
California Department of Health Services
Richmond, California
USA

Elaine Scallan
Enteric Diseases Epidemiology Branch
Centers for Disease Control and Prevention
Atlanta, Georgia
USA

Anne Schuchat
National Center for Immunization and
    Respiratory Diseases
Centers for Disease Control and Prevention
Atlanta, Georgia
USA

Edmund Seto
Environmental Health Sciences
School of Public Health
University of California
Berkeley, California
USA

Frederic E. Shaw
Public Health Law Program
Office of the Chief of Public Health Practice
Centers for Disease Control and Prevention
Atlanta, Georgia
USA

Tami H. Skoff
National Center for Immunization
    and Respiratory Diseases
Centers for Disease Control and Prevention
Atlanta, Georgia
USA

Perry F. Smith
Center for Community Heath
New York State Department of Health
Albany, New York
USA

Daniel M. Sosin
Coordinating Office for Terrorism Preparedness
    and Emergency Response
Centers for Disease Control and Prevention
Atlanta, Georgia
USA

Brian G. Southwell
School of Journalism and Mass Communication
University of Minnesota
Minneapolis, Minnesota
USA

Ron St. John
Center for Emergency Preparedness
    and Response
Public Health Agency of Canada
Ottawa, Ontario
Canada

Lauren J. Stockman
National Center for Immunization
    and Respiratory Diseases
Centers for Disease Control and Prevention
Atlanta, Georgia
USA

Maha Talaat
Disease Surveillance Program
US Naval Medical Research Unit, No. 3 (NAMRU-3)
Cairo
Egypt

Stephen B. Thacker
Office for Workforce and Career Development
Centers for Disease Control and Prevention
Atlanta, Georgia
USA

Thomas Tsang
Department of Health
Centre for Health Protection
Hong Kong SAR

Marta Valenciano
Institute Carlos III, EPIET
Centro Nacional de Epidemiologia
Sinesio Delgado
Madrid
Spain

Chris A. Van Beneden
National Center for Immunization and Respiratory
  Diseases
Centers for Disease Control and Prevention
Atlanta, Georgia
USA

Hans van Vliet
Epidemiology and Surveillance Unit
Centre for Infectious Disease Control
National Institute for Public Health and the
  Environment (RIVM)
Bilthoven
The Netherlands

Hillard Weinstock
Division of STD Prevention
Centers for Disease Control and Prevention
Atlanta, Georgia
USA

David P. Welliver
Information Technology Department
Penn State Milton S. Hershey Medical Center
Hershey, Pennsylvania
USA

Denise Werker
Epidemic and Pandemic Response Unit
World Health Organization
Geneva
Switzerland

Jean M. Whichard
Division of Foodborne, Bacterial
  and Mycotic Diseases
Centers for Disease Control and
  Prevention
Atlanta, Georgia
USA

David G. White
US Food and Drug Administration
Center for Veterinary Medicine
Division of Animal and Food Microbiology
Laurel, Maryland
USA

Cynthia G. Whitney
National Center for Immunization and Respiratory
  Diseases
Centers for Disease Control and Prevention
Atlanta, Georgia
USA

Elizabeth R. Zell
National Center for Immunization
  and Respiratory Diseases
Centers for Disease Control and Prevention
Atlanta, Georgia
USA

Foreword

A compendium of infectious disease surveillance must confront both the inevitable and the impossible. As long as the human host and microbial agents occupy the same environment, it is inevitable that infectious diseases will continue to occur and pose real challenges to public health programs and the populations they serve. Unlike classical surveillance for vital statistics, which tracks those constants of the human condition—birth and death—surveillance for infectious diseases tackles the impossibly diverse spectrum of illness that an evolving microbial world sets loose on the human population. In recent years, infectious disease surveillance is increasingly bridging the gap between human and animal worlds in order to track infections in the vectors that play important roles in the emergence and spread of new infectious diseases. Our surveillance systems are now tasked to extend to multiple host species in order to better monitor infectious threats to humans. Additionally, in recent years, authorities are interested in surveillance systems that can anticipate what has not yet happened: identify new infectious agents before they emerge, detect signals of exposure or prodromal symptoms before a disease has become manifest in large numbers of the population. Fortunately, the seemingly impossible scope and standards to which practitioners of surveillance for infectious disease must strive is often matched by innovation and execution equal to these challenges.

This new textbook on infectious disease surveillance features selected best practices and model surveillance programs that are being carried out on a local, state, national, or global scale, to address the infectious disease challenges of the twenty-first century. The book also contains lessons learned from surveillance of the past—in particular, the experience of surveillance targeted against the only infectious disease ever eradicated globally, smallpox. Public health practitioners and students approach infectious disease surveillance from a variety of backgrounds, and must assume a range of responsibilities in carrying out their mandates. For example,

today every public health practitioner has by necessity become a leader in their own community's efforts to prepare for future pandemics of influenza. This textbook can provide a strong grounding in infectious disease surveillance that is vital to these efforts.

Pathogens: Many infectious diseases caused by the major pathogens of the past century are now well controlled in several regions of the world and progress is being made in others—thanks to the advent of effective vaccines, sanitation, infection control, and improvements in food hygiene and nutrition. Surveillance for vaccine-preventable diseases and enteric pathogens highlights some of these success stories and guards against the complacency that can precede resurgences. However, an astounding number of new infectious diseases have emerged in the past 30 years, and some agents of the past such as tuberculosis have reemerged with more severe, multidrug-resistant forms that challenge traditional control programs. Each of these poses some unexpected challenges to surveillance approaches. The emergence of West Nile virus into new regions of the world brought surveillance in insects, birds, and horses into the mainstream of state and local public health efforts. The emergence of drug resistance among bacteria, parasites, and more recently viruses, and the recent diffusion of a new hypervirulent strain of *Clostridium difficile* in hospitals of North America and Europe are just a few timely examples of infectious disease surveillance needs that showcase the interdependence and synergy that occurs when laboratory characterization of strains is linked with epidemiologic analysis of disease patterns. Preparedness for pandemic influenza requires facile and flexible laboratory-based surveillance systems that can span the globe and detect new variants. The number of pathogens of interest to infectious disease surveillance programs is expanding, and the availability and usefulness of detailed pathogen information down to the genetic code has also increased.

People: In addition to the dynamic nature of the microbial world, infectious disease surveillance must address a changing human population. Globalization, increased life expectancy, major expansion of populations suffering from immune suppression (from pathogens like HIV, and from treatments for conditions such as cancer and organ transplantation) have resulted in larger numbers of susceptible people who have ample opportunities to encounter microbes that can do them harm. Add to these forces the often-surprising types of human behavior, and one finds surveillance requirements that may encompass what is personal, private, or at times political. Inclusion of sociological, ethical, and legal aspects of surveillance in a core infectious disease surveillance textbook is clear recognition of the reality that in the twenty-first century the term "surveillance" has taken on increasingly nuanced connotations.

Places: The evolving environment and its interaction with infectious agents, animals, and people play an increasingly recognized role in disease transmission and emerging infections. The places in which people live, travel, work, and recreate encompass very diverse conditions that influence how surveillance should be implemented at various levels. Monitoring the impact on infectious disease of climate change, extension of the range of several vectors of infectious disease such as dengue, West Nile virus, or Chickungunya virus, are among the many new environmental challenges for surveillance and public health response. The healthcare environment continues to serve as a hot bed for infectious disease transmission and requires attention in all countries, including those with limited resources. The 2003 epidemic of severe acute respiratory syndrome (SARS) was characterized by major amplification of the newly recognized SARS coronavirus in the healthcare environment. Sensitive and timely surveillance was vital to the global control of SARS, permitting the effective targeted use of traditional strategies such as infection control, quarantine, and social distancing in order to interrupt transmission.

Processing information: Confronting the need for information that is faster, more granular, and increasingly complex, a huge growth area for innovations in surveillance relates to the technologic processes required to share public health information. From pony express to the information highway, from telegraph to text messaging, technology has the potential to transform infectious disease surveillance. However, the promise is often frustratingly greater than our current realities can deliver. Much of the world's population now lives in a "24/7" media cycle where surveillance data may become dated before they are even issued. Assuring both scientific accuracy and public health relevance in this evolving social environment has always been important to infectious disease surveillance and shall remain so, but increasingly high expectations may become more and more difficult for local, state, or national public health authorities to meet. Despite the opportunities that technological advances have provided to enhance infectious disease surveillance, there have often been political constraints to information sharing of public health data that is construed to threaten tourism, economic, or political interests. However, major changes in the legal framework that underpins communicating urgent public health information to the World Health Organization (WHO) and among nations result from the new WHO International Health Regulations (2005) endorsed by 192 countries at the World Health Assembly in 2005 and scheduled to be implemented in June 2007. These regulations emphasize the need for transparency and timeliness in communicating selected public health events around the world and offer a new global standard for sharing critical surveillance information. This new standard implies, however, that each country develops a critical level of public health surveillance and response capacity to meet the challenges of the new regulations.

Principles: Given the dynamic nature of the pathogens, people, places, and processes associated with infectious disease surveillance, assembling a textbook on this broad subject might be considered an impossible task. Fortunately, the principles underlying surveillance for infectious diseases are surprisingly stable. The common threads woven through the chapters of this book should display to the reader the key principles of why, how, when, and where to employ infectious disease surveillance programs. These principles will serve the public health practitioner well for the foreseeable future. The diverse public health workforce engaged at local, state, national, and international levels in infectious disease surveillance activities can look to this textbook to emphasize the basics for those new to the field and expand horizons for those who have spent careers engaged in one or more aspect of this work.

Anne Schuchat and Jean-Claude Desenclos
July 2007

Preface

High quality national surveillance is the cornerstone of infectious disease prevention and control.
—World Health Organization, 2004

Major challenges to global and national public health systems during the past 30 years arising from both emerging and established pathogens demonstrate the need for reassessment of the commitment to infectious disease surveillance. The critical need for better surveillance became more urgent during the past decade with the threat of bioterrorism and the recognition of the potential for an influenza pandemic. Concurrently, changes in public health information infrastructure, especially the widespread use of computers and Internet-based systems, resulted in ongoing improvements in the conduct of surveillance. In addition, advances in laboratory and epidemiologic methods, including molecular diagnostic tests for organism identification, have expanded the surveillance toolset and knowledge base.

Inspired to support local and national public health efforts in infectious disease surveillance, we have collaborated to create a readily accessible resource inclusive of recent developments in the field. It contains 40 chapters drawn from experiences of over 100 authors involved in implementation of surveillance systems. We acknowledge the disproportionate representation of surveillance systems from North America and Europe, but when possible, we sought to include considerations for surveillance as it may be applied around the world.

We have organized the subjects into four sections based on major themes. Section I begins with an introductory chapter that highlights the critical role surveillance plays in public health and offers an overview of the rest of the book. The second chapter introduces the International Health Regulations (IHR 2005) and its emphasis on international reporting and strengthening surveillance capacities worldwide. The other chapters in the first section describe disease-specific or program-specific surveillance systems, such as foodborne and vector-borne disease surveillance.

Section II explores the use of information technology to advance infectious disease surveillance. The chapters discuss use of the Internet to facilitate disease reporting and dissemination of findings, electronic transfer of surveillance data from laboratories, and data management. Also, novel surveillance systems that use algorithms to assist in detection of cases in electronic laboratory data or use automated analyses to detect temporal and spatial clustering are introduced. Section III presents topics in surveillance methodology, including molecular epidemiology, data analyses, communication with the media and the public, and evaluation of surveillance systems.

Section IV addresses broad topics important in the conduct of public health surveillance for infectious diseases. Chapters discuss ethical considerations, the legal basis for conducting surveillance, and the legal considerations for isolation and quarantine. In addition, examples of surveillance-related training opportunities and partnerships in the private sector are presented. Lastly, Section V concludes with a review of historical lessons learned from application of surveillance in disease control—in the 1970s, smallpox, and more recently in 2003, the severe acute respiratory syndrome or SARS.

It is our hope that this book will serve as a practical guide for surveillance practitioners and key partners; it provides not just conceptual theories, but practical pearls from other practitioners who have been involved in implementation of public health programs. Illustrative examples are provided and referenced for further reading. This book can also serve as a textbook for public health students and for trainees in applied epidemiology and preventive medicine. Lastly, the book may also be of interest to academic and industry researchers in infectious disease and medical informatics.

Finally, we acknowledge with gratitude many individuals who made this book possible through their encouragement and support. In particular, we are indebted to the generosity of the contributors and external reviewers, and the patience and understanding of our families and friends. We are encouraged by the hope that this book, which grew out of the dedication and expertise of many collaborators, will strengthen, even in a small way, current efforts to enhance infectious disease surveillance.

Nkuchia M. M'ikanatha
Ruth Lynfield
Chris Van Beneden
Henriette de Valk
July 2007

Acknowledgments

This book could not have taken shape without the shared vision and work of many people. Over one hundred experts in public health put finger to keyboard at very late hours in order to share their expertise. We are truly grateful for their generosity.

In addition to the authors' labors on their chapters, a number of people put significant effort into reviewing various components of the book. In particular, we thank Sean Altekruse, June Bancroft, James Buehler, Grant (Roy) Campbell, Elliot Churchill, Scott Danos, Scott Dowell, Andrea Forde, Jaclyn Fox, Samuel Groseclose, Lee Harrison, D.A. Henderson, Kathleen Julian, Denise Koo, Sunny Mak, Martin Meltzer, Jennifer Morcone, Bob Pinner, Katherine Robinson, Dale Rohn, Stephen Rosenberry, Kathleen Shutt, Kirk Smith, Perry Smith, Wiley Souba, Brian Strom, Christina Tan, David Welliver, and Jacqueline Wyatt.

We specifically acknowledge Andrea Infuso, then Project Coordinator of EuroTB, who coordinated the surveillance of tuberculosis in the WHO European region based in the Insititut de Veille Sanitaire in St Maurice, France. Dr Infuso was very supportive of this venture. Sadly, he passed away on September 20, 2005. We have dedicated *Surveillance for Tuberculosis in Europe* in his memory.

We are grateful to our colleagues at Blackwell Publishing Ltd for their encouragement and assistance, in particular Maria Khan and Rebecca Huxley.

Finally, we extend our most sincere gratitude to each of our family members and friends who supported our commitment to this project, and enabled it to come to fruition.

Disclaimer

The findings and conclusions in chapters by authors from federal agencies (e.g., Centers for Disease Control and Prevention, Food and Drug Administration) are those of the authors and do not necessarily represent the views of the federal agencies.

Introduction and Program-Area Surveillance Systems

1

Infectious disease surveillance: a cornerstone for prevention and control

Nkuchia M. M'ikanatha, Ruth Lynfield, Kathleen G. Julian, Chris A. Van Beneden & Henriette de Valk

In view of the galloping pace of globalization that is transforming the world into a global village, close international co-operation is essential in the detection, prevention, and control of communicable diseases.

Leung Pak-yin, Centre for Health Protection, Hong Kong [1]

Introduction

Throughout human history, infectious diseases have been a major force—constantly changing in form as new human behaviors pose new risks, old pathogens adapt, and novel pathogens emerge. The widespread availability of vaccines and antibiotics led to a mistaken confidence that infectious diseases had been conquered, as expressed by some United States (US) public health leaders in the late 1960s [2]. In the following decades, this optimism was replaced by a realization of the enormity of infectious disease challenges. New pathogens, including human immunodeficiency virus, have erupted while known pathogens, including drug-resistant tuberculosis and malaria, continue to cause major morbidity and mortality. Globally, infectious diseases are the leading cause of morbidity and the second leading cause of death [2].

The economic consequences associated with infectious diseases are enormous. Even in a small country like England with a population of approximately 50 million persons, the direct cost of treating infectious diseases was estimated to be approximately £6 billion (US$11.5 billion) per year [3]. Disease epidemics can undermine national and even global economic stability. The economic ramifications of the 2003 outbreak of severe acute respiratory syndrome (SARS) were experienced not only in Asian countries, but also globally. Direct and indirect economic costs of SARS have been estimated at US$80 billion [4].

We will demonstrate in this chapter and throughout this book that to confront threats of endemic and emerging pathogens, systematic disease tracking is essential to inform disease prevention and control programs. The successful eradication of smallpox in the twentieth century (see Part 1 of Chapter 39, *The use of surveillance in the eradication of smallpox and poliomyelitis*) is a dramatic example of the central role played by surveillance in guiding disease control (Figure 1.1). Many other important, ongoing achievements in surveillance will be illustrated in this chapter. We will introduce the basic principles of infectious disease surveillance and present a glimpse into the vast array of innovative surveillance systems currently in place. To reinforce key concepts, examples will be chosen from real-life surveillance systems with reference to further details provided in subsequent chapters of this book.

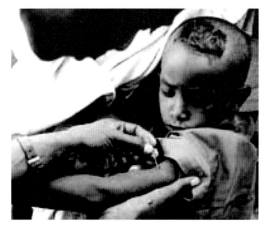

Fig 1.1 A child receiving smallpox vaccine. Surveillance data played a key role in smallpox eradication efforts by guiding vaccination campaigns.

Definition and scope of infectious disease surveillance

General principles of public health surveillance are used in programs to prevent and control infectious disease, chronic disease, and injury, and to insure occupational health. In this book we focus on infectious disease surveillance, primarily as communicable pathogens relate to human health but also with attention to pathogens in the closely interrelated animal realm and environment. The infectious diseases surveillance activities described in this book are primarily carried out by public health authorities or infection control entities in healthcare institutions; however, modern infectious disease surveillance requires collaboration with partners in a variety of fields, including wildlife biology, veterinary medicine, law, and information technology (IT).

The conduct of surveillance can be conceived as a "three-legged stool" consisting of three main integrated activities: (a) systematic collection of pertinent data (e.g., case reports of a specific disease); (b) analyses of these data (e.g., assessing trends in disease occurrences); and (c) timely dissemination of results to guide interventions (e.g., reports to public health teams implementing prevention programs or

to clinicians to guide empiric disease management). The three surveillance "legs" are contained both in the original 1969 *International Health Regulations* and the most recent definition of surveillance as is articulated in the *2005 International Health Regulations* (IHR 2005) [5]. IHR 2005 defines surveillance as "the systematic ongoing collection, collation and analysis of data for public health purposes and the timely dissemination of public health information for assessment and public health response as necessary." These components are considered central to every public health surveillance system and will be revisited in this book as they pertain to specific programs.

Besides the World Health Organization (WHO), local, regional, and national agencies have embraced surveillance as a means to characterize and address endemic and emerging infectious disease threats. Although many of the examples covered in this book are from North America and western Europe, infectious disease surveillance is conducted worldwide, albeit in varying degrees and forms.

What happens in the absence of infectious disease surveillance?

In considering the values of surveillance, it is instructive to ask, "What happens to public health in the absence of surveillance?" Where disease tracking is compromised, as occurs during protracted armed conflicts, previous progress made in disease control efforts can be reversed. For example, Somalia is one country where ongoing conflict has weakened the surveillance infrastructure necessary to identify and interrupt polio virus transmission [6]. Special investigations identified an outbreak of polio in Somalia that, between 2005–2006, resulted in an estimated 217 cases (www.emro.who.int/polio/). The resurgence of polio in one country threatens eradication efforts in neighboring countries.

Lack of surveillance and control programs contribute to resurgence of diseases like human African trypanosomiasis in the Democratic Republic of Congo in the 1990s [7]. Gains made earlier in the century were lost during war and socioeconomic deterioration. By the time public health teams were re-mobilized in 1993–1994, the incidence of trypanosomiasis was found to be 34,400, with neglected areas reporting the highest rates of the century. Impromptu surveillance and disease control measures can be expected to be much more difficult to implement in these and other countries that have suffered long-standing waves of violence and breakdown of the public sector infrastructure. Chapter 20 (*Communicable disease surveillance in complex emergencies*) offers practical considerations for conducting surveillance in complex emergency situations characterized by war or civil strife affecting large civilian populations. Examples are drawn from experiences in Albania, Basrah (Iraq), and the Greater Darfur region (Sudan).

Inadequate surveillance and consequent "blindness" to the health status of the population has contributed to the uncontrolled global spread of the human immunodeficiency virus/acquired immunodeficiency syndrome (HIV/AIDS), one of the worst pandemics in human history. Without accurate surveillance data to understand the true health status of their populations and to guide the use of limited public health resources, leaders can be grossly misinformed and, as in the case of HIV/AIDS, lose opportunities for early prevention and control before the virus becomes entrenched. Stigmatization,

discrimination, and marginalization—all fueled by ignorance—have contributed simultaneously to the denial and, paradoxically, to the explosion of the pandemic. As shown in Figure 1.2, in the 25 years since the first recognition of AIDS in the US, it is estimated that 65 million persons have been infected with HIV and more than 25 million have died of AIDS [8].

Complacency and diversion of resources have hindered maintenance of surveillance systems that are sensitive enough to detect smoldering epidemics. In the US during the mid-1980s, lack of support for tuberculosis surveillance and control is thought to have contributed to the subsequent multi-drug resistant tuberculosis outbreak which emerged in several geographic areas and resulted in more than $700 million in direct costs for tuberculosis treatment in 1991 alone [9]. (Also see Chapter 12, *Surveillance for tuberculosis in Europe*.) Deterioration of public health infrastructure, including capacity to detect diseases, is thought to have contributed to the reemergence of epidemic diphtheria in the Russian Federation in 1990 and its spread to all Newly Independent States and Baltic States by the end of 1994 [10]. In a statement that specifically addressed the resurgence of vector-borne diseases in Europe (but also applies to other infectious

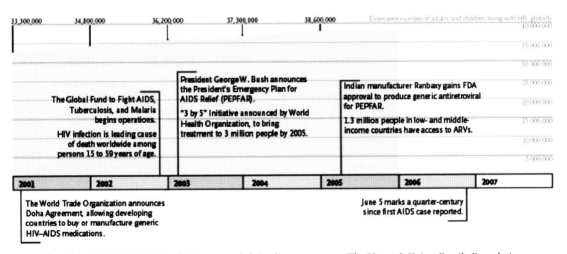

Fig 1.2 The Global HIV/AIDS Epidemic. For expanded timeline, see source: The Henry J. Kaiser Family Foundation, www.kff.org. Used with permission from the Henry J. Kaiser Family Foundation, Menlo Park, California [8].

diseases), WHO stated in 2004, "In the absence of major and dramatic outbreaks, health authorities often fail to allocate adequate funding for the surveillance and control of this group of diseases" [11].

In disease eradication programs, robust surveillance systems are necessary to detect every case. However, with low levels of disease, it is hard to convince decision makers to allocate sufficient resources for surveillance and a risk of undetected relapse remains. As a result of an ambitious plan to eradicate malaria in the mid-1950s, some countries (e.g., India) had sharp reductions in the number of cases followed by, after efforts ceased, increases to substantial levels [12].

The desire of societies to control the spread of highly contagious and virulent infectious pathogens (e.g., pandemic strains of influenza virus) may allow acceptance of quarantine by public health authorities even at the expense of individual liberty. However, without surveillance data, public health officials will have difficulties designing rational isolation and quarantine strategies and can expect to encounter legal obstacles and public disapproval. Chapter 35 (*Legal considerations in surveillance, isolation, and quarantine*) underscores the need to support isolation and quarantine decisions with sound medical and epidemiologic evidence.

The value of surveillance

Even with available surveillance data, what can public health programs realistically accomplish in terms of disease prevention and control? Merely collecting disease data for surveillance has little impact. However, successful surveillance programs also analyze and disseminate data to inform prevention and control activities. Specific programs, provided as examples here and further detailed later in this book, clearly illustrate the power of appropriately designed and utilized surveillance data.

Guide seasonal vaccine formulation

The WHO Global Influenza Surveillance Network, a network of 4 centers and 116 institutions in 87 countries, conducts annual surveillance for new strains of influenza (see Chapter 19, *Seasonal and pandemic influenza surveillance*). The results form the basis for WHO recommendations on the composition of influenza vaccine for the Northern and Southern hemispheres each year [13]. Use of surveillance data to guide production of influenza vaccine is critical because the vaccine is most effective when most antigenically similar to circulating viruses [14].

Guide vaccination strategies

Characterization of risk factors for bacterial infections such as invasive pneumococcal and meningococcal disease and data on circulating serotypes guide the development of vaccination recommendations. For example, in the US, data from active, population-based surveillance was used by public health advisory committees on immunization to help formulate the guidelines for vaccination of young children with a newly developed pneumococcal conjugate vaccine [15] and to recommend routine vaccination of incoming college students with meningococcal vaccine [16]. Further details are presented in Part 1 of Chapter 18 (*Surveillance for vaccine preventable diseases*).

Assess vaccine safety

Success of vaccination recommendations depends on their acceptance by the public and healthcare providers; an acceptable vaccine risk–benefit ratio is important in gaining this confidence. The establishment of surveillance for vaccine-associated adverse events has enabled ongoing assessment of vaccine safety. Exemplified by the US Vaccine Adverse Event Reporting System and the Yellow Card program used in the United Kingdom (UK) and other countries, this type of surveillance is important for detecting problems with vaccines (e.g., intussusception related to rotavirus vaccine) and, when supporting surveillance evidence exists, in promotion of vaccines with good safety records (see Part 2 of Chapter 18, *Vaccine adverse event reporting system*).

Guide clinical management in the face of evolving antimicrobial resistance

Surveillance for antimicrobial-resistant organisms can guide clinical management for these infections, as well as increase awareness of the consequences of antibiotic overuse. For example, surveillance for community-associated methicillin-resistant *Staphylococcus aureus* (CA-MRSA) in the US has demonstrated that CA-MRSA has become a common and serious problem and that the infecting strains are often resistant to prescribed antimicrobial agents [17]. Chapter 4 (*Surveillance for antimicrobial-resistant* Streptococcus pneumoniae) and Chapter 14 (*Surveillance for community-associated methicillin-resistant* Staphylococcus aureus) discuss bacterial antibiotic resistance. Global surveillance for chloroquine-resistant and other types of resistant malaria greatly impacts recommendations for treatment and prophylaxis for persons traveling to specific countries [18]. *International Travel and Health*, a publication by WHO, is updated every year and can be downloaded from http://www.who.int/ith/en/. Health travel information is also available on the Centers for Disease Control and Prevention (CDC) Web site http://www.cdc.gov/travel/.

Control emergence of antimicrobial-resistant organisms in domesticated animals

Widespread use of antimicrobial agents as growth promoters in animal husbandry is associated with increased resistance to antibiotics in bacteria isolated from animals and humans [19]. Surveillance for antimicrobial-resistant organisms in food animals is important to inform policies regarding use of antimicrobials outside human medicine. For example, the Danish Integrated Antimicrobial Resistance Monitoring and Research Programme (DANMAP) was established in 1995 to monitor antimicrobial resistance in bacteria from livestock, food, and humans, and to monitor use of antimicrobial agents [20]. Due to demonstration of rising antimicrobial resistance among bacteria isolated from food animals, Denmark banned use of certain antimicrobial agents as growth promoters in the 1990s (e.g., avoparcin, a glycopeptide similar to vancomycin, in 1995) [21]. For further discussions, see Chapter

7 (*Surveillance for antimicrobial-resistance among foodborne bacteria: the US approach*).

Guide allocation of resources for disease prevention and treatment programs

Surveillance data are used to guide allocation of resources to control infectious diseases at various levels. For example, in the US, over \$2 billion from the Ryan White federal emergency financial assistance program are allocated to support HIV/AIDS care facilities based on the number of AIDS cases reported [22]. Annual estimates of the burden of HIV/AIDS in different countries by the United Nations Program on HIV/AIDS has stimulated creation of organizations (e.g., Global Fund to Fight AIDS, Tuberculosis and Malaria; and the Bill and Melinda Gates Foundation) focused on securing resources to expand public health programs in the countries most affected by HIV/AIDS [23,24].

Identify outbreaks and guide disease control interventions

A major use of infectious disease surveillance data is to establish a baseline or reference point for detection of outbreaks requiring immediate investigation and intervention. Advancement in laboratory methods has enhanced usefulness of surveillance in outbreak detection by linking bacterial isolates obtained from geographically dispersed cases. For example, PulseNet is a national network of public health and food regulatory agency laboratories in the US that perform standardized molecular subtyping (or "fingerprinting") of disease-causing foodborne bacteria by pulsed-field gel electrophoresis (PFGE) [25]. PFGE patterns of isolates are compared with other patterns in the database to identify possible outbreaks. In a large multistate *Escherichia coli* O157:H7 outbreak in 1993, PFGE was used to link cases with consumption of hamburgers from a restaurant chain (Figure 1.3) [26]. Public health action in Washington state prevented consumption of over 250,000 potentially contaminated hamburgers, preventing an estimated 800 cases [27]. See Chapter 5 (*Surveillance for foodborne diseases*) for discussions on detection and investigation of foodborne disease outbreaks.

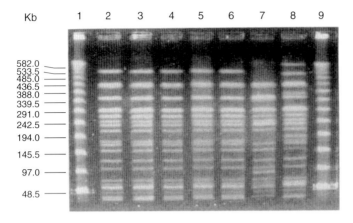

Fig 1.3 PFGE of *E. coli* O157:H7 strains associated with a multistate outbreak. Lanes 1 and 9, molecular weight markers (lambda ladder); lanes 2–5, patient isolates from Washington, Idaho, Nevada, and California, respectively; lane 6, isolate from an incriminated lot of hamburger meat; lanes 7 and 8, isolates from lots of hamburger meat unrelated to the outbreak [26]. (Used with permission from American Society of Microbiology Journals Department.)

Detect and respond to emerging infections

Surveillance is useful for detecting and controlling new or reemerging pathogens. The recent outbreak of SARS illustrates the role of surveillance in guiding response to an emerging global public health threat. First reported in Guangdong Province, China, in 2003, SARS resulted in 8098 probable cases with 774 deaths reported in 29 countries. Surveillance played a critical role in assessing the spread of the SARS epidemic and guiding quarantine recommendations and other control measures (see Chapter 39, Part 2, *SARS surveillance in Hong Kong and United States during the 2003 outbreak*).

The spectrum of infectious disease surveillance and disease-reporting systems

Students and newcomers to the practice of public health may perceive surveillance to be synonymous with mandatory healthcare-provider-based disease reporting systems. Although disease reporting is important, there are other components of surveillance. We will outline core disease reporting systems as exemplified in the US and other countries, and then introduce the breadth of other types of innovative systems used to monitor and respond to infectious diseases.

Disease reporters

In most countries, mandatory disease reporting relies upon physicians or other healthcare providers

both to diagnose diseases designated to be of public health importance and to report these cases to public health authorities. However, other professionals are also obligated to report specific diseases. For example, laboratory directors are given responsibilities to report cases when laboratory tests are indicative of a reportable disease. In some countries, directors of schools, homes for the elderly, prisons, or other institutions are required to notify public health officials of any clusters of disease, such as two or more cases of suspected food poisoning.

Despite being legally mandated, diseases are grossly underreported [28]. There are essentially no penalties for failing to report cases of disease. Health-care providers and other reporters are often unaware of which diseases to report, they may not believe in the utility of surveillance, and the logistics of reporting cases can become unmanageable for busy clinicians. Creative means to motivate and support disease reporters is essential, but often overlooked. As one example, in the UK, a (modest) financial compensation is offered to persons who report diseases [29]. To promote reporting of HIV, Michigan Department of Community Health (US) maintains an active relationship with HIV care specialists through an e-mail group that provides up-to-date information on HIV and other infectious disease news (see Chapter 16, *Surveillance for HIV/AIDS in the United States*).

Diseases selected for surveillance

In most European countries, diseases considered to be of public health significance and warranting

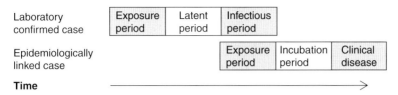

Fig 1.4 Guidance for defining an epidemiologically linked case prospectively. An epidemiological link is established when there is contact between two people involving a plausible mode of transmission at a time when (a) one of them is likely to be infectious and (b) the other has an illness onset within the incubation period after this contact. At least one case in the chain of epidemiologically linked cases (which may involve many cases) must be laboratory confirmed [32]. (Used with permission of the Australian Government – Department of Health and Aging.)

systematic surveillance are selected at a national level. Provisions often do allow, however, for regional adaptation (see Chapter 6, *Supranational surveillance in the European Union*). For example, chikungunya was made a mandatory notifiable condition in mainland France and the overseas departments in the Caribbean, but not in the department La Réunion in the Indian Ocean, where a massive epidemic involving over 100,000 persons in 2006 overwhelmed the disease reporting structure. In the US, the authority to require disease reporting is decentralized—states, territories, and independent local health departments legislate lists of reportable diseases, and these vary by state. For example, coccidiomycosis is reportable only in areas in the southwestern US where the fungus is endemic.

Case definitions

Case definitions are specific clinical and/or laboratory criteria used to standardize surveillance data from different health jurisdictions. Before being counted as a case, a disease report is investigated to ensure that these criteria are met. The Council of State and Territorial Epidemiologists (CSTE), a professional society of public health epidemiologists, establishes and periodically revises case definitions that are used in infectious disease surveillance in the US [30] and are available on the CDC Web site http://www.cdc.gov/epo/dphsi/casedef/. Case classifications range from "confirmed" to "probable", depending upon availability of supporting data.

For over 80% of nationally notifiable diseases in the US, positive laboratory test results are required for case confirmation, and many of the other dis-eases require an epidemiologic link to a laboratory-confirmed case [31] (Guidance on identifying "epidemiologically linked" cases is provided in Figure 1.4 based on Australian case definitions [32]). Case definitions for some diseases such as tetanus rely primarily on clinical criteria (e.g., an acute onset of hypertonia and/or painful muscular contractions, usually of the muscles of the jaw and neck, and generalized muscle spasms without other apparent medical cause). Case definitions are subject to evolution—this may be necessary in the face of a rapidly changing epidemic of a new disease (see Part 2 of Chapter 39) or more slowly as in the case of HIV/AIDS (see Chapter 16). When case definitions are changed, data can be expected to be altered merely as an artifact of the new criteria [33].

The sensitivity and specificity of a case definition are influenced by the availability of good laboratory diagnostic assays to support clinical criteria, and by epidemiologic goals. In an outbreak or in other settings where confirmatory laboratory assays do not exist or are not practical, sensitive but less specific case definitions may be selected. For example, a gastrointestinal illness can be counted as a case of salmonellosis if epidemiologically linked to a laboratory-confirmed case of *Salmonella*. By contrast, when a single case has major public health implications, the case definition may be quite rigorous with strict laboratory criteria (e.g., for vancomycin-resistant *S. aureus* or the reemergence of SARS).

Data flow

Reporters phone, fax, mail, or electronically transmit case reports to local health jurisdictions that investigate, ensure that case definitions are met, and initiate interventions as needed. All states in the US voluntarily contribute surveillance data to the national system. As determined by CSTE, with input from CDC, a subset of locally reportable diseases is deemed "nationally notifiable" and this subset of cases are forwarded to the National Notifiable Disease Surveillance System at the CDC. In many other countries where the disease reporting authority is centralized at the national level, all cases confirmed at the local jurisdiction are forwarded to the national surveillance system.

Dissemination of data

Surveillance data are compiled, analyzed, and presented at many levels. A prominent outlet in the US is the *Morbidity and Mortality Weekly Report*, where Surveillance Summaries on notifiable diseases are published on a freely accessible Web site, http://www.cdc.gov/mmwr/, and in printed copies that are mailed to subscribers. In the UK, surveillance data are published regularly in the *Communicable Disease Report Weekly*, available on the Health Protection Agency Web site http://www.hpa.org.uk/cdr/default.htm and by e-mail subscription. States, territories, and local health departments in the US have a variety of somewhat uneven methods to share surveillance data—use of the Web to support this data dissemination function is discussed in Chapter 21 (*Use of the World Wide Web to enhance infectious disease surveillance*). Of critical importance is sharing of information about infectious disease with the public. Chapter 32 (*Communication of information about surveillance*) covers this topic in two articles: Part 1 (*Media communication of surveillance information*) illustrates how the media conveys information and Part 2 (*Case study—a healthy response to increases in syphilis in San Francisco*) describes a public awareness campaign.

Internationally notifiable diseases—International Health Regulations

Public health agencies of most countries operate fairly independently. However, infectious pathogens do not respect country borders, and therefore some disease outbreaks are not solely the concern of the "index" country—intensified global public health response may become essential. IHR, as originally articulated by the World Health Assembly in 1969, has required countries to report cases of Yellow fever, plague, and cholera to the WHO. However, a 2005 revision broadens the scope of IHR to include not only an expanded list of known pathogens, but also as of yet undefined new or reemerging diseases which can spread rapidly with enormous health impact. International emergencies caused by noninfectious diseases are also addressed.

In the interests of the global community, the 2005 IHR addresses the need for an objective assessment of whether an event constitutes a public health emergency of international concern. As specified in the legal framework of the new regulations, WHO, with its extensive communications network, can rapidly assess information. Once it has determined that a particular event constitutes a public health emergency of international concern, IHR stipulates that WHO will make a "real-time" response to the emergency and recommend measures for implementation by the affected state as well as by other states. Official assessments from WHO, as an internationally prominent and neutral public health authority, can avoid unnecessary, uncoordinated interference with international traffic and trade that has previously made some countries reluctant to report significant events. For further discussion, see Chapter 2 (*Infectious disease surveillance and International Health Regulations*).

Additional examples of the spectrum of infectious disease surveillance programs

Some of the limitations encountered by disease reporting systems, including burden on reporters and subsequent underreporting, lack of representativeness, and focus on human diseases, are addressed by complementary systems. The principal alternate systems are described below.

Laboratory-based surveillance

Clinical microbiology and public health laboratories can be rich sources of information on pathogens causing disease within a population. Compared to individual healthcare providers who are often spread across multiple clinics and acute and chronic care facilities, laboratories may be a relatively consolidated source of data on reportable diseases. Many surveillance strategies involve collaborations with laboratories for sharing of data and isolates. For example, utilizing advancing information technologies, public health organizations have worked with clinical laboratories to enable electronic, automated transfer of information on reportable diseases to public health agencies (see Chapter 25, *Electronic reporting in infectious disease surveillance*, which offers electronic reporting examples from Germany and US). For an example of automated laboratory reporting using an Internet-based system, see Chapter 22 (*Infectious Diseases Surveillance Information System (ISIS) in the Netherlands: development and implementation*).

International surveillance systems

Although most surveillance systems are maintained by public health agencies within a given country, cooperation between countries have supported surveillance on a supranational and global scale. The international mandates of the IHR, as they apply to a small subset of exceptional diseases, have been discussed. An example of collaborative laboratory-based European surveillance is the European Antimicrobial Resistance Surveillance System (EARSS), which monitors seven major bacterial pathogens from 800 public health laboratories serving over 1300 hospitals in 31 European countries. EARSS was used to characterize methicillin-resistant *S. aureus* (MRSA) in participating European countries: during 1999–2000, MRSA prevalence varied from <1% of *S. aureus* isolates in northern Europe to >40% in southern and western Europe [34]. Facilitated by WHO, Global Salm-Surv is an example of an even larger global collaborative surveillance system. Five years after initiation, laboratories in 142 countries are sharing data on over 1 million *Salmonella* isolates, including 100,000 isolates from animals [35]. The WHO Global Influenza Surveillance Network, a network between 87 countries, is another example and is further described in Chapter 19.

Active surveillance

A misnomer used in describing surveillance is the term "passive" as this suggests minimal effort on anyone's part. Customarily, the intent of labeling some surveillance systems as "passive" and others as "active" is to distinguish the intensity of public health agency's effort in finding and investigating cases. State-mandated disease reporting systems in the US, while obviously relying on healthcare-provider energies, generally involve minimal public health effort to solicit case reports and thus are described as "passive." Underreporting is a major limitation of this type of surveillance data. It is also true that no surveillance system should be entirely "passive," even from the point of view of the public health agency, as regular communication and feedback to healthcare providers are necessary.

By contrast, "active" surveillance involves intensive public health involvement to seek reports of all diagnosed cases of a subset of reportable diseases, at least within defined regions, and to obtain additional epidemiologic and clinical information that may be missing from standard case reports. In actual practice, the distinction between both active and passive surveillance is not always so clear. An example is "enhanced passive" surveillance in which providers are actively solicited to assist in the identification of cases for a short-term surveillance study. For detailed discussions on active, population-based surveillance, including the Active Bacterial Core surveillance (ABCs) in the US and the Emerging Infections Program Network in Thailand, see Chapter 3 (*Population-based active surveillance for emerging infectious diseases*).

The Foodborne Disease Surveillance Network (FoodNET) established by the US CDC in collaboration with the US Department of Agriculture and the US Food and Drug Administration, and participating US Emerging Infection Program sites, is an active, laboratory-based surveillance program for foodborne pathogens [36]. Typically, only a small fraction of foodborne illnesses are reported to public health authorities, and often they lack accurate epidemiologic information (e.g., specific attributed causes, outcomes). To overcome these limitations, FoodNET investigators contact participating laboratories regularly to comprehensively identify all laboratory-confirmed cases of

Salmonella, Shigella, Campylobacter, E. coli O157, *Listeria monocytogenes, Yersinia enterocolitica, Vibrio, Cryptosporidium*, and *Cyclospora* among persons in the predefined catchment area. As part of FoodNET, dedicated resources are used to conduct epidemiologic investigations of these cases. Discussions on FoodNET's contribution to public health are presented in Chapter 5.

Sentinel surveillance

The intensive public health resources required to conduct population-based active surveillance are often not readily available; as an alternative strategy, sentinel surveillance involves collection of data from only a "sentinel" or subset of a larger population. The strategy of focusing only on a small population subset can be conceived as a type of "sampling." However, to be able to generalize these data to larger populations, it is necessary to ensure that the sentinel population is representative and that the sentinel data are linked to denominator information on a predefined population under surveillance (see discussion in Chapter 15, *Surveillance for viral hepatitis in Europe*).

The Gonococcal Isolate Surveillance Project systematically monitors antimicrobial resistance among *Neisseria gonorroheae* isolates collected from 25 to 30 sentinel US cities—antimicrobial susceptibility testing is performed on the first 25 isolates per month from male patients with gonococcal urethritis. In some states, rising resistance documented by this surveillance system has contributed to recommendations that fluoroquinolones should not be used to treat gonococcal infections (see Chapter 17, *Surveillance for sexually transmitted diseases*).

In France, a network of primary care physicians report information, at weekly intervals, on a selected group of health events that are relatively common in general practice: influenza-like illness, acute gastroenteritis, measles, mumps, chicken pox, male urethritis, hepatitis A, B, and C. Data are extrapolated to regional and national levels. The system detects and describes the occurrence and progression of regional and national outbreaks (available at: http://rhone.b3e.jussiue.fr/senti).

Multiple "sentinel" surveillance methods have been used to estimate the prevalence of HIV in Africa and other countries. A commonly used approach has been through routine HIV testing for women presenting for antenatal care. Although sentinel surveillance can be useful, unique features of the sampled population such as contraceptive use may prohibit generalization to other populations [37].

Animal reservoir and vector surveillance

Because of the central role of wildlife, domestic animals, and vectors (e.g., ticks and mosquitoes), zoonotic diseases cannot be adequately understood and controlled by only monitoring the disease in human populations. With increasing recognition of the importance of zoonotic diseases, surveillance systems have been designed to monitor pathogens as they circulate in various human and nonhuman hosts. Brucellosis control in the US has been successful because of the focus on animal health as a way to protect human health—comprehensive animal testing, vaccination of breeding animals, and depopulation of affected herds (see Chapter 8, *Surveillance for zoonotic diseases*). Although still requiring refinement, a major goal of surveillance for West Nile virus in the US is to be able to efficiently utilize dead bird, horse, or mosquito surveillance data to predict areas where transmission to humans is most likely to occur and therefore where vector control and other prevention efforts should be targeted (see West Nile virus case study in Chapter 9, *Surveillance for vector-borne diseases*).

Detection of pathogens in the environment

The identification of the fungus *Cryptococcus gattii* in British Columbia, Canada, illustrates the use of surveillance to detect and define an emerging pathogen intrinsically linked to the environment. This fungus was previously known only in tropical and subtropical climates, but the organism emerged around 1999 in Vancouver Island as a pathogen in humans and domestic and wild animals. Environmental sampling has identified the fungus on trees, in soil, in air samples, and in water (Plate 1.1), helping to define the evolving realm of this new pathogen [38].

Use of health services and administrative data for disease surveillance

Infectious disease surveillance systems have also incorporated administrative and vital statistics data already being collected for other purposes. For example, vital statistics data are a component of HIV/AIDS surveillance as data are linked to identify (at-risk) infants born to women with previously reported HIV infection (see Chapter 16). To bill for services, healthcare facilities in the US assign diagnosis codes (e.g., International Classification of Diseases, Tenth Revision (ICD-10)) to clinical care encounters—this is a potential data source for surveillance for a range of diseases (see Chapter 17). Hospital admission data can also complement routine surveillance data; in England, hospital admission data have been used to monitor end-stage liver disease where the underlying cause is chronic viral hepatitis (see Chapter 15). Monitoring of drug utilization and drug sales may be an indirect measure of disease activity. Pharmaceutical databases have been explored for a variety of syndromic surveillance systems. At the US CDC, where a supply of "orphan" drugs are housed for treatment of rare diseases, increased requests for pentamidine in the 1980s led to an investigation of a cluster of *Pneumocystis* pneumonia which, in turn, led to the first detection of AIDS in the world [39]. Hospital administrative data are also used to conduct surveillance for hospital-associated infections (see Chapter 13, *Surveillance for nosocomial infections*).

Use of media reports for disease surveillance

The availability and speed of information transmission over the Internet have allowed development of innovative electronic media-based surveillance systems. For example, the Global Public Health Intelligence Network (GPHIN) gathers, in seven languages on a real-time, 24/7 basis, electronic media reports of occurrence of diseases. Although the electronically gathered information requires further verification, GPHIN is used extensively as an early source of outbreak information by Health Canada, WHO, the US CDC, and others (see Chapter 23, *The Global Public Health Intelligence Network*).

Risk-factor surveillance

Although most surveillance systems focus on disease occurrences or circulation of pathogens causing disease, unique surveillance systems have focused on behaviors that pose risk for specific diseases. For example, the US National HIV Behavioral Surveillance system includes interviews of a sample of persons to assess the prevalence of sexual behaviors, drug use, and testing history for other sexually transmitted infections [40]. Data from this system examine the front end of the HIV/AIDS epidemic and may guide and assess prevention programs (see Chapter 29, *Analysis and interpretation of case-based HIV/AIDS surveillance data*). Similarly, Youth Risk Behavior Survey measures the prevalence of health-risk behaviors among adolescents through self-administered, school-based surveys. Reports of sex without condoms and sex associated with drug and alcohol use are among the data collected [41] (see Chapter 17).

Use of computer algorithms to conduct surveillance

A few surveillance systems have been developed that employ computer algorithms to screen electronic data sources for disease cases and apply automated statistical methods to assess data trends and changes in case activity. For example, a component of the Infectious Diseases Surveillance and Information System (ISIS) in the Netherlands runs automated algorithms on electronically-transmitted laboratory data to identify selected cases of public health interest (e.g., new positive *Neisseria gonorrhea* test results). Automated time-series analyses process these and other surveillance data to detect variations from expected rates; statistically significant changes automatically generate and distribute alerts (see Chapter 22). Syndromic surveillance systems use automated data extraction and analyses methods to detect aberrations from expected levels of various syndromes (see Chapter 26, *Implementing syndromic surveillance systems in the climate of bioterrorism*, for further discussion). Chapter 23 describes use of automated algorithms to scan 20,000 electronic news media sources for early reports of outbreaks around the world. Although these systems exhibit the powerful capacity of technologies to automatically process enormous quantities of data, humans must still verify, investigate, and prioritize these reports. Research is needed to refine these automated data processing systems and capitalize on their strengths.

Surveillance collaborations with partners outside traditional human public health systems

As illustrated by the broad variety of infectious disease surveillance systems, diverse sources of information can be utilized. The development of these systems relies upon new collaborations between human public health agencies and nontraditional partners. For example, domestic and wildlife animal health agencies have traditionally acted as separate entities apart from human health agencies. However, the increasing recognition of the importance of zoonotic diseases to human health has encouraged innovative collaborations. When West Nile virus emerged in the US, public health officials who customarily focused only on human diseases began forging collaborations with entomologists, veterinarians, and wildlife oversight agencies [42]. Human health agencies often do not have these diversely skilled personnel, but instead depend upon common goals and national agendas to facilitate collaborations.

In broad terms, surveillance requires consultations with legal partners to interpret laws as they relate to public health activities, for example, ensuring maintenance of patient confidentiality during collection of electronic data (see Chapter 35, Part 1, *Legal basis for infectious disease surveillance and control*). The need for review of public health surveillance practices from an ethicist's perspective is discussed in Chapter 34 (*Ethical considerations in infectious disease surveillance*). As described in Chapter 11 (*Surveillance for unexplained infectious disease related deaths*), medical examiners have the authority to investigate sudden, unattended, and unexplained deaths. Although the focus of these investigations has traditionally been on intentional or accidental deaths, public health agencies have collaborated with medical examiners to systematize specimen collection and diagnostic testing relevant for detection of reportable, emerging, or bioterrorism-related infectious diseases. Chapter 10 (*Surveillance for agents of bioterrorism in the United States*) also discusses collaboration with regional poison control centers in monitoring suspicious reports.

Syndromic surveillance systems use a variety of nontraditional data sources (e.g., employee absenteeism data, emergency department admission diagnoses). This has led to collaborations with academic institutions, healthcare institutions, and private sector IT specialists. Chapter 26 discusses some of the potential challenges faced in these collaborations, particularly in the investigation of surveillance data collected outside of public health jurisdictions (e.g., information not related to reportable diseases).

Today's increasingly complex surveillance systems require advanced data analysis and data management support. To adjust for missing data, account for confounders through multivariate modeling, and formally assess trends and clusters that may necessitate input from individuals with advanced training in biostatistics. Chapter 27 (*Informatics and software applications for data analyses*) and Chapter 28 (*Analyses and interpretation of reportable infectious disease data*) provide background on common software applications and analytic methods used in surveillance. Chapter 29 introduces issues in analysis and interpretation of case-based HIV/AIDS surveillance data. Collaborations with IT specialists have become essential and, for example, have enabled practical use of the Internet, ranging from posting practical disease reporting and surveillance information on the Web to development of Web-based means for reporting (see Chapter 21). Close collaborations between IT experts, stakeholders, and end users are critical in all phases of system design and testing to ensure the viability of these potentially multimillion dollar projects.

In the US and elsewhere, surveillance is not a wholly government function. For example, at their own cost, private hospital laboratories transmit large amounts of reportable disease information to health departments. Chapter 38 (*Public–private partnerships in infectious disease surveillance*) details the expanding role of the private sector in surveillance. Another example of public–private partnership is the US Vaccine Adverse Events Reporting System. While federal public health agencies set programmatic objectives and provide technical oversight, the for-profit Constella Group is contracted to support this surveillance system's data collection processes [43]. These types of "mixed model" partnerships may be able to harness private-sector energy and efficiency while remaining faithful to public health objectives.

Challenges and promises for the future of infectious disease surveillance

Progress in development of surveillance systems supports advances in disease prevention and control. However, public health challenges in surveillance and disease control continue to be faced around the globe. Despite IHR (2005) mandates [44], not all countries are able to devote adequate resources to surveillance. Countries are attempting to balance using limited resources to develop disease control and prevention programs (including surveillance as one important component) with the need to support struggling healthcare systems in the treatment of diseases. It may seem that the more pressing priority is to try to address the needs of persons who are already suffering from disease, rather than diverting resources towards surveillance and disease prevention. This sentiment is most acutely felt when countries cannot, because of lack of sufficiently trained workforces, maximize the benefits of surveillance and constructively use surveillance data for long-term disease prevention and control.

The gap between data collection and effective use of data for disease control and prevention is among the most formidable challenges faced by surveillance programs. An unfortunate reality of public health surveillance is that substantial efforts are spent on collection of data while sufficient resources are often not expended on timely dissemination and constructive use of the information. If these data are not appropriately analyzed, disseminated, and applied, surveillance will be perceived as categorically ineffective. As William Foege, former director of the CDC once remarked, "The reason for collecting, analyzing, and disseminating information on a disease is to control that disease. Collection and analysis should not be allowed to consume resources if action does not follow" [45].

Public health officials need to be sufficiently trained to be able to leverage benefits of surveillance. In many countries, workforce with adequate skills to carry out core surveillance activities including data collection, analysis, and use of data for disease prevention and control is limited (see Chapter 24, *National notifiable disease surveillance in Egypt*). While much of the practice of surveillance may be learned on the job as newly hired personnel begin careers in public health, selected epidemiology training programs (see Chapter 36, *Training in applied epidemiology and infectious disease surveillance: contributions of the Epidemic Intelligence Service*, and Chapter 37, *Surveillance training for Fogarty International Fellows from Eastern Europe and Central Asia*) have given special attention to surveillance. Through formal evaluations of in-use surveillance programs, EIS officers not only begin to understand real-life surveillance, but also bring fresh perspective to systems that may have become stagnant. In collaboration with many countries' Ministries of Health, the Field Epidemiology (and Laboratory) Training Program and Data for Decision Making program offer training around the world in applied epidemiology, including issues in surveillance (available on the CDC Web site at: http://www.cdc.gov/descd/). Practical training on actionable surveillance should also be an emphasis in schools of public health and other educational arenas.

Ongoing evaluations are repeatedly needed as a core component of living surveillance systems. Are components of a surveillance system operating as effectively as possible, and if not, what changes can be made? For an introduction to formal evaluation of surveillance, see Chapter 33 (*Evaluation of surveillance systems for early epidemic detection*). Surveillance systems face the challenges of chasing moving targets—as more is learned about the epidemiology of a disease, surveillance strategies must be adapted. Emerging pathogens add further complexities. Surveillance systems need to be regularly reviewed, refined, and reenergized.

On the promising frontiers of public health, technical advancements are assisting efforts to improve surveillance systems. Examples include sophisticated IT instruments mentioned previously. Molecular fingerprinting has the capacity to improve epidemiologic understanding of links between human cases, management of outbreaks, and links to animal reservoirs (see Chapter 30,

Use of molecular epidemiology in infectious disease surveillance). In the future, geographic information systems may hold new promises (see Chapter 31, *Use of geographic information systems and remote sensing for infectious disease surveillance*) to analyze multiple layers of geographical, ecological, and climatic information to assist in prediction of zoonotic and other diseases linked with the environment. New tools to enhance infectious disease surveillance continue to be developed; how to optimize the use of both old and new surveillance tools to inform disease prevention and control remains both an ongoing challenge and an opportunity.

References

1 Hong Kong Health Commitment Pledged in Sweden. Available from: http://www.news-medical.net/?id=5119. Accessed October 16, 2005.

2 Fauci AS. Infectious diseases: considerations for the 21st century. *Clin Infect Dis* 2001;**32**:675–85.

3 Health Protection Agency. Health protection in the 21st century. Available from: http://www.hpa.org.uk/ publications/2005/burden_disease/default.htm. Accessed November 1, 2006.

4 Knobler S, Mahmoud A, Lemon S, Mack, A, Sivitz L and Oberholtzer K (eds). Workshop summary. In: *Learning from SARS: Preparing for the Next Disease Outbreak*. Washington, DC: National Academies Press; 2004:11.

5 World Health Assembly. Revision of the International Health Regulations, WHA58.3. 2005. Available from: http://www.who.int/gb/ebwha/pdf_files/WHA58-REC1/english/Resolutions.pdf. Accessed on October 27, 2006.

6 Centers for Disease Control and Prevention. Progress toward poliomyelitis eradication—Eastern Mediterranean Region, January 2000–September 2001. *Morb Mortal Wkly Rep* 2001;**50**:1113–6.

7 Ekwanzala M, Pepin J, Khonde N, Molisho S, Bruneel H, De Wals P. In the heart of darkness: sleeping sickness in Zaire. *Lancet* November 23, 1996;**348**:1427–30.

8 Merson MH. The HIV-AIDS pandemic at 25—the global response. *N Engl J Med* 2006;**354**:2414–7.

9 Berkelman RL, Bryan RT, Osterholm MT, LeDuc JW, Hughes JM. Infectious disease surveillance: a crumbling foundation. *Science* 1994;**264**:368–70.

10 Dittmann S, Wharton M, Vitek C, *et al*. Successful control of epidemic diphtheria in the states of the Former Union of Soviet Socialist Republics: lessons learned. *J Infect Dis* 2000;**181**(suppl 1):S10–22.

11 World Health Organization. The vector-borne human infections of Europe: their distribution and burden on public health. Available from: http://www.euro.who.int/ document/E82481.pdf. Accessed November 7, 2006.

12 Sharma VP, Mehrotra KN. Malaria resurgence in India: a critical study. *Soc Sci Med* 1986;**22**:835–45.

13 World Health Assembly. Global influenza surveillance. Available from: http://www.who.int/csr/disease/influenza/influenzanetwork/en/index.html. Accessed November 3, 2006.

14 Centers for Disease Control and Prevention. Efficacy and Effectiveness of Inactivated Influenza Vaccine. Available from: http://www.cdc.gov/flu/professionals/vaccination/efficacy.htm. Accessed November 9, 2006.

15 Van Beneden CA, Whitney CG, Levine OS, for the Centers for Disease Control and Prevention. Preventing pneumococcal disease among infants and young children: recommendations of the Advisory Committee on Immunization Practices (ACIP). *MMWR* 2000;**49**(RR-9):1–38.

16 Bilukha OO, Rosenstein N; National Center for Infectious Diseases, Centers for Disease Control and Prevention (CDC). Prevention and control of meningococcal disease: recommendations of the Advisory Committee on Immunization Practices (ACIP). *MMWR Recomm Rep* 2005;**54**(RR-7):1–38.

17 Fridkin SK, Hageman JC, Morrison M, *et al*., Active Bacterial Core Surveillance Program of the Emerging Infections Program Network. Methicillin-resistant *Staphylococcus aureus* disease in three communities. *N Engl J Med* 2005;**352**:1436–44.

18 World Health Organization. Monitoring antimalarial drug resistance. Report of a WHO consultation, Geneva, Switzerland, December 3–5, 2001.

19 Fey PD, Safranek TJ, Rupp ME, *et al*. Ceftriaxone-resistant salmonella infection acquired by a child from cattle. *N Engl J Med* 2000;**342**:1242–9.

20 Danish Integrated Antimicrobial Resistance Monitoring and Research Programme. Monitoring antimicrobial resistance in Denmark. *Int J Antimicrob Agents* 2000;**14**:271–4.

21 Aarestrup FM, Seyfarth AM, Emborg HD, Pedersen K, Hendriksen RS, Bager F. Effect of abolishment of the use of antimicrobial agents for growth promotion on occurrence of antimicrobial resistance in fecal enterococci from food animals in Denmark. *Antimicrob Agents Chemother* 2001;**45**:2054–9.

22 Mokotoff ED, Glynn MK. Surveillance for HIV/AIDS in the United States. In: M'ikanatha NM, Lynfield R, Van Beneden CA, De Valk H (eds), *Infectious Disease Surveillance*. London: Blackwell; 2007:201–11.

23 United Nations Programs on HIV/AIDS. Uniting the World Against AIDS. Available from: http:// www.unaids.

org/en/HIV_data/default.asp. Accessed November 7, 2006.

24 Bill and Melinda Gates Foundation. Available from: http://www.gatesfoundation.org/default.htm. Accessed December 26, 2006.

25 Centers for Disease Control and Prevention. PulseNet. Available from: http://www.cdc.gov/pulsenet/index. htm. Accessed November 9, 2006.

26 Barrett, TJ, Lior, H, Green, JH, *et al*. Laboratory investigation of a multistate food-borne outbreak of *Escherichia coli* O157:H7 by using pulsed-field gel electrophoresis and phage typing. *J Clin Microbiol* 1994;**32**:3013–17.

27 Bell BP, Goldoft M, Griffin PM, *et al*. A multistate outbreak of *Escherichia coli* O157:H7-associated bloody diarrhea and hemolytic uremic syndrome from hamburgers: the Washington experience. *JAMA* 1994;**272**:1349–53.

28 Doyle TJ, Glynn MK, Groseclose SL. Completeness of notifiable infectious disease reporting in the United States: an analytical literature review. *Am J Epidemiol* 2002;**155**:866–74.

29 Bannister BA, Begg NT, Gillespie SH. *Infectious Diseases*. London: Blackwell Science; 1996:455.

30 Centers for Disease Control and Prevention. Case definitions for infectious conditions under public health surveillance. *MMWR Recomm Rep* 1997;**46**(RR-10):1–55.

31 Smith PF, Birkhead GS. Electronic clinical laboratory reporting for public health surveillance. In: M'ikanatha NM, Lynfield R, Van Beneden CA, De Valk H (eds), *Infectious Disease Surveillance*. London: Blackwell; 2007:Pt 2, 339–48.

32 Commonwealth of Australia. Australian notifiable diseases case definitions. Available from: http://www.health.gov.au/internet/wcms/publishing.nsf/Content/cda-surveil-nndss-casedefs-epilink.htm#epi. Accessed November 27, 2006.

33 Schwarcz SK, Hsu LC, Parisi MK, Katz MH. The impact of the 1993 AIDS case definition on the completeness and timeliness of AIDS surveillance. *AIDS* 1999;**13**:1109–14.

34 Tiemersma EW, Bronzwaer SL, Lyytikainen O, *et al*. European Antimicrobial Resistance Surveillance System Participants. Methicillin-resistant *Staphylococcus aureus* in Europe, 1999–2002. *Emerg Infect Dis* 2004;**10**:1627–34.

35 World Health Organization. Global Salm-Surv. Available from: http://www.who.int/salmsurv/en/ Accessed November 5, 2006.

36 Centers for Disease Control and Prevention. FoodNet Surveillance. Available from: http://www.cdc.gov/foodnet/surveillance.htm. Accessed November 5, 2006.

37 Gregson S, Terceira N, Kakowa M, *et al*. Study of bias in antenatal clinic HIV-1 surveillance data in a high contraceptive prevalence population in sub-Saharan Africa. *AIDS* 2002;**16**:643–52.

38 MacDougall L, Fyfe M. Emergence of *Cryptococcus gattii* in a novel environment provides clues to its incubation period. *J Clin Microbiol* 2006;**44**:1851–2.

39 Centers for Disease Control and Prevention (CDC). Pneumocystis pneumonia—Los Angeles. *MMWR Morb Mortal Wkly Rep* 1996;**45**:729–33.

40 Centers for Disease Control and Prevention. Human immunodeficiency virus (HIV) risk, prevention, and testing behaviors—United States, National HIV Behavioral Surveillance System: men who have sex with men, November 2003–April 2005. *MMWR Morb Mortal Wkly Rep* 2006;**55**(SS-6):1–16.

41 CDC. Youth Risk Behavior Surveillance—United States, 2001. *MMWR Morb Mortal Wkly Rep* 2002; **51**(SS04):1–64.

42 Fine A, Layton M. Lessons from the West Nile viral encephalitis outbreak in New York City, 1999: implications for bioterrorism preparedness. *Clin Infect Dis* 2001;**32**:277–82.

43 Constella Group. Constella Health Sciences Rewins CDC and FDA's $21 Million Vaccine Adverse Event Reporting System Contract. Available from: http://www.constellagroup.com/news/news_releases/2004/010404. shtml. Accessed November 27, 2006.

44 Hardiman BJM, González-Martin F, Rodier G. Infectious disease surveillance and the International Health Regulations. In: M'ikanatha NM, Lynfield R, Van Beneden CA, De Valk H (eds), *Infectious Disease Surveillance*. London: Blackwell; 2007:18–31.

45 Foege WH, Hogan RC, Newton LH. Surveillance projects for selected diseases. *Int J Epidemiol* 1976;**5**:29–37.

2

Infectious disease surveillance and the International Health Regulations

Bruce J. Plotkin, Max Hardiman, Fernando González-Martín & Guénaël Rodier

Background

For over 35 years, the World Health Organization's (WHO's) International Health Regulations ("IHR" or "Regulations") have been the primary legally binding global agreement addressing the risks of the international spread of infectious disease. However, the current 1969 Regulations ("IHR (1969)") [1]—which remain in force generally until June 2007—are quite limited, dealing primarily with a small number of infectious diseases. To address these and other shortcomings in the IHR (1969), the World Health Assembly in 1995 adopted resolution WHA48.7 that commenced the 10-year process of revising the Regulations to bring them up-to-date in policy and technology and to broaden their scope to address the transnational challenges presented by today's increasingly globalized movements of trade, transport, and travelers. These newly revised IHR (2005) were adopted by the Health Assembly on May 23, 2005 [2], and will enter into force on June 15, 2007, for all WHO Member States who have not rejected them, or made certain reservations to them, by December 15, 2006 (see Table 2.1).

The IHR (2005) completely revised and replaced the provisions concerning surveillance in the IHR (1969), providing broad new mandates and obligations for the "States Parties" to this new agreement and for WHO. The scope of coverage, including notification by States Parties and their obligations to respond to requests for verification by WHO, is expanded to include any event which may constitute a public health emergency of international concern (as well as certain other public health risks). Un-

derlying the entire instrument is the new "purpose and scope" provision in Article 2, stating that the IHR (2005) "are to prevent, protect against, control and provide a public health response to the international spread of disease in ways that are commensurate with and restricted to public health risks, and which avoid unnecessary interference with international traffic and trade."

A brief history of WHO and the IHR

The IHR evolved from efforts to address the threat posed by the international spread of epidemics; the use of quarantine procedures, for example, dates back at least to the Middle Ages. The more recent international sanitary agreements grew out of international conventions dating to the last half of the nineteenth century and the public health institutions founded in the first half of the twentieth century [3]. These international agreements and institutions (such as the Pan American Sanitary Bureau, the Office International d'Hygiene Publique [4], and the League of Nations' Health Organization [5]) established and coordinated related functions including limited notification obligations and surveillance for certain infectious diseases [6].

The World Health Organization

WHO was created in the aftermath of the Second World War in the effort to unify and provide increased public health efforts on a global scale. The WHO Constitution was adopted at an International

Table 2.1 Timeline: International Health Regulations.

1951	WHO adopts International Sanitary Regulations ("ISR") (rev. 1955–1956, 1960, 1963, 1965)
1969	ISR revised—renamed International Health Regulations ("IHR"; rev. 1973 and 1981)
1995	May: World Health Assembly resolves to revise and update the IHR (WHA48.7)
1998	First provisional draft of revised IHR
1999	Pilot testing of syndromic reporting approach
2001	World Health Assembly resolution on Global Health Security: epidemic alert and response (WHA54.14)
2003	May: World Health Assembly resolves to establish an Intergovernmental Working Group ("IGWG") to prepare revision of IHR and mandates WHO proactive response to SARS (WHA56.28 and 56.29)
2004	November: First IGWG session of global negotiations to revise IHR
2005	February/May: Second IGWG negotiation sessions revising IHR
	23 May: WHA adopts revised International Health Regulations (2005) (WHA58.3)
2006	May: World Health Assembly resolves to urge Member States to voluntarily comply with IHR (2005) prior to entry into force with regard to avian and pandemic influenza (WHA59.2)
2006	15 December: Deadline for Member States to reject or make reservations to IHR (2005)
2007	15 June: IHR (2005) entry into force
2009	Deadline for State Party assessments of the ability of their national structures and resources to meet the IHR (2005) minimum core public health capacities
2012/2014	Expiration of 2-year extensions to develop and maintain minimum core public health capacities

Health Conference in 1946 and entered into force on April 7, 1948, effectively establishing the new Organization [7].

Although the Constitution contains a range of fundamental provisions concerning global and individual health, several of these provisions emphasize WHO's broad mandate in the context of surveillance-related activities. Under Article 2 of the Constitution, these functions include acting as "the directing and co-ordinating authority on international health work"; assisting governments in "strengthening health services"; providing "technical assistance and, in emergencies, necessary aid"; establishing administrative and technical services such as epidemiological and statistical services; acting "to eradicate epidemic, endemic and other diseases"; making recommendations with respect to international health matters; and, particularly relevant for the IHR (2005), proposing "conventions, agreements and regulations[.]"

The Constitution specifically authorizes the World Health Assembly to adopt regulations such as the IHR, and, in an unusual provision, mandates that once the regulations are adopted, they bind all WHO Member States unless they take affirmative steps to opt out within a limited period of time as noted above.

International Sanitary Regulations (1951)/International Health Regulations (1969)

In 1951, the fourth World Health Assembly adopted the International Sanitary Regulations (ISR), the first of these WHO global agreements. In 1969, the ISR were replaced by the IHR which were revised in minor aspects in 1973 and 1981. The IHR (1969) focus on obligations of WHO Member States with regard to reporting of human cases and related hosts/vectors to WHO and implementation of public health response measures, primarily relating to three "quarantinable" diseases currently subject to the Regulations: cholera, plague, and yellow fever. There are also certain sanitary requirements for international ports and airports, as well as international maritime and air traffic, and a limited number of more generalized provisions.

The revision of the International Health Regulations

Weaknesses of the current IHR regarding surveillance

There is plainly limited value for overall disease surveillance from a reporting system focusing on only three diseases. The routine notification of even these three diseases has also often been incomplete, delayed, or otherwise lacking. The focus on these three diseases has also added to their effective stigmatization; at times, for example, countries have characterized cases of cholera in more generic terms, such as variations of acute/watery diarrhea, in order to avoid reporting.

Compliance with the notification obligations has also been undercut by the cycle of excessive or unjustified responses from trading and travel partners of the stricken country (e.g., in some contexts closing of borders to travelers and transport or rejection of imports with no role in transmission). In response to the 1991 arrival of cholera in parts of South America, trade and travel partners of affected countries at times rejected food imports and even some nonfood manufactured goods, or closed borders [8]. Some of these same problems arose again when some Asian countries experienced the severe acute respiratory syndrome (SARS) outbreaks in 2003.

In addition to technical shortcomings and obsolescence, the IHR (1969) have historically been subject to a number of additional detrimental factors, including the limitation on important WHO communications under the Regulations regarding outbreak information not officially reported by Member States and a tendency to ignore the legally binding nature of the IHR [8].

The changing world: emergence and reemergence of diseases

In 1995, noting the "continuous evolution in the public health threat posed by infectious diseases related to the agents themselves, to their easier transmission in changing physical and social environments, and to diagnostic and treatment capacities," the Health Assembly requested that the Director-General take steps to prepare a revision of the IHR [9]. By that time, it was already old news that infectious diseases were emerging and reemerging in every corner of the world in the course of globalized demographic and commercial activities, and that microbial agents travel from one country to another, often faster than the incubation periods of the diseases. By 1996, the WHO World Health Report noted that in the preceding 20 years, at least 30 diseases had emerged "to threaten the health of

hundreds of millions of people[,]" and that "[a]n outbreak anywhere must now be seen as a threat to virtually all countries, especially those that serve as major hubs of international travel" [10]. More recently, over a 5-year period, the WHO Alert and Response Operations group verified some 900 events of potential international public health importance. The variety of such events over the past decade is shown in Plate 2.1.

International travel and trade

The extent of international travel in the modern world presents an extraordinary opportunity for international disease transmission. According to the World Tourism Organization, international tourist arrivals reached "an all-time record" in 2005, exceeding 800 million, with growth in all regions [11]. Global trade in merchandise has similar implications in terms of potential foodborne or other goods-borne disease, from certain enteric diseases in fruits or vegetables to the agents of variant Creutzfeldt–Jakob disease carried in beef infected with bovine spongiform encephalopathy. In 2004, international exports of food products alone had a value of US$627 billion, and agricultural exports overall a value of US$783 billion [12]. When emergent infections enter the international trade network, their transmission is amplified, as is their potential impact in human and economic terms [13].

Drug resistance, environmental changes, and civil conflicts

The emergence and spread of drug-resistant strains of diseases are major challenges to the control and containment of globally significant infectious disease. Resistance to first-line drugs has been increasingly observed in a range of critical infectious diseases, including HIV/AIDS, diarrheal diseases, tuberculosis, and malaria. Such failures in treatment may also lead to longer periods of infectivity, which can increase the numbers of persons exposed to a drug-resistant infection. Under the newly revised IHR (2005), antibiotic resistance is one of the factors to be considered in assessing whether a public health "event" is one which "may constitute a public health emergency of international concern" and would hence be notifiable to WHO.

Regarding other developments associated with the emergence and reemergence processes, a recent Millennium Ecosystem Assessment report identified a number of environmental and related factors, including intensified human encroachment on natural environments, habitat alterations that lead to changes in vector breeding sites, reductions in biodiversity, particular livestock and poultry production methods, and environmental contamination by infectious disease agents [14]. As throughout history, wars, natural disasters, and other upheavals also continue to destroy public health infrastructure and cause mass migrations of persons in poor sanitary conditions across small and great distances, contributing to the transmission and emergence of disease in new areas or among new populations.

WHO's evolving role

Steps toward the new Regulations were accompanied by developments in the important role played by WHO's key alert and response (and other surveillance-related) activities [15,16]. As noted below, this trend reached a high point during the response to the SARS outbreaks. Together with other key proposals (such as the concept of public health emergencies of international concern) [17], these alert and response functions were to be key components of the IHR negotiations and would be reflected in the final text of the revised IHR (2005).

Naturally occurring, accidental, and deliberately caused events

The deliberate transmission of anthrax in the United States following the events of September 11, 2001, was a turning point in the perceived threat posed by infectious disease. The emergence of new infectious diseases had previously raised serious concerns about the negative social and economic impact of epidemics in modern societies, including their potential to become new threats to national security. The reality of bioterrorism brought the infectious disease threat directly to the attention of the security and defense communities, which became more interested in issues usually left to public health professionals, such as silent incubation periods, vaccine manufacturing capacity, and international measures to contain the international spread of diseases.

The healthcare system serves as the front line and main setting for public health response to naturally occurring, accidental, and deliberately caused epidemics. It is central to the detection of new cases, the confirmation of diagnosis, and the management of suspected or confirmed cases. The role of the public health sector is crucial in providing authoritative information on public health risk assessment and best control measures.

Against this background, the World Health Assembly in 2002 adopted a resolution explicitly acknowledging WHO's focus "on the possible public health consequences of an incident involving biological and chemical agents and radionuclear material, regardless of whether it is characterized as a natural occurrence, accidental release or a deliberate act" [18]. Incorporating this broad focus, and under their mandate to protect public health against international disease spread, the IHR (2005) have the potential to address health-related aspects of international public health risks that may also be seen as threats to national security, such as a bioterrorist attack as well as a severe influenza pandemic.

Defining *public health emergencies of international concern*

During the revision process, attention was focused on the problem of defining those events that should be required to be notified to WHO at the international level. In 2001, the Department for Epidemiology of the Swedish Institute for Infectious Disease Control was commissioned to carry out an expert consultation to establish criteria to define an urgent international public health event. Using a modified Delphi consultation process, the Swedish project resulted in the first draft of an algorithm or flowchart accompanied by more detailed indicators. This draft was then tested within WHO against events that were being identified through the Alert and Response Operations unit, and externally by epidemiologists who used it to evaluate a number of scenarios developed from actual events. After modification and further testing, the algorithm became the decision instrument contained in Annex 2 of the first draft of the IHR revision sent out by the WHO Secretariat for consultation in January 2004.

The term *public health emergency of international concern* became accepted as the label for those events that should be the major focus of notification and international response under the revised IHR. Thus, the Annex 2 decision instrument was formulated as a tool to assist the States Parties in identifying those events that may constitute public health emergencies of international concern, and therefore require notification to WHO (under Article 6 of the IHR (2005)). Further, the determination that an *actual* public health emergency of international concern is occurring became the starting point for a number of further actions within WHO, including specific information dissemination, coordination of response efforts, and guidance and support for States Parties, both those directly experiencing the emergency and others.

SARS and the global reaction

A further key development for WHO and the revision process was the SARS experience, including the central role played by WHO in control and containment efforts as well as surveillance [19] and the impetus it provided for formal negotiations on a revised IHR which began in late 2004 [20]. When SARS spread internationally in early 2003, the disease placed every country with an international airport at risk for an imported case. SARS spread from person to person, required no vector, displayed no particular geographical affinity, mimicked the symptoms of many other diseases, took its heaviest toll on hospital staff, and killed around 10% of those infected. In the absence of a vaccine or curative intervention, isolation and quarantine became the principal control measures. SARS caused great social disruption and economic losses far out of proportion to the number of cases and deaths and well beyond the outbreak sites. Projections for economic growth were revised downward. Commerce in distant countries dependent on Asian goods and manufacturing capacity suffered. Schools, hospitals, businesses, and some borders were closed. Broad access to electronic communications and extensive media coverage made the public deeply aware of SARS and fears about it spread. Travel to affected areas plummeted, causing airlines with Asian routes to lose an estimated US$10 billion. Fortunately, these consequences, apparent early on, brought political support at the highest level and increased pressure to contain the outbreak.

SARS revealed how much the world has changed in terms of increased and universal vulnerability to new disease threats. SARS challenged the assumption that wealthy nations, with their well-equipped hospitals and high standards of living, would be shielded from the amplification of cases seen when new diseases emerged in the developing world. Contrary to expectations, SARS spread most efficiently in sophisticated urban hospitals. SARS also redefined national responsibilities for outbreaks in two important ways. First, given the international repercussions of outbreaks in an interconnected and mobile world, governments are likely to be held accountable, by the international community as well as by their citizens, for failures in their response to an outbreak. Second, broad access to electronic communications—from mobile telephones to the Internet—has made it increasingly likely that official notification of an unusual disease event will be preempted by quickly spreading rumors that give national events an immediate international audience. It has accordingly made it almost impossible to conceal important outbreaks for any significant period of time. In February 2003, mobile telephone users sent millions of text messages about a fatal flu in Guangdong Province. SARS raised the profile of public health to new heights by demonstrating the severity of adverse effects that a health problem can have on economies, social stability, and political careers.

The negotiation process

Plans for a formal IHR negotiation process began with the adoption of resolution WHA56.28 by the World Health Assembly, which established an intergovernmental working group (IGWG), open to all WHO Member States, "to review and recommend a draft revision of the International Health Regulations for consideration by the Health Assembly under Article 21 of the WHO Constitution." In resolution WHA56.29 concerning SARS, adopted on the same day, Member States specifically requested the Director-General "to take into account evidence, experiences, knowledge and lessons acquired during the SARS response when revising the International Health Regulations." (Both resolutions are cited in the preceding section.)

A number of drafts of proposed revisions to the IHR (1969) were prepared prior to and during the course of the negotiations. Based upon initial comments and input, the WHO Secretariat prepared an initial draft which was made available on the WHO Web site in January 2004 [21]. Incorporating reports from a series of subsequent regional and subregional consultations and other comments received by WHO, the WHO Secretariat prepared a further draft disseminated on September 30, 2004 [22], together with information papers on issues raised in the consultations, including WHO's alert and response operations [23].

The first session of the IGWG met in November 2004 with delegates from 155 Member States registered; the second met in February and May 2005. At the request of the Health Assembly, the Director-General ensured that the participation of countries with limited resources was made a priority. Between the November and February meetings, a further draft revision [24] was prepared under the direction of the Chair of the IGWG, Irish ambassador Mary Whelan. After intensive negotiations, agreement on the draft revised IHR was reached at 4:20 on the morning of May 14. The IHR (2005) were adopted by the Health Assembly 9 days later.

A legally binding and globally accepted instrument

The global agreement to the revised WHO Regulations reflects an extraordinary collective consensus, and individual consent, to the instrument's legal norms. In a world marked by interdependence in terms of reciprocal needs to control diseases of international importance and where measures implemented by one State can affect the health and economies of so many others, the global agreement in favor of the IHR is of critical importance. Among international legal instruments generally, the IHR are one of the relatively few such binding agreements with such global acceptance. WHO Member States may opt out of the IHR; however, this has been fairly rare. Although predictions of future developments on the world stage are necessarily speculative, it appears at this time that the IHR (2005) are likely to be met with a very high level of international acceptance.

A further important characteristic of the Regulations is their legally binding nature. Although a complex issue, such binding international agreements can be associated with increased levels of compliance through greater expectations of compliance by the parties (as well as intergovernmental organizations and other important non-State actors in global health and politics), concerns about potential retributive responses by other parties in cases of noncompliance, and other factors.

Surveillance-related provisions in the IHR (2005)

National IHR Focal Points and WHO IHR Contact Points

Important procedural and institutional innovations under the IHR (2005) are the requirements under Article 4 that urgent IHR communications, including those concerning State Party reporting, are generally transmitted through specific National IHR Focal Points (for States Parties) and WHO IHR Contact Points (for WHO) in order to facilitate efficient and effective exchanges of event-related information. Where an existing governmental agency or unit can implement these functions, they must be officially designated accordingly; alternatively, new structures can be established.

Critical terms in the IHR (2005): disease and event

As with many other provisions in IHR (2005), the building blocks of alert and response obligations are the terms "disease" and "event." The disease-related scope of the IHR (2005) is extremely broad, including events where the underlying agent is not known (Table 2.2). There are no exceptions for events that may have originated in an intentional or deliberate act, or for events that may involve chemical, radiological, or infectious disease agents.

Role of WHO: surveillance, responding to State Party reports, use of unofficial sources, and verification

Under the IHR (2005), WHO is at the center of global surveillance of events with potential international implications. WHO's fundamental surveillance obligation is to "collect information regarding events through its surveillance activities and

Table 2.2 Key surveillance-related provisions in the IHR (2005).

New definitions
• Disease: "an illness or medical condition, irrespective of origin or source, that presents or could present significant harm to humans"
• Event: "a manifestation of disease or an occurrence that creates a potential for disease"
• Surveillance: "the systematic ongoing collection, collation and analysis of data for public health purposes and the timely dissemination of public health information for assessment and public health response as necessary"

States Parties
• Development and maintenance of core public health capacities for surveillance and response throughout territories
• Notification to WHO of: (i) all events which may constitute a public health emergency of international concern as determined by assessment using the decision instrument and additional guidance in Annex 2 of the IHR (2005); and (ii) all cases of four diseases–smallpox, poliomyelitis due to wild-type poliovirus, human influenza caused by a new subtype (including, for example, H5N1 in humans), and SARS
• Reporting to WHO of evidence of a public health risk identified outside of their territory which may cause international disease spread as manifested by imported/exported human cases, infected/contaminated vectors, and contaminated goods

WHO
• Collect and assess information about potential of events to cause international disease spread and possible interference with international traffic
• Obtain verification from States Parties of events which may constitute public health emergencies of international concern
• Collaborate with States Parties concerning notification and other reporting
• Support national capacity building for surveillance and response

assess their potential to cause international disease spread and possible interference with international traffic" (see Article 5.4). In addition to receiving and assessing notifications, reports, and consultations from States Parties, the revised Regulations expressly mandate that WHO seek verification from States Parties of information it has collected from unofficial sources or reports (e.g., the media, electronic mailing lists or networks, or non-governmental organizations) concerning potential events which may constitute public health emergencies of international concern. In turn, States are required to respond to WHO within 24 hours with an initial reply or acknowledgment, and the available public health information on the status of the referenced events (see Articles 9.1 and 10); they must also provide the detailed information required for assessments of such events (e.g., case definitions, laboratory results, numbers of cases and deaths). Although beyond the scope of this chapter on infectious disease surveillance, WHO has extensive additional responsibilities in the new Regulations, including public health response, related support

and coordination activities, as well as procedural and institutional functions.

Role of States Parties: notification, consultation, reports of imported and exported cases, and requests for assistance

Notification to WHO
Events which may constitute a public health emergency of international concern The critical State obligations for surveillance purposes arise in the range of event reports required under the IHR (2005). The primary reporting obligation under the revised IHR is the mandatory duty in Article 6 to "*assess*" "events" occurring within their territories according to the decision instrument and criteria in Annex 2, and then to *notify* WHO of all such "events which may constitute a public health emergency of international concern" within 24 hours of assessment. For State reporting, "events which may constitute a public health emergency of international concern" are effectively defined by the four criteria in the decision instrument and Annex 2 (see

Appendix to this chapter) that are tied to the specific context of the event at issue: whether the event has a serious public health impact, is unusual or unexpected, risks international spread, or risks restrictions on international traffic. If, upon application of the decision instrument by the State Party, an event within its territory fulfills two of the four listed criteria, the event qualifies as one that "may constitute" such an international emergency and must be notified by the State through its National IHR Focal Point. In addition to these criteria, there are 11 questions, and further indicative examples of factual contexts, to guide use of the decision instrument. The delegates agreed in the negotiations that the examples were not to be binding, but "are for indicative guidance purposes to assist in the interpretation of the decision instrument criteria" (see Appendix).

Consistent with the broad, nonspecific scope of the IHR (2005), the decision instrument—and hence State Party notification—does not require that the event involve a particular disease or kind of agent (i.e., biological, chemical, or nuclear) or even a known agent, nor does it exclude events based upon whether they may be accidental, natural, or intentional in nature.

Events that involve certain diseases and must always be analyzed under the decision instrument While the decision instrument and Annex 2 require that all events are subject to assessment as indicated, the IHR (2005) specifically provide that events involving a range of specific diseases that, as indicated above, "have demonstrated the ability to cause serious public health impact and to spread rapidly internationally" must always be analyzed utilizing the decision instrument (but only notified if fulfilling the same above requirements), including cholera, pneumonic plague, yellow fever, viral haemorrhagic fevers, West Nile fever, and other diseases that are of special national or regional concern (listing, e.g., dengue fever, Rift Valley fever, and meningococcal disease).

Diseases that always require notification Finally, the IHR (2005) identify four diseases that are "unusual or unexpected and may have serious public health impact" and hence always qualify as contexts which may constitute a public health emer-

gency of international concern. Accordingly, even one case of these diseases must be notified to WHO: smallpox, poliomyelitis due to wild-type poliovirus, human influenza caused by a new subtype (e.g., H5N1 in humans), and SARS.

Other reporting to WHO
Information sharing during unexpected or unusual public health events The IHR (2005) ultimately did not include a provision explicitly referring to reporting or information sharing concerning suspected intentional or deliberate releases of agents. As a result of related negotiations, the IHR (2005), however, do provide in Article 7 that "[i]f a State Party has evidence of an unexpected or unusual public health event within its territory, irrespective of origin or source, which may constitute a public health emergency of international concern, it shall provide to WHO all relevant public health information. In such a case, the provisions of Article 6 [requiring notification of detailed information on the event] shall apply in full." As a practical matter, it appears likely that reporting under this provision will overlap significantly with notification under Article 6.

Consultations As a complement to the obligation to notify, Article 8 provides an option for States Parties to keep WHO informed on a confidential basis regarding events within their territories that are apparently not notifiable under Article 6, and to consult with WHO on appropriate responsive health measures. This provision focuses "in particular [on] those events for which there is insufficient information available to complete the decision instrument[.]"

Reporting of foreign public health risks: imported and exported cases, vectors, and goods In addition to notification of events within their territories, States Parties are obligated under Article 9.2 to "inform WHO within 24 hours of receipt of evidence of a public health risk identified outside their territory that may cause international disease spread, as manifested by exported or imported: (a) human cases; (b) vectors which carry infection or contamination; or (c) goods that are contaminated." Unlike notifications under Article 6, this reporting obligation states that it is required "as far as practicable." It appears likely that many cases of disease in humans which are reportable under this provision will also be notifiable under Article 6.

Further surveillance-related provisions
Confidentiality and dissemination of information As part of an incentive to States Parties to notify and report events to WHO, the IHR (2005) in Article 11 provide that information in notifications under Article 6, reports under Article 9.2, and consultations under Article 8 is not to be made generally available to other States Parties, unless circumstances arise which justify dissemination generally in order to address the risk of international spread. The contexts justifying communication of the information to other States Parties are specified to include the situations where the Director-General has declared a public health emergency of international concern, where international spread has been confirmed, or where control measures are not likely to succeed or implementation of international control measures is required immediately. If WHO intends to make this information available to other States Parties, it will consult with the State Party experiencing the event.

WHO may also make it available to the public if other information about the event is already public and a related need exists for public availability of information that is authoritative and independent.

Development and maintenance of core surveillance capacities Separate from the above surveillance activities, a fundamental innovation in the IHR (2005) is the mandatory obligation for all States Parties to develop and maintain core public health capacities for surveillance (Article 5.1-.2) and response (Article 13.1-.2), both in accordance with Annex 1A, and to develop and maintain certain services and facilities at designated international ports, airports, and ground crossings (Article 19(a) and Annex 1B). These core public health capacities must be developed within 5 years of entry into force for each State Party, with options for two 2-year extensions under certain circumstances. Annex 1A delineates the domestic and international surveillance and response obligations in some detail for community, intermediate, and national levels of a country (see Table 2.3).

Table 2.3 Selected provisions: surveillance-related core capacity requirements.

4. At the local community level and/or primary public health response level
The capacities:
(a) to detect events involving disease or death above expected levels for the particular time and place in all areas within the territory of the State Party; and
(b) to report all available essential information immediately to the appropriate level of healthcare response. **** For the purposes of this Annex, essential information includes the following: clinical descriptions, laboratory results, sources and type of risk, numbers of human cases and deaths, conditions affecting the spread of the disease and the health measures employed; and
(c) ****
5. At the intermediate public health response levels
The capacities:
(a) to confirm the status of reported events and to support or implement additional control measures; and
(b) to assess reported events immediately and, if found urgent, to report all essential information to the national level. For the purposes of this Annex, the criteria for urgent events include serious public health impact and/or unusual or unexpected nature with high potential for spread.
6. At the national level
Assessment and notification. The capacities:
(a) to assess all reports of urgent events within 48 hours; and
(b) to notify WHO immediately through the National IHR Focal Point when the assessment indicates the event is notifiable pursuant to paragraph 1 of Article 6 and Annex 2 and to inform WHO as required pursuant to Article 7 and paragraph 2 of Article 9.

IHR (2005), Annex 1A (Response capacities omitted).

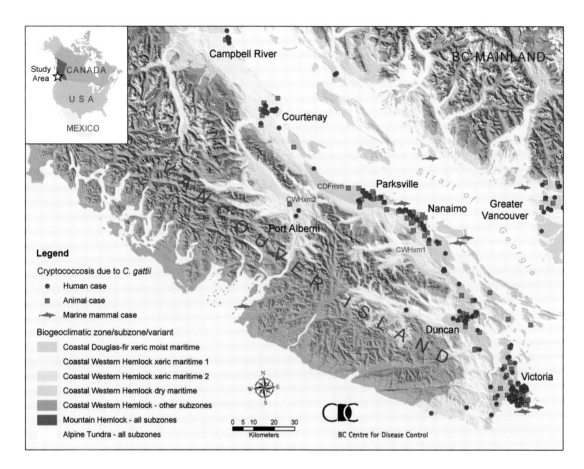

Plate 1.1 Geographic distribution of cryptococcal disease in humans and animals due to *Cryptococcus gattii* on Vancouver Island, Canada, from 1999 to 2004. Note that cases are mapped by place of residence, and the BC mainland cases are due to travel-related exposure on Vancouver Island.

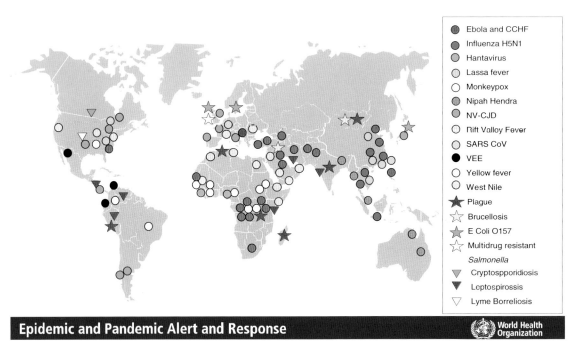

Epidemic and Pandemic Alert and Response

World Health Organization

Ebola and CCHF
Influenza H5N1
Hantavirus
Lassa fever
Monkeypox
Nipah Hendra
NV-CJD
Rift Valley Fever
SARS CoV
VEE
Yellow fever
West Nile
Plague
Brucellosis
E Coli O157
Multidrug resistant
Salmonella
Cryptospporidiosis
Leptospirossis
Lyme Borreliosis

Plate 2.1 Emerging and Re-emerging Infectious Diseases, 1996–2006. The boundaries and names shown and the designations used on this map do not imply the expression of any opinion whatsoever on the part of the WHO concerning the legal status of any country, territory, city, or area or of its authorities, or concerning the delimitation of its frontiers or boundaries. Dotted lines on maps represent approximate border lines for which there may not yet be full agreement.

Conclusion: the IHR (2005), implementation, and the future

Given the new Regulations' broadened scope and requirements, implementing the IHR (2005) is a challenge for both WHO and States, and efforts are underway to meet these challenges. For WHO, the IHR (2005) involve a range of technical areas, from epidemic-prone infectious diseases to chemical and nuclear agents, that will require involvement of many parts of WHO. In addition, implementation will require extensive coordination within an organization that operates globally, as well as at country and regional levels.

The implementation of the IHR (2005) will also be a challenge for many WHO Member States. The new rights and obligations established by the IHR (2005) for States Parties are extensive. It is in part for this reason that WHO's strategic implementation plan for the IHR (2005) builds on existing regional and national strategies for epidemic-prone diseases. Such strategies, however, are no substitute for the high level of commitment that will be needed at the individual country level and through international collaboration.

In light of the shortcomings of the current IHR (1969), important issues for the IHR (2005) will be how to deal with those concerns under the revised surveillance-related requirements. Cholera, plague, and yellow fever (particularly the first two) are likely to remain stigmatized for at least the foreseeable future; these diseases are all specifically referenced in the IHR (2005) as diseases that trigger use of the decision instrument to assess potential notification. Recent years have also brought new diseases that have become "stigmatized" to varying extents. There will still be pressures and fears of excessive restrictions on trade or travel from an affected State Party.

However, much has changed in the world and in the IHR (2005) that augur well for the future. The expanding scope of electronic media and tools such as the Global Public Health Information Network (Chapter 23) will ensure that, as a practical matter, countries will find it increasingly the best approach to be transparent about outbreaks or other public health events within their territories with potential international implications. Together with WHO's new mandate to seek verification and share information with other States Parties under certain circumstances, these developments will call for greater openness about these events.

Additional favorable factors for effective implementation of the IHR (2005) are the new expectations and resolve of Member States and WHO associated with the face-to-face negotiations and adoption of this unprecedented new public health instrument, awareness of its legally binding nature, the new sense of urgency associated with SARS and avian and human influenza, the extensive research and planning that went into development of the new surveillance provisions, and the unavoidable acknowledgment that this is an increasingly interdependent world in terms of international transport, trade, travel, and *public health*.

References

1 World Health Organization. *International Health Regulations (1969)*, 3rd edn. Geneva: World Health Organization; 1983.

2 World Health Assembly. Revision of the International Health Regulations, WHA58.3. May 23, 2005. Available from: http://www.who.int/csr/ihr/IHRWHA58_3-en.pdf. Accessed January 3, 2007.

3 Burci GL, Vignes CH. *World Health Organization*. The Hague: Kluwer Law International; 2004.

4 Office International d'Hygiène Publique. Vingt-cinq Ans d'Activité de l'Office International d'Hygiène Publique, 1909–1933, Paris: Office International d'Hygiène Publique; 1933. Available from: http://whqlibdoc.who.int/hist/chronicles/publique_hygiene_1909-1933.pdf. Accessed January 3, 2007.

5 Health Organization. League of Nations: Health Organization. Geneva: Health Organization; 1931. Available from: http://whqlibdoc.who.int/hist/chronicles/health_org_1931.pdf. Accessed January 3, 2007.

6 Aginam O. International law and communicable diseases. *Bull World Health Organ* 2002; **80**(12):946–51.

7 Constitution of the World Health Organization, July 22, 1946. In: *Basic Documents*, 45th edn. Geneva: World Health Organization; 2005:1–18.

8 Plotkin BJ, Kimball AM. Designing an international policy and legal framework for the control of emerging infectious diseases: first steps. *Emerging Infect Dis* 1997;3(1):1–9.

9 World Health Assembly. Revision and updating of the International Health Regulations, WHA48.7. May 12, 1995.

10 World Health Organization. *World Health Report 1996: Fighting Disease, Fostering Development*. Geneva: World Health Organization; 1996.

11 World Tourism Organization. Tourism highlights 2006 edition: overview international tourism 2005. Madrid: World Tourism Organization; 2006. Available from: http://www.unwto.org/facts/eng/pdf/highlights/highlights_06_eng_hr.pdf. Accessed January 2, 2007.

12 World Trade Organization. International Trade Statistics 2005. Geneva: World Trade Organization; 2005. Available from: http://www.wto.org/english/res_e/statis_e/its2005_e/section4_e/iv01.xls. Accessed January 2, 2007.

13 Kimball AM, Arima Y, Hodges JR. Trade related infections: farther, faster, quieter. Globalization and Health [serial on the Internet]. April 22, 2005. Available from: http://www.globalizationandhealth.com/content/1/1/3. Accessed January 2, 2007.

14 Corvalan C, Hales S, McMichael A [core writing team]. Ecosystems and human well being: health synthesis: a report of the Millennium Ecosystem Assessment. Geneva: World Health Organization. Available from: http://www.who.int/globalchange/ecosystems/ecosysbegin.pdf. Accessed January 3, 2007.

15 World Health Assembly. Communicable diseases prevention and control: new, emerging, and reemerging infectious diseases, WHA48.13. May 12, 1995.

16 World Health Assembly. Global health security: epidemic alert and response, WHA54.14. May 21, 2001.

17 World Health Organization. Global crises—global solutions: managing public health emergencies of international concern through the revised International Health Regulations. Geneva: World Health Organization; 2002. Available from: http://www.who.int/csr/resources/publications/ihr/en/whocdsgar20024.pdf. Accessed January 2, 2007.

18 World Health Assembly. Global health response to natural occurrence, accidental release or deliberate use of biological and chemical agents or radionuclear material that affect health, WHA55.16. May 18, 2002.

19 World Health Assembly. Severe acute respiratory syndrome (SARS), WHA56.29. May 28, 2003.

20 World Health Assembly. Revision of the International Health Regulations, WHA56.28. May 28, 2003.

21 World Health Organization. International Health Regulations: working paper for regional consultations. Geneva: World Health Organization; 2004. Available from: http://www.who.int/csr/resources/publications/IGWG_IHR_WP12_03-en.pdf. Accessed January 3, 2007.

22 World Health Organization. Review and approval of proposed amendments to the International Health Regulations: draft revision. Geneva: World Health Organization; 2004. Available from: http://www.who.int/gb/ghs/pdf/A_IHR_IGWG_3-en.pdf. Accessed January 2, 2007.

23 World Health Organization. Review and approval of proposed amendments to the International Health Regulations: alert and response operations: report by the Secretariat. Geneva: World Health Organization; 2005. Available from: http://www.who.int/gb/ghs/pdf/IHR_IGWG2_ID1-en.pdf. Accessed January 2, 2007.

24 World Health Organization. Review and approval of proposed amendments to the International Health Regulations: proposal by the chair. Geneva: World Health Organization; 2005. Available from: http://www.who.int/gb/ghs/pdf/IHR_IGWG2_2-en.pdf. Accessed January 3, 2007.

Appendix: Annex 2 of International Health Regulations (2005)

ANNEX 2

DECISION INSTRUMENT FOR THE ASSESSMENT AND NOTIFICATION OF EVENTS THAT
MAY CONSTITUTE A PUBLIC HEALTH EMERGENCY OF INTERNATIONAL CONCERN

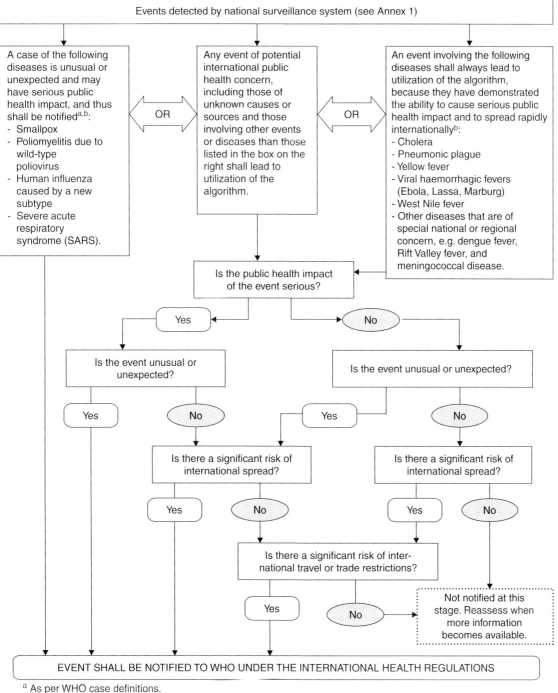

EXAMPLES FOR THE APPLICATION OF THE DECISION INSTRUMENT FOR THE ASSESSMENT AND NOTIFICATION OF EVENTS THAT MAY CONSTITUTE A PUBLIC HEALTH EMERGENCY OF INTERNATIONAL CONCERN

The examples appearing in this Annex are not binding and are for indicative guidance purposes to assist in the interpretation of the decision instrument criteria.

DOES THE EVENT MEET AT LEAST TWO OF THE FOLLOWING CRITERIA?

	I. Is the public health impact of the event serious?
	1. *Is the number of cases and/or number of deaths for this type of event large for the given place, time or population?*
	2. *Has the event the potential to have a high public health impact?*
	THE FOLLOWING ARE EXAMPLES OF CIRCUMSTANCES THAT CONTRIBUTE TO HIGH PUBLIC HEALTH IMPACT:
	✓ Event caused by a pathogen with high potential to cause epidemic (infectiousness of the agent, high case fatality, multiple transmission routes or healthy carrier).
	✓ Indication of treatment failure (new or emerging antibiotic resistance, vaccine failure, antidote resistance or failure).
	✓ Event represents a significant public health risk even if no or very few human cases have yet been identified.
	✓ Cases reported among health staff.
	✓ The population at risk is especially vulnerable (refugees, low level of immunization, children, elderly, low immunity, undernourished, etc.).
	✓ Concomitant factors that may hinder or delay the public health response (natural catastrophes, armed conflicts, unfavourable weather conditions, multiple foci in the State Party).
	✓ Event in an area with high population density.
	✓ Spread of toxic, infectious or otherwise hazardous materials that may be occurring naturally or otherwise that has contaminated or has the potential to contaminate a population and/or a large geographical area.
	3. *Is external assistance needed to detect, investigate, respond and control the current event, or prevent new cases?*
	THE FOLLOWING ARE EXAMPLES OF WHEN ASSISTANCE MAY BE REQUIRED:
	✓ Inadequate human, financial, material or technical resources – in particular:
	– Insufficient laboratory or epidemiological capacity to investigate the event (equipment, personnel, financial resources)
	– Insufficient antidotes, drugs and/or vaccine and/or protective equipment, decontamination equipment, or supportive equipment to cover estimated needs
	– Existing surveillance system is inadequate to detect new cases in a timely manner.
	IS THE PUBLIC HEALTH IMPACT OF THE EVENT SERIOUS?
	Answer "yes" if you have answered "yes" to questions 1, 2 or 3 above.

Is the public health impact of the event serious?

	II. Is the event unusual or unexpected?
Is the event unusual or unexpected?	4. *Is the event unusual?*
	THE FOLLOWING ARE EXAMPLES OF UNUSUAL EVENTS:
	✓ The event is caused by an unknown agent or the source, vehicle, route of transmission is unusual or unknown.
	✓ Evolution of cases more severe than expected (including morbidity or case-fatality) or with unusual symptoms.
	✓ Occurrence of the event itself unusual for the area, season or population.
	5. *Is the event unexpected from a public health perspective?*
	THE FOLLOWING ARE EXAMPLES OF UNEXPECTED EVENTS:
	✓ Event caused by a disease/agent that had already been eliminated or eradicated from the State Party or not previously reported.
	IS THE EVENT UNUSUAL OR UNEXPECTED? **Answer "yes" if you have answered "yes" to questions 4 or 5 above.**

	III. Is there a significant risk of international spread?
Is there a significant risk of international spread?	6. *Is there evidence of an epidemiological link to similar events in other States?*
	7. *Is there any factor that should alert us to the potential for cross border movement of the agent, vehicle or host?*
	THE FOLLOWING ARE EXAMPLES OF CIRCUMSTANCES THAT MAY PREDISPOSE TO INTERNATIONAL SPREAD:
	✓ Where there is evidence of local spread, an index case (or other linked cases) with a history within the previous month of:
	– international travel (or time equivalent to the incubation period if the pathogen is known)
	– participation in an international gathering (pilgrimage, sports event, conference, etc.)
	– close contact with an international traveller or a highly mobile population.
	✓ Event caused by an environmental contamination that has the potential to spread across international borders.
	✓ Event in an area of intense international traffic with limited capacity for sanitary control or environmental detection or decontamination.
	IS THERE A SIGNIFICANT RISK OF INTERNATIONAL SPREAD? **Answer "yes" if you have answered "yes" to questions 6 or 7 above.**

	IV. Is there a significant risk of international travel or trade restrictions?
Risk of international restrictions ?	8. *Have similar events in the past resulted in international restriction on trade and/or travel?*
	9. *Is the source suspected or known to be a food product, water or any other goods that might be contaminated that has been exported/imported to/from other States?*
	10. *Has the event occurred in association with an international gathering or in an area of intense international tourism?*
	11. *Has the event caused requests for more information by foreign officials or international media?*
	IS THERE A SIGNIFICANT RISK OF INTERNATIONAL TRADE OR TRAVEL RESTRICTIONS? **Answer "yes" if you have answered "yes" to questions 8, 9, 10 or 11 above.**

States Parties that answer "yes" to the question whether the event meets any two of the four criteria (I-IV) above, shall notify WHO under Article 6 of the International Health Regulations.

31

3

Active, population-based surveillance for infectious diseases

Chris A. Van Beneden, Sonja J. Olsen, Tami H. Skoff &
Ruth Lynfield

Introduction

Active, population-based surveillance can be a powerful surveillance tool for monitoring infectious diseases and evaluating disease prevention strategies. As will be described in this chapter, one of the main strengths of this intensive type of surveillance is its potential to provide comprehensive, accurate data on disease incidence that are generalizable to larger populations. We will illustrate the key components of active, population-based surveillance as it is implemented in two disparate settings—the Active Bacterial Core surveillance (ABCs) in the United States (US), a program within the US Centers for Disease Control and Prevention's (CDC) Emerging Infections Program Network (EIP), and the Thailand International Emerging Infections Program (IEIP), a collaboration between the Thailand Ministry of Public Health and CDC. IEIP sites are core components of CDC's Global Disease Detection Program, the agency's principal and most visible program developing strengthened global capacity to identify and respond to emerging infections around the world. Both these programs address emerging infections.

Emerging infections programs: an overview

In 1992, the Institute of Medicine issued the report *Emerging Infections: Microbial Threats to Health in the United States* [1]. In it, emerging infections are defined as "new, re-emerging, or drug-resistant infections whose incidence in humans has increased within the past two decades or whose incidence threatens to increase in the near future." In late 1994, CDC established EIP, a collaboration among CDC, state health departments, academic institutions and partners, including local health departments, public health and clinical laboratories, infection control professionals, healthcare providers, and other federal agencies. The objectives of EIP are to assess the impact of emerging infections on public health and to evaluate methods for their prevention and control. In 2001, the first international EIP site was developed in Thailand.

Active Bacterial Core surveillance

One of the core components of the US EIP is ABCs [2]. The Foodborne Diseases Active Surveillance Network (FoodNet), another core component, is described in Chapter 5. Since its inception in 1994, ABCs has grown to include 10 geographically disparate surveillance areas in the US: California (the 3-county San Francisco Bay area), Colorado (5-county Denver area), New York (15-county Rochester and Albany areas), Tennessee (11-urban counties), and the entire states of Connecticut, Georgia, Maryland, Minnesota, New Mexico, and Oregon (Figure 3.1). In 2006, the population under surveillance was approximately 39 million people and represented 13% of the US population (see http://www.cdc.gov/ abcs/). ABCs includes surveillance for a number of invasive bacterial diseases: group A *Streptococcus*, group B *Streptococcus*, *Streptococcus pneumoniae*, *Haemophilus*

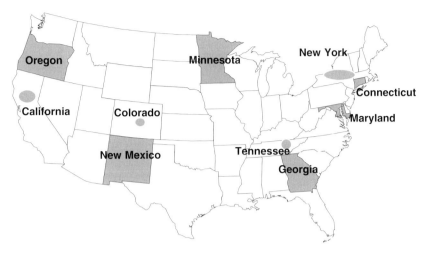

Fig 3.1 Active Bacterial Core surveillance sites, 2006.

influenzae, Neisseria meningitidis, and methicillin-resistant *Staphylococcus aureus*.

ABCs documents the disease burden and epidemiology of ABCs pathogens, tracks antimicrobial resistance, and contributes to development of vaccines and vaccine recommendations. ABCs also serves as a base from which applied epidemiological research can be performed, including case-control studies to determine risk factors for disease, evaluation of different strategies for prevention and control of disease, and measurement of the postlicensure vaccine impact on disease.

International Emerging Infections Programs

As of 2006, the US Health and Human Services and CDC, in collaboration with Ministries of Health, have established collaborations to address emerging infections in five countries: Thailand, Kenya, China, Guatemala, and Egypt (Figure 3.2). The first IEIP began in Thailand in late 2001 and built upon a collaboration between the Thailand Ministry of Public Health and the US CDC that had commenced in 1980 [3]. The four pillars of these programs are active population-based surveillance, applied public health research, outbreak support, and capacity building. Priority areas of focus for the population-based surveillance component of IEIP include diseases of both local and international importance, such as pneumonia and diarrhea, for

which there may be opportunities for vaccine or other interventions.

Definition and rationale for active, population-based surveillance

In general, *passive* surveillance is provider-initiated surveillance that relies on a healthcare provider or laboratory personnel to report an infectious disease to public health authorities. In contrast, *active* surveillance is initiated by a local, state, or national public health agency. In *active* surveillance, public health personnel actively solicit reports of the disease of interest directly from a provider who has recognized a suspected or confirmed infection in a patient or from a laboratory that has identified the infectious agent. Population-based surveillance is surveillance conducted among an entire or a representative sample of a predefined population.

Active, population-based surveillance is often considered the "gold standard" of surveillance because it theoretically captures 100% of diagnosed cases in a well-defined population. The health data collected from active, population-based surveillance can be used to estimate the burden of disease (morbidity) and deaths (mortality) in both the population under surveillance and a larger geographic area with similar population characteristics and epidemiologic setting, to calculate age- and sex-specific disease incidence rates, to monitor disease trends

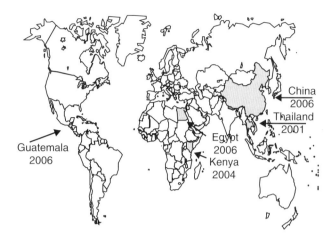

Fig 3.2 Location and inception date for the five International Emerging Infections Programs.

over time, and to evaluate the impact of various public health interventions.

Methodology: setting up active, population-based surveillance

When setting up an active, population-based surveillance system, several factors need to be addressed proactively. These include the choice of the particular disease or pathogen to be monitored, engaging partners, ensuring data quality, and the approach taken to analyze and disseminate data. In addition, the components that must be in place to ensure data reliability include a clear case definition, appropriate pairing of cases and the denominator, closely monitored collection and management of data and isolates, and methods for auditing the reporting system to ensure completeness of case ascertainment. These key elements of establishing high-quality active and population-based surveillance are described below.

Selection of diseases under surveillance

Because the resources required to set up and maintain any surveillance system are invariably limited, careful thought must go into selecting the infectious disease for which surveillance should be performed. This may be especially critical in the design of active, population-based surveillance that may require especially intensive use of resources. Some

issues to take into account include the impact of the infectious disease on the population:
• Does the disease have a high morbidity and mortality?
• Is the disease very communicable?
• Do effective disease prevention measures exist?
• Does prevention or treatment consume significant resources?
• Are surveillance data needed to develop vaccines or other disease prevention measures, and to assess the impact of these prevention measures?

Engaging surveillance partners

Engaging potential partners early in the development of a new active, population-based surveillance system allows for a more thorough understanding of the needs for surveillance and the possible resource, personnel and political constraints. In addition to dedicated staff (i.e., surveillance officers) at the level of the public health agency responsible for the surveillance, surveillance often depends upon the cooperation of many others including local public health personnel, infection control professionals, laboratorians, clinicians, and government and academic partners. International EIP collaborations are usually a bilateral relationship between the Ministry of Health and the US Department of Health and Human Services' CDC. Additional partners can also be found in the World Health Organization (WHO) or nongovernmental organizations.

It may take years for a surveillance system to be fully functional and provide data useful for decision makers. Local support from public health officials and clinicians is paramount to the successful integration of the system into the existing public health structure and its long-term sustainability. At all times it is important to understand potential barriers to surveillance, including an increase in workload and training needed for implementation of new information systems, and to work with partners to determine solutions. Another major component of the partnership, the dissemination and use of data, will be discussed later in the chapter, but this component must be considered in the earliest stages of the development of any surveillance system.

Case definition

As with all surveillance, the case definitions for diseases tracked in an active, population-based surveillance system must include person, place, and time. Specific to this type of surveillance is the need for an objective means of disease confirmation to maintain a measurable, standardized case definition. These programs have aspired to high degrees of precision, and have tended to focus on diseases that can be more readily and objectively diagnosed. The optimal case definition includes a diagnostic test for the disease under surveillance that is widely and readily available and has a high degree of sensitivity and specificity. Many current active, population-based surveillance systems, including ABCs, are laboratory-based and rely on confirmation of the presence of a bacterium or virus through positive culture, identification of nucleic acid, or a rise in a specific antibody. Infectious diseases that rely on clinical judgment are more difficult to monitor accurately, as are diseases for which laboratory testing is not adequately sensitive, specific, or standardized across multiple clinics or laboratories comprising the surveillance area.

In some situations it may be important to conduct active, population-based surveillance for diseases for which a suitable laboratory test is unavailable or is not widely used. Despite the challenges with clinical surveillance for a disease syndrome, this approach may be necessary in the international arena where laboratory capacity may be less well developed and less routinely used. In this setting it is critical to develop a standard clinical case definition that removes clinical judgment. In Thailand's pneumonia surveillance, chest radiographs interpreted by a panel of radiologists blinded to clinical information except age and sex are used to enhance the clinical criteria to define a case [4]. In this situation, laboratory testing of a subset of patients should accompany clinical surveillance, where feasible.

For other diseases or settings, laboratory diagnostic tests may be available but the approach toward testing and the specific tests used lack uniformity. For example, the US EIP sites are now conducting population-based surveillance for individuals hospitalized with laboratory-confirmed influenza. Laboratory tests employed clinically include rapid diagnostics with differing sensitivities and specificities. In addition, many patients are not tested for influenza but are treated empirically. As a result influenza surveillance is not as accurate as population-based surveillance for culture-confirmed bacterial disease. Nevertheless, it does provide insight into the burden of influenza and serves as a platform to assess vaccine effectiveness among specific subgroups [5].

The residence or geographic location of the case patient is a critical part of the case definition of population-based surveillance. Challenges include categorization of residence of transient populations such as temporary migrant workers and college students attending school outside of their hometown jurisdiction. Although the specific rules for handling these situations may be made by the public health personnel who are establishing or developing the system, the most important principle to follow is the need to be consistent when applying rules for categorization.

Calculations of disease incidence: importance of numerators and denominators

An essential aspect of population-based surveillance—regardless whether syndrome- or laboratory-based, active or passive—is the accurate description and matching of both the numerator and denominator data regarding the population under surveillance. Both cases of disease (the numerator) and the surveillance population (denominator) should be residents of the predefined surveillance area. To capture the numerator data, it is important to assess where the population under surveillance tends to seek healthcare services to ensure that the providers who treat patients from the geographic area under surveillance and the laboratories that process clinical specimens from these patients are contacted to detect potential cases. Residents of a county or state may travel to a neighboring county or state for medical care. Similarly, clinical specimens might be sent outside of the surveillance area for testing at a reference laboratory. It is important to be able to include these cases.

It is also essential to choose a surveillance population or catchment area for which one can obtain reliable denominator data. In the US, census data (typically by counties under surveillance) are most commonly used to establish denominator data. Alternatively, for pathogens causing neonatal disease such as group B *Streptococcus*, live birth data obtained from birth certificates or birth registries can be used for the denominator. Thailand also has comprehensive census data that can be used to accurately define the population denominator.

Case ascertainment

The trigger for case detection and reporting is the identification of a case of interest by a healthcare provider or laboratory. In countries with a robust laboratory infrastructure like the US, the most efficient method of capturing all cases of a laboratory-confirmed infection is to maintain routine contact with the laboratory processing patient samples. In ABCs, a network of surveillance personnel, infection control professionals, and local health department staff are the "eyes and ears" of the surveillance system. They routinely visit or make contact with participating laboratories to capture all cases of interest. This process is labor- and time-intensive, especially when travel is required to laboratories spread out over a large geographic area. However, with the increasing use of electronic databases, this task has become easier. Once surveillance staff have established good relationships with laboratories where electronic reporting capabilities exist, laboratories may routinely generate and send electronic summaries of case information to the surveillance staff.

In countries where laboratory capacity is not well developed, case ascertainment for active, population-based surveillance is conducted differently than in the US. In rural Thailand, most hospitals conduct routine clinical testing such as chemistry and hematology but lack resources necessary for bacteriological testing. The initial disease under surveillance in the Thailand IEIP was severe (requiring hospitalization) pneumonia with radiographic confirmation. Surveillance officers use a standard clinical case definition to identify cases of pneumonia at the time of admission to 1 of 20 acute care hospitals (18 public health and 2 military) in two provinces [6]. Chest radiographs are digitized and sent to Bangkok to be interpreted by a panel of radiologists using standard criteria based on WHO guidelines [4]. In the second year of clinical surveillance, the pneumonia patients were enrolled into a research study to identify the etiologies for which routine testing was not available. In this and similar surveillance systems, hospital-based surveillance can appropriately be considered population-based if the case definition requires hospitalization (as a marker of severity) and it is known that patients in the population who have severe disease seek care only at the hospital for which the surveillance is established.

Data collection

Once a case is identified, data collection includes completion of a standardized form that collects demographic information such as age, race and ethnicity, type of infection, disease outcome (e.g., hospitalization, death), and underlying comorbidities (e.g., diabetes, heart disease, HIV infection). Other potential variables include risk factors for infection and vaccination history (Table 3.1) (see example, ABCs case report form: http://www.cdc.gov/ncidod/dbmd/abcs/files/ABCs 2005-2006_CaseReportForm.pdf). In ABCs, data are obtained through review of patient medical records; to protect patient confidentiality, identifiable information such as name and address are removed before data are transmitted and aggregated at the national level. Alternative strategies may include patient and provider interview. In order to limit individual interpretations in the data collection phase, standardized data collection instruments, written instruction

Table 3.1 Typical data elements collected on case report forms.

Key data elements or variables

- Person (unique identifier or name)
- Place (patient's address or other geographic location, e.g., city, county, province, state)
- Age (or date of birth)
- Sex or gender
- Race
- Time (e.g., date of illness onset, date of confirmatory laboratory test)
- Clinical illness or disease presentation (e.g., bacteremia, pneumonia, meningitis)*
- Outcome (e.g., hospitalization, death)

Optional variables
- Disease risk factor information (e.g., presence of underlying diseases or conditions such as diabetes, HIV infection, exposure to disease vector)
- History of vaccination (if applicable)
- Further pathogen characterization[†]: result of antimicrobial susceptibility testing, subtyping (e.g., serotype of *S. pneumoniae, emm* or M-type of group A streptococcus)

*For clinical disease surveillance, this section will be more detailed and collect information on admission signs and symptoms.

[†]Laboratory testing results may be found in patient charts but more frequently are obtained from reference laboratories and eventually merged with case report form data.

manuals, and standard operating procedures or protocols should be developed and accompany staff training [7].

In a laboratory-based surveillance system such as ABCs, bacterial isolates are collected and sent to reference laboratories for microbiological confirmation and further characterization (e.g., antimicrobial susceptibilities, serotype) as shown in Figure 3.3. Frequent contact (e.g., monthly) with participating clinical laboratories is important not only for case detection but also for isolate collection as bacterial isolates are often discarded by laboratories within days to a few weeks of collection. The incorporation of case-isolate characterization is a powerful component that expands the value of surveillance, e.g., facilitating description of antimicrobial resistance trends or an evaluation of the impact of

vaccine targeted against particular serotypes. In the international setting where such laboratory testing may not be routine, specimen collection and testing can occur through a research protocol.

Data management

Surveillance data should be maintained in a common electronic database. Surveillance personnel can complete a paper case report form or enter data directly into the database. The data flow within the ABCs system is shown schematically in Figure 3.3. Moves toward more automated data entry systems, such as scannable forms or handheld computers, may help to limit the number of data entry errors. When establishing a data management system, careful thought and consideration should go into the creation of database elements. The format and coding of individual variables, the size and manageability of data files, and the compatibility of the data with other data sources (e.g., census files) are some of the issues that need to be considered. Proper management of surveillance data is critical and can often become quite complex.

System monitoring and evaluation

Because complete case detection and collection of accurate demographic and clinical information are essential in active, population-based surveillance, methods for monitoring and evaluation of the surveillance system should be developed and standardized. Strategies for system monitoring begin with evaluation of data accuracy and completeness. Internal data checks, through automated data entry validation (looking for internal inconsistencies), double data entry, or manual review by staff of their records, should occur frequently.

Systematic audits assure complete case detection. In ABCs, if a laboratory is not able to routinely report all positive cultures of the pathogens under surveillance via an electronic printout, an on-site laboratory audit is performed biannually to capture any missed cases identified in the previous 6 months. Surveillance staff review laboratory logbooks or electronic lists of testing results to detect ABCs pathogens; the subsequent list is compared to a list of cases reported through routine ABCs surveillance to detect any missed cases. Even

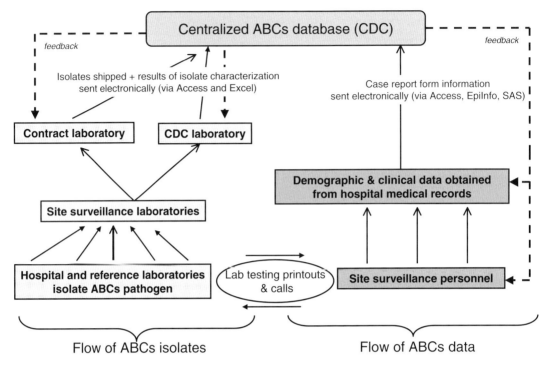

Fig 3.3 Data, isolate, and feedback pathways, Active Bacterial Core surveillance (ABCs).

if the participating laboratory routinely reports all cultures of interest via computer printouts, ABCs surveillance staff still periodically review the laboratory's testing results to ensure complete case detection. For cases newly identified through an audit, ABCs staff review the medical record and complete a case report form, and bacterial isolates are collected, if available.

Surveillance staff should routinely assess data completeness. If essential variables (e.g., age, outcome) are frequently found to be incomplete, the method of data collection should be reviewed and modified to correct the problem. Performance indicators are measures used to quantify the objectives of a surveillance system and to reflect the performance of the system. They are also used to motivate surveillance staff to improve quality of their work and to communicate achievements to partners in the public health arena and to policy makers in the larger community. ABCs uses the following performance measures to indicate the accuracy of the system: sensitivity of >90% for routine surveillance (as confirmed by laboratory audit) and collection of >85% of bacterial isolates from reported cases.

In the IEIPs, yearly audits are conducted by staff not associated with the day-to-day operations in the province. In Thailand, staff at the Bureau of Epidemiology perform audits using performance indicators to assess completeness of reporting and coverage of screening criteria through a manual review of inpatient admission logbooks, medical records, and discharge diagnoses (Table 3.2).

Data analysis and feedback

In addition to audits and use of performance indicators, periodic review and analysis of data are necessary to (a) maximize data quality, (b) detect important disease trends, and (c) provide timely feedback and motivation to surveillance participants. Although rigorous, detailed and formal analysis of the available surveillance data should be completed after surveillance is well-established, regular and periodic review of all interim data is critical. Periodic data review increases the potential

Table 3.2 Audit procedures used in pneumonia surveillance, Thailand IEIP.

Performance measure	Methods	Target
Completeness of case reporting	• Review inpatient logbooks for 1 month (30 days) • Identify patients that meet the screening criteria (cases) • Compare names to those reported for that month • Calculate completeness (%) of reporting	Number of cases reported in surveillance is ≥90% of number identified by audit of logbooks
Completeness of case capture by screening criteria	• Review hospital discharge data for 1 month (30 days) • Identify patients discharged with pneumonia (ICD10 codes J12.9 through J18.9) • Review charts to determine whether community or nosocomially acquired* • Compare patient names to those reported to surveillance for that month • Determine proportion (%) captured by screening criteria	Number reported in surveillance is ≥80% of the number identified by audit of admit and discharge data
Patients with chest radiograph taken within 48 hours of admission	• Review suspect pneumonia patients who have not had chest radiograph • Determine % of patients with suspect pneumonia who have had chest radiograph taken >48 hours after admission	Number of suspect pneumonia patients with chest radiograph taken >48 hours after admission is ≤20% the total number of suspect cases

*Community-acquired: pneumonia acquired in the community as defined by (1) patient entered hospital with evidence of acute infection and signs/symptoms of respiratory illness and (2) patient not hospitalized within 3 days prior to admission; Nosocomially acquired: pneumonia acquired in the hospital as defined by (1) patient hospitalized for ≥3 days before developing evidence of acute infection and signs/symptoms of respiratory illness or (2) patient hospitalized within 3 days prior to current admission.

for detection of disease outbreaks, identifies possible changes in the epidemiology of the disease under surveillance (i.e., increased antimicrobial resistance), and highlights trends (i.e., seasonal variation in influenza) that may be used to guide vaccine recommendations [8]. More detailed discussion of analysis of surveillance data is provided in Chapters 27–29.

Engaging partners in periodic review and analysis of surveillance data is vital to the continued success of a surveillance program. This begins with feedback to participating epidemiologists, surveillance and laboratory staff using multiple formats including: data integrity checks, basic summary tables of key descriptive variables and completeness of data, summary of laboratory results from reference laboratories, and sharing of data through newsletters or other types of data summaries. Involvement of part-

ners also includes coauthoring publications when criteria for authorship are met.

Key advantages, disadvantages, and ongoing challenges of active, population-based surveillance

The primary benefit of population-based surveillance is the ability to calculate reliable disease rates across selected age groups, race, and sex, when the appropriate information is also available for the denominator, allowing both the development of public health policies for disease prevention aimed at higher risk groups and measurement of the impact of vaccine and other prevention efforts. If laboratory-based, this system also allows detection of the emergence of rare isolates or serotypes among a population under surveillance that is of adequate size.

Another advantage is that the resulting infrastructure can be used to assess other emerging public health issues. For example, in response to reports of severe illnesses among children with laboratory-confirmed influenza early in the 2003–2004 influenza season, US EIP sites rapidly developed and issued surveys to assess the burden of disease in their states [5]. The results led to development of a surveillance system for children hospitalized with laboratory-confirmed influenza. Central reference laboratories can be utilized to improve detection and diagnosis of important or novel pathogens both inside and outside the surveillance area. This may be particularly true in the international setting. For example, the US CDC recently transferred technology to the Thailand National Institute of Health (NIH) to rapidly detect viral pathogens causing pneumonia by real-time reverse transcriptase polymerase chain reaction. These assays can be used to detect a number of respiratory viruses, including influenza virus, from specimens sent to the Thailand NIH from anywhere in the country.

Chief among the disadvantages are the resource requirements; population-based surveillance is an expensive endeavor in terms of monetary resources and personnel. The activities in the US and Thailand would not be sustainable without the additional federal resources allocated to EIP. Because of this cost, it is imperative that public health personnel periodically review the information gleaned from surveillance to determine if objectives have been reached on a particular disease, so that surveillance can be modified or discontinued in order to conduct surveillance for a new emerging disease. Advantages and disadvantages are outlined in Table 3.3.

Examples of the use and impact of active, population-based surveillance

As summarized above, data from active, population-based surveillance are powerful

Table 3.3 Advantages and disadvantages of active, population-based surveillance.

Advantages	Disadvantages/challenges
• "Gold standard" surveillance system: calculate age-, sex-, race-specific disease rates • Monitor disease trends over time • Compare disease rates with those from other active, population-based surveillance systems using similar case definition when access to care and diagnostic services are similar (regardless of geographic location) • Estimate national rates and disease burden using surveillance and national census data when area under surveillance is representative of the country • Measure effectiveness of public health interventions (e.g., vaccines, antibiotic prophylaxis) • Infrastructure in place to better enable investigation of outbreaks and new public health threats • May be used as a platform for additional studies (e.g., risk factor studies) *If bacterial or viral isolates collected:* • Detect antimicrobial susceptibility patterns • Aid vaccine development using patterns of bacterial or viral strain distribution • Detect emergence of rare bacterial isolates or strains (e.g., pneumococcal serotypes)	• Resource intensive: significant personnel time and costs, training requirements, and (*if laboratory-based*) laboratory supplies • Data not always timely • Systematic, periodic evaluation of system is necessary to achieve 100% case detection and quality data collection • Participation and commitment of all laboratories or providers in surveillance area is imperative • Requires consistent approach to diagnosis by healthcare providers • Audits needed to ensure complete case reporting, and to monitor changes in reporting structure (i.e., change in laboratories serving surveillance population) • Not as flexible as simpler systems

tools that should be used to quantify the burden of disease in areas where prevention measures can be applied and their impact measured. Surveillance partners and stakeholders need to have regular access to the data so that decisions on allocation of resources or determination of control measures are data-driven. More specific, local information on diseases can be used for local prioritization of resources and influence local policies and practices, whereas national data can be used to impact national policies. Examples of the use of ABCs and IEIP data are illustrated below:

A. *Early-onset neonatal group B streptococcal disease: use of routine active, population-based US surveillance data and information from supplementary surveillance-based studies to guide disease prevention*

Invasive group B streptococcal disease (GBS) is a major cause of invasive infections in newborns. Consensus guidelines for the prevention of early-onset (EO) GBS published in 1996 recommended that prenatal care providers follow one of two approaches to determine use of intrapartum antibiotic prophylaxis to prevent EO-GBS infection. The risk-based approach identifies women with an increased risk for GBS (e.g., prolonged rupture of membranes); in the screening approach, women are cultured at 35–37 weeks' gestation to determine if colonized with GBS.

In 2000, ABCs reviewed randomly selected labor and delivery records from 5144 births in 1998 and 1999 in eight surveillance areas. The review included all EO-GBS cases in these areas (312 cases); births without documented GBS screening were considered exposed to the risk-based approach. Screening identified colonized women without established risk factors who still might have a baby with GBS. With use of a universal screening approach the relative risk of EO-GBS was approximately half of that of the risk-based approach [9].

The consensus guidelines for the prevention of EO-GBS were critically reviewed and modified in 2002 to recommend a universal screening-based approach [10]. ABCs surveillance data have documented the decrease in EO GBS infections from a projected national annual incidence of 2600 EO cases in 1997 (0.7 cases/1000 live births) to 1325 EO cases in 2004 (0.3 cases/1000 live births) [11] (Figure 3.4).

Local data can be analyzed, disseminated, and used. For example, in Minnesota, ABCs data on the incidence of EO-GBS, information from GBS laboratory and prenatal provider practices surveys, and the Minnesota data from the 2000 project have all been disseminated through publications [12,13], conferences, newsletters, and information posted on the Minnesota Department of Health Web site. Surveys done on prenatal practices in 2003

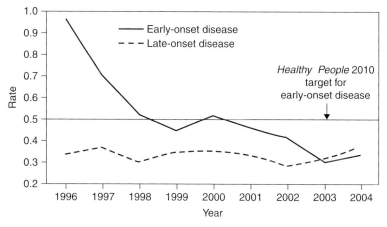

Fig 3.4 Rate (cases per 1000 live births) of early-onset and late-onset invasive group B streptococcal disease in infants by year. Data from the Active Bacterial Core surveillance system, United States, 1996–2004 [11].

compared with 1998 found significant changes in practice [14].

B. *Impact of introduction of pneumococcal conjugate vaccine (PCV7) on invasive pneumococcal disease*

Pneumococcus is a leading cause of bacterial meningitis, bacteremia, and otitis media in young children. It also causes disease in older individuals and those with comorbidities. Prior to use of PCV7, more than 50,000 cases of bacteremia, 3000–6000 cases of meningitis, and 175,000 hospitalizations for pneumonia due to pneumococcus occurred each year in the US in all age groups.

ABCs has documented the direct and indirect effects of PCV7 on the incidence of invasive pneumococcal disease by collecting and analyzing surveillance data before and after vaccine introduction. From 1998–1999 to 2003 the incidence of invasive pneumococcal disease in children under 5 years dropped 75% and the rate of disease due to vaccine serotypes dropped 94%. In age groups over 5 years the overall rate dropped 29% with the highest drop occurring in individuals 65 years and older [15] (Figure 3.5). Ongoing surveillance is needed to monitor the incidence of pneumococcal disease caused by serotypes not included in the conjugate vaccine. In fact, review of ABCs data in 2004 and 2005 has found that disease caused by nonvaccine

serotypes has increased, particularly that disease due to serotype 19A [16].

C. *Establishing the incidence and cost of seasonal influenza to guide vaccine decisions in Thailand*

In the tropics, seasonal influenza is generally considered to be a mild disease of little importance that occurs at a low-level year round; the vaccine, which is expensive, is rarely used. Recent outbreaks of avian influenza A (H5N1) have resulted in renewed interest in seasonal influenza and recognition that data from Southeast Asia are needed for decision making. Using data from active, population-based pneumonia surveillance in Thailand, together with data from outpatients with influenza-like illness in the same province, Thai and US researchers established that the incidence of influenza in Thailand was 43 times greater than the rate identified through the passive surveillance system [8]. The annual incidence of hospitalized influenza-related pneumonia may be as high as 111 per 100,000 persons and outpatient influenza 1420 per 100,000 persons. The burden, or cost, of influenza was also substantial, up to US$63 million per year, particularly in terms of lost productivity. The data also highlight a clear seasonal distribution, with peaks between June and October each year. These findings have important implications on the timing of yearly influenza vaccine distribution. An additional study of risk factors

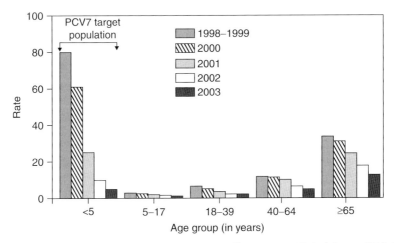

Fig 3.5 Rate (cases per 100,000 population) of vaccine-type (VT) invasive pneumococcal disease (IPD) before and after introduction of pneumococcal conjugate vaccine (PCV7) by age group and year. Data from the Active Bacterial Core surveillance system, United States, 1998–2003. For each age group, the decrease in VT IPD rate for 2003 compared with the 1998–1999 baseline is statistically significant ($p < 0.05$). [15].

for influenza-pneumonia identified young children, the elderly, and those with chronic respiratory disease as those at greatest risk for severe disease and for whom the vaccine might be recommended [17].

Summary and recommendations

Active and population-based surveillance has the potential to be an accurate and powerful tool for monitoring emerging infections and for obtaining the detailed information necessary to develop and monitor disease prevention strategies. When implemented properly and carefully maintained, this type of surveillance can quantify disease burden, capture changes in its epidemiology, and provide reliable measurements of the impact of public health and provider-initiated disease interventions. However, this system is resource-intensive; therefore the disease chosen for surveillance should provide important, actionable information. Data need to be shared with partners and disseminated to public policy decision makers and the general public. The infrastructure and partnerships developed to create a surveillance system are often a useful investment for pubic health preparedness and practice.

References

1 Lederberg J, Shope RE, Oaks SCJ. *Emerging Infections: Microbial Threats to Health in the United States*. Washington, DC: National Academy Press; 1992.

2 Schuchat A, Hilger T, Zell E, *et al*. Update from the Active Bacterial Core surveillance of the Emerging Infections Program Network. *Emerg Infect Dis* 2001;7(1):92–9.

3 Dowell SF, Chunsuttiwat S, Olsen SJ, *et al*. The International Emerging Infections Program, Thailand—an early report. *Emerg Infect* 2003;6:191–203.

4 Javadi M, Subhannachart P, Levine S, *et al*. Diagnosing pneumonia in rural Thailand: digital cameras versus film digitizers for chest radiograph teleradiology. *Int J Infect Dis* 2006;10(2):129–35.

5 Schrag SJ, Shay DK, Gershman K, *et al*. Multistate surveillance for laboratory-confirmed, influenza-associated hospitalizations in children: 2003–2004. *Pediatr Infect Dis J* 2006;25:395–400.

6 Olsen SJ, Laosiritaworn Y, Siasiriwattana S, Chunsuttiwat S, Dowell SF. The incidence of pneumonia in rural Thailand. *Int J Infect Dis* 2006;10(6):439–45.

7 Fischer JE, Olsen SJ, Wongjindanon W, Dowell SF, Peruski L. Population-based surveillance for microbial agents of pneumonia and sepsis with detection of *Streptococcus pneumoniae*: standard operating procedure for clinical and laboratory staff. Available from: http://www.cdc.gov/ncidod/global/ieip/pdf/ieip_sop.pdf.

8 Simmerman JM, Lertiendumrong J, Dowell SF, *et al*. The cost of influenza in Thailand. *Vaccine* 2006;24: 4417–26.

9 Schrag SJ, Zell ER, Lynfield R, *et al*. A population-based comparison of strategies to prevent early-onset group B streptococcal disease in neonates. *N Engl J Med* 2002;347:233–9.

10 Centers for Disease Control and Prevention. Prevention of perinatal group B streptococcal disease. *MMWR* 2002;51(RR-11):1–22.

11 Centers for Disease Control and Prevention. Early-onset and late-onset neonatal group B streptococcal disease—United States, 1996–2004. *MMWR* 2005;54(47):1205–8.

12 Centers for Disease Control and Prevention. Adoption of perinatal group B streptococcal disease prevention recommendations by prenatal care providers—Connecticut and Minnesota, 1998. *MMWR* 2000;49: 228–32.

13 Prevention of perinatal group B streptococcal disease in Minnesota: results from a retrospective cohort study and new prevention guidelines. *Minn Med* 2003;86: 40–5.

14 Morin CA, White K, Schuchat A, Danila RN, Lynfield R. Perinatal group B streptococcal disease prevention, Minnesota. *Emerg Infect Dis* 2005;11:1467–9.

15 Centers for Disease Control and Prevention. Direct and indirect effects of routine vaccination of hildren with 7-valent pneumococcal conjugate vaccine on incidence of invasive pneumococcal disease—United States, 1998–2003. *MMWR* 2005;54(36):893–7.

16 Pai R, Moore MR, Pilishvili T, Gertz RE, Whitney CG, Beall B. Postvaccine genetic structure of *Streptococcus pneumoniae* serotype 19A from children in the United States. *J Infect Dis* 2005;192:1988–95.

17 Katz MA, Tharmaphornpilas P, Chantra S, *et al*. Who gets hospitalized for influenza pneumonia in Thailand? Implications for vaccine policy. *Vaccine* 2007;25(19):3827–33.

Additional Web resources

Emerging Infections Programs: http://www.cdc.gov/ncidod/osr/site/eip/

Active Bacterial Core surveillance: http://www.cdc.gov/abcs/

International Emerging Infections Program: http://www.cdc.gov/ncidod/global/ieip/

FoodNet—Foodborne Diseases Active Surveillance Network: http://www.cdc.gov/foodnet/

Antibiotic resistance surveillance toolkit for *Streptococcus pneumoniae*: http://www.cdc.gov/drspsurveillancetoolkit/

4

Surveillance for antimicrobial-resistant *Streptococcus pneumoniae*

Matthew R. Moore, Ruth Lynfield & Cynthia G. Whitney

Introduction

Streptococcus pneumoniae (pneumococcus) is a leading cause of otitis media, sinusitis, bacteremia, pneumonia, and meningitis worldwide. The World Health Organization estimates that over 1.6 million deaths annually, including 716,000 deaths among children aged less than 5 years, are attributable to pneumococcal disease [1]. Because some of this burden is vaccine-preventable and because some pneumococcal infections are resistant to antibiotics, surveillance for pneumococcal disease is an important public health activity.

With the availability of antibiotics since the 1940s, the case-fatality rate from pneumococcal infections declined precipitously. However, within a few decades, pneumococci began to adapt to antibiotic pressures and to demonstrate resistance to certain antibiotics, including penicillin [2]. The incidence of infections caused by antibiotic-resistant *S. pneumoniae* increased markedly during the mid-to-late 1990s [3]. This increase meant that surveillance for pneumococcal infections, and antibiotic-resistant infections in particular, assumed greater importance. In response to this increase, as well as the increasing incidence of other antibiotic-resistant infections, a task force comprising 10 federal agencies developed a plan to respond to the growing threat of antibiotic resistance [4]. That task force identified surveillance as one of the four focus areas and, within that area, the development and implementation of a coordinated national surveillance plan was named as the first priority goal.

The purpose of this chapter is to describe practical approaches to surveillance for antibiotic-resistant infections caused by *S. pneumoniae*; these approaches also apply to surveillance for other antibiotic-resistant infections [5]. Surveillance for resistant foodborne infections is discussed in Chapter 7, community-associated methicillin-resistant *Staphylococcus aureus* infections in Chapter 14, multidrug resistant tuberculosis in Chapter 12, and resistant *Neisseria gonorrhoeae* infections in Chapter 17. The details of pneumococcal epidemiology, methods for susceptibility testing, and detection of resistance mechanisms are available elsewhere [6–8]. Particular emphasis will be placed on the implementation, advantages, and disadvantages of various surveillance strategies.

The role of surveillance

Surveillance for antibiotic-resistant pneumococcal infections can play several roles in preventing the spread of resistance. First, the dissemination of surveillance data can raise local awareness of the problem of antibiotic resistance. Clinicians who are aware of the magnitude of the local problem are more likely to consider their role in preventing the spread of resistant bacteria. Second, resistance varies geographically [9]. Therefore, knowledge of areas with increased prevalence of resistance can lead to interventions specific to those areas, as well as an assessment of the impact of those interventions (e.g., vaccination programs or appropriate antibiotic use campaigns) [10]. Third, surveillance data can be used to monitor trends over time and to detect the emergence of new resistance profiles [11,12]. Finally, in some instances, surveillance for antibiotic-resistant pneumococcal infection can steer the development of national or local clinical management guidelines [13].

A framework for pneumococcal surveillance

Similar to other conditions of public health importance, surveillance for antibiotic-resistant pneumococcal disease fits into a paradigm of public health prevention. Surveillance serves the dual functions of case enumeration, important for following trends over time, and case characterization, and is critical to understanding the populations at risk. Examination of surveillance data can and should stimulate the formulation of hypotheses about transmission of the disease in the underlying population. For example, an increase in the rate of antibiotic-resistant disease among preschool-aged children might suggest an outbreak among day care attendees [14]. By identifying individual cases, a surveillance system can serve as a platform for special studies, such as case-control studies that identify risk factors for antibiotic-resistant pneumococcal disease [15] or studies evaluating the effectiveness of a new vaccine in preventing pneumococcal disease [16]. In this way, a surveillance system can be used not only to stimulate hypotheses but also to test them. Once the findings of an investigation are known—when one knows the risk factors for drug-resistant pneumococcal disease, for example—a policy or pro-

gram can be implemented and the impact of that policy can be evaluated using the surveillance system [14,17,18].

Pneumococcal syndromes

A thorough understanding of pneumococcal syndromes is important for appreciating the limitations of surveillance for certain types of antibiotic-resistant pneumococcal infections (Figure 4.1). Upper respiratory tract infections, including acute otitis media and sinusitis, are among the most common manifestations of pneumococcal disease. Because most pneumococcal upper respiratory infections occur among children and because upper respiratory infections account for the majority of antibiotic prescriptions, children are at particularly high risk of upper respiratory infections caused by antibiotic-resistant *S. pneumoniae*. However, surveillance that is specific for pneumococcal otitis or sinusitis is challenging given that most clinicians in the United States (US) do not routinely collect middle ear fluid or sinus aspirates for bacterial culture. Without clinical isolates, susceptibility testing cannot be performed. Furthermore, asymptomatic carriage of pneumococci occurs among 30% of children; therefore, the presence of pneumococci in the upper respiratory tract does not necessarily represent a disease state. Carriage poses a particular problem in diagnosing pneumococcal pneumonia—the most common form of bacterial pneumonia in most countries—because identification of pneumococci in the sputum cannot be used to distinguish

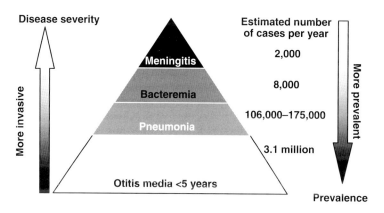

Fig 4.1 The burden of pneumococcal disease in the US [19].

between carriage and disease. Surveillance for pneumococcal pneumonia without infection in the bloodstream, whether occurring among children or adults, is challenging because it is a common occurrence but one which is difficult to diagnose reliably.

Surveillance for antibiotic-resistant pneumococcal infections is most feasible for the invasive syndromes, (i.e., those characterized by isolation of pneumococcus from a normally sterile site, such as blood or cerebrospinal fluid). Invasive pneumococcal disease syndromes are appropriate for surveillance for four reasons. First, because they are typically severe, they represent important causes of morbidity and mortality. Second, clinical laboratories routinely evaluate clinical specimens from sterile sites for the presence of *S. pneumoniae*. Third, when pneumococcus is found in a sterile site it virtually always represents a disease state. Fourth, susceptibility testing is routinely performed on sterile site isolates and the clinical relevance of resistance is generally documented, particularly for meningitis [20] and, to a lesser extent, bacteremia [20,21].

The meaning and measurement of antibiotic resistance

Antibiotic resistance, in the strictest sense, means that a given infection caused by a particular pathogen cannot be successfully treated with an antibiotic to which that pathogen is resistant. In practice, however, it is challenging to predict with certainty whether a particular infection can be treated successfully with a particular antibiotic. The underlying health status of the host, virulence factors specific to the pathogen, and environmental factors all play a role in determining the severity of an individual's illness. Other factors, such as the site of the infection, the dose, route, and timing of administration of an antibiotic, and the physiologic distribution of that antibiotic in a particular patient all play important roles in determining the success or failure of treatment. For the purposes of public health surveillance, antibiotic resistance is represented by the results of laboratory testing performed on an isolate from a patient (i.e., *in vitro* testing) and does not incorporate the patient's clinical response to antibiotic treatment.

Antibiotic resistance can be identified using several laboratory methods. What these methods have in common is that they use an *in vitro* assay with one or more known concentrations of an antibiotic to estimate the ability of the organism—pneumococcus, in this case—to grow in the presence of that antibiotic. The simplest method, Kirby-Bauer disk diffusion, involves the uniform inoculation of an agar plate with a pneumococcal strain followed by the placement on the plate of a paper disk containing a fixed amount of antibiotic. After incubating the organism and antibiotic together for 24 hours or more, the agar is inspected for the growth of the organism near the disk. If the antibiotic inhibits the growth of the organism, a "zone of inhibition" will be present around the disk. If the organism is resistant to the antibiotic, the bacteria will grow immediately adjacent to the disk. Depending on the size of the zone of inhibition, the organism is considered to be susceptible, intermediate, or resistant to the antibiotic. For pneumococcus, an oxacillin disk is sometimes used for screening for penicillin resistance, with a zone of inhibition of ≤19 mm suggestive of resistance to β-lactam antibiotics. Isolates resistant to oxacillin generally undergo specific testing for resistance to penicillin or the cephalosporins using other methods. For invasive isolates, laboratories generally immediately use definitive testing methods rather than oxacillin screening, as the oxacillin-screening step can add considerably to the time needed to obtain a final susceptibility testing result. The β-lactams are the only drugs for which Kirby-Bauer testing is considered a screen for resistance; for other antibiotics, isolates can be classified as susceptible, intermediate, or resistant by measuring the zone of inhibition without a need for testing with a second method.

Most other susceptibility methods involve varying the concentration of an antibiotic over a predetermined range, e.g., 0.025–16 μg/mL for penicillin, and identifying the minimum concentration at which the organism is incapable of growth. This minimum inhibitory concentration (MIC) is then assigned an interpretation of susceptible, intermediate, or resistant, identical to those used for the disk diffusion method. Intermediate or resistant isolates are considered "nonsusceptible." The most commonly used MIC methods are broth microdilution, agar dilution, and antimicrobial gradient strips (Etest®). For the dilution methods, an organism is placed in wells or on plates of media that contain a range of antibiotic concentrations, and the MIC is the lowest concentration of antibiotic that inhibits the growth of the organism. Antimicrobial gradient strips are hybrids between the dilution methods and disk diffusion. Each strip contains a graded concentration of a particular antibiotic. The strips are labeled with the concentrations and the MIC can be read from the strip as the organism grows up to the level on strip containing the inhibitory concentration of antibiotic.

Because antibiotic resistance is a phenomenon identified by microbiology laboratories, the laboratories play a central role in surveillance for antibiotic-resistant pneumococcal disease. Clinical microbiology laboratories are typically affiliated with individual hospitals or hospital systems although commercial reference laboratories often provide testing services for outpatient clinics and hospitals, especially smaller community-based hospitals. Knowing which laboratories serve the hospitals and clinics in a particular area is important because that knowledge guides which laboratories—and therefore, which populations—are targeted for inclusion in a surveillance program.

Microbiology laboratories in the US are regulated by the Clinical Laboratory Improvement Amendments (CLIA), passed by Congress in 1988 to establish quality standards for all laboratory testing performed on patient specimens, regardless of where the test is performed [22]. Whereas CLIA establishes quality standards, a separate nonprofit, nongovernmental organization, the Clinical and Laboratory Standards Institute (CLSI, formerly known as the National Committee for Clinical Laboratory Standards or NCCLS) establishes by consensus the laboratory interpretations of specific Kirby-Bauer zone sizes or MICs. The details of this process are beyond the scope of this text, but it is important to understand that standards exist whereby all laboratories that estimate a particular zone size or MIC assign the same susceptibility category to that strain of pneumococcus. Furthermore, CLSI routinely reevaluates these standards against new clinical and microbiologic data and, if necessary, modifies the standards [23].

Case definitions

Regardless of the pneumococcal syndrome of interest, a surveillance program must have clear, unambiguous case definitions. The critical elements of any case definition include person, place, and time, but the specifics of those elements depend on the specific goals of surveillance.

A surveillance case definition is developed for either or both of the two reasons—to count a particular event or to take action in response to an unusual event. For example, a small, county health department may want to raise awareness among clinicians of the problem of antibiotic-resistant pneumococcal infections. The health department would likely require reporting of all cases of invasive disease caused by penicillin-resistant pneumococcal strains and subsequently summarize those data for its clinicians. Clinicians simply want to know whether their community is experiencing a higher, lower, or stable prevalence of penicillin resistance among invasive pneumococcal cases and how this prevalence compares to other parts of the county or state. In this scenario, the event of interest is penicillin-resistant invasive pneumococcal disease (person), the population under surveillance includes residents of the county (place), and each case is recorded based on the date on which pneumococcus was isolated from the patient (time). Because the proportion of cases that demonstrates resistance to penicillin is unlikely to change rapidly, the county health department might gather and disseminate these data quarterly, semiannually, or annually.

On the other hand, if a particular country was experiencing an outbreak of vancomycin-resistant pneumococcal meningitis, a phenomenon that has never been reported, it would cause great concern. Given the importance of vancomycin in the treatment of pneumococcal meningitis, this country would likely search aggressively for all cases so that it could develop a strategy for limiting the spread of these organisms. In addition, the ministry of health might seek extensive information from all patients, such as their clinical course, preceding antibiotic use, and whether they had received one or more doses of a pneumococcal vaccine. Here, the event of interest is vancomycin-resistant pneumococcal meningitis (person), the population of interest includes all residents of a country (place), and again, cases would be recorded based on the date of isolation of pneumococcus (time). However, because of the public health implications of identifying additional cases, the frequency of monitoring for this event might be much greater (e.g., weekly or monthly).

These two examples demonstrate the importance of clearly defining the goals for surveillance. In the first instance, it is only necessary to count cases of invasive pneumococcal disease that demonstrate resistance to penicillin. In the second example, the goal is to identify a much smaller number of cases characterized by resistance to vancomycin. Furthermore, the vancomycin-resistant cases need to be identified much more rapidly than the penicillin-resistant cases so that the epidemic can be interrupted. These two scenarios have very different goals, different approaches, and different resource implications.

Approaches to surveillance

There are several methodological considerations when deciding how exactly to conduct surveillance for antibiotic-resistant pneumococcal disease (Table 4.1). In the end, the specific goals of surveillance and the available resources largely determine

Table 4.1 Advantages and disadvantages of different methods for conducting surveillance for infections caused by antibiotic-resistant *Streptococcus pneumoniae*.

Method	Advantages	Disadvantages	References
Population-based	• If case capture is relatively complete, can calculate rates of disease and compare across age, sex, geographic regions, and other epidemiologic factors • Surveillance sites capture all cases in a geographic region. Therefore, they are representative and no extrapolation is necessary • Better at detecting emerging resistance	• Most resource intensive, especially if data are captured on cases individually rather than in an aggregated format	[11,24]
Sentinel surveillance	• Can conserve resources by limiting participation to a few institutions • Limiting the volume of cases may allow resources to be used to gather more data on each individual case • Data are often specific to individual or small groups of hospitals and therefore might be preferred by clinicians	• Surveillance sites chosen might not be representative of all sites in a geographic region • Cannot typically calculate rates of disease	[25]
Aggregated antibiograms	• Least resource intensive • Data are routinely generated by hospital microbiology laboratories; therefore, data are readily available • Closely approximates the prevalence of resistance estimated by other methods • Includes most clinically relevant antibiotics • Data are often specific to individual or small groups of hospitals and therefore might be preferred by clinicians	• Typically includes duplicates and nonsterile site isolates • Individual antibiograms may not include the total number of isolates; therefore, may not be amenable to aggregation • Cannot analyze data by age, sex, or other epidemiologic features • Cannot calculate rates of disease	[26–28]

which approach is most suitable (see Chapters 3 and 14 for further discussions of surveillance methods).

Passive surveillance means that a health department waits for reporting entities (e.g., clinical microbiology laboratories or healthcare providers) to report their data. Clinical laboratories need to know what sort of data are required, how frequently the data should be reported, and by what means (e.g., electronically, mail), but once that reporting structure is established, passive reporting implies that the health department does little to encourage the clinical laboratories to submit their data.

Active surveillance suggests that the health department deliberately and routinely requests the data. Some health departments might remind clinical laboratories by telephone, fax, or e-mail on a monthly basis. In other scenarios, health department personnel might have direct access to laboratory log books or electronic data managed by clinical microbiology laboratories. Active surveillance is much more labor intensive; however, the data are usually more complete and of higher quality. Active surveillance, by definition, also demands greater cooperation on the part of infection control practitioners, clinicians, and laboratorians because they are expected to report their cases on a predetermined schedule. To ensure that reporting is complete, some surveillance programs will perform regular audits of reporting laboratories. Such an audit might involve a quarterly review of all laboratory data to ensure that all cases have actually been reported.

Surveillance can be population-based or it can rely on sentinel sites. Surveillance that is population-based means that one can clearly enumerate and describe the population that gives rise to the cases. If the population under surveillance includes all residents of a county or group of counties, then the surveillance program must determine the county of residence of every case captured. This means that some episodes of antibiotic-resistant pneumococcal disease captured by surveillance will not be cases because they are not residents of the surveillance area. However, it also means that the surveillance program must have information on which clinical microbiology laboratories, hospitals, and clinics serve residents of the surveillance area, knowing that some residents might seek care at fa-

cilities outside their counties of residence. The principal strength of population-based surveillance is that one can calculate rates of disease that can be compared to rates of disease in other surveillance areas, whether in the US or abroad. In addition, one may be able to calculate age-, sex-, and race-specific rates within the surveillance area, if such information is collected for each case. Individual rates for these specific groups can then be compared to determine which groups are at highest risk of disease and, therefore, might be amenable to specific intervention programs. The principal disadvantage of population-based surveillance is that it is labor-intensive because it requires gathering additional information about every case of disease, information that is not always readily available.

The most resource-intensive method for conducting surveillance for antibiotic-resistant infections is active, population-based surveillance. Because this approach involves program personnel routinely contacting clinical microbiology laboratories in a given surveillance area, one assumes that all cases have been captured: 20 cases means 20 cases, not 19 or 21, and zero cases means zero. Because this approach is population-based, one can assume that the population from which the cases arise is well-characterized and can therefore be used to estimate rates of disease, often stratified by age, sex, race, and ethnicity [24,29]. The Centers for Disease Control and Prevention's Active Bacterial Core surveillance (ABCs) part of the Emerging Infections Program, is an example of active, population-based surveillance that has tracked changes in antibiotic-resistant invasive pneumococcal disease [17].

Despite these advantages, active, population-based surveillance poses several challenges. First, the resources needed to maintain such a program are large, not only in terms of monetary funds but also in terms of human capital and energy needed to sustain continuous participation from all clinical microbiology laboratories. Second, despite complete case ascertainment, information about each case is often incomplete because most cases do not have a single source of complete information from which surveillance personnel can extract data. For example, without directly interviewing each case, it is challenging to determine unequivocally the race and ethnicity of an individual patient. Similarly,

49

patients admitted to hospital have frequently received antibiotics before admission, but the precise antibiotic, dosing, and dates of use are often not available from the inpatient medical record.

Sentinel site surveillance means that a program captures cases from a sample of healthcare facilities that serve a particular population or region. For example, a local health department might choose 3 hospitals from among the 10 that serve a large, metropolitan area. The cases captured by those hospitals would be counted as the only cases and they would be included regardless of the geographic areas in which they reside. If a large, academic referral hospital is included as a sentinel site, then cases might be included if they arise from counties, or even states, other than the one in which the hospital is situated. Likewise, if residents of that same county seek healthcare at hospitals not included in the surveillance network, including those in other counties, then cases occurring among those residents would not be captured by the surveillance system.

The sample of hospitals and laboratories included in a sentinel site surveillance program can dramatically influence the reported incidence of antibiotic-resistant pneumococcal disease. This principle was demonstrated clearly in an evaluation of surveillance data captured by an active, population-based, laboratory-based surveillance program for invasive pneumococcal disease [25]. Because all clinical microbiology laboratories serving well-defined surveillance populations were included, the investigators were able to simulate the surveillance data that would be obtained if random combinations of three, four, or five laboratories were included in a hypothetical sentinel network. This approach allowed the investigators to compare the proportion of invasive pneumococcal cases that were antibiotic-resistant across the surveillance area to proportions that would be expected with different combinations of laboratories. The investigators were also able to determine whether trends in the proportion of cases that were antibiotic-resistant could be reliably determined and whether the emergence of new resistance profiles could be detected.

This study showed that sentinel surveillance sites could be used to reliably estimate the true prevalence of antibiotic-resistant pneumococcal disease depending on the sites chosen. Information on the number of cases detected by each laboratory and the variability in the prevalence of antibiotic-resistant pneumococcal cases between laboratories can help predict the performance of a sentinel system. For example, if the proportion of cases that are antibiotic-resistant in five different laboratories varies from 10 to 15%, then any sample of two or three laboratories will provide a reasonable estimate of the prevalence of resistance across all five laboratories. On the other hand, if the prevalence of resistance among 20 laboratories varies from 10 to 45%, then one must exercise great care in choosing which laboratories to include in surveillance, as the choice of any two or three laboratories could influence greatly the estimated prevalence of resistance. A simple albeit more resource-intensive way of reducing the influence of individual laboratories is to simply include more of them. Again, however, the decision to invest more resources in a system must be balanced against the resources available to sustain that system.

Finally, this study determined that sentinel laboratories have varying abilities to detect newly emerging antibiotic resistance. The investigators randomly chose five laboratories from each of the five surveillance areas and then asked what proportion of those groups of five laboratories would have captured fluoroquinolone-resistant isolates that emerged in each area during the period of observation. Given that only one or two fluoroquinolone-resistant isolates were identified in each area, it is not surprising that the ability to detect those rare events varied depending on what proportion of all laboratories were included in each group of five laboratories: when the five laboratories were the only five in a surveillance area, they were able to detect the one resistant isolate. When the total number of laboratories in an area was much larger than five, the proportion of sentinel groups of five laboratories capturing the one resistant isolate was as low as 42%. The important lesson from this study is that more than one surveillance approach may be necessary if one of the goals of surveillance is the detection of rare events like the emergence of new resistance profiles.

Another approach to surveillance for antibiotic-resistant pneumococcal infections involves the use of antibiograms [26–28]. Antibiograms are tabular summaries of the proportions of common bacterial pathogens determined to be susceptible, intermediate, or fully resistant to a variety of antibiotics. Many hospital microbiology laboratories generate pocket-sized antibiograms for their clinicians who need hospital-specific data to make treatment decisions. While individual antibiograms are not sufficient for performing surveillance for antibiotic-resistant pneumococcal infections in a geographical area, one can combine, or aggregate, antibiograms from individual hospitals to estimate the prevalence of antibiotic resistance among pneumococcal strains from that region (see Chapter 14).

The accuracy of antibiograms in estimating the prevalence of antibiotic-resistant pneumococcal infections has been estimated by comparing the prevalence of resistance estimated from antibiograms to the prevalence estimated from population-based, laboratory-based, active surveillance [28]. While the prevalence of resistance estimated by each method was similar, antibiograms had two major shortcomings. First, most hospitals include all pneumococcal susceptibility results in a single antibiogram. This is problematic because the prevalence of resistance varies widely among age groups and among isolates from different specimen sources. For example, the prevalence of resistance among upper respiratory tract isolates of pneumococci from children is generally higher than that among blood isolates recovered from adults. Therefore, surveillance programs that rely solely on antibiograms are unable to disaggregate their resistance data to evaluate the prevalence of resistance in subsets of cases. Second, antibiograms are useful for estimating the prevalence of resistance to penicillin, cefotaxime, ceftriaxone, and erythromycin. Susceptibility data for other antibiotics of public health interest are included in antibiograms less frequently; therefore, antibiograms cannot be used to estimate the prevalence of resistance to those antibiotics. Conversely, surveillance using antibiograms is an attractive option for health departments because antibiograms are readily available from most hospitals and gathering them and aggregating the data can be done with very limited resources. A consideration for communities interested in aggregated antibiograms is to standardize antibiotics included on susceptibility panels. A detailed discussion of antibiograms used for surveillance for antibiotic-resistant pneumococcus can be found at http://www.cdc.gov/drspsurveillancetoolkit.

The role of routine isolates collection

All the approaches to surveillance described above can rely exclusively on susceptibility data generated by clinical microbiology laboratories and without any confirmation or additional testing of clinical isolates (e.g., serotyping, DNA fingerprinting) [30]. There are certain advantages, however, to having pneumococcal isolates submitted along with the surveillance data. For example, clinical isolates can be tested by reference laboratories against a standard panel of antibiotics, including some that might not be included routinely in a hospital antibiogram. Reference laboratories can sometimes perform pneumococcal serotyping, which can have important implications for assessing the impact of pneumococcal vaccines [31]. Collections of pneumococcal strains with diverse resistance patterns can also be distributed back to clinical laboratories for quality assurance purposes.

All these benefits need to be weighed against certain epidemiologic and logistical considerations. For example, if the only isolates available are obtained from the most severe cases, then they might not be representative of the underlying population; interpretation of additional testing of those isolates would have to be done cautiously. Shipping, processing, and storing isolates are expensive, so routine isolate collection has important resource implications. Like all other decisions related to managing an antibiotic-resistant pneumococcal surveillance program, decisions regarding isolate collection must be made in the context of the goals of the program.

Interactions with partners

As with any surveillance program, the data obtained from an antibiotic-resistant pneumococcal surveillance program should be managed in a way that recognizes appropriately the source of the data. Public health departments rarely have funds to support the work required of clinical partners to maintain accurate collection and timely reporting of surveillance data. Therefore, the sustainability of such a program depends in large part on the willingness of reporting entities to continue reporting and on their understanding of the importance of the activity. To the extent possible, health departments work diligently to provide feedback to their clinical microbiology laboratories, infection control practitioners, and clinicians. This feedback can take the form of regular newsletters or reports, electronic mail distributions, or regular symposia sponsored by the state or local health department. In Minnesota, where active, population-based, laboratory-based surveillance occurs, case isolates are submitted to the public health laboratory and undergo susceptibility testing and serotyping. A yearly, state-based antibiogram, including pneumococcal disease and other reported infectious diseases, is created and distributed widely to

Table 4.2 Minnesota Department of Health antibiogram.

Antimicrobial Susceptibilities of Selected Pathogens, 2005 — MINNESOTA DEPARTMENT of HEALTH (MDH)

Sampling Methodology
† all isolates tested
‡ ~10% sample of statewide isolates received at MDH
# ~20% sample of statewide isolates received at MDH
§ isolates from a normally sterile site

	Campylobacter spp. [1‡]	Salmonella Typhimurium [2†]	Other Salmonella serotypes (non-typhoidal) [2‡]	Shigella spp. [#]	Neisseria gonorrhoeae [3]	Neisseria meningitidis [4†§]	Group A Streptococcus [5†§]	Group B Streptococcus [6†§]	Streptococcus pneumoniae [7†§]	Haemophilus influenzae [8†§]	Mycobacterium tuberculosis [9†]
Number of Isolates Tested	79	112	45	10	392	16	111	293	532	46	151
% Susceptible											
β-lactam antibiotics											
amoxicillin									94		
ampicillin		68	93	60			100	100		63	
penicillin					3	88	100	100	77		
cefixime					100						
cefuroxime sodium									87	96	
cefotaxime							100	100	90	100	
ceftriaxone		94	98	100	100	100			92		
meropenem						100			90	100	
Other antibiotics											
ciprofloxacin	79[1]	100	100	100	92	100				100	
levofloxacin							100	100	99	99	
azithromycin					32					98	
erythromycin	100						92	67	77		
clindamycin							99/92[5]	83/74[6]	91		
chloramphenicol		76	96	60		100			99	100	
gentamicin	97										
spectinomycin					100						
tetracycline	44				34			89	90	100	
trimethoprim/sulfamethoxazole		96	96	50			63	89	77	89	
vancomycin							100	100	100		
TB antibiotics											
ethambutol											97
isoniazid											91
pyrazinamide											97
rifampin						100				100	97

Table 4.2 (*Continued*)

	Trends, Comments and Other Pathogens
[1] *Campylobacter* spp.	Ciprofloxacin susceptibility was determined for all isolates (n=746). Only 34% of isolates from patients returning from foreign travel were susceptible to quinolones. Susceptibilities were determined using 2005 CLSI (formerly NCCLS) breakpoints for *Enterobacteriaceae*. Susceptibility for erythromycin was based on an MIC < 4.0 µg/ml.
[2] *Salmonella enterica* (non-typhoidal)	Antimicrobial treatment for enteric salmonellosis generally is not recommended.
[3] *Neisseria gonorrhoeae*	In 2005, we tested 392 *Neisseria gonorrhoeae* isolates for antibiotic resistance including 286 (73%) from a Minneapolis STD clinic and 106 (27%) from a St. Paul STD clinic.
[4] *Neisseria meningitidis*	One isolate had intermediate susceptibility (MIC of 0.12 µg/ml) and one was resistant (MIC of 0.5 µg/ml) to penicillin per the newly established CLSI (formerly NCCLS) breakpoints for *N. meningitidis*. CLSI suggests that MICs $\geq$ 8 µg/ml for nalidixic acid may correlate with diminished fluoroquinolone susceptibliity. None of our isolates had an MIC > 2 µg/ml.
[5] Group A *Streptococcus*	Of 9 isolates that were resistant to erythromycin, 1 was also resistant to clindamycin. The other 8 were susceptible but each had inducible clindamycin resistance by D-test.
[6] Group B *Streptococcus*	100% (15/15) of early-onset infant, 94% (16/17) of late-onset infant, 58% (7/12) of maternal, and 90% (257/287) of other invasive GBS cases were tested. Among 48 erythromycin-resistant, clindamycin-susceptible strains, 26 (54%) had inducible resistance to clindamycin by D-test. Overall, 74% (217/293) were susceptible to clindamycin and were D-test negative (where applicable). 56% (22/39) of infant and maternal cases were susceptible to clindamycin and were D-test negative (where applicable).
[7] *Streptococcus pneumoniae*	The 532 isolates tested represented 89% of 596 total cases. Of these, 14% (75/532) had intermediate susceptibility and 9% (46/532) were resistant to penicillin. Reported above are the proportions of case-isolates susceptible by meningitis breakpoints for cefotaxime and ceftriaxone (intermediate = 1.0 µg/ml, resistant $\geq$ 2.0 µg/ml). By nonmeningitis breakpoints (intermediate = 2.0µg/ml, resistant $\geq$ 4.0 µg/ml) 96% (509/532) and 99% (526/532) of isolates were susceptible to cefotaxime and ceftriaxone, respectively. Isolates were screened for high-level resistance to rifampin at a single MIC; all were $\leq$ 2.0 µg/ml. 17% (92/532) of isolates were resistant to two or more antibiotic classes and 12% (65/532) were resistant to 3 or more antibiotic classes.
[8] *Haemophilus influenzae*	All ampicillin-resistant isolates produced ß-lactamase and were susceptible to amoxicillin-clavulanate, which contains a ß-lactamase inhibitor. Four percent of the isolates were ampicillin-intermediate and ß-lactamase negative. Only one isolate was resistant to 2 or more antibiotics.
[9] *Mycobacterium tuberculosis* (TB)	National guidelines recommend initial four-drug therapy for TB disease, at least until first-line drug susceptibility results are known. In 2005, both resistance to isoniazid and multidrug-resistant TB (MDR-TB) were more common among U.S.-born TB cases than among foreign-born cases (10% versus 8%, and 5% versus 2%, respectively). One of the four MDR-TB cases was resistant to all four first-line TB drugs.
Community-associated Methicillin Resistant *Staphylococcus aureus* (CA-MRSA)	998 CA-MRSA cases were reported in 2005. 93% (925/998) had an isolate submitted and antimicrobial susceptibility testing was conducted on 80% (285/355) of the isolates with culture dates from January – June. 13% were susceptible to erythromycin, 60% were susceptible to ciprofloxacin, 93% were susceptible to tetracycline, 98% were susceptible to mupirocin, and 99% were susceptible to gentamicin and trimethoprim/sulfamethoxazole. All isolates were susceptible to linezolid, synercid, rifampin, and vancomycin. 14% (31/215) of erythromycin-resistant, clindamycin-susceptible isolates tested positive for inducible clindamycin resistance using the D-test. Overall 78% (221/285) were susceptible to clindamycin and D-test negative (where applicable).
Bordetella pertussis	160/161 isolates tested were susceptible to erythromycin using provisional CDC breakpoints. One isolate appeared to have reduced susceptibility to erythromycin. This isolate is undergoing further investigation.
Escherichia coli O157:H7	Antimicrobial treatment for *E. coli* O157:H7 infection is not recommended.

clinicians, infection control practitioners, and microbiologists (Table 4.2). In addition, information on pneumococcal disease, including resistant pneumococcal infections, is available on the Minnesota Department of Health Web site. Data are also disseminated through oral and written presentations, and individualized slides on surveillance data are created by request. On an international scale, public health officials and researchers collaborate to track specific antibiotic-resistant pneumococcal clones as they circulate around the world (http://www.sph.emory.edu/PMEN/). In short, because surveillance for antibiotic-resistant infections often requires more detailed reporting than other types of surveillance, public health agencies often have to work harder to maintain the interest and support of their reporting partners.

Monitoring, evaluation, and modification

A surveillance program focused on antibiotic-resistant pneumococcal infections requires regular monitoring similar to other types of surveillance activities. Because clinical microbiology laboratories are critical components of such a program, the surveillance area should be evaluated regularly to confirm that all relevant laboratories are participating in the program. Similarly, the program as a whole should be evaluated regularly [32] to confirm that reporting is timely, complete, and accurate; to reaffirm the goals and objectives of the program; to ensure that all partners understand what is expected; and to clarify instructions for processing and shipping of isolates, if indicated.

Use of antibiotic-resistant pneumococcal surveillance data

The occurrence of antibiotic-resistant pneumococci is related to antibiotic use. In Iceland, a dramatic increase in the prevalence of pneumococci that were nonsusceptible to penicillin was observed in the early 1990s. Following the initiation of physician and public education campaigns, investigators documented reductions in both antimicrobial use and the prevalence of penicillin-resistant pneumococci among children attending day care centers [33]. In recent years, Get Smart (http://www.cdc.gov/drugresistance/community/campaign_info.htm), a CDC-sponsored program, as well as state and locally sponsored judicious antibiotic use programs, have routinely used data on the prevalence of antibiotic-resistant pneumococci to communicate the dangers of antibiotic overuse. Local surveillance data are particularly useful in educating physicians and the public.

Immunization with the pediatric pneumococcal conjugate vaccine is a tool that has been extremely important in decreasing the incidence of antibiotic-resistant pneumococcal infections. The seven serotypes included in the pneumococcal conjugate vaccine, which was licensed in 2000 in

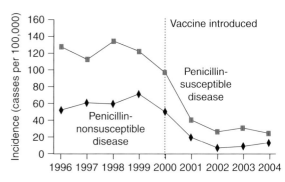

Fig 4.2 The impact of pneumococcal conjugate vaccination. The incidence of invasive pneumococcal disease caused by penicillin-nonsusceptible strains in children less than 2 years (cases per 100,000 children) from the years 1996–2004 is plotted [17]. The pneumococcal vaccine was introduced in 2000 and rates of both penicillin-susceptible (squares) and nonsusceptible (diamonds) disease dropped dramatically. (From Reference [17]. Copyright © 2006 Massachusetts Medical Society. Used with permission.)

the US, accounted for approximately 80% of the nonsusceptible pneumococcal infections observed among young children before introduction of the vaccine. Population-based surveillance conducted as part of CDC's ABC system during 1996–2004 has documented a 59% reduction in the incidence of invasive pneumococcal infections not susceptible to three or more classes of antibiotics among all age groups and an 84% reduction among children aged less than 2 years (Figure 4.2) [17]. However, continued surveillance is needed because antibiotic-resistant disease is beginning to emerge among serotypes not included in the seven-valent conjugate vaccine [34].

Lessons learned

Surveillance for antibiotic-resistant pneumococcal infections is an important public health activity because it can provide useful information for treatment and prevention of a major cause of morbidity and mortality. A variety of options (Table 4.1) are available for conducting this type of surveillance but all require a clear articulation of goals early in the process of planning such a program and reassessment of the goals once the program is established. Depending on the design, a surveillance program for antibiotic-resistant pneumococcal infections can require substantial resources to maintain the program and to provide the necessary feedback to partners to reinforce its importance. If done properly, this same surveillance program can be used to test important hypotheses and to implement key public health interventions to reduce the public health burden of antibiotic-resistant pneumococcal infections.

References

1 World Health Organization. *2004 Global Immunization Data*. Geneva: World Health Organization; 2005.

2 Kislak JW, Razavi LM, Daly AK, Finland M. Susceptibility of pneumococci to nine antibiotics. *Am J Med Sci* 1965;**250**(3):261–8.

3 Whitney CG, Farley MM, Hadler J, *et al*. Increasing prevalence of multidrug-resistant *Streptococcus pneumoniae* in the United States. *N Engl J Med* 2000;**343**(26):1917–24.

4 Interagency Task Force on Antimicrobial Resistance. *A Public Health Action Plan to Combat Antimicrobial Resistance*. Washington, DC: Interagency Task Force on Antimicrobial Resistance; 1999.

5 Noggle B, Iwamoto M, Chiller T, *et al*. Tracking resistant organisms: Workshop for improving state-based surveillance programs [conference summary]. Available from: http://www.cdc.gov/ncidod/eid/vol12no03/05-1335.htm. Accessed April 26, 2007.

6 Butler JC, Dowell SF, Breiman RF. Epidemiology of emerging pneumococcal drug resistance: implications for treatment and prevention. *Vaccine* 1998;**16**(18):1693–7.

7 Mandell LA. Relationship of penicillin resistance to mortality in pneumococcal pneumonia. *Curr Infect Dis Rep* 2001;**3**(1):9–12.

8 Klugman KP. Bacteriological evidence of antibiotic failure in pneumococcal lower respiratory tract infections. *Eur Respir J Suppl* 2002;**36**:3s–8s.

9 Geographic variation in penicillin resistance in *Streptococcus pneumoniae*—selected sites, United States, 1997. *MMWR Morb Mortal Wkly Rep* 1999;**48**(30):656–61.

10 Bhavnani SM, Hammel JP, Jones RN, Ambrose PG. Relationship between increased levofloxacin use and decreased susceptibility of *Streptococcus pneumoniae* in the United States. *Diagn Microbiol Infect Dis* 2005;**51**(1):31–7.

11 Chen DK, McGeer A, de Azavedo JC, Low DE. Decreased susceptibility of *Streptococcus pneumoniae* to fluoroquinolones in Canada. Canadian Bacterial Surveillance Network. *N Engl J Med* 1999;**341**(4):233–9.

12 Wolter N, Smith AM, Farrell DJ, *et al*. Novel mechanism of resistance to oxazolidinones, macrolides, and chloramphenicol in ribosomal protein L4 of the pneumococcus. *Antimicrob Agents Chemother* 2005;**49**(8):3554–7.

13 Mandell LA, Bartlett JG, Dowell SF, File TM, Jr, Musher DM, Whitney C. Update of practice guidelines for the management of community-acquired pneumonia in immunocompetent adults. *Clin Infect Dis* 2003;**37**(11):1405–33.

14 Craig AS, Erwin PC, Schaffner W, *et al*. Carriage of multidrug-resistant *Streptococcus pneumoniae* and impact of chemoprophylaxis during an outbreak of meningitis at a day care center [see comments]. *Clin Infect Dis* 1999;**29**(5):1257–64.

15 Beekmann SE, Diekema DJ, Heilmann KP, Richter SS, Doern GV. Macrolide use identified as risk factor for macrolide-resistant *Streptococcus pneumoniae* in a 17-center case-control study. *Eur J Clin Microbiol Infect Dis* 2006;**25**(5):335–9.

16 Whitney CG, Pilishvili T, Farley MM, *et al*. Effectiveness of seven-valent pneumococcal conjugate vaccine against invasive pneumococcal disease: a matched case-control study. *Lancet* 2006;**368**(9546):1495–502.

17 Kyaw MH, Lynfield R, Schaffner W, *et al*. Effect of introduction of the pneumococcal conjugate vaccine on drug-resistant *Streptococcus pneumoniae*. *N Engl J Med* 2006;**354**(14):1455–63.

18 Gonzales R, Camargo CA, Jr, MacKenzie T, *et al*. Antibiotic treatment of acute respiratory infections in acute care settings. *Acad Emerg Med* 2006;**13**(3):288–94.

19 Pilishvili T, Noggle B, Moore MR. Pneumococcal disease. In: Roush ST, Wharton MK (eds.), *Manual for the Surveillance of Vaccine-Preventable Diseases*, 4th edn. Atlanta, GA: Centers for Disease Control and Prevention. Available from: http://cdc.gov/nip/publications.

20 Klugman KP, Friedland IR. Antibiotic-resistant pneumococci in pediatric disease. *Microb Drug Resist* 1995;**1**(1): 5–8.

21 Tleyjeh IM, Tlaygeh HM, Hejal R, Montori VM, Baddour LM. The impact of penicillin resistance on short-term mortality in hospitalized adults with pneumococcal pneumonia: a systematic review and meta-analysis. *Clin Infect Dis* 2006;**42**(6):788–97.

22 *100th Congress. Clinical Laboratory Improvement Amendments of 1988*. United States Government; 1988.

23 Effect of new susceptibility breakpoints on reporting of resistance in *Streptococcus pneumoniae*—United States, 2003. *MMWR Morb Mortal Wkly Rep* 2004;**53**(7):152–4.

24 Schuchat A, Hilger T, Zell E, *et al*. Active bacterial core survcillance of the emerging infections program network. *Emerg Infect Dis* 2001;**7**(1):92–9.

25 Schrag SJ, Zell ER, Schuchat A, Whitney CG. Sentinel surveillance: a reliable way to track antibiotic resistance in communities? *Emerg Infect Dis* 2002;**8**(5):496–502.

26 Chin AE, Hedberg K, Cieslak PR, Cassidy M, Stefonek KR, Fleming DW. Tracking drug-resistant *Streptococcus pneumoniae* in Oregon: an alternative surveillance method. *Emerg Infect Dis* 1999;**5**(5):688–93.

27 Stein CR, Weber DJ, Kelley M. Using hospital antibiogram data to assess regional pneumococcal resistance to antibiotics. *Emerg Infect Dis* 2003;**9**(2):211–6.

28 Van Beneden CA, Lexau C, Baughman W, *et al.* Aggregated antibiograms and monitoring of drug-resistant *Streptococcus pneumoniae*. *Emerg Infect Dis* 2003;**9**(9): 1089–95.

29 Flannery B, Schrag S, Bennett NM, *et al.* Impact of childhood vaccination on racial disparities in invasive *Streptococcus pneumoniae* infections. *JAMA* 2004; **291**(18):2197–203.

30 Morrisscy I, Robbins M, Viljoen L, Brown DFJ. Antimicrobial susceptibility of community-acquired respiratory tract pathogens in the UK during 2002/3 determined locally and centrally by BSAC methods. *J Antimicrob Chemother* 2005;**55**(2):200–8.

31 Whitney CG, Farley MM, Hadler J, *et al.* Decline in invasive pneumococcal disease after the introduction of protein-polysaccharide conjugate vaccine. *N Engl J Med* 2003;**348**(18):1737–46.

32 Centers for Disease Control and Prevention. Updated guidelines for evaluating public health surveillance systems: recommendations from the guidelines working group. *MMWR Morb Mortal Wkly Rep* 2001;**50**(RR-13):1–51.

33 Kristinsson KG. Effect of antimicrobial use and other risk factors on antimicrobial resistance in pneumococci. *Microb Drug Resist* 1997;**3**(2):117–23.

34 Pai R, Moore MR, Pilishvili T, Gertz RE, Whitney CG, Beall B. Postvaccine genetic structure of *Streptococcus pneumoniae* serotype 19A from children in the United States. *J Infect Dis* 2005;**192**(11):1988–95.

5 Surveillance for foodborne diseases

Elaine Scallan & Frederick J. Angulo

Introduction

Food may become contaminated by a variety of different agents, resulting in over 250 different foodborne diseases. Most foodborne diseases are infectious, caused by bacteria, viruses, and parasites (Table 5.1). Noninfectious causes are harmful toxins or chemicals. Although ingested agents commonly cause vomiting and diarrhea, there is no single clinical syndrome attributable to all foodborne disease. Some pathogens, such as *Listeria monocytogenes*, are predominantly foodborne, while others have multiple transmission routes. *Escherichia coli* O157:H7 infections, for example, can be acquired by ingesting contaminated food or water, or following contact with farm animals or infected persons. An understanding of the epidemiology of a particular disease is necessary to judge the contribution of contaminated food.

Foodborne illness is an important public health problem worldwide. In countries with poor sanitary conditions, diarrheal illness is a leading cause of mortality and malnutrition in young children. While most infections are acquired from contaminated drinking water, food is an important route of transmission. In developed countries, although improvements in water sanitation, hygiene, and the safety of the food supply have greatly reduced the number of deaths due to foodborne disease, morbidity remains high. In 1999, it was estimated that foodborne diseases caused 76 million illness, 325,000 hospitalizations, and 5,000 deaths each year in the United States (US) [1]. Preventing foodborne disease, therefore, continues to be a challenging but critical public health priority. Foodborne disease surveillance facilitates interventions aimed at preventing foodborne diseases.

The purpose of this chapter is to assist public health professionals to enhance human foodborne disease surveillance by describing various surveillance methods and strategies and outlining their advantages, disadvantages, and relevance for meeting different public health objectives. Opportunities for improving foodborne disease surveillance capacity and infrastructure are discussed.

Objectives of foodborne disease surveillance

Surveillance is essential to efforts to define, control, and prevent foodborne disease [2]. Information on the burden and trends in specific foodborne diseases can assist policy makers in prioritizing, monitoring, and evaluating prevention strategies. Information on high-risk populations can help target prevention strategies more effectively. Surveillance activities lead to epidemiological investigations which improve our understanding of disease by identifying new agents or novel foods vehicles. Much of what we know about specific agents and how they enter the food supply is gained during the course of outbreak investigations. The early detection of foodborne outbreaks and their sources can lead to the control of acute public health threats, for example, removing a contaminated product from the market. Epidemiological investigations can also help identify gaps in knowledge, leading to applied research

Table 5.1 Common etiologic agents causing foodborne disease.

Etiologic agent	Clinical syndrome
Bacterial	
Bacillus cereus	
Vomiting toxin	Vomiting; some patients with diarrhea; fever uncommon
Diarrheal toxin	Diarrhea, abdominal cramps, and vomiting in some patients; fever uncommon
Brucella	Weakness, fever, headache, sweats, chills, arthralgia, weight loss, splenomegaly
Campylobacter	Diarrhea (often bloody), abdominal pain, fever
Clostridium botulinum	Variable severity; common symptoms are diplopia, blurred vision, and bulbar weakness; paralysis, which is usually descending and bilateral, might progress rapidly
Clostridium perfringens	Diarrhea, abdominal cramps; vomiting and fever uncommon
Escherichia coli	
Enterohemorrhagic (*E. coli* O157:H7 and others)	Diarrhea (often bloody), abdominal cramps (often severe), little or no fever
Enterotoxigenic (ETEC)	Diarrhea, abdominal cramps, nausea; vomiting and fever less common
Enteropathogenic (EPEC)	Diarrhea, fever, abdominal cramps
Enteroinvasive (EIEC)	Diarrhea (might be bloody), fever, abdominal cramps
Listeria monocytogenes	
Invasive disease	Meningitis, neonatal sepsis, fever
Diarrheal disease	Diarrhea, abdominal cramps, fever
Nontyphoidal *Salmonella*	Diarrhea, often with fever and abdominal cramps
Salmonella **Typhi**	Fever, anorexia, malaise, headache, and myalgia; sometimes diarrhea or constipation
Shigella **spp.**	Diarrhea (often bloody), often accompanied by fever and abdominal cramps
Staphylococcus aureus	Vomiting, diarrhea
Streptococcus, group A	Fever, pharyngitis, scarlet fever, upper respiratory infection
Vibrio cholerae	
O1 or O139	Watery diarrhea, often accompanied by vomiting
Non-O1 and non-O139	Watery diarrhea
Vibrio parahaemolyticus	Diarrhea
Yersinia enterocolitica	Diarrhea, abdominal pain (often severe)
Parasitic	
Cryptosporidium spp.	Diarrhea, nausea, vomiting; fever
Cyclospora cayetanensis	Diarrhea, nausea, anorexia, weight loss, cramps, gas, fatigue, low-grade fever; may be relapsing or protracted
Giardia intestinalis	Diarrhea, gas, cramps, nausea, fatigue
Toxoplasma gondii	Swollen lymph glands, muscle aches, retinitis, encephalitis
Trichinella spp.	Fever, myalgia, periorbital edema, high eosinophil count
Viral	
Hepatitis A	Jaundice, dark urine, fatigue, anorexia, nausea
Norovirus	Diarrhea, vomiting, nausea, abdominal cramps, low-grade fever
Astrovirus	Diarrhea, vomiting, nausea, abdominal cramps, low-grade fever
Chemical	
Marine toxins	
Ciguatoxin	Usually gastrointestinal symptoms followed by neurologic symptoms (including paresthesia of lips, tongue, throat, or extremities) and reversal of hot and cold sensation
Scombroid toxin (histamine)	Flushing, dizziness, burning of mouth and throat, headache, gastrointestinal symptoms, urticaria, and generalized pruritis

Table 5.1 (Continued)

Etiologic agent	Clinical syndrome
Paralytic or neurotoxic shellfish poison	Paresthesia of lips, mouth or face, and extremities; intestinal symptoms or weakness, including respiratory difficulty
Puffer fish, tetrodotoxin	Paresthesia of lips, tongue, face, or extremities, often following numbness; loss of proprioception, floating sensations
Heavy metals (Antimony, cadmium, copper, iron, tin, zinc)	Vomiting, often metallic taste
Monosodium glutamate (MSG)	Burning sensation in chest, neck, abdomen, or extremities; sensation of lightness and pressure over face or heavy feeling in chest
Mushroom toxins	
Shorter-acting toxins	Usually vomiting and diarrhea; other symptoms differ with toxin
Longer-acting toxins (e.g., *Amanita* spp.)	Diarrhea and abdominal cramps for 24 h followed by hepatic and renal failure

and the identification of new food safety hazards or unsafe food handling practices, findings which, in turn, will lead to new prevention measures. Once in place, continued surveillance can monitor and evaluate the effectiveness of preventive strategies and indicate the need for further investigation or research.

Objectives of foodborne disease surveillance

• Determine the human health burden and etiology of disease
• Monitor trends
• Identify high-risk populations
• Detect outbreaks
• Attribute illness to specific foods, practices or settings
• Prioritize interventions
• Monitor and evaluate effectiveness of preventive strategies

---

General methods in foodborne disease surveillance

It is useful to consider foodborne disease surveillance as a spectrum with four distinct levels, each becoming progressively more complex and resulting in enhanced capacity for controlling and detecting disease, but requiring more resources and infrastructure [3]. At one end of the spectrum, no formal foodborne disease surveillance system exists and outbreaks are detected only if they are very large. The next level is syndromic surveillance, followed by laboratory-based surveillance, and integrated food-chain surveillance. While a country may be primarily within one category, it may have surveillance elements from more than one category. Outbreak detection may occur at any level; however, the sensitivity to detect outbreaks varies considerably.

Syndromic surveillance

Syndromes related to foodborne disease include diarrhea, acute gastroenteritis, and "food poisoning". Systems that receive reports of syndromic conditions may function with or without diagnostic laboratory capacity, but there is often no formal laboratory-based surveillance. The use of standard case definitions and report forms are vital. The World Health Organization's (WHO's) definition of diarrhea, three or more loose stools in 24-hours, is often employed in countries collecting these data. In countries where clinicians have been asked to report cases of "food poisoning", the lack of a clear definition has led to reporting difficulties, as food poisoning itself is not a disease but a mode of transmission [4]. While syndromic surveillance may identify large localized outbreaks, this approach is often not specific enough for most surveillance needs and is not generally recommended if resources allow a component of laboratory diagnosis.

Laboratory-based surveillance

Surveillance based on laboratory diagnosis provides higher quality data than surveillance based on syndromes. Laboratory-based surveillance combines epidemiological data about the ill person with microbiological information about the infecting organism. Since many foodborne pathogens cause illness with similar signs and symptoms, laboratory-diagnosis can help identify the pathogens causing disease and determine pathogen-specific trends. Laboratory-based surveillance should also use standard case definitions and laboratories should use standardized methods for pathogen identification. Laboratory-based surveillance can identify both point source and diffuse national outbreaks. Surveillance has been enhanced for some infections by further characterization of the infecting pathogen (see section on *Laboratory subtyping of pathogens*).

Integrated food-chain surveillance

Integrated food-chain surveillance involves the collection, analysis, and interpretation of data from humans, animals, and food, including subtyped, pathogen-specific case counts for human infections and data of the prevalence of pathogen contamination in animals and food. Data can be used to generate hypotheses about the causes of human disease and to estimate the burden of foodborne disease due to specific food-pathogen combinations. Thus, integrated food-chain surveillance can increase our ability to assess the effectiveness of specific food safety interventions. By comparing routine laboratory-based surveillance in human, animals, and food, Denmark has been able to identify specific food–pathogen associations and has evaluated control measures directed at animals and food [5].

Strategies for foodborne disease surveillance

Strategies for foodborne disease surveillance include (1) outbreak investigations and surveillance, (2) routine surveillance for notifiable diseases, (3) laboratory subtyping of pathogens, (4) sentinel site surveillance, and (5) use of death registration and hospital discharge records. One strategy may be more appropriate than another for meeting different public health objectives. Strategies may be used alone or in combination.

Outbreak investigations and surveillance

Public health surveillance assists in the early detection of outbreaks of foodborne illness [6]. Although national reporting systems often exist, most foodborne outbreaks are investigated at the local level. Information gained through the outbreak investigations includes the nature of the pathogen or toxin, size and impact of the outbreak (i.e., number ill, hospitalized, type and severity of symptoms), and if determined, the implicated food vehicle and factors contributing to the outbreak (e.g., cross-contamination events).

As with other voluntary surveillance systems, underreporting of outbreaks does occur. In the US, the CDC has collected reports of outbreaks of foodborne illness investigated by local, state, and national health authorities since 1967. Prior to 1998, these reports were collected on paper, reviewed, and compiled. The introduction of an improved reporting form, active solicitation of reports from states, and the development of a Web-based reporting system (eFORS, the electronic Foodborne Outbreak Reporting System) increased the number of reports from an average of 500 to 1300 annually [6]. Common-source outbreaks of foodborne disease may be unrecognized, and therefore, underreported. The detection of low-level, geographically diffuse outbreaks has been enhanced by the introduction of a molecular subtyping surveillance network for foodborne infections, called PulseNet (see section on *Molecular subtyping*).

Despite underreporting, information gathered by outbreak investigation and reporting is important for monitoring long-term trends in foodborne pathogens, particularly those for which other sources of surveillance data are not available. Outbreak surveillance also provides important information on the link between specific pathogens and foods, as well as summarizing the foods most frequently associated with illness, and factors contributing to the outbreaks. In England and Wales, data from national foodborne outbreak surveillance was used, in conjunction with data from population-based studies, to estimate the burden of foodborne disease associated with different food types [7]. It was estimated that consumption of contaminated chicken meat and eggs accounted for nearly a third of all cases of indigenous foodborne diseases.

Routine surveillance for notifiable diseases

Surveillance systems for foodborne disease are frequently part of broader surveillance that requires clinicians or clinical laboratories to report cases of notifiable conditions to the relevant public health authorities [8]. In some countries, notifications may be legally required from clinicians. The information collected may be syndromic or laboratory-based and includes the diagnosis, date of diagnosis, and patient demographic information, such as age, sex and area of residence. Enhanced surveillance systems that capture additional information on disease severity and symptoms, and food and other exposures (e.g., travel) are often used for more severe, low-incidence diseases such as foodborne botulism.

Surveillance of notifiable conditions captures infections in persons who seek medical attention. These case reports provide useful information on local and national disease trends, high-risk populations, and the impact of prevention activities. Timely notification of cases can alert local, state, and national health authorities to potential outbreaks of foodborne illnesses. An outbreak may only be recognized when case reports from multiple facilities in the region are collated by a single public health agency. Rapid reporting, in the case of outbreaks, can occur electronically through health alert systems (for example, EpiX in the US). Summaries of reported cases are often published at the national level on a weekly and annual schedule (for example, *Morbidity and Mortality Weekly Report* in the US).

Reporting delays and undernotification are common. The clinician or clinical laboratory must recognize that the disease is notifiable and have an incentive to notify. Clinicians may be more likely to notify if required by law or if the report will result in public health action. Reporting is often more complete for more serious conditions or those considered to pose an immediate public health threat.

Providing clinicians and clinical laboratories with summaries of disease notifications and details of any public health action taken is important to engage their participation [9].

Laboratory subtyping of pathogens

Further characterization of disease-causing organisms is critical for detecting many outbreaks. Subtyping of pathogens provides important information on the epidemiology of a pathogen and clues about the source and the risk factors for infection.

Serotyping

In 1962, clinical laboratories in the US that isolated *Salmonella* from humans began to send strains to their state public health laboratories for serotyping; results were then mailed to CDC [10]. These serotyped data have been critical to the detection of many outbreaks of *Salmonella* and have helped to unravel the epidemiology of this important pathogen. Since 1995, CDC has routinely used an automated statistical outbreak detection algorithm that compares current reports with the preceding 5-year mean number of cases for the same geographic area and week of the year to look for unusual clusters of infection [11]. The usefulness of the outbreak algorithm is limited by the timeliness of reporting and the background rate of reporting for more common serotypes, such as *S. typhimurium* and *S. enteriditis*. The sensitivity of *Salmonella* serotyping to detect meaningful clusters is greatest for rare serotypes; further subtyping of the isolate is necessary for more common serotypes. The utility of serotyping as an international designation for *Salmonella* subtypes has led to its widespread adoption [12].

Molecular subtyping

Today, a new generation of subtyping methods is emerging, increasing the specificity and power to detect outbreaks [13]. In the US, pulsed-field gel electrophoresis (PFGE) has been introduced for routine subtyping of *E. coli* O157, *Salmonella*, and other enteric pathogens. By comparing the molecular "fingerprint" of bacterial strains in real time through PulseNet, the national molecular subtyping network for foodborne infections, public health officials can rapidly identify geographically diffuse clusters that are potential foodborne disease outbreaks [14]. The ability to identify geographically diffuse outbreaks has become increasingly important, as more foods are mass-produced and widely distributed. Following the launch of PulseNet in 1996, the number of *E. coli* O157:H7 outbreaks reported nationwide increased dramatically, demonstrating the utility of the subtyping approach [15]. Similar networks are being developed in Canada, Europe, the Asia-Pacific region, and Latin America, providing a unique opportunity for the detection of multiregional clusters. The usefulness of PFGE analysis depends on prompt submission of isolates to public health laboratories, timely processing by trained laboratorians, and appropriate analysis.

Antibiotic resistance

Antimicrobial susceptibility testing is another form of subtype-based surveillance and is used to help monitor the prevalence of antimicrobial resistance in enteric bacteria. In the US, the National Antimicrobial Resistance Monitoring System (NARMS), a collaborative effort between CDC, the US Department of Agriculture (USDA), and the US Food and Drug Administration (FDA), monitors the prevalence of resistance in *Salmonella*, *Campylobacter*, and other foodborne pathogens from humans, animals, and foods (see Chapter 7). NARMS data provide information to public health professionals involved in controlling highly resistant strains, clinicians making treatment decisions, and regulators responsible for evaluating the association between antibiotics used in animals or present in the environment and resistance developing in human pathogens [16].

Sentinel sites surveillance

Surveillance for foodborne diseases, syndromes, or complications of foodborne disease in selected sites or healthcare facilities can provide useful information of disease burden and trends, particularly when no reliable national data are available or more detailed information is required. Sentinel surveillance areas or facilities should be selected to be representative of the general population, although this may not always be possible. The population of the catchment area comprising the sentinel sites or facilities should be clearly defined so that population-based incidence can be calculated from case counts. The usefulness of sentinel networks in detecting outbreaks is limited unless they occur within the surveillance area.

FoodNet: an example of enhanced sentinel surveillance

The Foodborne Diseases Active Surveillance Network (FoodNet) was established in 1996 after a request from the USDA for a system to ascertain the public health impact of USDA's Pathogen Reduction: Hazard Analysis and Critical Control Point Final Rule (PR/HACCP rule) [17]. The principal foodborne disease component of CDC's Emerging Infections Program, FoodNet is a collaborative project among CDC, USDA, FDA, and 10 state health departments (www.cdc.gov/foodnet). In 2005, FoodNet catchment area comprised 15% of the US population. This surveillance network has had a major role in food safety in the US by conducting population-based, active surveillance for laboratory-confirmed infections from pathogens commonly transmitted through food (*Campylobacter*, *Cryptosporidium* and *Cyclospora*, *L. monocytogenes*, *Salmonella*, *Shigella*, Shiga toxin-producing *E. coli*, *Vibrio*, *Yersinia enterocolitica*) and one syndrome (hemolytic uremic syndrome (HUS), a serious complication of *E. coli* O157 infections).

FoodNet personnel routinely contact clinical laboratories to ascertain laboratory-confirmed cases occurring within the surveillance area. All clinical laboratories serving the FoodNet catchment area are contacted, including larger reference laboratories receiving specimens from, but geographically located outside, the FoodNet sites. Each clinical laboratory is audited at least twice yearly to ensure that all cases are ascertained and that changes in incidence are not due to surveillance artifacts. In 2005, there were >650 clinical laboratories serving the catchment area. Surveys of clinical laboratories serving the FoodNet catchment area are periodically conducted to detect temporal or geographical differences in clinical laboratory practices, which may contribute to variations in pathogen isolation rates [18].

Each year in April, preliminary FoodNet data for the preceding calendar year are published in CDC's *Morbidity and Mortality Weekly Report*.

This report has become known as the "National Report Card on Food Safety" and is used by regulatory agencies, industry, consumer groups, and public health personnel to prioritize and evaluate food safety interventions and monitor progress toward national health objectives. For example, since 2003, FoodNet has reported significant declines in the incidence of infection due to *E. coli* O157 [19]. This decline is likely due to a major initiative by USDA and the meat industry to reduce *E. coli* O157 in ground beef. Conversely, the lack of a decline in the incidence of *Salmonella* in recent years supports the need for initiatives to reduce the presence of *Salmonella* in raw meat and poultry products.

FoodNet also conducts related epidemiological studies. FoodNet routinely surveys the general population and clinical laboratories to estimate the frequency with which cases of foodborne disease go undetected at each surveillance step (seeking medical care, stool specimen submission, laboratory testing) (Figure 5.1) [20,21]. Surveys of the general population also collect baseline information on consumption patterns for "risky" foods, useful for hypotheses generation during outbreak investigations. Data are also collected on consumer knowledge, attitudes, and practices related to a range of foodborne-related topics [22]. FoodNet has been able to use its surveillance platform to conduct case-control and other epidemiologic studies to determine the proportion of foodborne diseases that are

caused by specific foods or preparation and handling practices [17].

Use of death registration and hospital discharge records

Death registration is usually based on the death certificate completed by a physician at the time of death. Information on the cause of death may be accompanied by data on the date of death and basic demographic characteristics, such as age, sex, and residence. Hospital discharge data are also available in many countries and may provide information on diagnosis, length of stay, and patient demographics. Because hospital discharge data include information on a patient's condition at discharge, they can also be used as a source of information on in-hospital deaths. In most countries, mortality data are summarized annually by a central vital statistics office. Hospital discharge data may also be routinely summarized by hospitals or available on a regional or national basis.

Causes of death or hospitalization are usually coded using the International Classification of Diseases (ICD), which facilitates international comparisons. Published by the WHO, the 10th Revision (ICD-10) is the latest in this series, although many countries still use ICD-9 codes (www.who.int/classifications/icd/en/). Classifications of interest to foodborne disease surveillance include nontyphoidal *Salmonella* (ICD-10 code A02), *Campylobacter* (ICD-10 code A04.5), and foodborne *Bacillus cereus* intoxication (ICD-10 code A05.4). Some foodborne diseases will, however, be coded using more general classifications not specific enough for foodborne disease surveillance, e.g., diarrhea and gastroenteritis of presumed infectious origin (ICD-10 code A09).

Coverage of death certificate data is limited to those persons whose death was medically certified, and completeness and accuracy may be low. When there are multiple causes of death (e.g., an elderly patient with comorbidities), the data most significant for foodborne disease surveillance may not be recorded. For hospital discharge data, coverage is limited to persons admitted to a hospital where a system for recording hospital discharge information is in place. It is important to note that most systems recording information on reasons for hospital

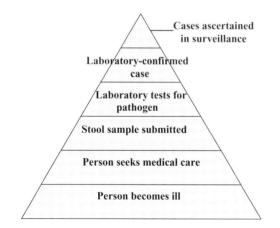

Fig 5.1 Surveillance steps that must occur for laboratory-confirmed cases to be ascertained through active in surveillance.

discharge were created not for disease surveillance but to document hospital activity and billing. The sensitivity of hospital discharge data may be affected by availability of diagnostic services (e.g., microbiologic assays), clinicians' laboratory test ordering practices, and coding practices in individual institutions.

Strategies for foodborne disease surveillance

- Outbreak investigations and surveillance
  - Information on link between specific pathogens and specific foods
  - Identifies foods most frequently associated with illness and factors contributing to outbreaks
  - Useful for monitoring long-term trends
- Routine surveillance for notifiable diseases
  - Information on local and national disease trends, high-risk populations, and impact of prevention activities
  - Timely notification can alert public health authorities to potential outbreaks
- Laboratory subtyping of pathogens
  - Critical for detecting outbreaks
  - Molecular subtyping methods, such as PFGE, have the power to detect geographically diffuse clusters
  - Provides clues about the source of the pathogen and risk factors for acquiring illness
- Sentinel site surveillance
  - Useful when no reliable national data are available or more detailed information is required
- Use of death registration and hospital discharge records
  - Contribute in a limited way to understanding severe illnesses; may be useful in monitoring trends in severe disease

---

Estimating the overall burden of foodborne illness

Cases ascertained in surveillance represent a fraction of the total number of cases in the community. Several "surveillance steps" are necessary for a case to be ascertained by laboratory-based surveillance: the ill person must seek medical care, a stool specimen must be submitted, and the laboratory must test for the pathogen and report the case to public health (Figure 5.1). Several countries have augmented surveillance with epidemiological studies in order to better understand the overall human health impact of foodborne illness [23,24]. These epidemiological studies fall into two broad categories: (i) prospective cohort studies and (ii) cross-sectional surveys.

Examples of prospective cohort studies include the Infectious Intestinal Disease Study (IID study) in England and the Sensor Study in the Netherlands [25,26]. Both studies followed a cohort of persons in the community for a defined time period, asking them to report weekly on the presence or absence of gastrointestinal symptoms. Those meeting the case definition were asked to submit a stool specimen for extensive laboratory testing for a range of bacteria, viruses, and parasites to determine the incidence and etiology of disease. Although relatively expensive and complex, cohort studies have the advantage of providing community incidence by pathogen. Community incidence can be compared to incidence derived from the national surveillance and the rate of surveillance case ascertainment can be estimated. The percentage of persons seeking medical care for specific syndromes or pathogens can be calculated, and the factors associated with seeking medical care and the frequency of stool specimen testing can be assessed [27].

In England, it was estimated that 20% of the population suffered from acute gastroenteritis each year. The most common etiologic agents identified were Norovirus, *Campylobacter*, Rotavirus, and nontyphoidal *Salmonella*. Data from this study were used in conjunction with data from national surveillance and special studies to estimate trends in the foodborne disease [28]. Investigators estimated that domestically acquired foodborne disease resulted in 2.9 million cases in 1992 and 1.3 million cases in 2000. *Campylobacter* infection accounted for most health service usage while salmonellosis caused most deaths. As described previously, this information was then used in conjunction with outbreak data to determine the burden and risk of foodborne disease associated with different foods [7].

Cross-sectional surveys have been used to estimate the overall human health impact of foodborne disease by estimating the frequency with which cases go underreported at each surveillance step, thereby extrapolating from laboratory-confirmed cases (at the top of the burden of illness pyramid—Figure 5.1) to estimate the overall burden of disease in the community (at the bottom of the burden of illness pyramid) [21,29]. Surveys of the general population have been used to estimate the prevalence of acute diarrheal illness and the frequency with which ill persons seek medical care and submit a stool culture. These surveys are often conducted by telephone over a 12-month period, to account for seasonal variation. The advantage of this study design is its relative simplicity and lower cost, compared to cohort studies, making it easily repeatable in different populations or time periods. Cross-sectional surveys of clinical diagnostic laboratories have been conducted to determine the frequency with which cases of foodborne diseases go undetected because of laboratory testing practices. By augmenting surveillance with information from laboratory surveys and surveys of the general population, FoodNet estimated that in 2004, for each laboratory-confirmed case of *Salmonella*, there were 38 cases in the community [21].

Enhancing surveillance internationally

The globalization of the food industry and the rise in air travel have presented new challenges for food safety, making foodborne disease surveillance a global priority. Begun in 2000, WHO Global Salm-Surv (www.who.int/salmsurv/en/) is a network of institutions and individuals involved in *Salmonella* surveillance, serotyping, and antimicrobial resistance testing [30]. The program, which aims to strengthen laboratory-based surveillance worldwide, is coordinated by the WHO, CDC, FDA, the Danish Institute for Food and Veterinary Research, Reseau International des Instituts Pasteur, Health Canada, Animal Sciences Group-Netherlands, OzFoodNet, and Enter-net. The core elements of WHO Global Salm-Surv include international training courses, a moderated electronic discussion group, an external quality assurance system, a country databank of the top 15 annual *Salmonella*

serotypes, and reference testing services (Figure 5.2). Through 2005, 34 training courses for microbiologists, epidemiologists, and managers have involved more than 700 participants from more than 130 countries from all six WHO designated regions. By enhancing laboratory-based surveillance, WHO Global Salm-Surv is helping those countries establish a foundation upon which studies to estimate the burden of foodborne illnesses can be conducted.

Recommendations for foodborne surveillance

At minimum, countries should systematically investigate outbreaks that meet predefined prioritization criteria (e.g., threshold number of cases, severity of illness, high-risk settings such as long-term care facilities). Many countries would benefit from improving their capacity to identify, investigate, and control foodborne outbreaks. Improved communication between healthcare providers, laboratories, and public health authorities is important as it can facilitate an increase in the number of cases that are reported, which can increase the potential for identifying outbreaks of foodborne illness. Once outbreaks have been identified, the formation of joint investigation teams will further develop interdisciplinary networks. Findings from outbreak investigations should guide prevention interventions. Outbreak investigation exercises offer an opportunity for multidisciplinary training and open lines of communication between key organizations. Summary information on outbreaks is important when advocating for resources for foodborne disease surveillance. Centralized reporting and collection of outbreak data in a database allows information to be easily summarized and reported. Findings should be disseminated widely to the government, industry, and the general population. The public health and economic impact (e.g., impact on trade or tourism) should be emphasized and success stories highlighted.

While syndromic surveillance is usually not specific enough for most foodborne surveillance needs, it may be useful in countries with insufficient resources to establish laboratory-based surveillance. Syndromic surveillance for foodborne diseases should be developed based on the priority

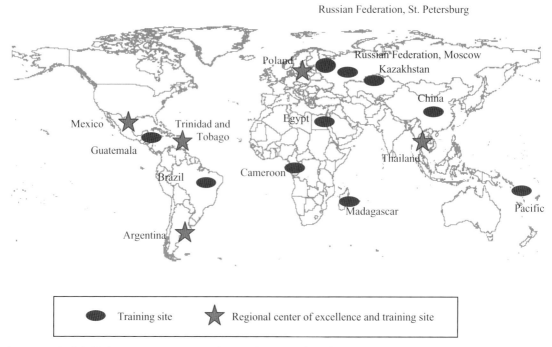

Fig 5.2 WHO global Salm-Surv training sites and regional centers of excellence.

diseases in that country. The flow of data from patient to district to national level should be delineated and case definitions, report forms, and a description of the process disseminated to public health authorities and medical personnel responsible for collecting these data. Collected data should be analyzed, interpreted, and summarized on a regular basis and findings communicated so that control measures can be implemented. Routine data analysis will allow investigators to gain a better understanding of baseline numbers, follow trends, and promptly identify outbreaks. Syndromic surveillance data may be more useful if supplemented with data collected from hospital discharge data reviews or existing laboratory data from hospitals or private laboratories as these data can provide important supplemental information of the common organisms and subtypes isolated. Whenever possible, incorporation of more specific diagnostic information may increase the yield of syndromic surveillance.

Countries moving toward a laboratory-based surveillance for foodborne diseases should encour-age physicians to request stool cultures by highlighting the benefits of knowing the pathogen and antibiotic resistance profile in treatment success rates. Such a system can begin with collection of culture specimens from sentinel clinics and those that are part of outbreaks, rather than attempting to collect all isolates. A systematic sampling scheme provides better data than a more haphazard attempt at universal reporting. A survey of clinical laboratories is useful to better understand current testing practices and capacity in terms of the number of stools tested annually and the number of isolates positive for enteric organisms. Clinical laboratories should be encouraged to report existing data centrally to the National Public Health Laboratory. The importance of good communication between public health laboratories and epidemiologists cannot be understated. Regular meetings facilitate rapid sharing of information and the identification of outbreaks. During outbreak investigations, hypotheses from epidemiological investigations can be shared and used to help guide laboratory investigations. Laboratory-based surveillance will be greatly enhanced with the introduction of new subtyping methods.

Studies assessing the overall human health impact of foodborne disease can provide important information for policy formation and disease prevention. The stage of development of a country's surveillance systems will influence a country's ability to conduct an assessment of disease burden. The more sophisticated the surveillance system is, the more specific the outcomes of the study will be in regard to etiology. The cost and complexity of these studies varies considerably depending on the study design and setting in which they are conducted. Besides providing estimates of the burden of foodborne pathogens in the community, burden of illness studies can improve our understanding of how the current surveillance system works. Studies can promote cooperation and collaboration among various government sectors.

Summary

Globally, the benefits of mass production, distribution, and importation of food have been accompanied by the rapid spread and dissemination of pathogens, creating new challenges for the detection, investigation, control, and prevention of foodborne diseases. In the future, it is likely that new pathogens will be recognized, new diagnostic strategies will identify some pathogens that currently are often or completely undetected, and novel food vehicles will continue to be described. Enhanced public health surveillance for human foodborne illness will be vital to identify and investigate these new challenges, and provide needed information for control strategies aimed at preventing foodborne diseases.

References

1 Mead PS, Slutsker L, Dietz V, *et al*. Food-related illness and death in the United States. *Emerg Infect Dis* 1999;5(5):607–25.

2 Borgdorff MW, Motarjemi Y. Surveillance of foodborne diseases: what are the options? *World Health Stat Q* 1997;50(1–2):12–23.

3 World Health Organization, *Methods for Foodborne Disease Surveillance in Selected Sites: Report on a WHO con-*

sultation. Leipzig, Germany: World Health Organization; March 18–21, 2002.

4 Cowden JM. Food poisoning notification: time for a rethink. *Health Bull (Edinb)* 2000;58(4):328–31.

5 Hald T, *et al*. A Bayesian approach to quantify the contribution of animal-food sources to human salmonellosis. *Risk Anal* 2004;24(1):255–69.

6 Lynch M, *et al*. Surveillance for foodborne-disease outbreaks—United States, 1998–2002. *MMWR Surveill Summ* 2006;55(10):1–42.

7 Adak GK, *et al*. Disease risks from foods, England and Wales, 1996–2000. *Emerg Infect Dis* 2005;11(3):365–72.

8 Roush S, *et al*. Mandatory reporting of diseases and conditions by health care professionals and laboratories. *JAMA* 1999;282(2):164–70.

9 Allen CJ, Ferson MJ. Notification of infectious diseases by general practitioners: a quantitative and qualitative study. *Med J Aust* 2000;172(7):325–8.

10 Thacker S. Historical development. In: C.R. Teutsch S (ed.), *Principles and Practice of Public Health Surveillance*. New York: Oxford University Press; 2000.

11 Hutwagner LC, *et al*. Using laboratory-based surveillance data for prevention: an algorithm for detecting *Salmonella* outbreaks. *Emerg Infect Dis* 1997;3(3):395–400.

12 Herikstad H, Motarjemi Y, Tauxe RV. *Salmonella* surveillance: a global survey of public health serotyping. *Epidemiol Infect* 2002;129(1):1–8.

13 Tauxe RV. Molecular subtyping and the transformation of public health. *Foodborne Pathog Dis* 2006;3(1):4–8.

14 Gerner-Smidt P, *et al*. PulseNet USA: a 5-year update. *Foodborne Pathog Dis* 2006;3(1):9–19.

15 Rangel JM, *et al*. Epidemiology of *Escherichia coli* O157:H7 outbreaks, United States, 1982–2002. *Emerg Infect Dis* 2005;11(4):603–9.

16 Anderson AD, *et al*. Public health consequences of use of antimicrobial agents in food animals in the United States. *Microb Drug Resist* 2003;9(4):373–9.

17 Scallan E. Activities, achievements and lessons learned during the first 10 years of FoodNet, 1996–2005. *Clin Infect Dis*, 2007;44(5):718–25.

18 Voetsch AC, *et al*. Laboratory practices for stool-specimen culture for bacterial pathogens, including *Escherichia coli* O157:H7, in the FoodNet sites, 1995–2000. *Clin Infect Dis* 2004;38(suppl 3):S190–7.

19 Preliminary FoodNet data on the incidence of infection with pathogens transmitted commonly through food—10 States, United States, 2005. *MMWR Morb Mortal Wkly Rep* 2006;55(14):392–5.

20 Jones TF, McMillian MB, Scallan E, *et al*. A population-based estimate of the substantial burden of diarrheal

be recognized in two ways. First, one country may recognize an outbreak and inform the network and, members may recognize a similar occurrence in their countries. This was the case in an outbreak of *Salmonella* Oranienburg in 2001, when contaminated chocolate from Germany led to 462 cases in Germany and additional cases in Austria, Belgium, Denmark, Finland, the Netherlands, and Sweden. In Canada, the chocolate was taken off the shelf before cases occurred [13]. Alternatively, outbreaks may be identified by analyzing the international database for unusually high levels of infection [14]. When international outbreaks are recognized, the coordination of their investigation is managed following principles that have been agreed upon by the network participants [15].

Apart from short-term actions, surveillance data can generate hypotheses for targeted epidemiological studies. Time-series analyses of long-term trends can reveal shifts in risk-groups or regions that can trigger subsequent actions. For example, Chapter 12 describes the steep increase in TB notification rates in the non-Baltic former Soviet Union countries, that coincided with the socio-political changes associated with the break-up of the Soviet Union. It also describes the high frequency of drug-resistant TB in these countries, partly a result of the imprudent use of antibiotic treatment.

Continuous monitoring of quality

As surveillance systems vary widely in scope, objectives, and methods, performance indicators (sensitivity, predictive value, representativeness, timeliness, simplicity, flexibility, acceptability, and efficient resource utilization) that are important to one surveillance system may be less important to another. Timeliness, for example, is of great importance for outbreak-prone diseases such as listeriosis or salmonellosis, but of less importance for chronic infections such as HIV or tuberculosis. Each surveillance system should identify the performance indicators that are most important to its objectives. Efforts to strengthen certain attributes—such as the ability of a system to detect every health event (sensitivity)—may detract from other attributes, such as simplicity or timeliness. Furthermore, expanding surveillance objectives to be addressed by

the system may compromise the performance of the system in relation to its primary objectives.

Procedures to check and validate the data should be built into the information technology (IT) components of the supranational systems. These procedures should be automated as much as possible—this requires an intensive discussion between the supranational coordination and the contact points in the participating countries. Quality assurance schemes also need to be set up for the relevant national reference laboratories, and for methods that are not included in national quality assurance systems.

Lessons learned and recommendations

With the creation of the ECDC, surveillance in the EU is in a transition period. Surveillance activities of the past years operated through the DSN need to be consolidated and integrated into a coordinated surveillance strategy. Important lessons can be learned from the experience of the DSN over the last decade working with countries with pre-existing surveillance systems, sometimes with long traditions. Common case definitions and use of standardized methods for data collection and laboratory analysis are prerequisites for supranational surveillance. Choosing standardized methods requires intensive baseline work to assess each country's practices, and the constraints and possibilities to adapt to standardized methods. Implementation of pilot tests is necessary to identify appropriate, acceptable, and feasible methodologies.

To win acceptance, it is important to clearly formulate a convincing rationale for supranational reporting that explains what data are needed to answer which questions. The added value of supranational surveillance, not replacing national systems but providing an additional, coordinated overview perspective that no individual country can have on its own, should be made explicit to data providers and users.

Successful collaboration requires a clearly defined set of rules by which to work. Standard operating procedures, memoranda of understanding, and principles of collaboration have to be established and continuously adapted to ensure that all participants are aware of their rights and their responsibilities as members of the international network. Issues of data ownership, confidentiality, and freedom of information legislation need to be addressed and agreed upon.

The principal determinant of the effectiveness of supranational surveillance is the quality of contributing national surveillance systems. Continuous monitoring of quality and predefined performance indicators are essential both at the supranational level and in the individual countries. Supranational surveillance should encourage and support the strengthening of national surveillance systems in the Member States.

References

1 Käferstein FK, Motarjemi Y, Bettcher DW. Foodborne disease control: a transnational challenge. *EID* 1997;**3**(4):503–10.

2 Frank C, Walter J, Muehlen M, *et al*. Large outbreak of hepatitis A in tourists staying at a hotel in Hurghada, Egypt, 2004—orange juice implicated. *Euro Surveill Wkly* June 9, 2005;**10**:6.

3 Decision No 2119/98/EC of the European Parliament and of the Council of 24 September 1998 setting up a network for the epidemiological surveillance and control of communicable diseases in the Community. *OJE* 1998;**L268**:1–6.

4 Commission Decision of 22 December 1999 (2000/ 96/EC) on the communicable diseases to be progressively covered by the Community network under Decision No 2119/98/EC of the European Parliament and the Council. *OJE* 2000;**L28**:50–53.

5 Commission Decision of 22 December 1999 (2000/ 57/EC) on the early warning and response system for the prevention and control of communicable diseases under Decision 2119/98/EC of the European Parliament and of the Council. *OJE* 2000;**L21**:32–35.

6 Ammon A, fellows of the European Programme for Intervention Epidemiology Training (EPIET), Members of the National Public Health Institutes and Laboratories. Surveillance of enterohaemorrhagic *E. coli* (EHEC) infections and haemolytic uraemic syndrome (HUS) in Europe. *Euro Surveill* 1997;**2**(12):91–6.

7 Takkinen J, Ammon A, Robstad O, Breuer T, and the Campylobacter Working Group. European survey on *Campylobacter* surveillance and diagnosis, 2001. *Euro Surveill* 2003;**8**(11):207–13.

8 de Valk H, Jacquet C, Goulet V, *et al*. Surveillance of *Listeria* infections in Europe. *Euro Surveill* 2005;**10**(10): 251–5.

9 Martin P, Jacquet C, Goulet V, Vaillant V, de Valk H, and participants in the Pulsenet Europe Feasibility Study. Pulse-field gel electrophoresis of *Listeria monocytogenes* strains: the PulseNet Europe Feasibility Study. *Foodborne Pathog Dis* Fall 2006;**3**(3):303–8.

10 Regulation (EC) No 851/2004 of the European Parliament and of the Council of 21 April 2004, establishing a European centre for disease prevention and control. *Off J Eur Union* 2004;**L142**:1–11.

11 Wheeler JG, Sethi D, Cowden JM, *et al*, for the Infectious Intestinal Disease Study Executive. Study of infectious intestinal disease in England: rates in the community, presenting to general practice, and reported to national surveillance. *BMJ* 1999;**318**(7190):1046–50.

12 Fisher IST on behalf of the Enter-net participants. The Enter-net international surveillance network—how it works. *Euro Surveill* 1999;**4**:52–5.

13 Werber D, Dreesman J, Feil F, *et al*. International outbreak of *Salmonella* Oranienburg due to German chocolate. *BMC Infect Dis* 2005;**5**:7.

14 Fisher I, Crowcroft N. Enter-net/EPIET investigation into the multinational cluster of *Salmonella* Livingstone. *Euro Surveill Wkly* 1998;**2**:980115. Available from: http://www.eurosurveillance.org/ew/1998/980115.asp#2.

15 Desenclos JC, Fisher IST, Gill N. Management of the investigation by Enter-net of international foodborne outbreaks of gastrointestinal organisms. *Euro Surveill* 1999;**4**(5):58–62.

Appendix: Communicable diseases and special health issues to be covered by the community network*

DISEASES

Diseases preventable by vaccination
Diphtheria
Infections with *Haemophilus influenza* group B[†]
Influenza[†]
Measles[†]
Mumps
Pertussis[†]
Poliomyelitis
Rubella
Smallpox
Tetanus
Sexually transmitted diseases
Chlamydia infections
Gonococcal infections
HIV-infection[†]
Syphilis

Viral hepatitis
Hepatitis A
Hepatitis B
Hepatitis C
Food- and waterborne diseases and diseases of environmental origin
Anthrax
Botulism
Campylobacteriosis
Cryptosporidiosis
Giardiasis
Infection with enterohaemorrhagic *E. coli*[†]
Leptospirosis
Listeriosis
Salmonellosis[†]
Shigellosis
Toxoplasmosis
Trichinosis
Yersinosis
Diseases transmitted by nonconventional agents
Transmissible spongiform encephalopathies, variant Creutzfeldt—Jakob disease[†]
Airborne diseases
Legionellosis[†]
Meningococcal disease[†]
Pneumococcal infections
Tuberculosis[†]

Zoonoses
Brucellosis
Echinococcosis
Rabies
Q-fever
Tularaemia
Serious imported diseases
Cholera
Malaria
Plague
Viral haemorrhagic fevers

SPECIAL HEALTH ISSUES
Nosocomial infections
Antimicrobial resistance[†]

---

[*]Commission decision of July 12, 2003, amending Decision 2000/96/EC as regards the operation of dedicated surveillance networks (2003/542/EC) , Official Journal of the European Union L185/55–58. For the communicable diseases and special health issues listed, epidemiological surveillance is to be performed by the standardized collection and analysis of data in a way that is to be determined for each communicable disease and special health issue when specific dedicated surveillance networks are put in place.

[†]Those communicable diseases and special health issues for which a dedicated surveillance network is in place as of 2006.

7 Surveillance for antimicrobial resistance among foodborne bacteria: the US approach

Jean M. Whichard, Kathryn Gay, David G. White & Tom M. Chiller

Summary

Several countries have made significant strides toward establishing surveillance systems for tracking antimicrobial resistance among foodborne bacteria. This chapter will describe the development and evolution of antimicrobial resistance surveillance among foodborne bacteria in the United States (US) as conducted by the National Antimicrobial Resistance Monitoring System (NARMS). The key aspects of sampling and testing bacterial isolates from humans, retail meats, and animals will be defined. Knowledge gained through implementation and execution of NARMS applicable to other surveillance systems development will also be presented, as will strengths and weaknesses of current surveillance efforts. Finally, specific examples will be presented that highlight the achievements and continued challenges to overcome in antimicrobial resistance surveillance of foodborne bacteria in the US.

Introduction

Antimicrobial agents are one of the main therapeutic tools in human and veterinary medicine to control a wide range of bacterial infectious diseases. However, the development of antimicrobial resistance, particularly to critically important antimicrobials, has become an omnipresent problem. Antimicrobial-resistant bacteria are not only a significant medical problem, but they also exert a large economic impact because of prolonged and some-

times unsuccessful treatment. There is also much concern that these bacteria act as "reservoirs" of antimicrobial resistance. The nature of this concern is that resistant commensal and environmental bacteria, although not typically causing disease themselves, can function as reservoirs for resistance genes that can be transferred to bacteria that cause disease.

Antimicrobial agents have greatly benefited human health and animal health. In animal agriculture, introduction of antimicrobial agents corresponded with significant improvements in productivity [1]. In food animals, antimicrobial agents are used for the control, prevention, and treatment of infectious diseases, as well as for enhancing growth and feed efficiency. As early as the 1960s, recognition that antimicrobial use in food animals was associated with transmissible drug resistance among zoonotic foodborne bacteria prompted public health authorities to evaluate the human consequences of antimicrobial use in agriculture [2,3]. Recognizing this potential health hazard, the World Health Organization (WHO), the Food and Agriculture Organization (FAO), and the World Organization for Animal Health (OIE) recommended that each country implement a monitoring program on both the usage of antimicrobials in animals and on the occurrence of antimicrobial resistance in bacteria from animals and from food of animal origin [4]. The increased international concern over transfer of bacterial foodborne pathogens and resistant variants between animals and humans helped spur the development of numerous surveillance systems and networks worldwide [5].

Components of antimicrobial resistance surveillance for foodborne pathogens in the US

Antimicrobial resistance is spread by complex inter-actions at various stages of animal and food pro-duction, and coordinated efforts are required for surveillance. In the US, food producers, the US De-partment of Agriculture (USDA), and US Food and Drug Administration (FDA) are responsible for the safety of the nation's food supply. The Centers for Disease Control and Prevention (CDC), in close collaboration with State and Territorial Depart-ments of Health, is responsible for human health surveillance and, at the invitation of the states, in-vestigating human illness. For example, outbreaks of egg-associated human *Salmonella* ser. Enteridi-tis infections prompted the egg industry to initi-ate egg quality assurance programs. Partnering with state and federal agencies, these programs have re-duced the incidence of egg-associated salmonellosis [6]. Although antimicrobial resistance was not ad-dressed in these programs, this partnership set an important precedent for these stakeholders to unite despite their differences. Given the recent increase in the prevalence of quinolone resistance among *Salmonella* ser. Enteriditis isolated from ill people, there are renewed opportunities for these groups to work together to control and mitigate the public health impact of resistance.

The ultimate goal of antimicrobial resistance surveillance of foodborne bacteria is to maintain clinical efficacy of antimicrobial agents used to combat human and animal disease. The specific ob-jectives toward achieving this goal include:

• Collect descriptive data on the extent and tempo-ral trends of antimicrobial susceptibility in enteric foodborne bacteria isolated from farms, farm ani-mals, animal slaughter and food processing plants, retail meats, and healthy and ill humans.

• Conduct applied research studies to better under-stand the emergence and transfer of antimicrobial resistance among foodborne bacteria.

• Provide information to physicians, public health authorities, veterinarians, and other stakeholders on antimicrobial resistance so that timely action can be taken to protect public health.

Risk modeling and assessment using surveillance and other data forms the foundation of science-

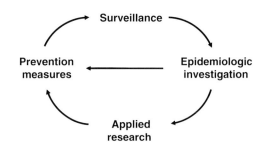

Fig 7.1 The cycle of foodborne disease control and prevention.

based mitigation. Continued monitoring, in turn, is essential to evaluate risk management strategies and public actions (Figure 7.1).

In addition to antimicrobial susceptibility data, subtyping and molecular studies may be conducted for selected bacterial strains to more fully under-stand the nature of antimicrobial resistance. For example, serotyping is critical for the surveillance of *Salmonella* and can help put antimicrobial re-sistance patterns into appropriate subtype con-text [7]. Further molecular characterization might include whole genome strain typing by pulsed-field gel electrophoresis (PFGE). These data are used along with susceptibility information to as-sess strain relatedness, source, and subtype dis-semination. Increasingly, PFGE data on NARMS strains is submitted to PulseNet, the national molec-ular subtyping network for foodborne diseases [8].

In the US, national surveillance for antimicro-bial resistance among foodborne bacteria was es-tablished in 1996 with the formation of NARMS [9]. This system is the result of collaborative ef-forts of CDC, the US Food and Drug Administra-tion Center for Veterinary Medicine (FDA-CVM), and USDA, and was designed to prospectively mon-itor changes in susceptibility to antimicrobial agents of human and veterinary importance [10]. The es-tablishment of NARMS was prompted by a 1994 FDA joint Veterinary Medicine and Anti-Infective Drugs Advisory Committee convened to consider the proposed first approval of fluoroquinolone use in food animals in the US. The Committee recom-mended that a national surveillance system be es-tablished to monitor resistance trends among hu-man and animal foodborne bacteria. Today, CDC,

FDA, and USDA conduct the human, retail meat, and animal components of NARMS, respectively. Over the years, NARMS has adapted to changing needs by increasing the number of bacteria under surveillance and adjusting the antimicrobial agents it evaluates (Figure 7.2).

Since antimicrobial susceptibility testing is not routinely performed by clinical laboratories on the bacteria included in NARMS, and since standardized, quality controlled susceptibility testing can more efficiently be conducted at fewer laboratories, NARMS uses three central laboratories for susceptibility testing. Human isolates are tested at CDC in Atlanta, GA; retail meat isolates are tested at FDA in Laurel, Maryland; and food animal isolates are tested at USDA in Athens, GA. Bacterial isolates are collected from several sources using various sampling strategies. Given the variety of foodborne bacteria included in NARMS, surveillance and sampling strategies are tailored to the specific bacteria. Important considerations used for developing the sampling strategies have included the number and representative nature of isolates available, and the cost and workload involved in shipping the isolates to a central laboratory for susceptibility testing. Most isolates submitted to NARMS are derived through existing surveillance or monitoring programs. Participating sites are shown in Figure 7.3. Currently, isolates are received for testing as follows.

Human isolates, CDC (Atlanta, GA), nationwide surveillance

As part of routine surveillance, clinical laboratories send isolates of *Salmonella, Shigella*, and *Escherichia coli* O157 to state public health laboratories. In each of the 50 states in the US, the state public health laboratory sends bacterial isolates they receive from clinical laboratories to CDC for susceptibility testing.
• Every 20th isolate of non-Typhi *Salmonella*, *Shigella*, and *E. coli* O157:H7 received is submitted. Every isolate of *Salmonella* ser. Typhi is submitted.
• For *Campylobacter*, a frequency-based sample of isolates received by the state public health laboratory in each of 10 Foodborne Diseases Active Surveillance Network (FoodNet) sites is submitted [11].

• Enterococci Resistance Study: five states submit commensal bacteria (enterococci and generic *E. coli*) isolated from the stool specimens collected from outpatients or healthy volunteers.

Retail meat isolates, FDA (Laurel, MD)

NARMS retail meat surveillance is an ongoing collaboration between the US FDA, CDC, and all 10 of the current FoodNet laboratories: California, Colorado, Connecticut, Georgia, Maryland, Minnesota, New Mexico, New York, Oregon, and Tennessee.
• FoodNet Retail Meat Study: 40 retail meats each month are purchased from a random sample of 5 grocery stores selected from a commercially available list from each FoodNet site. Two samples each of chicken breast, ground turkey, ground beef, and pork chops are purchased from each store. Each site cultures the rinsate from each meat sample for the presence of *Salmonella* and *Campylobacter*. In addition, four states culture all rinsates for generic *E. coli* and *Enterococcus*. Bacterial isolates are sent to FDA/CVM for confirmation of species, antimicrobial susceptibility testing, and genetic analysis.

Animal isolates, USDA (Athens, GA)

• Veterinary Diagnostic Laboratories: *Salmonella* isolated from specimens collected from ill animals submitted to 12 diagnostic laboratories and the National Veterinary Services Laboratory (NVSL) in Ames, IA, are submitted to USDA for susceptibility testing.
• National Animal Health Monitoring System (NAHMS): *Salmonella* are isolated from specimens collected on farms as part of NAHMS, which collects animal specimens from beef, catfish, dairy, equine, poultry, sheep, and swine operations approximately every 5 years [12].
• Hazard Analysis and Critical Control Points (HACCP) verification program: *Salmonella* are isolated from specimens collected at food animal slaughter and processing plants as part of the Food Safety and Inspection Service (FSIS) HACCP program. *Campylobacter*, generic *E. coli*, and enterococci are isolated from the chicken carcass rinsates FSIS collects at poultry processing plants for the HACCP program.

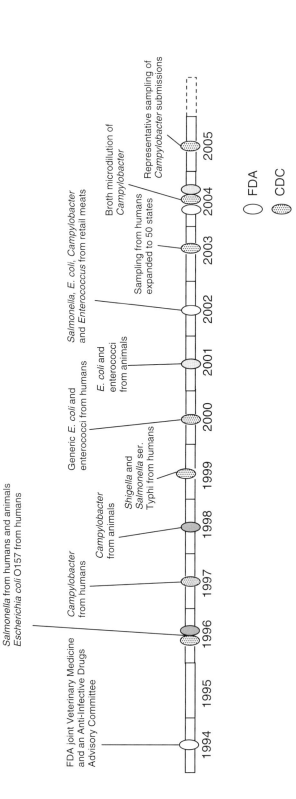

Fig 7.2 Significant events in NARMS project development.

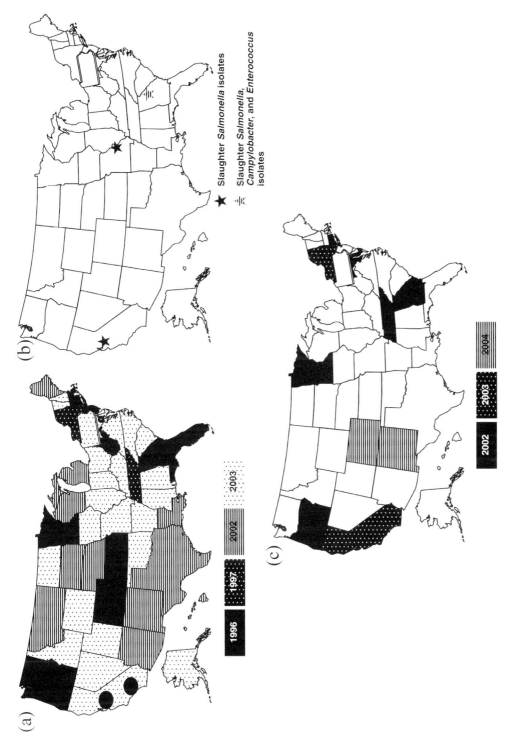

Fig 7.3 Sequence and extent of NARMS participation: (a) human isolate monitoring; (b) animal slaughter isolate monitoring; (c) retail meats monitoring.

food animal components highlights the unique challenges of each part of the surveillance. However, the uniform nature of the susceptibility testing methods and reporting facilitates comprehensive comparable surveillance data collection. This section describes how NARMS was developed and how it evolved to the techniques employed today.

Human sampling evolution

The human NARMS program was based in large part on pilot projects that estimated the prevalence of resistance. For non-Typhi *Salmonella*, the CDC NARMS program was preceded by four surveys of antimicrobial resistance conducted in 1979–1980, 1984–1985, 1989–1990, and 1994–1995 [19]. In the first three surveys, a random sample of counties throughout the US representing rural and urban areas was selected for inclusion, and isolates from all culture-confirmed cases of salmonellosis were requested from these counties. Counties were selected and recruited to participation until a target of 5% of the annual nationwide estimated culture-confirmed cases of salmonellosis was reached. Patient questionnaires were used to ascertain demographic details and risk factors for infection. All states participated in the 1994–1995 survey during which state public health laboratories submitted 10% of non-Typhi *Salmonella* isolates they received. Susceptibility testing was performed at CDC using a disk diffusion method [20,21]. These studies helped demonstrate what was needed for surveillance in a broader geographic area. Issues central to development of the surveillance program included logistics of isolate storage, shipment and testing, data acquisition, analysis, and management.

From 1989 to 1990, a similar sentinel county study was performed to assess antimicrobial resistance among *Campylobacter* isolated from humans [22]. During the study period, 19 counties in the US forwarded the first five *Campylobacter* isolated each month to CDC for susceptibility testing. Susceptibility was determined for eight antimicrobial agents using a broth microdilution method [23]. This study helped establish the one isolate per week submission scheme employed when NARMS began *Campylobacter* sampling in a broader geographic area (5 states) in 1997.

Surveillance for antimicrobial resistance among *Salmonella* ser. Typhi and *Shigella* is specific to the NARMS human isolate program, and strategies for sampling these two pathogens were also based on preliminary studies that addressed prevalence of antimicrobial resistance, risk factors, and clinical outcomes. A 1-year survey of antimicrobial resistance among *Salmonella* ser. Typhi was conducted in 1996–1997. Isolates and patient questionnaires were available for 293 of the 364 culture-confirmed cases (80%) reported in 45 US states and territories during that period and were included in the analysis [24]. One-year surveys of resistance among *Shigella* species were conducted in 1985–1986 and 1995–1996 [18,25]. Counties were stratified to form two groups (east and west) based on location with respect to the Mississippi River. Counties were enrolled from those that had reported five or more cases of *Shigella* in 1983 until 10% of the total number of reported cases in each stratum was represented. Much like the non-Typhi *Salmonella* sentinel county studies, disk diffusion methods were used to determine antimicrobial susceptibility for both *Salmonella* ser. Typhi and *Shigella*. Results from these studies helped determine the sampling scheme used when the NARMS human isolate program for these pathogens commenced in 1999: every isolate of *Salmonella* ser. Typhi and every tenth *Shigella* isolate.

Consideration of data from the sentinel county studies led to the conclusion that prospective frequency-based sampling would be best for capturing resistance prevalence changes over time. However, *Campylobacter* prevalence, isolation rates, and viability were less predictable, so a weekly sampling strategy was initially used. Sampling frequency decisions were designed to maximize sensitivity given the resources available for isolate disposition and testing. For instance, as NARMS expanded to become nationwide, the sampling frequency for non-Typhi *Salmonella* and *Shigella* was changed from every tenth isolate to every twentieth isolate received at participating state public health laboratories (Figure 7.3). In 2004, based on recommendations from a 2003 external review, *Campylobacter* surveillance (now in 10 FoodNet sites) was changed from one isolate per week to a proportional sampling model based on prevalence of *Campylobacter* in each site.

Retail meat sampling evolution

Before adding the retail meat component to NARMS, a year-long statistically robust pilot study was conducted throughout the state of Iowa. This study allowed evaluation of methodologies, workload, workflow, costs, and data (prevalence, susceptibility, seasonality, etc.) for a retail meat surveillance system. Many conclusions from the Iowa study were later applied to the NARMS retail meat program, such as determination of meat types consistently available for purchase, and refinement of bacterial culture methods. Moreover, this pre-NARMS study determined the frequency at which a single meat sample was contaminated by multiple strain types. The pilot study also allowed determination of baseline contamination and antimicrobial resistance prevalence using a statistically designed sampling scheme. Experience gained from the Iowa study was instrumental in the final design of the NARMS retail meat program, which began in January 2002 and became the third component of NARMS. Six FoodNet sites were initially involved in 2002; two additional FoodNet sites joined in 2003; and the last two remaining FoodNet sites joined in 2004 (Figure 7.3). In 2005, based on recommendations from an internal review, the NARMS retail meat surveillance program transitioned from a convenience sampling scheme to a more statistically robust randomized sampling scheme for collection of retail meats, using a census of grocery stores obtained from a commercial source.

Food animal sampling evolution

The animal component of NARMS collects isolates from diagnostic specimens and on-farm and slaughter/processing sources. Due to resource limitations and existing sampling infrastructures, there was less flexibility in sample selection compared with the other NARMS components. Diagnostic isolate sampling relies on voluntary submissions and referrals to veterinary bacteriology laboratories including the national referral facility, the National Veterinary Services Laboratory (NVSL). Nondiagnostic isolate submissions from farm operations have depended on the design and collection strategies of the National Animal Health Monitoring System (NAHMS), a national sampling of food animal operations that studies each commodity every 5 years based on the National Agricultural Statistics Service design. NARMS slaughter isolate sampling has always depended on the USDA FSIS verification isolates for *Salmonella*, and on FSIS-provided carcass rinsates for *Campylobacter*, *Enterococcus*, and *E. coli*. From its inception to the present time, the food animal monitoring program has tested all isolates received from these sources rather than adopting a frequency-based sampling scheme.

Development of susceptibility testing methods and reporting

Although disk diffusion methods were used for some pre-NARMS studies, [20] a broth microdilution method was adopted for NARMS testing. Reasons for this included ease of standardization, reproducibility, and ability to capture numerical MIC data for many antimicrobial agents. When testing began, there were no semiautomated platforms nor CLSI breakpoints available for *Campylobacter*. For these reasons and because of the microaerophilic conditions necessary to cultivate this organism, different methods had to be employed. The FDA laboratory determined *Campylobacter* MICs by agar dilution while CDC and USDA used Etest® (AB Biodisk), a diffusion method from which an MIC can be read. As described above, a new CLSI *Campylobacter* broth microdilution testing method was adopted by all NARMS participating laboratories in 2005. Numerical MIC distributions have always been reported in addition to susceptible, intermediate, and resistant categories since qualitative definitions are not as sensitive to changes as MIC shifts.

Validation and system modifications

In any ongoing surveillance project, periodic evaluation of data quality, robustness, and relevance is necessary. NARMS is no exception. Specific areas of focus for NARMS evaluation include sampling scheme validation, susceptibility test performance, and data management and reporting. Modifications to the surveillance system are made based on joint decisions by NARMS partners.

isolates with this or a very similar resistance profile, but further molecular subtyping of NARMS isolates confirmed cattle products as a major source for these infections [27,28]. This strain resulted in morbidity and mortality among cattle, and several large outbreaks were linked to dairy cattle and ground beef [29]. The ability to detect this emerging strain allowed public health and animal health authorities to act rapidly and put into place interventions to attempt to curb the spread of this multidrug resistant strain. Since 2001, the prevalence of this *Salmonella* ser. Newport strain among human isolates in NARMS appears to be declining.

Fluoroquinolone-resistant *Campylobacter* and the withdrawal of approval of these drugs for use in poultry in the US

NARMS identified an increase in the proportion of human *Campylobacter* isolates that were fluoroquinolone-resistant from 1997 to 2000. This increase was noted soon after the approval of enrofloxacin for use in poultry in the US [18]. Fluoroquinolones (including ciprofloxacin and enrofloxacin) are highly efficacious antimicrobial agents commonly used in human medicine, and for certain bacterial diseases in animals, including acute bovine respiratory disease and avian colibacillosis [30]. However, a growing number of studies worldwide document an association between the emergence of fluoroquinolone-resistant zoonotic pathogens, such as *Salmonella*, *E. coli*, and *Campylobacter*, and the approval and use of these agents in veterinary medicine [31–33]. These observations, along with data from NARMS, prompted FDA to propose to withdraw approval of fluoroquinolones for use in poultry in 2000. An order to withdraw approval of enrofloxacin for use in poultry became effective in September 2005. This was based on evidence that poultry was a source of *Campylobacter* infections; that the use of enrofloxacin in poultry resulted in emergence and dissemination of fluoroquinolone-resistant *Campylobacter*; that fluoroquinolone-resistant *Campylobacter* in poultry can be transferred to humans and "can contribute to" fluoroquinolone-resistant *Campylobacter* infections in humans; and that fluoroquinolone-resistant *Campylobacter* infections in humans "have the potential to adversely affect human

health." [34] This ruling did not affect the other approved uses of enrofloxacin (bovine respiratory disease). FDA subsequently revised their regulatory approach for managing the potential risks associated with use of antimicrobial drugs in food-producing animals. This regulatory approach includes use of risk assessment to quantify the human health impact of antimicrobial use in animals as well as implementation of robust monitoring and targeted research.

Lessons learned and recommendations

Our participation in the development and evolution of a national antimicrobial resistance surveillance system has provided insights as to the utility and appropriate design of this type of surveillance system. NARMS data are widely used. NARMS isolate collections have become an important resource for numerous studies pertinent to our understanding of the emergence and dissemination of antimicrobial resistance among foodborne bacteria and resulting disease. These include projects that address risk factors, clinical outcomes, environmental reservoirs, transmission of pathogens, as well as horizontal gene transfer. These outcomes highlight the need for careful, consistent approaches to surveillance so that they may stand the test of time. In designing national surveillance systems, these lessons would lead us to design a program such that data would be easily comparable over time (e.g., with as few changes to antimicrobials and dilutions as possible), and easily comparable across programs (e.g., by either combining data in one platform or at minimum in "mirror databases" based on the same data architecture). Likewise, we would strongly recommend simultaneous collection of other ancillary data, such as antimicrobial use information, so that the antimicrobial resistance data would be more meaningful in terms of exposures and selective pressures.

Considering the magnitude of international travel and agricultural product trade, global surveillance of foodborne pathogens is increasingly important to national interests. Antimicrobial resistance monitoring is an important part of this surveillance. In order to understand the consequences of the global movement of these bacteria and their mobile genetic resistance elements, it will be critical to develop national surveillance systems for antimicrobial resistance among foodborne bacteria that lend themselves to international comparison.

References

1 Piddock LJ. Does the use of antimicrobial agents in veterinary medicine and animal husbandry select antibiotic-resistant bacteria that infect man and compromise antimicrobial chemotherapy? *J Antimicrob Chemother* 1996;**38**(1):1–3.

2 Swann MM. *Report on the use of Antibiotics in Animal Husbandry and Veterinary Medicine*. London, UK: Her Majesty's Stationery Office; November 1969.

3 National Research Council; Institute of Medicine. *The Use of Drugs in Food Animals: Benefits and Risks*. Washington, DC: National Academy Press; 1999.

4 Food and Agriculture Organization of the United Nations WHO, World Organization for Animal Health. Joint FAO/OIE/WHO expert workshop on non-human antimicrobial usage and antimicrobial resistance: scientific assessment [monograph on the Internet]. Geneva, Switzerland: FAO, OIE, WHO; 2003. Available from: http://whqlibdoc.who.int/hq/2004/WHO_CDS_CPE_ZFK_2004.7.pdf. Accessed November 17, 2006.

5 Aarestrup FM (ed). *Antimicrobial Resistance in Bacteria of Animal Origin*. Washington, DC: ASM Press; 2006.

6 Mumma GA, Griffin PM, Meltzer MI, Braden CR, Tauxe RV. Egg quality assurance programs and egg-associated *Salmonella* enteritidis infections, United States. *Emerg Infect Dis* 2004;**10**(10):1782–9.

7 Herikstad H, Motarjemi Y, Tauxe RV. *Salmonella* surveillance: a global survey of public health serotyping. *Epidemiol Infect* 2002;**129**(1):1–8.

8 Swaminathan B, Barrett TJ, Hunter SB, Tauxe RV. PulseNet: the molecular subtyping network for foodborne bacterial disease surveillance, United States. *Emerg Infect Dis* 2001;7(3):382–9.

9 Tollefson L, Angulo FJ, Fedorka-Cray PJ. National surveillance for antibiotic resistance in zoonotic enteric pathogens. *Vet Clin North Am Food Anim Pract* 1998;**14**(1):141–50.

10 Tollefson L, Flynn WT. Impact of antimicrobial resistance on regulatory policies in veterinary medicine: status report. *AAPS PharmSci* 2002;**4**(4):E37.

11 Preliminary FoodNet data on the incidence of infection with pathogens transmitted commonly through food—10 States, United States, 2005. *MMWR Morb Mortal Wkly Rep* 2006;**55**(14):392–5.

12 Wineland N, Marshall K. NAHMS plays key role in surveillance efforts. NAHSS Outlook 2006;10(April).

13 NCCLS. *Performance Standards for Antimicrobial Disk Diffusion and Dilution Susceptibility Tests for Bacteria Isolated from Animals; Approved Standard*, 2nd edn. Wayne, PA: NCCLS; 2002.

14 NCCLS. *Methods for Dilution Antimicrobial Susceptibility Tests for Bacteria that Grow Aerobically; Approved Standard*, 6th edn. Wayne, PA: NCCLS; 2003.

15 CLSI. *Performance Standards for Antimicrobial Susceptibility Testing*, Sixteenth Informational Supplement (M100-S16). Wayne, PA: CLSI; 2006.

16 Fritsch T, McDermott PF, Knapp C, Bodeis-Jones C, Killian S, Jones R. Wild-type MIC distributions for *Campylobacter* spp. Testing against nine antimicrobials using recently approved CLSI broth microdilution (BMD) methods (2005). In: *Interscience Conference on Antimicrobial Agents and Chemotherapy*. Washington, DC: American Society for Microbiology; 2005.

17 Danish Integrated Antimicrobial Resistance Monitoring and Research Programme (DANMAP) 2005. *Use of Antimicrobial Agents and Occurrence of Antimicrobial Resistance in Bacteria from Food Animals, Foods and Humans in Denmark*; Denmark: DANMAP; 2006.

18 Centers for Disease Control and Prevention. NARMS Human Isolates Final Report, 2003. In: Division of Bacterial and Mycotic Diseases; 2006.

19 Centers for Disease Control and Prevention. NARMS Human Isolates Final Report, 2000. In: Division of Bacterial and Mycotic Diseases; 2002.

20 MacDonald KL, Cohen ML, Hargrett-Bean NT, *et al*. Changes in antimicrobial resistance of *Salmonella* isolated from humans in the United States. *JAMA* 1987;**258**(11):1496–9.

21 NCCLS. *Performance Standards for Antimicrobial Disk Susceptibility Tests; Approved Standard*, 7th edn. Wayne, PA: NCCLS; 2000.

22 Gupta A, Nelson JM, Barrett TJ, *et al*. Antimicrobial resistance among *Campylobacter* strains, United States, 1997–2001. *Emerg Infect Dis* 2004;**10**(6):1102–9.

23 Tenover FC, Baker CN, Fennell CL, Ryan CA. Antimicrobial resistance in *Campylobacter* species. In: Nachamkin I, Blaser MJ, Tompkins LS (eds.), Campylobacter jejuni *Current Status and Future Trends*. Washington, DC: American Society for Microbiology; 1992: 66–73.

24 Ackers ML, Puhr ND, Tauxe RV, Mintz ED. Laboratory-based surveillance of *Salmonella* serotype Typhi infections in the United States: antimicrobial resistance on the rise. *JAMA* 2000;**283**(20):2668–73.

25 Tauxe RV, Puhr ND, Wells JG, Hargrett-Bean N, Blake PA. Antimicrobial resistance of *Shigella* isolates in the USA: the importance of international travelers. *J Infect Dis* 1990;**162**(5):1107–11.

26 Centers for Disease Control and Prevention. PHLIS *Salmonella* Annual Summary 2003 [monograph on the Internet]. Atlanta, GA: US Department of Health and Human Services; 2004. Available from: http://www.cdc.gov/ncidod/dbmd/phlisdata/salmonella.htm. Accessed November 17, 2006.

27 Harbottle H, White DG, McDermott PF, Walker RD, Zhao S. Comparison of multilocus sequence typing, pulsed-field gel electrophoresis, and antimicrobial susceptibility typing for characterization of *Salmonella enterica* serotype Newport isolates. *J Clin Microbiol* 2006;**44**(7):2449–57.

28 Zhao S, Qaiyumi S, Friedman S, *et al*. Characterization of *Salmonella enterica* serotype Newport isolated from humans and food animals. *J Clin Microbiol* 2003;**41**(12):5366–71.

29 Gupta A, Fontana J, Crowe C, *et al*. Emergence of multidrug-resistant *Salmonella enterica* serotype Newport infections resistant to expanded-spectrum cephalosporins in the United States. *J Infect Dis* 2003; **188**(11):1707–16.

30 White DG, Piddock LJ, Maurer JJ, Zhao S, Ricci V, Thayer SG. Characterization of fluoroquinolone resistance among veterinary isolates of avian *Escherichia coli*. *Antimicrob Agents Chemother* 2000;**44**(10):2897–9.

31 Zhao S, Maurer JJ, Hubert S, *et al*. Antimicrobial susceptibility and molecular characterization of avian pathogenic *Escherichia coli* isolates. *Vet Microbiol* 2005;**107**(3–4):215–24.

32 Zhang Q, Sahin O, McDermott PF, Payot S. Fitness of antimicrobial-resistant *Campylobacter* and *Salmonella*. *Microbes Infect* 2006;**8**(7):1972–8.

33 Collignon P. Fluoroquinolone use in food animals. *Emerg Infect Dis* 2005;**11**(11):1789–90; author reply: 1790–2.

34 US Food and Drug Administration. Final Decision of the Commissioner. Withdrawal of approval of the new animal drug application for enrofloxacin in poultry [monograph on the Internet]. Washington, DC: US Department of Health and Human Services; 2005. Available from: http://www.fda.gov/oc/antimicrobial/baytril.html#order. Accessed November 17, 2006.

8 Surveillance for zoonotic diseases

Mira J. Leslie & Jennifer H. McQuiston

Introduction

Zoonotic infections (zoonoses) involve pathogens that are sustained in animal populations but can be transmitted to and cause disease in humans. Zoonoses encompass some of the most ancient communicable diseases, such as rabies and plague, as well as newly recognized emerging infections, such as hantavirus pulmonary syndrome (HPS) and severe acute respiratory syndrome (SARS). A recent review of agents known to infect humans identified 61% (868/1415) as zoonotic in origin; furthermore, 75% (132/175) of human diseases classified as emerging were zoonotic [1]. The global distribution, diversity, clinical severity, and potential use as bioweapons all contribute to the importance of zoonotic pathogens in public health. In this chapter, we describe key host and transmission attributes of zoonotic infections and discuss some strategies for surveillance of zoonotic pathogens. We also discuss ongoing surveillance for rabies in the United States (US) and enhanced surveillance during a monkeypox outbreak.

Overview of zoonotic diseases

Zoonoses constitute a diverse group of viral, bacterial, rickettsial, fungal, parasitic, and prion diseases with a variety of animal reservoirs, including wildlife, livestock, domestic pets, and birds (Table 8.1). Some zoonotic pathogens, such as ra-

bies virus and *Coxiella burnetii* (Q fever), can infect a broad spectrum of animal hosts that may each serve as a source of infection to humans. Other zoonotic pathogens, such as rodent-borne hantaviruses and arenaviruses, are found in a narrower range of reservoir hosts.

Transmission

Many common zoonotic pathogens are excreted in animal feces and fecal-oral transmission (ingestion) plays an important role in foodborne and waterborne infections due to enteric pathogens (e.g., *Escherichia coli*, *Salmonella*; see also Chapter 5). Other diseases caused by zoonotic pathogens are transmitted by inoculation of infected animal tissue or contaminated products (e.g., cutaneous anthrax, rabies); inhalation of small droplets or aerosols (e.g., HPS, Q fever, psittacosis); or by an arthropod vector (e.g., Lyme disease, Rocky Mountain spotted fever; see also Chapter 9). Anthrax, plague, and many other zoonoses have multiple routes of transmission.

For most zoonoses, the pathogen is maintained in one or more animal reservoirs with occasional transmission to humans but without subsequent human-to-human spread (e.g., anthrax, HPS, tularemia, Q fever). However, in some cases, initial zoonotic transmissions are responsible for significant disease epidemics that are sustained by subsequent person-to-person transmission (e.g., pandemic influenza, SARS).

Table 8.1 Selected important zoonotic diseases.

Organism	Disease	Primary reservoir or host	Transmission to human
Bacterial			
Bacillus anthracis	Anthrax	Livestock	Cutaneous inoculation; ingestion; inhalation
Bartonella henselae/quintana	Cat scratch disease	Cats	Inoculation
Brucella abortus, B. melitensis, B. canis, B. suis	Brucellosis	Cattle, sheep, goats, dogs, swine	Ingestion; inoculation; inhalation
Burkholderia mallei	Glanders	Equine	Inoculation
Chlamydophila psittaci	Psittacosis	Birds	Inhalation
Coxiella burnettii	Q fever	Livestock	Inhalation; ingestion
Escherichia coli O157:H7	Hemolytic uremic syndrome/*E. coli* infection	Livestock, wild ruminants	Ingestion
Francisella tularensis (var *tularensis* and *palaeartica*)	Tularemia	Rabbits, hares, voles, muskrat, beaver, rodents	Inoculation; inhalation; vector-borne; ingestion
Leptospira interrogans (multiple serovars)	Leptospirosis	Wild and domestic animals	Inoculation; ingestion
Salmonella spp. (multiple serovars)	Salmonellosis	Birds, mammals, reptiles, amphibians	Ingestion
Yersinia pestis	Plague	Rodents	Inoculation; inhalation; vector-borne
Viral			
Arenaviruses	Lymphocytic choriomeningitis virus, Bolivian (Machupo), Brazilian (Sabia), Argentine (Junin), African (Lassa) hemorrhagic fevers	Rodents	Inhalation
Filoviruses	Ebola, Marburg	Unknown (possibly bats)	Inoculation
Hantaviruses (Bunyavirus)	Hantavirus pulmonary syndrome, hemorrhagic fever with renal syndrome, hantaviral illness	Rodents	Inhalation
Influenza A	Avian influenza, swine influenza	Wild birds, swine	Inhalation
Lyssaviruses	Rabies	Dogs, wild carnivores, bats	Inoculation
Orthopoxviruses	Monkeypox, cowpox	Rodents, cattle	Direct contact
Prion			
Prion	New variant Creutzfeldt–Jakob disease in humans; Bovine Spongioform Encephalopathy (BSE, mad cow disease) in cattle	Cattle	Ingestion

Table 8.1 (*Continued*)

Organism	Disease	Primary reservoir or host	Transmission to human
Protozoal			
Cryptosporidium parvum	Cryptosporidiosis	Wild and domestic animals	Ingestion
Giardia lambia	Giardiasis	Wild and domestic animals	Ingestion
Toxoplasma gondii	Toxoplasmosis	Felids	Ingestion
Parasitic Nematodes			
Toxocara canis, T. cati, Baylisascaris procyonis	Larval migrans	Dogs, cats, raccoons	Ingestion
Ancylostoma spp., Strongyloides spp.	Cutaneous larval migrans		Inoculation; direct contact
Trichinella spp.	Trichinosis	Swine, rodents, wild carnivores	Ingestion
Fungal			
Microsporum canis, Trichophyton	Dermatophytosis (ringworm)	Mammals, some birds	Direct contact

Host factors

In humans, host factors such as occupation, age, immune status, and recreational activities may facilitate exposure or susceptibility to zoonotic pathogens. For example, occupations that involve handling of animals or animal carcasses such as veterinary work, farming, aviary work, zookeeping, and slaughterhouse work may expose workers to zoonotic pathogens. Persons with immune compromising conditions such as HIV/AIDS may be more susceptible to some zoonotic pathogens [2]. Recreational and peridomestic activities that involve animals or animal product handling such as hunting, cleaning rodent infested buildings, owning exotic pets, visiting petting zoos, and ecotourism, also put people at risk for exposure to zoonotic pathogens.

Environmental factors

Zoonoses are sustained in epizootic and enzootic cycles in reservoir animals. These cycles are influenced by environmental factors such as biome, climate, land use, and the presence and behaviors of appropriate hosts. Interactions between human populations, domestic animals, and wildlife facilitate transmission of infections among these groups in what has been described as a host–pathogen continuum (Figure 8.1) [3]. In North America, zoonoses such as rabies, plague, hantavirus, and tularemia are widespread in wildlife, posing an ongoing risk to human health. The emergence of a zoonotic disease often results from encroachment of human and domestic animal populations into wildlife habitat [3,4]. For example, recent serosurveys show evidence of novel viral infections with as yet unknown consequences in humans that hunt and trap native populations of nonhuman primates [5,6]. The global trade in wildlife shows how environmental and social factors combine to create a high risk for zoonotic disease emergence in susceptible human populations [7]. In this example, animals of unknown health status are trapped in the wild to be sold for human consumption, traditional medicine, or the commercial pet trade. Disease transmission may occur when humans have contact with infected animals. Activities involving the sale and consumption of infected wildlife in China likely resulted in the initial transmission of SARS-coronavirus to humans [8].

Prevention and control

In the US, successful surveillance and control programs have been developed for some zoonoses associated with domesticated animals. For example, a

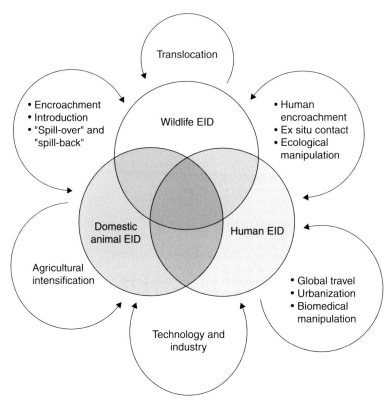

Fig 8.1 The host–pathogen ecological continuum for emerging infectious diseases (EIDs) of zoonotic origin. (Reprinted with permission from [3]. Copyright 2000 AAAS.)

national brucellosis-eradication campaign in livestock conducted by state and federal agriculture departments has included comprehensive animal testing, vaccination of breeding animals, and depopulation of affected herds. The program reduced infected herds from 124,000 in 1956 to only 5 herds nationally in 2000 [9]. Concurrently, reported brucellosis in humans plummeted from a high of approximately 6300 reported cases in 1947 to 114 cases in 2004 [10]. In the early 1900s, approximately 10,000 rabid dogs were reported annually in the US. Widespread canine rabies vaccination programs and stray animal control in the 1940s and 1950s allowed elimination of circulating canine variant of rabies virus, and in 2005 only 76 cases of rabies were reported in dogs following contact with rabid wildlife [11]. Successful programs such as these require enormous resources. As a result, there are no eradication programs for the majority of zoonotic pathogens, especially those with wildlife reservoirs.

Surveillance for zoonoses

The interconnected roles of wildlife, domestic animals, the environment, and human populations in zoonotic disease pathogenesis pose distinct challenges for surveillance. In contrast to those diseases that only affect humans, zoonotic diseases cannot be adequately studied or controlled without an understanding of the influences and dynamics of infection in animal hosts. Therefore, the approach to zoonotic disease surveillance involves flexibility, innovation, and interdisciplinary strategies. Four essential objectives of zoonotic disease surveillance include (1) designing systems for early identification of a human and animal health threat; (2) describing the epidemiological and ecological factors influencing zoonoses; (3) guiding and evaluating prevention, education, and control measures; and (4) describing the public health burden.

Surveillance and reporting of human infections

With the exception of rabies, zoonotic diseases are usually first recognized when human illness is reported. Surveillance depends on timely reporting of suspected and confirmed zoonotic infections by healthcare providers and laboratories to public health authorities. Depending on the pathogen and available resources, the animal source may be identified as part of the public health investigation. Linking human infection to the animal source is often more feasible with pets or livestock than with wildlife, as they may be more accessible to investigators for testing. For example, several outbreaks of human salmonellosis have been linked to contact with infected domestic and exotic pets, including cats, pet rodents, baby chicks, and reptiles [12,13]. In 2004 and 2005, three separate outbreaks identified over 170 people infected with *E. coli* O157:H7 who had visited livestock pens in petting zoos [14]. In 2005, lymphocytic choriomeningitis virus infection in four organ transplant recipients was traced to a donor who acquired infection from a pet hamster [15]. Determining whether there is ongoing risk to the public from a suspected animal source influences how much investigation is warranted.

Surveillance and reporting of animal diseases

In the US, veterinarians are required to report certain animal diseases to animal health and agriculture officials. Diseases under surveillance include diseases of livestock and poultry with serious economic implications and suspected foreign animal diseases [16]. Though many of these diseases do not infect humans, anthrax, rabies, and brucellosis are among the reportable animal diseases that also cause disease in humans (Table 8.2). Recent recognition of emerging zoonotic diseases and bioterrorism preparedness initiatives has bolstered public health's outreach to veterinarians. Some state and local public health agencies, such as those in New York City and Washington State, have developed

Table 8.2 Selected reportable zoonotic diseases in humans and animals, United States, 2006.

Disease	Reportable in humans	Reportable in animals
Anthrax	Yes	Yes
Brucellosis	Yes	Yes (cattle)
Cryptosporidiosis	Yes	No
Escherichia coli O157:H7; HUS	Yes	No
Hantavirus pulmonary syndrome	Yes	No
Leptospirosis	In some states	Yes
Lyme disease	Yes	No
Plague	Yes	In some western states
Prion diseases	In some states	Yes (BSE)
Psittacosis	Yes	Yes
Q fever	Yes	Yes
Rabies	Yes	Yes
Salmonellosis	Yes	In some states
Tularemia	Yes	Yes
Trichinosis	Yes	Yes

additional reporting regulations for zoonoses in animals that more commonly infect humans [17,18].

To more effectively monitor zoonotic diseases, animal and human disease data from public health and animal health agencies and laboratories should be integrated. Currently, the sharing of disease surveillance information in most states depends largely on interpersonal relationships, legal agreements such as memoranda of understanding, and agency priorities. As electronic databases become more widely utilized in public health and animal health agencies, coordination of disparate systems should be a primary goal.

Strategies for surveillance of zoonoses

Several strategies may be useful for surveillance of zoonotic pathogens in animals, including veterinary surveillance, sentinel surveillance, longitudinal surveillance, and laboratory-based surveillance.

Veterinary surveillance

As frontline healthcare providers, veterinarians assist with the recognition, diagnosis, reporting, and control of zoonotic disease in animals. When an unusual zoonotic disease trend or outbreak is recognized, veterinarians can assist the investigation through enhanced surveillance for animal disease. Many states, through cooperation of state veterinary medical associations, agricultural and public health agencies, have developed veterinary alert systems for rapid notification of zoonotic or animal disease outbreaks. Health alerts typically include information on veterinary occupational risks as well as symptoms, diagnosis, and reporting protocols for the disease in animals.

Sentinel surveillance
Monitoring animals for zoonotic pathogens can provide early recognition of human health risks and may allow for control efforts prior to the transmission of disease to humans. Mortality events are particularly important and some data on wildlife mortality is monitored and compiled nationally by the National Wildlife Health Center [19]. As one example, prairie dog colonies in northern Arizona experience periodic die-offs caused by enzootic cycles of plague (*Yersinia pestis*). Sentinel surveillance involves routine visual observation of prairie dog colonies to detect any increases in mortality. When plague is confirmed as the cause of a die-off, human disease prevention measures are initiated, including public education campaigns, posting of signs in the affected area, pesticide dusting of burrows to kill infected fleas, and warnings to pet owners to confine pets and use flea control.

Longitudinal surveillance
Where resources are available, meaningful surveillance to elucidate disease patterns in animal reservoirs includes ongoing systematic data collection. For example, prospective longitudinal studies at sites in Arizona, Montana, and Colorado involve serial monthly trapping of *Peromyscus* spp. of mice and serological testing for antibody to Sin Nombre virus [20,21]. Data from these studies show that the prevalence of infection in mice is influenced by local seasonal and climatic events that affect food supply and mouse population density. Trends observed assist in predicting human disease risk.

Laboratory-based surveillance
Effective surveillance for zoonotic pathogens requires diagnostic laboratory capacity for both hu-

man and animal specimens. In some states, commercial clinical laboratories are required to report positive findings for zoonotic pathogens to public health authorities. Diagnosis often requires specialized confirmatory testing that is available only in state or federal veterinary, agriculture, or public health laboratories. Advanced laboratory techniques are increasingly able to confirm genetic relationships among pathogens infecting humans and animals. This information, combined with epidemiological data, is useful for establishing zoonotic transmission events. For example, PulseNet, a national network of public health and food regulatory agency laboratories coordinated by the Center for Disease Control and Prevention (CDC), maintains a national database of molecular fingerprints of foodborne pathogens submitted from laboratories throughout the US. This system has proven very successful in detecting disease outbreaks associated with zoonotic pathogens such as *E. coli* and *Salmonella* [22]. PulseNet was used to determine that infected rodents distributed in commercial pet stores were the cause of a multistate outbreak of salmonellosis in humans [13].

Examples of zoonotic disease surveillance

The following two descriptions of zoonotic disease surveillance systems in the US illustrate some of the key ideas explained in this chapter, including the interconnected roles of human and animal disease surveillance and partnerships between human and animal health agencies. The first example describes routine disease surveillance for rabies and the second describes surveillance instituted during an outbreak of monkeypox.

Surveillance for rabies in the US

Background
Rabies is a viral disease of the central nervous system that, after the onset of clinical symptoms, is almost universally fatal—thus, rabies is a serious public health threat. Although all mammals are susceptible to rabies, the disease is efficiently maintained in enzootic cycles by specific animal reservoirs including raccoons, skunks, foxes, and several

species of insectivorous bats in North America. These wildlife reservoirs account for over 90% of confirmed rabid animals and sporadic domestic animal and human rabies cases in the US result primarily from interactions with these wildlife reservoirs [11].

Despite its high mortality rate, rabies infection can be prevented in most domestic pets and livestock with appropriate vaccination before and after exposure. Furthermore, infection in humans can be prevented after exposure through the timely administration of rabies postexposure prophylaxis (PEP) that usually consists of a series of vaccinations and administration of rabies immune globulin. Several million animal bites occur annually in the US and it is estimated that more than 35,000 people bitten by animals receive PEP every year [23]. Examples of potential human rabies exposures include bats found in houses, stray dog and feral cat bites, and wild animal bites. National guidance for human rabies exposure management is found in the Advisory Committee on Immunization Practices (ACIP) Rabies Prevention document [24].

Overview of rabies surveillance
Rabies surveillance in the US integrates human and animal zoonotic disease detection and prevention. Surveillance provides epidemiologic information to assist human PEP decisions and focus prevention and control programs. Animal bites to humans must be reported to public health authorities and each reported event is investigated. In addition, laboratory-confirmed rabies infection in both humans and animals is reportable. Because rabies poses a significant human health threat, in most areas animal rabies surveillance is primarily under the jurisdiction of local and state (human) public health agencies rather than animal health agencies. An example of a model rabies surveillance and control program is shown in Figure 8.2.

Goals and objectives of surveillance
A primary goal of rabies surveillance is to quickly evaluate and mitigate any risk of rabies; in the event of possible human exposure, this includes proper and timely administration of PEP. State and local health departments support 24/7 availability for consultation with healthcare providers and their

patients to assist in animal bite assessment, describe local and regional rabies epidemiology and risk, and facilitate correct administration of rabies PEP to prevent human rabies infection. When the biting animal is available, testing or observation periods for rabies may be initiated; however, in situations where the biting animal is not available, it is important to have robust epidemiological animal surveillance data to guide medical decisions.

Other goals of rabies surveillance include defining enzootic and epizootic status of rabies in a region, directing prevention efforts such as public education campaigns and animal control policies, detecting changes in disease patterns, and identifying unusual or novel disease events such as new modes of transmission or the evolutionary emergence of rabies virus variants. Notable recent examples in the US include the discovery of rabies transmission via organ transplantation [25] and the emergence of bat-associated rabies transmitted among skunks in an area previously free of terrestrial rabies [26].

Finally, rabies surveillance is used to evaluate the efficacy of animal vaccination in rabies control. For example, a thorough investigation of rare cases of rabies occurring in vaccinated dogs helps assess the efficacy of rabies vaccines [27]. Programs distributing oral rabies vaccine baits to control rabies in raccoons also benefit from post baiting surveillance to assess program efficacy [28].

Surveillance in animal populations
In the US, wild carnivores and bats are the most important potential source of rabies infection for humans and domestic animals. All states except Hawaii report annual cases of rabies in animals [11]. Rabies surveillance in animals includes identifying the disease in both domestic animals and wildlife. Rabies surveillance is enhanced significantly when public awareness is raised by media reports of unusual animal rabies cases, a human rabies case, or local epizootic rabies activity. The number of animals tested and those found rabid depends on the rabies reservoirs in the area, the human population base, and whether animal control, diagnostic laboratory infrastructure, and resources are available. During 2005, five states reported less than 11 rabid animals each (Alaska, Louisiana, Mississippi, New Mexico, and Oregon), and five

an Internet-accessible centralized database called RabID is being developed to map, compile, and disseminate rabies data in real time [34]. Surveillance using GIS is described in Chapter 31.

Partners

Surveillance for rabies relies on an extensive network of partnerships, including healthcare providers, veterinarians, animal control officers, public health officials (local, state, and federal), agriculture and wildlife officials, laboratories, wildlife rehabilitators, humane organizations, pharmaceutical companies, and the general public. This framework can also be adapted and used to address other zoonoses. In many areas, interagency advisory committees and task force groups are organized to coordinate rabies issues. Risk communication skills and public information officers are essential to public health messaging about rabies. Rapid surveillance efforts are often assisted by the media especially during attempts to identify people who may not be aware that they were potentially exposed to rabies, for example, by contact with a rabid animal in a petting zoo, campground, or pet store.

Strengths and weaknesses

Several limitations affect the efficacy of rabies surveillance. Clinical rabies infection in both humans and domestic animals may be underrecognized since it resembles several other encephalitic diseases. Many fatal cases of unexplained viral encephalitis in humans do not undergo postmortem autopsy. Antemortem rabies tests for animals are not available and definitive diagnosis requires public health resources for specialized laboratory testing of fresh brain tissues. Where resources are limited, rabies testing is often offered only for animals that have potentially exposed pets or people. Thus, the data generated are incomplete and biased by the degree of human and pet interaction with a particular species. The number of confirmed cases of animal rabies does not approximate the true incidence of disease, since many infected wild, stray, and feral animals are not observed or submitted for testing.

A primary strength of the system is that the results of surveillance (animal test results) are used to guide human treatment options and prevent hu-

man infection and death. As a result, very few human cases are reported each year in the US with many potential cases avoided through appropriate and timely administration of PEP.

Surveillance for monkeypox during an outbreak

Background

In 2003, an outbreak of monkeypox occurred in the US, representing the first time this disease had been recognized in humans outside of Africa where the disease is endemic [35]. Monkeypox is in the orthopoxvirus group of viruses (as is smallpox) and is capable of causing severe or fatal illness in humans. Some strains of monkeypox may be transmissible between humans and associated with higher mortality. Fortunately, the virus associated with the 2003 outbreak in the US was a less virulent West African strain of virus.

During the US outbreak, disease transmission was linked to contact with infected prairie dogs distributed in the commercial pet trade through an Illinois animal dealer. Over 70 persons in several Midwestern states were infected [36]. Extensive investigations of the implicated prairie dogs revealed that the Illinois dealer also bought and sold African rodents and epidemiologic evidence suggested that the prairie dogs were infected at this location. Traceback investigations of the African rodents linked them to a shipment from Ghana that contained over 800 small mammals [36]. Laboratory testing showed that several of the imported African rodent species were infected with monkeypox virus. The investigation was complicated by inadequate record keeping and widespread dissemination of the imported animals.

In the following section we will describe the enhanced surveillance for monkeypox virus infection in humans and animals that enabled characterization of the outbreak and guided containment of disease. Early identification of cases offered the possibility of reducing the clinical impact. Additionally, rapid control of the outbreak was needed to prevent the establishment of an enzootic cycle of monkeypox in native US wildlife. Federal emergency orders restricting the movement, trade, and importation of implicated species of animals contributed to control of the outbreak [37].

Goals of surveillance

A primary goal of surveillance was to define the extent and magnitude of the outbreak in humans and animals. The number of infected animals and their distribution was unknown initially, as was the clinical spectrum of illness in prairie dogs. Therefore, surveillance to detect human infection was the most effective way to define the extent and magnitude of the outbreak initially. Effective control of the outbreak required identification of close contacts to infected humans to monitor for and prevent human-to-human transmission of virus. An important objective of surveillance in animals was to identify infected and exposed animals so they could be removed from situations where they could transmit the infection to humans or other animals. Surveillance in animals also facilitated traceback investigations to identify the source of infection and to determine how many animals were potentially involved. Surveillance in native and captive wild rodents and other mammals was initiated to determine whether monkeypox had been introduced to, and spread among, native US wildlife species.

Surveillance in humans

Because human monkeypox had never been previously reported outside of continental Africa and it was considered implausible that the virus could affect the US, it was not a reportable disease at the time of the outbreak. However, its public health significance, clinical resemblance to smallpox, and the fact that it was not an endemic disease, allowed surveillance and reporting to be implemented under state regulations that address public health emergencies due to bioterrorism or novel agents. Retrospective surveillance included contacting and interviewing people who had handled potentially infected animals and reviewing patients with recent clinically compatible illnesses in outbreak-affected areas. Prospective surveillance involved identifying suspected cases meeting the clinical and epidemiologic case definition through reports from healthcare providers. Surveillance was facilitated by dissemination of outbreak updates and reporting guidelines through Internet-based systems (e.g., Health Alert Network, Epidemic Information Exchange (Epi-X) and *Morbidity and Mortality Weekly Report* (*MMWR*) [36,38–40].

Human cases identified during the investigation were classified as either suspect, probable, or confirmed monkeypox infections depending on the clinical presentation (presence of rash, fever, and lymphadenopathy) and epidemiological information available [37]. Confirmed cases required laboratory demonstration of the presence of virus through culture, electron microscopy, or nucleic acid detection techniques in the absence of another potential poxvirus [37]. Because laboratory testing for monkeypox is highly specialized, it was initially primarily conducted at CDC. However, through the healthcare worker smallpox vaccination program preparations, the Laboratory Response Network (LRN) laboratories had the capacity to screen clinical rash-derived samples for orthopoxvirus nucleic acid signatures; these facilities were used to aid in the triage and initial testing of samples, largely derived from the Midwestern states.

The investigations and case follow-up required extensive local, state, and federal resources and personnel and in many cases these resources were diverted from other important public health issues to accommodate outbreak needs. Coordination among affected states, confirmatory testing, and communication was facilitated by the CDC with daily national conference calls. This ensured consistency of case investigations and reporting, appropriate laboratory submissions, and rapid dissemination of current information and case numbers.

Surveillance in animals

In 2003, although many studies of experimental infection of animals existed, scientific information about the natural history of monkeypox in animals was sparse. Unknown factors included the range of susceptible animal species, the spectrum of clinical syndromes, and the possibility of viral shedding from asymptomatic animals. Therefore, surveillance focused on identifying animals with potential exposure to infected or exposed animals. The histories of infected animals were meticulously investigated, including their points of sale and shipments to identify additional exposed animals, and to reveal the source of infection for the animals. Clinical presentations were compiled to generate an animal case definition [37]. The investigation involved site visits to animal dealers and traders, pet shops, pet owners' homes, and the examination of written records or verbal interviews. Known clinical symptoms such as lethargy, cough, conjunctivitis, and skin lesions were useful in identifying potentially infected animals [37]. Because CDC and LRN laboratory testing was prioritized for human illness, there were inadequate laboratory resources for processing and testing animal specimens. Additionally, tests had not been fully evaluated with any of the animal specimen types submitted for analysis. Viral and serologic testing at CDC was conducted to confirm the initial infections in prairie dogs, to investigate possible infections in African rodents from the implicated shipment, and to investigate reports of diseased/suspect case animals in new locations.

A coalition of federal and state agriculture officials, state and local public health officials, and practicing veterinarians conducted the animal surveillance and investigations. Involved federal agencies included CDC, the Food and Drug Administration (FDA), and the United States Department of Agriculture (USDA)/Animal and Plant Health Inspection Service (APHIS). Animal breeders licensed by the USDA were visited and provided information about the outbreak. Educational materials were developed and disseminated to pet stores and veterinarians. National conference calls were held several times a week between federal and state agency personnel to coordinate activities.

Surveillance to determine whether monkeypox had exposed native wild rodents was coordinated by USDA-APHIS Wildlife Services. Traps were set on and near premises holding infected prairie dogs or African rodents. Blood collected on trapped wildlife was tested for antibodies to assess whether infection had been transmitted to native species. This surveillance found no evidence of infection in native rodents.

Strengths and weaknesses

A weakness of human and animal surveillance associated with this outbreak is that the systems were necessarily largely reactive and were implemented during the height of the outbreak. Because the initial infections in prairie dogs were not recognized as significant and reported to authorities, recognition of the outbreak was delayed until the first human cases were diagnosed. Thus, health authorities missed an early opportunity to control the outbreak. Educating animal dealers and veterinarians to quickly report unusual or suspicious illnesses in animals to authorities, and ensuring that state agriculture, wildlife, and human health agencies have the capacity to respond could facilitate a more rapid response in the future.

A primary strength of the surveillance system is the collaborative efforts that evolved between state and federal partners for human health and animal health. Although this emerged out of necessity during the emergency response, the relationships that were forged proved to be effective and have continued during subsequent zoonotic disease outbreaks and preparedness activities. Bioterrorism preparedness initiatives related to the detection and diagnosis of orthopoxviruses (due to smallpox concerns) greatly assisted in the response to this outbreak at both CDC and affiliated LRN laboratories. Additional benefits of the investigation include an enhanced understanding of the natural history of monkeypox virus and the development of testing strategies that may be used to identify monkeypox in various animal species.

Discussion

Surveillance for zoonotic diseases involves many challenges and offers opportunities for early detection of disease threats, improved assessment of risks posed by enzootic pathogens, and targeting effective prevention and control measures (see Chapter 10). In addition to providing direction for immediate public health actions, surveillance systems for zoonoses can provide vital insight into the factors influencing disease emergence, persistence, and spread. The importance of good communication and multidisciplinary participation in monitoring zoonoses is highlighted by the examples of rabies and monkeypox surveillance, and also through programs such as ProMED-mail, an Internet-based reporting system dedicated to rapid global dissemination of information on outbreaks of infectious diseases in humans, animals, and plants (available at: www.promedmail.org). ProMED-mail, a program of the International Society of Infectious Diseases, is widely used by public health agencies, animal health agencies, scientists, and medical and veterinary providers to provide early warnings of zoonotic disease issues that might benefit from enhanced surveillance efforts [41].

The close association of humans and animals in modern society, including the globalization of agriculture, the pet trade, tourism and recreation, combined with ecologic pressures such as habitat transformation, climate change, and human overpopulation, will continue to facilitate unpredictable zoonotic disease threats [42]. Whether dealing with the persistence of ancient zoonoses, or the mysteries of newly recognized diseases, astute, innovative, and vigilant disease surveillance is imperative to reduce morbidity and mortality among humans and animals.

Acknowledgments

The authors thank Charles Rupprecht, Inger Damon, and Russ Regnery from the Centers for Disease Control and Prevention (CDC) for assistance in developing the content matter of this chapter. The authors also thank Doug Beckner for technical assistance.

References

1 Taylor LH, Latham SM, Woolhouse MEJ. Risk factors for human disease emergence. *Philos Trans R Soc Lond B* 2001;**356**:983–9.

2 Glaser CA, Angulo FJ, Rooney J. Animal associated opportunistic infections in HIV-infected persons. *Clin Infect Dis* 1994;**18**:14–24.

3 Daszak P, Cunningham AA, Hyatt AD. Emerging infectious diseases of wildlife—threats to biodiversity and human health. *Science* 2000;**287**:443–9.

4 Blancou J, Chomel BB, Belotto A, Meslin FX. Emerging or re-emerging bacterial zoonoses: factors of emergence, surveillance and control. *Vet Res* 2005;**36**(3):507–22.

5 Wolfe ND, Heneine W, Carr JK, *et al.* Emergence of unique primate T-lymphotropic viruses among central African bushmeat hunters. *Proc Natl Acad Sci U S A* May 31,2005;**102**(22):7994–9.

6 Peeters M, Courgnaud V, Abela B, *et al.* Risk to human health from a plethora of simian immunodeficiency viruses in primate bushmeat. *Emerg Infect Dis* 2002;**8**(5):451–7.

7 Karesh WB, Cook RA, Bennett EL, Newcomb J. Wildlife trade and global disease emergence. *Emerg Infect Dis* 2005;**11**:1000–2.

8 Song HD, Tu CC, Zhang GW, *et al.* Cross-host evolution of severe acute respiratory syndrome coronavirus in palm civet and human. *Proc Natl Acad Sci U S A* 2005;**102**:2430–5.

9 United States Department of Agriculture, Animal and Plant Health Inspection Services, Veterinary Services. Facts about Brucellosis. Available from: http:// www.aphis.usda.gov/vs/nahps/brucellosis/. Accessed November 21, 2006.

10 Centers for Disease Control and Prevention. Summary of notifiable diseases—United States, 2004. *MMWR Morb Mortal Wkly Rep* 2006;**53**:1–79.

11 Blanton JD, Krebs JW, Hanlon CA, Rupprecht CE. Rabies surveillance in the United States during 2005. *J Am Vet Med Assoc* 2006;**229**:1897–911.

12 National Association of State Public Health Veterinarians. Compendium of measures to prevent disease associated with animals in public settings, 2006. Available from: http://www.nasphv.org/documentsCompendia. html. Accessed October 30, 2006.

13 Centers for Disease Control and Prevention. Outbreak of multidrug resistant *Salmonella* Typhimurium associated with rodents purchased at pet stores—United States—December 2003–October 2004. *MMWR Morb Mortal Wkly Rep* 2005;**54**:429–33.

14 Centers for Disease Control and Prevention. Outbreaks of *Escherichia coli* O157:H7 associated with petting zoos—North Carolina, Florida, and Arizona, 2004 and 2005. *MMWR Morb Mortal Wkly Rep* 2005;**54**;1277–80.

15 Centers for Disease Control and Prevention. Lymphocytic choriomeningitis virus infection in organ transplant recipients—Massachusetts, Rhode Island. *MMWR Morb Mortal Wkly Rep* 2005;**54**(21):537–9.

16 List of Animal Diseases Notifiable to USDA and OIE. Available from: http://www.oie.int/eng/maladies/ en_classification.htm. Accessed October 17, 2006.

17 New York City Department of Health and Hygiene: Reporting Zoonoses in animals. Available from: http:// home2.nyc.gov/html/doh/html/zoo/zoo-reporting.shtml. Accessed October 17, 2006.

18 Washington Department of Health. Notifiable condition for the veterinarian. Available from: http://apps.leg. wa.gov/WAC/default.aspx?cite=246-101-405. Accessed January 10, 2007.

19 United States Geological Survey, National Wildlife Health Center Disease Information. Mortality events in wildlife. Available from: http://www.nwhc.usgs.gov/ disease_information/mortality_events/index.jsp. Accessed November 2, 2006.

20 Abbott K, Ksiazek T, Mills JN. Long-term hantavirus persistence in rodent populations in Central Arizona. *Emerg Infect Dis* 1999;**5**:102–12.

21 Calisher CH, Root JJ, Mills JN, *et al.* Epizootiology of Sin Nombre and El Moro Canyon viruses, southeastern Colorado 1995–2000. *J Wildl Dis* 2005;**41**(1):1–11.

22 Swaminathan B, Barrett TJ, Fields P. Surveillance for human *Salmonella* infections in the United States. *J AOAC Int* 2006;**89**:553–9.

23 Krebs JW, Long-Marin SC, Childs JE. Causes, costs, and estimates of rabies postexposure prophylaxis treatment in the United States. *J Public Health Manag Pract* 1998;**4**:56–62.

24 Human Rabies Prevention—United States, 1999. Recommendations of the Advisory Committee on Immunization Practices (ACIP). Available from: http://www.cdc.gov/MMWR/preview/mmwrhtml/00056176.htm. Accessed October 30, 2006.

25 Srinivasan A, Burton EC, Kuehnert MJ, *et al*, Rabies in Transplant Recipients Investigation Team. Transmission of rabies virus from an organ donor to four transplant recipients. *N Engl J Med* 2005;**352**(11):1103–11.

26 Leslie MJ, Messenger S, Rohde RE, *et al.* Bat-associated rabies virus in skunks. *Emerg Infect Dis* 2006;**12**:1274–7.

27 McQuiston JH, Yager PA, Smith JS, Rupprecht CE. Epidemiologic characteristics of rabies virus variants in dogs and cats in the United States, 1999. *J Am Vet Med Assoc* 2001;**218**(12):1939–42.

28 Slate D, Rupprecht CE, Rooney JA, Donovan D, Lein DH, Chipman RB. Status of oral rabies vaccination in wild carnivores in the United States. *Virus Res* 2005;**111**:68–76.

29 Centers for Disease Control and Prevention. Rabies diagnosis. Available from: http://www.cdc.gov/ncidod/dvrd/rabies/Diagnosis/diagnosi.htm. Accessed November 15, 2006.

30 National Association of State Public Health Veterinarians. Compendium of animal rabies prevention and control, 2006. *J Am Vet Med Assoc* 2006;**228**(6):858–64.

31 Lembo T, Niezgoda M, Velasco-Villa A, Cleaveland S, Ernset E, Rupprecht CE. Evaluation of a direct rapid immunohistochemical test for rabies diagnosis. *Emerg Infect Dis* 2006;**12**(2):310–3.

32 Chapman AS, Hanlon CA, McQuiston J, *et al.* Epidemiology of human rabies in the United States, 1997 to 2004. Abstract #337, presented at *International Conference on Emerging Infectious Diseases.* Atlanta, GA, March 19–22, 2006.

33 Noah DL, Drenzek CL, Smith JS, *et al.* Epidemiology of human rabies in the United States, 1980–1996. *Ann Intern Med* 1998;**126**(11):922–30.

34 Blanton JD, Managan A, Managan J, Hanlon CA, Slate D, Rupprecht CE. Development of a GIS based, real-time Internet mapping tool for rabies surveillance. *Int J Health Geogr* 2006;**5**:47.

35 Reed KD, Melski JW, Graham MB, *et al.* The detection of monkeypox in humans in the Western hemisphere. *N Engl J Med* 2004;**350**:342–50.

36 Centers for Disease Control and Prevention. Update: multistate outbreak of monkeypox—Illinois, Indiana, Kansas, Missouri, Ohio, and Wisconsin. *MMWR Morb Mortal Wkly Rep* 2003;**52**:642–6.

37 Centers for Disease Control and Prevention. Monkeypox website http://www.cdc.gov/ncidod/monkeypox/index.htm. Accessed October 30, 2006; Human Case definition: http://www.cdc.gov/ncidod/monkeypox/casedefinition.htm; Animal Case definition: http://www.cdc.gov/ncidod/monkeypox/animalcasedefinition.htm.

38 Centers for Disease Control and Prevention. Health Alert Network. Available from: http://www2a.cdc.gov/HAN/Index.asp. Accessed November 1, 2006.

39 Centers for Disease Control and Prevention. Epi-X http://www.cdc.gov/epix/. Accessed November 1, 2006.

40 Centers for Disease Control and Prevention. Morbidity and Mortality Weekly Report (MMWR). Available from: http://www.cdc.gov/mmwr/. Accessed January 9, 2007.

41 Cowen P, Garland T, Hugh-Jones ME, *et al.* Evaluation of ProMED-mail as an electronic early warning system for emerging animal diseases: 1996 to 2004. *J Am Vet Med Assoc* 2006;**229**:1090–9.

42 Gibbs EPJ. Emerging zoonotic epidemics in the interconnected global community. *Vet Rec* 2005;**157**:673–9.

Additional resources

Centers for Disease Control and Prevention–Healthy Pets/ Healthy People: http://www.cdc.gov/healthypets/

Rabies Professional Resources: http://www.cdc.gov/ncidod/dvrd/rabies/Professional/professi.htm

Health Topics Alphabetical List: http://www.cdc.gov/az.do

Emerging Infectious Disease Journal: http:/www.cdc.gov/ncidod/EID/.

National Association of State Public Health Veterinarians Documents: http://www.nasphv.org/ documentsCompendia.html

United States Department of Agriculture, Animal Plant and Health Inspection Service–National Animal Health Surveillance System: http://www.aphis.usda.gov/vs/nahss

National Annual Animal Disease Summary report: http://www.aphis.usda.gov/vs/ceah/ncahs/index.htm

ProMED-mail: http://www.promedmail.org/

Hugh-Jones ME, Hubbert WMT, Hagstad HV. *Zoonoses Recognition, Control, and Prevention.* Iowa: Iowa State University Press; 1995.

9

Surveillance for vector-borne diseases

James L. Hadler & Lyle R. Petersen

Introduction

Vector-borne infections, acquired through the bite of infected blood-sucking arthropods, are major global public health problems (Table 9.1). Increasing travel and trade, changes in land use patterns, and urbanization of areas where natural enzootic cycles exist are increasing the geographic distribution and incidence of these infections. The introduction of West Nile virus and its subsequent spread throughout the Americas is a striking recent example [1].

This chapter provides a practical overview of surveillance methods related to monitoring and control of vector-borne diseases, emphasizing those occurring in the United States (US). However, the methods described apply to vector-borne diseases occurring globally. This chapter begins with an overview of the biology, epidemiology, and prevention strategies of vector-borne diseases relevant to their surveillance. The chapter then discusses surveillance objectives and methods and concludes with case studies involving West Nile virus and Lyme disease in the US. As will become evident, surveillance for vector-borne diseases can be complex and involves expertise from a number of different disciplines with a need for public health coordination and leadership.

Overview of vector-borne diseases

Vector-borne pathogens are maintained in enzootic cycles between susceptible primary vertebrate hosts and specific hematophageous arthropod vectors (Figure 9.1; Table 9.1). Primary vertebrate hosts are usually unaffected and the enzootic cycle continues silently in nature, although there are notable exceptions discussed later. Vector-borne disease incidence often varies seasonally, corresponding to temperature or rainfall fluctuations that influence vector and host abundance. Human behaviors may alter the natural effects of temperature and rainfall. For example, peridomestic surface water storage may create mosquito breeding sites during dry seasons. Large epidemics or epizootics occur when environmental conditions favor significant amplification of the pathogen in its natural enzootic cycle. Under these conditions, amplification can be logarithmic, causing explosive outbreaks that occur with little warning. The epidemic potential of many vector-borne pathogens is indicated in Table 9.1.

Humans are usually dead-end hosts and do not contribute to the pathogen's maintenance in nature; however, dengue, malaria, and filariasis are important exceptions as humans are the primary vertebrate hosts for the pathogens that cause these diseases. Occasionally, a secondary cycle may be important for amplification of the pathogen in certain settings (Figure 9.1). For example, wading birds are the primary vertebrate hosts for maintaining the Japanese encephalitis virus but pigs serve as important amplifying, secondary vertebrate hosts in the peridomestic environment.

Mosquitoes, ticks, and fleas are the most important arthropod vectors. Each pathogen usually depends on a limited range of vector species that are capable of maintaining the pathogen in natural

Table 9.1 Selected, important vector-borne diseases.

Organism	Vector	Vertebrate host	Geographic distribution	Epidemics
Togaviridae				
Chikungunya	Mosquitoes	Humans, primates	Africa, Asia	Yes
Eastern equine encephalitis	Mosquitoes	Birds	Americas	Yes
Venezuelan equine encephalitis	Mosquitoes	Rodents	Americas	Yes
Flaviviridae				
Dengue 1–4	Mosquitoes	Humans, primates	Worldwide in tropics	Yes
Yellow fever	Mosquitoes	Humans, primates	Africa, South America	Yes
Japanese encephalitis	Mosquitoes	Birds	Asia	Yes
St. Louis encephalitis	Mosquitoes	Birds	Americas	Yes
West Nile encephalitis	Mosquitoes	Birds	Asia, Africa, North America, Europe	Yes
Tick-borne encephalitis	Ticks	Rodents	Europe, Asia	No
Bunyaviridae				
Rift Valley fever	Mosquitoes	Humans, domestic ruminants	Africa	
La Crosse encephalitis	Mosquitoes	Rodents	North America	No
Crimean-congo hemorrhagic fever	Ticks	Rodents	Europe, Asia, Africa	Yes
Protozoa				
Plasmodium vivax, P. malariae, P. ovale, P. falciparum	Mosquitoes	Humans	Worldwide in tropics	Yes
Babesia microti	Ticks	Rodents	North America, Europe	No
Leishmania (multiple species)	Sandflies	Rodents, dogs	Africa, India, Middle East, Africa, Europe, Central and South America	No
Nematodes (round worms)				
Wuchereria bancrofti	Mosquitoes	Humans, primates	South America, Africa, Asia	No
Onchocerciasis	Black flies, midges	Humans, cattle, horses, deer	South America, Africa	No
Bacteria				
Borrelia burgdorferi, B. garinii, B. afzelii	Ticks	Rodents	North America, Eurasia	No
Yersinia pestis	Fleas	Rodents	Worldwide	Yes
Francisella tularensis	Ticks	Rodents, lagomorphs	Worldwide	Yes
Rickettsia rickettsii	Ticks	Rodents, small mammals	Americas	No

enzootic cycles. A secondary vector may be involved in a secondary cycle, and so-called bridge vectors may be important for transmission to humans. Bridge vectors feed on the pathogen's primary or secondary vertebrate hosts, but may also feed upon humans. An example is the *Culex salinarius* mosquito, which feeds on birds, the primary vertebrate hosts for West Nile virus, but also readily feeds on humans.

Many vector-borne pathogens may be transmitted by non-vector-borne routes, such as via aerosols, blood transfusion, organ transplantation, or direct contact. Although these transmission modes are usually of minor public health significance, they have the potential to become a formidable problem. For example, after it was recognized that West Nile virus could be transmitted through blood transfusion, enormous effort

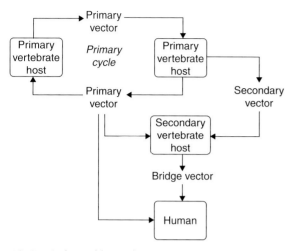

Fig 9.1 Arthropod-borne disease maintenance cycle.

was expended to implement routine blood–donor screening for West Nile virus in the US and Canada. The lethality following aerosol exposure has made some of these pathogens, such as plague, tularemia, and Venezuelan equine encephalitis virus, potential agents of bioterrorism; considerable epidemiologic investigation is required to differentiate naturally acquired from intentional infections.

Prevention of vector-borne diseases primarily focuses on minimizing human exposure to vectors by reducing vector populations and by promotion of avoidance and protective behaviors. For some vector-borne diseases, it is possible to prevent illness even after exposure to the pathogen. Integrated pest management is recommended to reduce vector populations. This method incorporates multiple vector control strategies such as elimination of breeding sites and use of larvicides and adulticides. The use of the latter is driven by surveillance data and local conditions. Behavioral interventions may include avoidance of areas with vectors and use of protective clothing, mosquito nets, window screens, and insect repellents. Methods to prevent illness in settings where pathogen exposure may be unavoidable include vaccination (e.g., for yellow fever and Japanese encephalitis) and prophylactic antibiotics (e.g., for travelers to malaria endemic areas). When surveillance data indicate a threatened or ongoing epidemic, emergency control measures may include wide area aerial or ground-based application of pes-

ticides, enhanced public communication efforts to increase the use of personal protection measures, and vaccination campaigns.

Surveillance objectives

Three main objectives for surveillance related to vector-borne diseases include (1) evaluating potential public health threats, (2) guiding and evaluating prevention and control measures, and (3) defining public health burden.

Evaluating potential and emerging public health threats

Vector-borne disease pathogens are localized to geographic areas where competent vector species and primary vertebrate hosts are present, and where environmental conditions allow maintenance of the pathogen in an enzootic cycle. Nevertheless, the geographic distributions of many vector-borne pathogens are evolving through expansion of known endemic areas or introduction into suitable habitats remote from their normal geographic distributions. Monitoring vector prevalence and distribution (e.g., competent mosquito or tick populations) may help evaluate potential geographic expansion of a pathogen should it be introduced. Examples include monitoring the expanding distribution of *Ixodes* ticks capable of maintenance of *Borrelia burgdorferi*, the agent of Lyme disease, or of competent flea vectors for plague.

Once competent vectors are identified, monitoring the presence of the pathogen in primary vertebrate hosts (e.g., West Nile virus in birds, *B. burgdorferi* in mice or deer, plague in ground squirrels) and its prevalence in vectors (e.g., percentage of vector mosquitoes infected with West Nile virus, percentage of ticks infected with *B. burgdorferi*) can help to evaluate a vector-borne pathogen's potential threat to humans. In addition, human and ecological surveillance data can help monitor a rapidly evolving vector-borne infectious disease threat if knowledge of the principal vectors and amplifying hosts, eventual distribution, and public health impact are incomplete, as illustrated by two examples regarding West Nile virus surveillance in North America discussed later in this chapter.

109

Guiding and evaluating prevention and control efforts

Surveillance data can focus on prevention and control measures to evaluate and improve efficacy, reduce costs, minimize inconvenience, and reduce environmental toxicity from pesticides. For example, surveillance of vector populations may focus prevention efforts on geographic areas of greatest risk. Surveillance data indicating substantially elevated vector populations and vector infection rates may dictate implementation of emergency control efforts even before a human outbreak occurs. Subsequent monitoring of vector populations will determine efficacy of those control measures. Other examples of the use of surveillance data to guide prevention and control efforts include monitoring of insecticide and antibiotic resistance (both essential for malaria prevention and control) and determining uptake of behavioral interventions (e.g., insect repellent use, use of bed nets).

Defining public health burden

Ultimately, resources committed to disease prevention and control depends on human disease incidence, morbidity, and mortality. Most commonly, as will be discussed in the section on *Human surveillance*, public health authorities assess the burden of human disease by evaluating mandated reporting of specifically diagnosed laboratory findings and/or of cases with clinical evidence strongly suggestive of disease. This method has been used for both Lyme disease and West Nile virus surveillance. For diseases such as malaria, which can result in chronic infection and infectiousness, information on the prevalence of chronic infection can be important.

Methods of surveillance for vector-borne diseases

The complexity of vector-borne disease maintenance and transmission cycles provides a variety of opportunities for measuring different components of a pathogen's activity that relates to the risk of human infection. Vector-borne disease surveillance can be categorized into human and ecologic surveillance. Human surveillance may include monitoring of infections, disease, or behaviors. Ecologic surveillance includes monitoring of infection or disease in primary vertebrate hosts, other affected animals, sentinel animals, and vectors. Institution of ecologic surveillance systems requires the involvement of wildlife experts, veterinarians, and entomologists [2]. The human and ecologic surveillance modalities incorporated into the surveillance system for each pathogen depend on the surveillance system's objectives, the pathogen's potential for geographic spread and epidemic potential, the existence of important natural enzootic cycles, the ease and cost of monitoring enzootic cycles, and whether other important indicator animals are affected. Thus, while many possible surveillance methodologies exist, those used must be adapted to the specific disease, the situation, and the resources available.

Human surveillance

Disease incidence, morbidity, mortality
Monitoring human disease incidence, morbidity, and mortality is the most direct method of assessing health impact of a vector-borne disease. These conditions can be made reportable to public health authorities. Case definitions can be applied consistently, demographic and risk information obtained, population-based rates calculated, and trends monitored over time. Nationally notifiable vector-borne diseases in the US are listed in Table 9.2. Plague and yellow fever are internationally notifiable in accordance with the International Health Regulations (IHR) issued by the World Health Organization. Revised regulations, which will be effective in June 2007, changed notifiability to include pneumonic plague, yellow fever, and West Nile fever, as well as other conditions or events constituting a public health emergency of international concern [3].

Disease incidence, morbidity, and mortality data are often the most compelling for gathering support for prevention and control programs and can be used directly to evaluate them. For emerging vector-borne diseases such as West Nile virus, surveillance of human disease can result in discovery of a multitude of new clinical syndromes and modes of transmission. However, these data have several important limitations. Vector-borne disease outbreaks may be explosive and delays in diagnosis

Table 9.2 US nationally notifiable vector-borne disease conditions, 2006.

Arboviral neuroinvasive and non-neuroinvasive diseases

• California serogroup virus disease
• Eastern equine encephalitis virus disease
• Powassan virus disease
• St. Louis encephalitis virus disease
• West Nile virus disease
• Western equine encephalitis virus disease
Ehrlichiosis

• Human granulocytic
• Human monocytic
• Human, other or unspecified agent

Lyme disease
Malaria
Plague
Rocky Mountain spotted fever
Tularemia
Yellow fever

and reporting of clinical cases in humans often mean that an outbreak is well underway before it is recognized and control measures implemented. Since most vector-borne diseases have a high proportion of asymptomatic or mildly symptomatic infections, reported cases often represent a grossly undercounted incidence of true infection. Many vector-borne diseases are clinically indistinguishable from other similar illnesses and diagnostics are either unavailable or not sensitive during early infection. For example, diagnostics for dengue are unavailable or unaffordable in much of the world and antibody tests are often negative in early infection. Finally, even when the disease is recognized, clinicians may not bother to report it, especially if the disease is common and readily treated [4].

Surveillance case definitions also have limitations. The surveillance case definition for Lyme disease has focused on a relatively specific clinical indicator of acute infection, erythema migrans [5]. Although this definition has proved useful for determining the descriptive epidemiology of incident Lyme disease and for monitoring trends over time, it has been less helpful for determining the extent and trends in later manifestations such as arthritis and chronic neurological disease.

To overcome some of these difficulties, the surveillance case definition for West Nile virus provides measures of both the more severe and likely confirmed cases of neuroinvasive disease and the less severe and more variably confirmed cases of West Nile virus fever [6]. Monitoring reports of neuroinvasive West Nile virus disease enables determination of trends over time by providing a relatively reliable tip of the iceberg. The West Nile fever case definition includes a larger array of human infections, and thus may enable earlier detection of outbreaks.

Infection incidence, cumulative incidence, and prevalence

Since most vector-borne infections are asymptomatic or mildly symptomatic, conducting serosurveys to detect the whole spectrum of infection is compelling. Because vector-borne diseases have seasonal incidence, cumulative incidence over a transmission season can be measured by IgM or IgG antibody prevalences at the end of the transmission season in a cross-sectional survey. However, this approach has several limitations. Most vector-borne diseases do not have high population incidences, thus requiring large sample sizes for precise seroprevalence estimates [7]. Voluntary surveys are also subject to participation bias, potentially resulting in nonrepresentative sampling. Because it is difficult to conduct repeated annual seroprevalence studies, this method is more amenable to one-time studies or research cohorts rather than a yearly surveillance system. Also, by its retrospective nature, this method does little to guide prevention and control efforts. For chronic and highly prevalent infections such as malaria and filariasis, serial prevalence surveys in endemic areas are useful for determining burden of infection and for evaluating the impact of intensive control measures [8,9].

Behaviors

In order to evaluate behavioral intervention prevention programs, some surveillance systems are based on serial prevalence surveys to monitor risk reduction behaviors, such as use of insect repellents or bed nets (see Appendix). Interview and telephone surveys should use validated questions to determine that they are measuring what they intend to

111

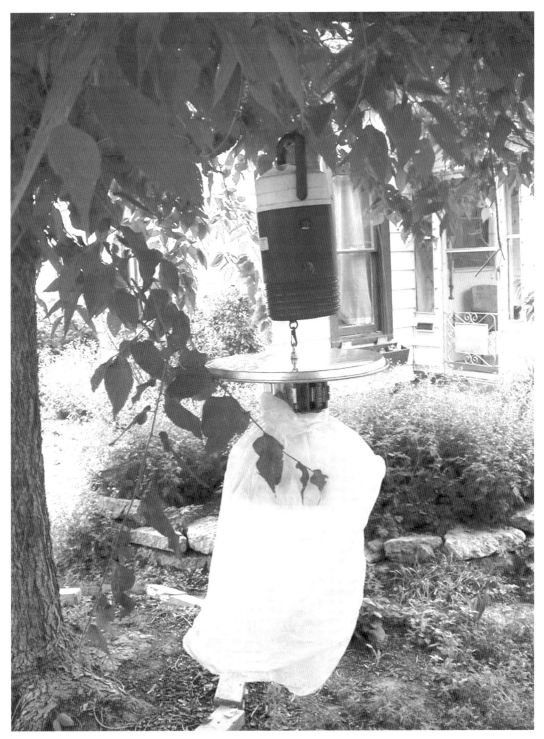

Fig 9.2 A light source baited with a carbon dioxide source (dry ice), to simulate the exhaled respiratory gases of birds or mammals, attracts mosquitoes or other species of insects under surveillance. Insects attracted to the trap are pushed into the collection net (white device) by a fan located above the net.

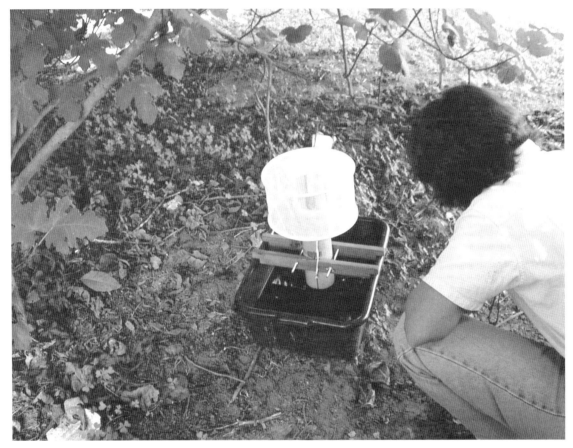

Fig 9.3 A gravid trap with nutrient rich pool of water used to attract female mosquitoes looking to deposit their eggs. Mosquitoes are blown into the collection bag (in white) by an upward current of air from within the confines of the trap.

seasons in a given area with actual extent of human disease is needed.

Pathogens

Vector-borne pathogens can be isolated from humans, other infected animals, and vectors using the surveillance methods described above. These pathogens can be further characterized for insecticide and antibiotic resistance and genetically fingerprinted. The amount of insecticide resistance relates to insect species involved, and the volume and frequency of applications. Insecticide resistance in mosquitoes was first noted for DDT when used for malaria control and, more recently, organophosphates and pyrethroids [20]. Antibiotic resistance has not been significant for most bacterial vector-borne pathogens since humans are not the primary vertebrate hosts, so there is little selective pressure for antibiotic resistance. However, for malaria, where humans are the primary vertebrate hosts, antibiotic resistance has proven to be a significant public health problem [21].

Genetic characterization of the pathogen can help determine its geographic origin. Techniques such as multiple-locus variable tandem repeat analysis and pulse field gel electrophoresis are being applied to isolates collected as part of plague and tularemia surveillance. Genetic characterization can be helpful to distinguish between natural and possible intentional (i.e., bioterrorism) infection with plague and tularemia [22].

115

Examples of vector-borne disease surveillance

Several new vector-borne diseases have been recognized in the US within the past three decades, two of these—West Nile virus and Lyme disease—now have the highest incidence by far of all the vector-borne pathogens in that country. Each has presented several challenges to surveillance, including establishing initial surveillance systems to identify the geographic scope and magnitude of the human health problem and maintaining surveillance as the diseases spread and become endemic. The remainder of this chapter will highlight several specific examples of these surveillance challenges.

West Nile virus—dead crow surveillance

West Nile virus was first recognized in the Americas in September 1999 when it caused an outbreak of encephalitis among residents of New York City and surrounding counties, as well as die-offs of birds in a larger geographic area [23]. Widespread insecticide spraying of areas with human cases was the main control measure; this proved controversial but called national attention to the need for establishing prospective surveillance. After the mosquito season ended in late November, concern remained that the virus would return next year and cause an even larger outbreak.

The observation that several North American bird species were highly susceptible to West Nile virus, particularly crows, suggested that bird die-offs might be sentinel indicators for viral reemergence and circulation, and for determining its geographic spread and potential human risk. Surveillance, which called for public telephone or Internet-based reporting of dead bird sightings, courier services to pick up dead birds, and subsequent laboratory testing for West Nile virus, was initiated. The main outcome measures were the number of dead crows in any geographic area and the number and percentage that tested positive for West Nile virus. It was not known whether the magnitude of crow die-offs or percentage positive would be predictive of increased human risk. Intensive dead bird surveillance and testing, as well as mosquito trapping and testing, was made pos-

sible in large part by a special Congressional appropriation to the Centers for Disease Control and Prevention to support state-based West Nile virus surveillance efforts.

Results from the four surveillance areas in the region (New York City, New York State, New Jersey, and Connecticut) showed that West Nile virus did reemerge and affected a much larger geographic area than in 1999 (Figure 9.4). Although mosquito, horse, and human surveillance systems were also established, the first indicator of West Nile virus circulation in each geographical area was dead crows that tested positive for West Nile virus. This finding preceded any human cases by at least several weeks. As the summer progressed, the number and percentage of all dead crows testing positive increased to the point that by September, nearly 70% of all dead crows were infected with West Nile virus, although this varied by county [19,24]. The total number of dead crows counted was high, with 4,335 in Connecticut and 17,571 in New York [10,24].

Human disease was more widely scattered than in 1999 (Figure 9.4), but fewer cases occurred. A total of 21 human cases were identified, compared to 62 total cases in 1999. All cases occurred in areas of high population density. The geographic area where humans were affected was much smaller than the areas in which West Nile virus-positive crows were identified.

Efforts were made to correlate ecological surveillance indicators with human infection risk. It was found that higher density of dead crows (number reported per square mile per week) in a state, county, or city borough was strongly associated with subsequent risk of two or more cases of human infection in that area in the subsequent few weeks [25]. In addition, cluster analysis of the dead bird reports in New York City showed that clusters correlated with subsequent human risk within the area defined by cluster analysis [26]. Dead crow density and cluster analysis have since been used to define areas in New York City where preemptive insecticide spraying should be done to reduce vector mosquito populations.

This experience was used to initiate a national surveillance effort using crow die-offs as a sentinel indicator of the movement of West Nile virus into new geographic areas [1]. This surveillance system proved to be a most sensitive indicator of the

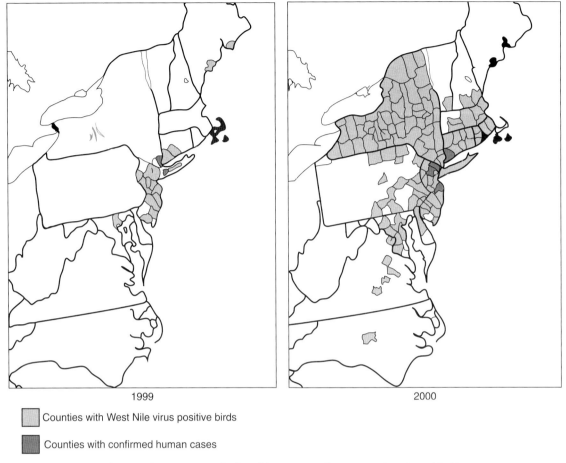

1999

2000

■ Counties with West Nile virus positive birds

■ Counties with confirmed human cases

Fig 9.4 Distribution of West Nile virus positive birds and human cases, by county, US, 1999 and 2000.

spread of West Nile virus across the US and Canada and illustrated the utility of monitoring morbidity and mortality of susceptible host species to track a newly introduced vector-borne pathogen. A similar system has been developed in Europe to monitor the spread of Usutu virus, a flavivirus introduced into Vienna, Austria, that kills blackbirds [27].

Mosquito surveillance for West Nile virus

As described above, regional and then national entomological surveillance for West Nile virus was established after the initial 1999 New York City area outbreak. It was not initially clear whether the virus

would successfully overwinter and become enzootic in North America, but a search began for potential amplifying and bridge vectors. The West Nile virus was soon identified in overwintering *Culex* mosquitoes in New York City [28]. These data increased the vigilance for the likely emergence of the virus in the spring. Methodology was soon established to detect viral RNA in mosquito pools. In 2000, mosquito trapping and testing data from New York City and surrounding states detected viral RNA in pools of *C. pipiens*, *C. restuans*, and *C. salinarius* mosquitoes. The finding of West Nile virus in large numbers of *C. restuans and pipiens*, both ornithophilic mosquitoes, suggested that they were important amplifying vectors. *C. pipiens* and *C. salinarius* also feed on humans and were thought

117

to be important avenues of transmission to humans. Positive mosquito pools in proximity to human cases were often found at the same time or later than human cases. Studies in New York suggested that *Culex* mosquito infection rates correlated with the percentage of dead crows testing positive for West Nile virus [19]. Thus, vector control efforts focused on *Culex* mosquito control. Nevertheless, the utility of mosquito surveillance to guide control efforts was limited by scant capacity to conduct the surveillance and lack of timeliness relative to human or bird surveillance. Nevertheless, mosquito surveillance detected infection prevalences as high as 5%, indicating that the virus had great epidemic potential. Infection prevalences of other mosquito-borne pathogens such as St. Louis encephalitis virus typically are less than 1 per 1000. In 2002, the West Nile virus caused the largest epidemic of arboviral encephalitis ever in North America. As the West Nile virus spread across the US, surveillance identified more than 60 infected mosquito species, although the main amplifying vectors in the northeastern, southern, and western US are *C. pipiens*, *C. quinquefasciatus*, and *C. tarsalis*, respectively. Thus, surveillance now focuses on these species.

Evolving roles of West Nile virus dead bird and mosquito surveillance

The role of mosquito surveillance for West Nile virus is evolving as nationwide entomological surveillance capacity is increasing, the utility of bird surveillance is decreasing, and funding is no longer sufficient to support both systems in all states. Dead bird surveillance has been hampered by reductions of crow and other indicator species populations and, possibly public complacence with dead bird reporting. Thus, it is increasingly difficult to correlate indicators such as dead bird densities with the degree of viral amplification in the bird–mosquito cycle and subsequent human risk. Research efforts to correlate vector mosquito densities and West Nile virus infection prevalences in vectors with degree of human risk may eventually create reliable indices to predict the risk and magnitude of human outbreaks.

The experience with West Nile virus is perhaps the best documented example of the role of entomo-

logical surveillance of an emerging mosquito-borne disease. This example showed that with a concerted effort, key ecological questions could be quickly answered. However, this example also showed that the role and nature of entomological surveillance in guiding prevention efforts evolved over time as surveillance capacity increased and a scientific foundation to fully interpret the gathered data developed. Entomological surveillance is likely to replace dead bird surveillance as the main system for prospectively determining local current human West Nile virus risk in most of the US.

Lyme disease surveillance

Lyme disease was first recognized in 1975 when a cluster of acute arthritis cases in residents of Lyme, Connecticut, was investigated, and cases were found to be preceded by erythema migrans and tick exposure [29]. Subsequent investigations established that human infection results from bites of *Ixodes* ticks infected with *B. burgdorferi* and that the ticks are the vector component of a maintenance cycle involving white-footed mice and deer host species.

Connecticut began human surveillance for Lyme disease in 1984. At the time, Lyme disease was a new and ongoing challenge for clinicians and public health. Newly developed serologic antibody-based diagnostic tests showed that early treatment, critical for preventing arthritis and neurological complications, blunted the immune response and often caused false-negative test results. Further, most patients had not recognized an antecedent tick bite as *Ixodes* ticks are tiny; thus, a negative history of tick bite could not rule out Lyme disease. Initial surveillance objectives were broad: to describe the epidemiology in person, place, and time (season); to monitor incidence trends, particularly in geographic range; and to identify risk factors for acquiring Lyme disease.

Lyme disease initially was not a reportable condition. However, the work of several Connecticut laboratories to develop and standardize serologic testing provided an opportunity for surveillance. It was decided to offer free serologic testing statewide. Notice of availability of free testing was promoted to primary care providers through an article in the bimonthly Department of Public Health publication, the *Connecticut Epidemiologist*, sent to all licensed physicians with a primary care specialty. For every person for whom testing was done, a form with clinical information about the patient's illness was requested. A case was defined as a person clinically diagnosed with erythema migrans or a person with neurologic or joint disease with a positive serologic test for *Borrelia*. Feedback was provided through subsequent reports in the *Connecticut Epidemiologist*.

A key finding from this surveillance initiative was that disease rates by town ranged widely, from 1 to 156 cases per 100,000, with the highest rates in the area around Lyme [30,31]. Although most patients were tested because they had erythema migrans, only 25% of such cases had positive serologic tests. It became apparent that if ongoing surveillance were to be conducted, surveillance for erythema mi-

grans should be the basis. In addition, a standardized definition for erythema migrans was needed.

Beginning in 1987, Lyme disease became a physician reportable condition in Connecticut. A national case definition of erythema migrans was developed; this definition was intended to be more specific, but was also less sensitive. For a case to be counted, the largest erythema migrans lesion needed to be at least 5 centimeters in diameter [5]. To enable counting of cases without recognized erythema migrans but with later manifestations, persons with a clinically compatible illness with laboratory evidence of *Borrelia* infection were also reportable.

Results of ongoing surveillance in Connecticut showed that Lyme disease gradually spread to and increased in other parts of the state to the point where the greater Lyme area no longer had the highest incidence (Figure 9.5). Over the years, erythema

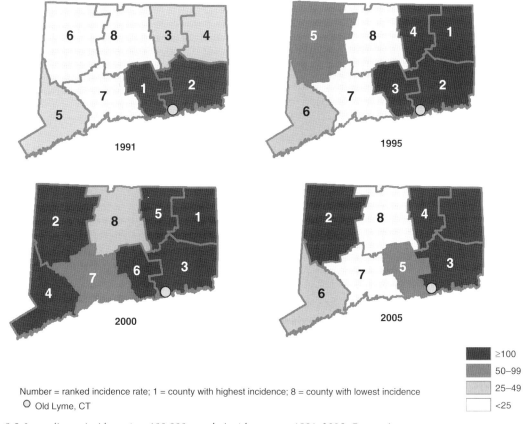

Number = ranked incidence rate; 1 = county with highest incidence; 8 = county with lowest incidence
○ Old Lyme, CT

≥100
50–99
25–49
<25

Fig 9.5 Lyme disease incidence (per 100,000 population) by county, 1991–2005, Connecticut.

migrans has consistently accounted for 70–80% of cases. Cases identified through surveillance have been the basis for several important risk and natural disease history studies. One case study demonstrated that most Lyme disease is acquired peridomestically and that risk is highest in residential settings abutting areas with forests, meadows, and a high prevalence of deer [32]. Another found no long-term health consequences from standard antibiotic treatment of erythema migrans [33]. A further study showed that the results from human and vector infection prevalence had a strong correlation [17].

The experience with Lyme disease surveillance in Connecticut demonstrates that human surveillance can be effectively initiated in the short-term without a reporting requirement. Data gathering can be tied to offering an experimental test that would not have otherwise been available. This approach was also used in Connecticut for another vector-borne disease, cat-scratch disease [34]. Conversely, longitudinal Lyme disease surveillance is an example of a system that is based on an imprecise clinical case definition to determine incident cases rather than a laboratory test that in this case is neither sensitive nor specific. Finally, even with an imprecise case definition and underreporting [4], longitudinal surveillance using a consistent framework was able to clearly detect changing geographic risk over time. To encourage consistency of awareness of reporting over time, annual surveillance updates have been reported in the *Connecticut Epidemiologist* [35] and statistics are readily available on the Department of Public Health Web site [36].

Conclusion

Surveillance for vector-borne disease will continue to be important in a world characterized by increasing travel and trade, changes in land use patterns, urbanization of areas where natural enzootic cycles exist, and climate change. A rich range of methods have been developed to attempt to characterize disease epidemiology and outbreak risk to human and animal populations. Surveillance for any one disease is best conducted using several mutually reinforcing methods at a time. Given the sometimes complex maintenance cycles and changing ecology, future surveillance for the known vector-borne dis-

eases and for not-yet recognized diseases will offer opportunities for creative approaches to application of proven methodologies.

References

1 Petersen L, Hayes EB. Westward ho? The spread of West Nile virus. *N Engl J Med* 2004;**351**:2257–9.

2 Fine A, Layton M. Lessons from the West Nile viral encephalitis outbreak in New York City, 1999: implications for bioterrorism preparedness. *Clin Infect Dis* 2001; **32**:277–82.

3 World Health Organization. Third report of Committee A, Annex 2. Available from: http://www.who.int/gb/ebwha/pdf_files/WHA58/A58_4-en.pdf. Accessed April 24, 2007.

4 Meek JI, Roberts CL, Smith EV, Jr, Cartter ML. Underreporting of Lyme disease by Connecticut physicians, 1992. *J Public Health Manag Pract* 1996;**2**:61–5.

5 Centers for Disease Control and Prevention. Case definitions for infectious conditions under public health surveillance. *MMWR* 1997;**46**(RR-10):20–1. Available from: http://www.cdc.gov/mmwr/PDF/rr/rr4610.pdf. Accessed April 24, 2007.

6 Centers for Disease Control and Prevention. Case definitions—arboviral diseases, neuroinvasive and non-neuroinvasive, 2004. Available from: http://www.cdc.gov/epo/dphsi/casedef/case_definitions.htm. Accessed April 24, 2007.

7 Centers for Disease Control and Prevention. Serosurveys for West Nile virus infection—New York and Connecticut counties—2000. *MMWR Morb Mortal Wkly Rep* 2001;**50**:37–9.

8 Mas J, Ascaso C, Escaramis G, *et al.* Reduction in the prevalence of infection in *Onchocerca volvulus* microfilariae according to ethnicity and community after 8 years of ivermectin treatment on the island of Bioko, Equatorial Guinea. *Trop Med Int Health* 2006;**11**:1082–91.

9 Rajendran R, Sunish IP, Mani TR, *et al.* Community-based study to assess the efficacy of DEC plus ALB against DEC alone on bancroftian filarial infection in endemic areas in Tamil Nadu, south India. *Trop Med Int Health* 2006;**11**:851–61.

10 Eidson M, Kramer L, Stone W, Hagiwara Y, Schmit K, and the New York State Avian Surveillance Team. Dead bird surveillance as an early warning system for West Nile virus. *Emerg Infect Dis* 2001;**7**:631–5.

11 Stafford KC, Massung RF, Magnarelli LA, Ijdo JW, Anderson JF. Infection with agents of human granulocytic ehrlichiosis, Lyme disease, and babesiosis in wild white-footed mice (*Peromyscus leucopus*) in Connecticut. *J Clin Micro* 1999;**37**:2887–92.

12 Reisen WK, Lundstrom JO, Scott TW, *et al.* Patterns of avian seroprevalence to western equine encephalomyelitis and Saint Louis encephalitis viruses in California, USA. *J Med Entomol* 2000;**37**:507–27.

13 Broom AK. Sentinel chicken surveillance program in Australia, July 2002to June 2003. *Commun Dis Intell* 2003;**27**:367–9.

14 Buckley A, Dawson A, Gould EA. Detection of seroconversion to West Nile virus, Usutu virus and Sindbis birus in UK sentinel chickens. *J Virol* 2006;**4**:71.

15 McCardle PW, Webb RE, Norden BB, Aldrich JR. Evaluation of five trapping systems for the surveillance of gravid mosquitoes in Prince Georges County, Maryland. *J Am Mosq Control Assoc* 2004;**20**:254–60.

16 Reisen WK, Pfuntner AR. Effectiveness of five methods for sampling adult Culex mosquitoes in rural and urban habitats in San Bernardino County, California. *J Am Mosq Control Assoc* 1987;**3**:601–6.

17 Stafford KC, III, Cartter ML, Magnarelli LA, Ertel S, Mshar PA. Temporal correlations between tick abundance and prevalence of ticks infected with *Borrelia burgdorferi* and increasing incidence of Lyme disease. *J Clin Microbiol* 1998;36:1240–4.

18 Biggerstaff, BJ. PooledInfRate: a Microsoft ExcelAdd-In to compute prevalence estimates from pooled samples. Centers for Disease Control and Prevention, Ft. Collins, Colorado. Available from: http://www.cdc.gov/ ncidod/ dvbid/westnile/software.htm. Accessed April 24, 2007.

19 Bernard KA, Maffei JG, Jones SA, *et al.* West Nile virus infection in birds and mosquitoes, New York State, 2000. *Emerg Inf Dis* 2001;7:679–85.

20 Hemingway J, Ranson H. Insecticide resistance in insect vectors of human disease. *Annu Rev Entomol* 2000;**45**:371–91.

21 Plowe CV. Antimalarial drug resistance in Africa: strategies for monitoring and deterrence. *Curr Top Microbiol Immunol* 2005;**295**:55–79.

22 Centers for Disease Control and Prevention. Imported plague—New York City, 2002. *MMWR Morb Mortal Wkly Rep* 2003;**52**:725–8.

23 Centers for Disease Control and Prevention. Update: West Nile encephalitis—New York, 1999. *MMWR Morb Mortal Wkly Rep* 1999;48:944–6, 955.

24 Hadler J, Nelson R, McCarthy T, *et al.* West Nile virus surveillance in Connecticut in 2000: an intense epizootic without high risk for severe human disease. *Emerg Infect Dis* 2001;7:636–42.

25 Eidson M, Miller J, Kramer L, Cherry B, Hagiwara Y, and the West Nile Virus Bird Mortality Analysis Group. Dead crow densities and human cases of West Nile virus. *Emerg Infect Dis* 2001;7:662–4.

26 Mostashari F, Kulldorff M, Hartman JJ, Miller JR, Kulasekera V. Dead bird clusters as an early warning system for West Nile virus activity. *Emerg Infect Dis* 2003;9:641–6.

27 Weisssenbock H, Kolodziejek J, Fragner K, Kuhn R, Pfeffer M, Nowotny N. Usutu virus activity in Austria, 2001–2002. *Microbes Infect* 2003;**5**:1132–6.

28 Centers for Disease Control and Prevention. Update: surveillance for West Nile virus in overwintering mosquitoes—New York, 2000. *MMWR Morb Mortal Wkly Rep* 2000;**49**:178–9.

29 Steere AC, Malawista SE, Snydman DR, *et al.* Lyme arthritis: an epidemic of oligoarticular arthritis in children and adults in three Connecticut communities. *Arthritis Rheum* 1977;**20**:7–17.

30 Petersen LR, Sweeney AH, Checko PJ, *et al.* Epidemiological and clinical features of 1149 persons with Lyme disease identified by laboratory-based surveillance in Connecticut. *Yale J Biol Med* 1989;**62**: 253–62.

31 Centers for Disease Control. Lyme disease—Connecticut. *MMWR Morb Mortal Wkly Rep* 1988;**37**:1–3.

32 Cromley EK, Cartter ML, Mrozinski RD, Ertel SH. Residential setting as a risk factor for Lyme disease in a hyperendemic region. *Am J Epidemiol* 1998;**147**: 472–7.

33 Seltzer EG, Gerber MA, Cartter ML, Freudigman K, Shapiro ED. Long-term outcomes of persons with Lyme disease. *JAMA* 2000;**283**:609–16.

34 Hamilton DH, Zangwill KM, Hadler JL, Cartter ML. Cat-scratch disease in Connecticut, 1992–1993. *JID* 1995;**172**:570–3.

35 Connecticut Department of Public Health. Connecticut Epidemiologist issues, 1998–2006. Available from: http://www.dph.state.ct.us/BCH/infectiousdise/cenl.htm. Accessed April 24, 2007.

36 Connecticut Department of Public Health. Lyme disease cases and rates per 100,000 population, 1991–1995, 1996–2000, and 2001–2005. Available from: http://www.dph.state.ct.us/BCH/infectiousdise/pdf/ld_webdata_1991_1995.pdf; http://www.dph.state.ct.us/BCH/infectiousdise/pdf/ld_webdata_1996_2000.pdf; and http://www.dph.state.ct.us/v bch/infectiousdisve/pdf/LD01_05web.pdf. Accessed April 24, 2007.

Additional resources

Vector-borne diseases and their ecology

1 Eldridge BF, Edman JD (eds.). *Medical Entomology.* Dortrecht: Klumer Academic Publishers; 2000.

2 Service MW (ed.). *The Encyclopedia of Arthropod-Transmitted Infections.* Oxon: CABI Publishing; 2001.

3 Gubler DJ. The global emergence/resurgence of arboviral diseases as public health problems. *Arch Med Res* 2002;**33**:330–42.

4 Perry RD, Fetherston JD. *Yersinia pestis*—etiologic agent of plague. *Clin Microbiol Rev* 1997;**10**:35–66.

5 Wilske B. The epidemiology and clinical diagnosis of *Lyme borreliosis*. *Ann Med* 2005;**37**:568–70.

6 Centers for Disease Control and Prevention. Eastern equine encephalitis—New Hampshire and Massachusetts, August–September 2005. *MMWR Morb Mortal Wkly Rep* 2006;**55**:697–700.

7 Weaver SC. Host range, amplification and arboviral disease emergence. *Arch Virol Suppl* 2005;**19**: 33–44.

8 Guinovart C, Navia MM, Tanner M, Alonso PL. Malaria: burden of disease. *Curr Mol Med* 2006;**6**: 137–40

Integrated pest management and disease control

1 Rose RI. Pesticides and public health: integrated methods of mosquito management. *Emerg Infect Dis* 2001;**7**: 17–23.

2 Dennis DT, Gage KL, Gratz N, Poland JD, Tikhomirov E. *Plague Manual: Epidemiology, Distribution, Surveillance and Control*. WHO/CDS/EDC/99.2. Geneva: World Health Organization; 1999.

3 Tripathi RP, Mishra RC, Dwivedi N, Tewari N, Verma SS. Current status of malaria control. *Curr Med Chem* 2005;**12**:2643–59.

Vector-borne disease surveillance

1 O'Leary DR, Marfin AA, Montgomery SP, *et al.* The epidemic of West Nile virus in the United States, 2002. *Vector borne Zoonotic Dis* 2004;**4**:61–70.

2 Chen H, White DJ, Caraco TB, Stratton HH. Epidemic and spatial dynamics of Lyme disease in New York State, 1990–2000. *J Med Entomol* 2005;**42**:899–908.

Web sites

Centers for Disease Control and Prevention, Division of Vector-borne Diseases: http://www.cdc.gov/ncidod/dvbid/. Accessed April 24, 2007.

Connecticut Agricultural Experiment Station: http://www.caes.state.ct.us/. Accessed April 24, 2007.

California Vectorborne Disease Surveillance System. http://vector.ucdavis.edu/. Accessed April 24, 2007.

Purdue University program in vector biology and vector-borne diseases: http://www.entm.purdue.edu/publichealth/. Accessed April 24, 2007.

Appendix

CDC Questionnaire: West Nile virus protective
behaviors among organ transplant recipients
(Baseline—Summer 2006)

		Please mark "x" in appropriate box or write in the answer if indicated
1.	What is your date of birth? *(month/day/year)*	__ __ /__ __/__ __
2.	What is your gender?	☐ Male ☐ Female
3.	In what county and state do you live?	*(Please write in your county below)*
4.	In your home, are the windows and doors that you usually leave open covered by intact screens?	☐Yes on all ☐ Yes on some ☐None
5.	What kind of air-cooling system do you have in your house?	***(Mark an "x" all that apply)*** ☐ Central air-conditioning ☐ Air-conditioning window units ☐ Swamp (evaporative) cooler ☐ Fans ☐ None
6.	Before this questionnaire, had you heard of West Nile virus?	☐ YES ☐ NO ☐ Don't Know
7.	Have you ever been told by a health care provider that you had a West Nile virus infection?	☐ YES ☐ NO If yes, when? (please write in month/year)

8. How concerned are you about getting sick because of West Nile virus during the summer or fall of 2006?

☐ Not at all concerned
☐ A little concerned
☐ Somewhat concerned
☐ Very concerned

How often did you do the following actions during summer and fall of last year (2005)?

9. I used an insect repellent when outdoors …

☐ Always ☐ Often ☐ Sometimes ☐ Rarely ☐ Never

10. I wore long sleeves or long pants when outdoors to avoid mosquito bites…

☐ Always ☐ Often ☐ Sometimes ☐ Rarely ☐ Never

11. I avoided being outdoors from dusk to dawn when mosquitoes are most likely to bite…

☐ Always ☐ Often ☐ Sometimes ☐ Rarely ☐ Never

12. I emptied containers with standing water around my home to prevent mosquitoes from breeding…

☐ Always ☐ Often ☐ Sometimes ☐ Rarely ☐ Never

13. How long do you spend outdoors after dusk or before dawn on an average WEEKDAY when the weather is warm?

☐ Less than 1 hour after dusk or before dawn
☐ 1–2 hours after dusk or before dawn
☐ More than 2 hours after dusk or before dawn

14. How long do you spend outdoors after dusk or before dawn on an average WEEKEND DAY when the weather is warm?

☐ Less than 1 hour after dusk or before dawn
☐ 1-2 hours after dusk or before dawn
☐ More than 2 hours after dusk or before dawn

15. When you didn't use an insect repellent, which of the following reasons describe why not?

("X" ALL THAT APPLY)
☐ Concerned about bad health effects of repellents
☐ Felt that I was outdoors too short a time to use repellent
☐ Repellent was not convenient when I needed it
☐ Repellents cost too much
☐ Do not like the smell/feel of repellents
☐ Not concerned about being bitten
☐ Do not have enough information about repellents
☐ Forgot/did not think about it
☐ Do not think repellents keep mosquitoes away

16. Have you ever heard information about protecting yourself against West Nile virus or mosquito bites?

☐ YES ☐ NO ☐ Don't Know

17. If yes, where did you hear this information?

Please mark all that apply
☐ General practitioner
☐ Medical specialist
☐ Transplant coordinator
☐ Pamphlet/brochure
☐ Newspaper article
☐ Radio
☐ TV news
☐ TV public service announcement
☐ Friend
☐ Family
☐ Other (Please specify) _____

18. Prior to receiving these materials (letter and this questionnaire), were you aware that you as an organ transplant recipient, are at increased risk for developing severe illness if you become infected with West Nile virus?

☐ YES ☐ NO
If yes, where did you get this information?

10 Surveillance for agents of bioterrorism in the United States

Richard N. Danila & Aaron T. Fleischauer

Introduction

Bioterrorism involves the intentional or threatened use of biological agents (bacteria, viruses, or toxins) to produce death or disease in humans, animals, or plants. In the United States (US) over the previous 25 years, several crimes have involved the intentional use of biological agents. These events include intentional food contamination with *Salmonella typhimurium* by the Rajneeshees in The Dalles, Oregon, and the deliberate infection of hospital coworkers with *Shigella dysenteriae* by a fellow employee in Dallas, Texas [1,2]. Epidemiologic investigations of these incidents emphasized the need for investigation by public health personnel, often in collaboration with law enforcement, to consider alternative mechanisms of exposure; as whether an outbreak is the result of a nefarious act may not be easy to determine.

In 2001, anthrax-spore-laden threat letters were mailed to a number of high-profile individuals in media and in government. These attacks stressed the need for development and implementation of innovative surveillance methods for rapid detection of bioterrorism events [3]. Although experts in public health continue to research and develop surveillance systems for bioterrorism, the level of suspicion and diligence in identifying a biological attack must remain high among public health professionals; a small outbreak of illness or a case of rare disease or unexplained death may be an early warning of a bioterror attack, and timely recognition could save thousands of lives [4]. In this chapter we will review surveillance for bioterrorism.

The category A agents

In 1999, the US Centers for Disease Control and Prevention (CDC) convened a multidisciplinary workgroup to provide guidance for strengthening public health to prepare for and respond to bioterrorism. The category A agents (Table 10.1) are those considered the most serious threats ([5]; http://www.bt.cdc.gov/agent/agentlist-category .asp), as (1) the disease may result in high mortality rates; (2) intentional dissemination has potential for major public health impact and may cause public panic or social disruption; (3) pathogens can be easily disseminated or have potential for person-to-person transmission; and (4) treatment requires special action for public health preparedness. Although new surveillance systems have been designed primarily for the rapid detection of the category A agents, preparedness efforts have also included enhanced surveillance activities for category B and C agents and diseases (Table 10.2), including naturally occurring outbreaks caused by these agents.

Legal authority for bioterrorism disease surveillance

All US states and territories have laws, statutes, or other regulations that mandate the reporting of communicable or infectious diseases ([6,7]; see also Chapter 35, Part 1). All category A agent diseases are nationally notifiable. Most states or entities also require reporting of unusual cases of disease,

Table 10.1 Category A bioterrorism agents/diseases.

Category A*	
Disease	Agent or Toxin
Anthrax	*Bacillus anthracis*
Botulism	*Clostridium botulinum* toxin
Plague	*Yersinia pestis*
Smallpox	*Variola major*
Tularemia	*Francisella tularensis*
Viral hemorrhagic fevers	Filoviruses[†], arenaviruses[‡]

*High priority agents pose a risk to national security.
[†]Includes Ebola and Marburg viruses.
[‡]Includes Lassa and Machupo viruses.

cases of public health significance, or clusters of cases of disease whether specifically diagnosed or not [8]. Thus, even if not specifically listed, in most instances, there is a legal mandate to report a disease that is suspected to be due to an agent of bioterrorism.

The state has the authority to monitor a central repository of disease cases where patterns, clusters, and outbreaks may be detected. This authority is due to the police powers afforded to states by the 10th Amendment of the US Constitution [8].

The federal role in disease surveillance takes place when data, without case-patient identifiers, are sent to CDC. Regarding bioterrorism-related disease or outbreaks, CDC's legal authority rests with the national defense mandate of the federal government to protect citizens from terrorists. Also, the federal government has isolation and quarantine authority for certain diseases and general authority to prevent interstate spread of disease (see Chapter 35, Part 2). In practice as well as in historical context, however, the names and identifying information of individual cases of disease are retained at the state level. Because legal authority rests with individual states and localities, one possible disadvantage is that small disease clusters crossing geographic lines or borders could conceivably be missed or their recognition delayed. State health departments need to develop data-sharing protocols with bordering states in advance.

Epidemiologic clues to bioterrorism

Bioterrorism is an infectious disease event characterized by the deliberate introduction of a causative pathogen versus a naturally occurring outbreak resulting from an inadvertent exposure. Epidemiologic clues to consider in designing a

Table 10.2 Category B and C agents/diseases.

Category B* diseases (Agent or Toxin)	
Brucellosis (*Brucella* species)	Melioidosis (*Burkholderia pseudomallei*)
Epsilon toxin (*Clostridium perfringens*)	Psittacosis (*Chlamydia psittaci*)
Food safety threats (*Salmonella* species, *Escherichia coli* O157:H7, *Shigella*)	Q fever (*Coxiella burnetii*)
Glanders (*Burkholderia mallei*)	Ricin toxin (*Ricinus communis*, castor beans)
Staphylococcal enterotoxin B	Typhus fever (*Rickettsia prowazekii*)
Viral encephalitis (alphaviruses)	Water safety threats (*Vibrio cholerae*, *Cryptosporidium parvum*)

Category C diseases[†]
Emerging infectious diseases such as Nipah virus and hantavirus

*Second highest priority agents that require enhancements of diagnostic capacity and enhanced disease surveillance.
[†]Third highest priority agents include emerging pathogens that could be engineered for mass dissemination in the future.

surveillance system to detect a covert bioterrorism event may include the following [4,9]:
• Higher morbidity or mortality than expected for a common disease or syndrome
• A common outcome with an unusual geographic or seasonal distribution
• The presence of a large epidemic or multiple simultaneous outbreaks in discrete population(s)
• Illness in persons, suggesting a common or unusual exposure (e.g., workplace, major public event)
• Unusual, atypical, or antiquated agent strain
• A rare disease typically observed in previously defined populations

However, even with the presence of the aforementioned characteristics, determining whether cases of disease or an outbreak is the result of terrorism or is naturally occurring may be difficult and requires a sound epidemiologic investigation in collaboration with law enforcement, emergency management, and the intelligence community.

Special considerations for surveillance for agents of bioterrorism

Conventional bombings and attacks with poisonous chemicals will be overt; their effects will be noticed immediately or within a short period of time. A biological release, generally even if announced afterward, is covert due to the delay between exposure (release of agent) and clinical manifestations [10]. The first cases of disease will appear in doctor's offices, clinics, and emergency rooms. Depending on the specific organism, the dose, and route of exposure, the incubation period may be short as that for botulinum toxin or relatively long as for smallpox. Public health authorities will need to quickly establish the etiology of the disease, that a bioterrorism attack has occurred, and the extent of the exposed population in order to prevent more casualties through prophylaxis of the exposed population (if prophylaxis is available), providing recommendations for early treatment (if treatment is available), vaccination of the exposed (if available), and isolation of the ill and quarantine of the exposed (if these are useful countermeasures).

Disease reporting by clinicians

A major challenge in reducing disease diagnosis and detection time is that the initial signs and symptoms of disease for many potential bioterrorism agents are nonspecific. For example, fever, malaise, cough, fatigue, and anorexia are early signs and symptoms for plague, anthrax, tularemia, brucellosis, and smallpox. Clinical acumen is critical for early detection. On October 2, 2001, Dr Larry Bush at J.F.K. Medical Center in Atlantis, Florida, examined a 63-year-old man admitted with fever, emesis, and confusion. The patient's initial chest radiograph showed evidence of basilar infiltrates and a widened mediastinum. A Gram stain of cerebrospinal fluid revealed many polymorphonuclear white cells and many large gram-positive bacilli, both singly and in chains. The Florida Department of Health was contacted for laboratory assistance, and an investigation started. This case was the first case of inhalational anthrax due to bioterrorism [11].

Even though multiple surveys and studies have shown that physicians are not the main source of infectious disease reports received by health departments, they are the main source of reports of diseases of public health significance. Completeness of disease reporting is generally better for diseases with severe clinical illness than with mild illness [12]. Clinician reporting led to the recognition of hantavirus in southwestern US in 1993, West Nile virus in 1999, anthrax in 2001, and SARS in 2003 [6,13].

CDC conducted a retrospective review of all outbreaks investigated by its Epidemic Intelligence Service from 1988 to 1999. Forty-four (4.0%) of 1099 outbreaks were caused by an agent with potential for bioterrorism including cholera, plague, and viral hemorrhagic fever. Intentional use of infectious agents to cause harm to civilians was considered in six investigations [14].

Failure of reporting may lead to delays that result in unnecessary illness and death. For example, in 2000, one of two sentinel cases of tularemia that represented the beginning of a naturally occurring outbreak of tularemia on Martha's Vineyard was misdiagnosed by a Connecticut family physician [15]. A chest radiograph showed a right middle-lobe infiltrate consistent with bronchopneumonia. The patient was treated with antimicrobials. Nearly

2 months later, the patient, who was now asymptomatic, recognized from media attention about the Martha's Vineyard outbreak that he might have had tularemia, and he contacted the state health department. A serological diagnosis of tularemia was then made. Earlier recognition and reporting may have prevented some cases.

During the anthrax bioterrorism outbreak of 2001, one New Jersey physician empirically treated a case of cutaneous anthrax several weeks before he reported it to the New Jersey Department of Health and Human Services. The case was in a postal worker who had been exposed at the Trenton Postal Processing and Distribution Center. It was only after an announcement was made that anthrax cases in other states were associated with letters that originated at the Trenton facility that the physician reported the case to the health department. The facility was immediately closed; earlier reporting might have led to prompter closing and prevention of cases [16].

Physicians need to be trained to recognize an unusual case or cluster of unusual cases and report them immediately. Clinicians may be unfamiliar with their role in reporting diseases or how to report [17]. Public health departments need to enhance clinician awareness of bioterrorism agents and how to report to a public health agency. Clinician education can be through traditional lectures or through more novel ways. In 2000, the Minnesota Department of Health (MDH) developed and distributed thousands of copies of an eye-catching poster to healthcare facilities and clinicians statewide (Figure 10.1). The theme of the poster was to turn around the medical adage of not looking for zebras when hearing hoof beats, but to look for horses. Clinicians were instructed to think of diseases of bioterrorism as zebras and to start looking for them. If they heard certain "hoof beats" such as a widened mediastinum on thoracic radiograph, influenza-like illness in summer months, or vesicular rash that started on the extremities, they should consider the "zebras" of anthrax, tularemia, or smallpox and most importantly they were to call the state health department. Patients infected with bioterrorism agents may first come to the attention of specialists such as dermatologists, radiologists, or intensivists. Because these clinicians are less likely to report infectious diseases or deal with public health

on a routine basis, they should be targeted for training. Health departments should consider collaboration with medical societies, and conduct targeted grand rounds for these specialists [13] in addition to primary care physicians.

Health departments need to remove barriers to disease reporting. Ideally, reporting should be done by telephone, toll-free, and on a 24/7 basis. One-half of health departments lacked this ability in 2002 [6]. Routine reporting by mail, facsimile machine, e-mail, and telephone should be allowed for diseases with consequences less urgent, but for surveillance for diseases due to bioterrorism to be successful, all barriers must be removed. Access to epidemiological expertise, infectious disease expertise, and public health laboratory consultation should be available on a 24/7 basis.

Special reporting systems: unexplained deaths and critical illnesses

Clinicians may encounter a patient with a critical or fatal illness that has hallmarks of infection but is unexplained because either laboratory evaluation has not been conducted or routine laboratory tests have not revealed a diagnosis. As part of its Emerging Infections Program, CDC funded four sites beginning in 1994 to participate in an Unexplained Deaths and Critical Illnesses Project ([18]; see also Chapter 11). Health agencies established active surveillance with hospital intensive care units and intensivists, infectious disease specialists, medical examiners/coroners, and pathologists. Enhanced laboratory diagnostics, including molecular testing and immunohistochemistry, are offered. A similar epidemiology and laboratory collaboration may be a tool that more health departments can promote to improve reporting, which in turn may lead to detection of a bioterrorism agent.

State health departments should enlist medical examiners and coroners as active disease reporting participants ([19]; see also Chapter 11). These professionals often evaluate fatalities among persons who have not sought medical attention. They also investigate, for medicolegal purposes, deaths of suspicious origin or sudden nature. Deaths due to bioterrorism might initially appear at the state or local medical examiner's office.

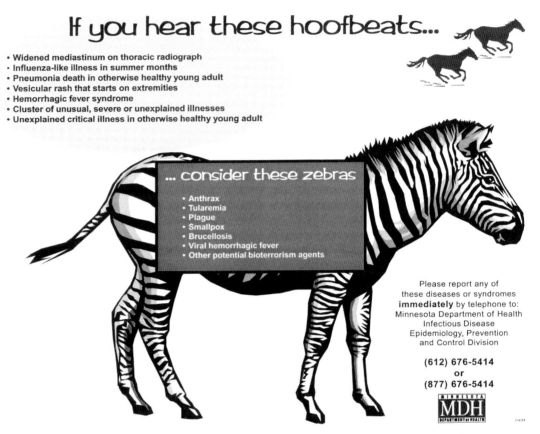

If you hear these hoofbeats...

- Widened mediastinum on thoracic radiograph
- Influenza-like illness in summer months
- Pneumonia death in otherwise healthy young adult
- Vesicular rash that starts on extremities
- Hemorrhagic fever syndrome
- Cluster of unusual, severe or unexplained illnesses
- Unexplained critical illness in otherwise healthy young adult

... consider these zebras

- Anthrax
- Tularemia
- Plague
- Smallpox
- Brucellosis
- Viral hemorrhagic fever
- Other potential bioterrorism agents

Please report any of
these diseases or syndromes
immediately by telephone to:
Minnesota Department of Health
Infectious Disease
Epidemiology, Prevention
and Control Division

**(612) 676-5414
or
(877) 676-5414**

MDH
DEPARTMENT of HEALTH

Fig 10.1 Zebra poster suggesting that these slightly unusual symptoms may indicate very unusual diseases (details available at the Minnesota Department of Health Web site: www.health.state.mn.us/bioterrorism/hcp/index.html). (Used with permission from the Minnesota Department of Health.)

Novel sources of disease reports

Symptoms of some bioterrorism agents, particularly of toxins such as botulinum toxin, staphylococcal enterotoxin B, or ricin, may mimic poisoning and prompt calls from patients or clinicians to a centralized poison control center. It behooves health departments to establish relationships with their state or regional poison control center, so that reports of suspicious nature can be forwarded. For example, MDH receives by facsimile all routine reports of foodborne illness that originate with the Minnesota Poison Center. Also, computerized intake reports at the center are collated into syndromes and electronically sent to MDH for geotemporal clustering analyses. Statistically significant clusters automatically generate an alert back to the Minnesota Poison Center to begin an investigation. It has proven useful for identification of clusters of environmental poisoning (i.e., widespread mercury contamination, ethylene glycol water supply contamination) and has the potential to be the initial report of a bioterrorism event.

Since many of the agents of bioterrorism are zoonoses or can affect animals, an environmental release of a biological agent could initially present with illness in animals [20]; therefore, partnering with veterinarians and veterinary diagnostic laboratories are important steps in building capacity for bioterrorism detection. Prior to the confirmation of West Nile virus being the cause of human illness in New York City in 1999, it was suspected of being the cause of wild and exotic bird die-offs, which preceded human illness by several weeks. Laboratory confirmation of West Nile virus in brain tissue of dead crows and zoo birds was first done by the National Veterinary Service Laboratory in Ames, Iowa [13].

Laboratory-based surveillance

In February 2006, a New York City resident traveling in Pennsylvania with his dance troupe collapsed with rigors, shortness of breath, and dry cough. The patient was admitted to a local hospital where blood cultures grew gram-positive rods (GPRs). Isolates were sent to the Pennsylvania Department of Health Laboratory and confirmed as *Bacillus anthracis*. In accordance with the Public Health Laboratory's surveillance and reporting policy, the Pennsylvania Department of Health and CDC were immediately notified of the results [21].

Prompt laboratory surveillance led to a coordinated epidemiologic investigation to (1) determine the source of exposure, (2) identify others who were potentially exposed and required postexposure prophylaxis, and (3) enhance surveillance for additional cases through outreach to the medical community. The investigation rapidly determined the source of exposure as mechanical manipulation of goat hides by the index case patient to make traditional African drums. Although other persons were exposed, no additional cases were observed through surveillance. This was the first naturally acquired inhalation anthrax case in the US over 30 years, and while this was an isolated and rare event, laboratory surveillance was essential in triggering a timely public health response [21].

This case-example exemplifies two laboratory surveillance methods: 24-hour passive reporting by clinical laboratories with GPR blood culture results, a screening test for *B. anthracis*, and surveillance through the Laboratory Response Network or LRN (LRN Web site: http://www.bt.cdc.gov/lrn/). Blood cultures are likely to be routine for patients with fever and severe respiratory illness, and *B. anthracis* grows readily in culture; therefore, the effectiveness of GPR surveillance is currently being pilot tested [22]. The LRN, established in 1999, is an international network of clinical and reference

Table 10.3 Services provided to LRN partners: products to ensure an effective laboratory network.

- Agent-specific protocols*
- Standardized reagents and controls
- Training and technology transfer
- Laboratory referral directory
- Secure communications and electronic reporting
- Proficiency testing
- Guidance for biosafety and biosecurity
- Appropriate vaccinations for workers

*Protocols for the biosafety, biosecurity, testing, and response for each category A agent.

laboratories (including state public health, veterinary, agriculture, and US government laboratories) with standardized methods, referral and reporting mechanisms, and communications [23]. The success of LRN is a testament to the multidisciplinary collaboration across local, state, national, and international boundaries. Table 10.3 shows the services provided to LRN partners, which have been integral in building a laboratory surveillance system capable of rapidly responding to a bioterrorism event. The LRN has demonstrated that the capacity to respond to a public health emergency can be enhanced through laboratory standards and coordinated communication.

During the 2001 anthrax attacks, public health officials and laboratories were overwhelmed by requests for evaluation of powders and other environmental samples thought to be contaminated with anthrax spores. Requests for testing came from clinical laboratories, clinicians, emergency responders, including fire fighters and police, and the general public. For example, from October through December 2001, the New York City Bioterrorism Response Laboratory processed >3200 environmental specimens [24]. Two months after the discovery of anthrax in the Trenton Postal Processing and Distribution Center, state police responded to >3500 false alarms involving suspected anthrax powders [24]. A public health laboratory system to detect bioterrorism agents in environmental samples is in many ways as important as one to detect agents in clinical samples. A rapid but reliable system with high sensitivity and specificity can rule out hoaxes and confirm actual bioterrorism agent releases. However, to conserve resources, health departments should develop and institute a triage and priority system for assessing the risk and likelihood that the powder or environmental sample truly does contain a bioterrorism agent before agreeing to test it. This system should be developed in collaboration with local FBI and state and local law enforcement officials. MDH developed such a system in 2001 and tested fewer than 30 samples from hundreds of requests.

Overview of syndromic surveillance

The concept underlying syndromic surveillance—the monitoring and identification of prodromes prior to disease diagnosis or laboratory confirmation—is not new to public health. Syndrome surveillance was an essential tool used during the successful Global Smallpox Eradication Program [25]. For example, in rural India active surveillance was conducted by public health field staff for early signs and symptoms of smallpox (e.g., rash) among weekly market attendees [26]. Syndromic surveillance functions as an integral component of the US Influenza Sentinel Provider Surveillance Network; sentinel primary care clinicians report weekly case totals of patients with influenza-like illness, defined by fever with cough and/or sore throat [27] (see also Chapter 26).

Even prior to the 2001 anthrax attacks, advances in syndromic surveillance specifically designed for the early detection of bioterrorism-related diseases were being implemented in US cities. These systems generally involved daily-automated data collection from local hospital emergency departments. More specifically, syndromic surveillance systems have been designed to collect electronic health information from novel data sources (e.g., emergency departments, 911 call centers, poison control hotlines) coupled with statistical methods, termed aberration detection, to identify increasing trends, clusters, and rare cases. Syndromic surveillance is described in detail in Chapter 26. In brief, the basic methods used in syndromic surveillance require prediagnostic data, such as patient's chief complaint, to be categorized in syndrome categories (e.g., respiratory illness, acute gastroenteritis, rash illness) based on *a priori* case definitions originally derived from the prodromes of category A agents. Daily syndrome rates or counts are then compared with baseline expected values using aberration detection for significant trends or events. The nonspecific syndromic case definitions also allow for detection of trends of naturally occurring infectious diseases (e.g., seasonal influenza, diarrhea illness clusters) [28–30].

Electronic hospital-based syndromic surveillance is a local process, where local data are collected and analyzed by city, county, and state health departments. Recently, national level electronic syndromic surveillance operated by CDC and other federal partners has garnered attention. BioSense, for example, collects and analyzes both national databases (e.g., laboratory test ordering databases, Veteran's Affairs and Department of Defense healthcare systems) and local level (e.g., hospital) information in an integrated syndromic surveillance system ([31]; http://www.cdc.gov/biosense). These data are available as a service to local public health departments.

Whether or not syndromic surveillance systems will detect a bioterrorism event sooner than individual reporting by an alert clinician is unknown. Some suggest that astute clinicians will be aware of a presumptive diagnosis just as soon as or sooner than syndromic data analyses are completed [32]. Agent-specific characteristics influence the likelihood that a clinician will recognize the disease and suspect bioterrorism. Small-scale attacks would not be detected by syndromic systems. For anthrax, a relatively broad incubation might occur with a nonspecific prodrome, thus leading to less likelihood of detection through syndromic systems. On the other hand, a widened mediastinum on chest radiograph or Gram stain of cerebrospinal fluid or pleural fluid will lead a knowledgeable physician to consider anthrax. Furthermore, *B. anthracis* grows rapidly in blood cultures. Others have argued that it may never be scientifically possible to show that syndromic surveillance detected an outbreak due to bioterrorism earlier than traditional clinician/laboratory reporting, and that practical issues such as responding to false-positive alarms and the intense resources needed to develop syndromic surveillance systems led one to question their ongoing establishment and existence [33].

Environmental monitoring: early warning systems

Some systems are designed to detect the release of a biological agent before the onset of symptoms in exposed persons. Such systems have been developed for indoor and outdoor use. The systems use rapid testing technology such as real-time polymerase chain reaction (PCR). Systems such as BioWatch pull air samples through a filter; the filter is retrieved and analyzed for the presence of nucleic acid coding for a specific agent. By reducing the detection time, theoretically, the time to treatment is reduced, thereby preventing more disease and death. In 2003, the US Department of Homeland Security in conjunction with the Environmental Protection Agency and the US Department of Health and Human Services deployed a national system of outdoor environmental monitors in large metropolitan areas to detect bioterrorism agents. The collection devices are located on existing Environmental Protection Agency air quality monitors. The filters from 24-hour samples are collected daily and delivered to an LRN laboratory for PCR testing [34,35]. A positive result is an early warning to be investigated, and clinical detecting and reporting can be primed. If enough environmental information is available, theoretically, an event/agent release can be reconstructed to determine the extent of the exposed population. This in turn might focus mass prophylaxis and treatment efforts. Thus far the systems have performed well with high sensitivity. In fact, detection of apparently very low levels of nucleic acid from naturally occurring organisms (tularemia and brucellosis) has occurred multiple times in multiple cities, leading to initial confusion and concern. The specificity is very high as well with several million tests having been run with no false positives [36]. Reliability, though, is affected by collection efficiency, weather patterns, and placement of the monitors. Indoor siting of these collection devices is ongoing in places where large numbers of people congregate. The BioWatch program and similar systems will probably proliferate in the near future, as automation of these systems reduces costs.

Another monitoring system is the Biohazard Detection System (BDS) used by the US Postal Service, currently testing only for anthrax. BDS is called an autonomous detection system in that automatic air sampling and testing are combined [37]. The BDS is at 283 mail processing and distribution centers nationwide. These are installed on or near high-speed mail processing devices (advanced facer-canceller system machines) that might mechanically aerosolize *B. anthracis* spores contained within envelopes. Sixty- or 90-minute samples are taken and analyzed by PCR on-site. Confirmation of positive tests is conducted at an LRN laboratory. Exposed workers can be placed on prophylactic antibiotics immediately, well before any symptoms of anthrax develop.

Collaboration with law enforcement

By definition, a disease case due to bioterrorism represents an illegal activity. As such, as soon as a suspect case is reported to a health department, health officials need to contact local law enforcement and the Federal Bureau of Investigation (FBI). Preestablished protocols should be followed that allow for exchange of private health data and a joint investigation to proceed. The FBI will not interfere with disease surveillance or disease control activities, but needs to be a key partner in a joint command structure overseeing the event. As such the FBI may need case report data in order for it to investigate possible culprits in a terrorist-associated agent release and to retain evidence. In turn, FBI and other joint law enforcement task force agencies may have intelligence or other information of use to the health department to determine the type of exposure, extent of exposure, agent characteristics, etc.

Postevent health department recognition of bioterrorism

Many of the possible bioterrorism agents are naturally occurring in the US, including those for anthrax, botulism, brucellosis, cholera, plague, tularemia, Q fever, and selected viral encephalitis. Diseases caused by critical bioterrorism agents have occurred at very low levels, with tularemia and brucellosis occurring at about 100 cases annually from 1992 to 1999. Anthrax, eastern equine encephalitis, western equine encephalitis, and plague are so rare that a single case reported in most areas of the US is of concern [38]. However, some of these microorganisms are endemic in various geographic areas, for example plague in the southwestern portion of the US; therefore, it is imperative for local public health officials to know the local epidemiology of these pathogens.

Several factors could distinguish patients infected naturally or a naturally occurring outbreak from one caused by bioterrorism, including law enforcement intelligence data (or an overt announced release of an agent), unusual clinical presentation or a presentation that is atypically severe, environmental evidence of the organism, an unusual mode of transmission, occurrence in a specific population or group, or unusual geographic location or seasonality of the cases [9,36,39]. There may be a shorter incubation period due to higher exposure amounts, or a compressed epidemic curve rather than a gradual rise in cases since all persons may be exposed at same time. Other clues indicative of a bioterrorism attack would be a geographic dispersal of cases downwind from a presumed release site or a natural vector-borne disease that lacks known vectors for that area. The organism may have evidence of genetic manipulation for increased virulence or antibiotic resistance.

Once cases have been identified as part of a bioterrorism event, the health department should investigate as it would any other outbreak. A case definition should be set, intensive surveillance for additional cases should begin, and data should be collected in an organized fashion, analyzed, and reviewed. Of immediate concern is a rapid delineation of time, place, and person to establish who was exposed in order to target prophylaxis and/or treatment or other countermeasures. Rapid epidemiology data collection forms might be developed and used as initial patients are seen in emergency rooms and urgent care clinics. A preestablished method of communicating with hospital emergency rooms and intensive care units could be used to facilitate reporting and two-way communication of suspect cases and case reports.

Following the detection of a bioterrorism event, a coordinated (federal, state, and local level) public health response will include rapidly deployable agent-specific surveillance methods targeted to (1) identify additional cases and predict the course of the event, (2) monitor compliance to and adverse outcomes from interventions, and to (3) monitor the health status of those in isolation and quarantine (if these measures are indicated). The term "situational awareness" can be loosely defined as monitoring the status of a public health emergency through interpretation of real-time surveillance and epidemiologic information.

As time and resources permit, a variety of surveillance systems and methods might be tapped to look for cases. For instance, once cutaneous anthrax had been confirmed in two New Jersey postal workers and the Trenton Postal Processing and Distribution Center closed, the New Jersey Department of Health and Human Services instituted "stimulated passive" hospital-based surveillance for inhalational anthrax. Infection control practitioners at 61 hospitals completed suspect case forms and a daily report of hospital emergency room visits and intensive care unit admissions for review and possible follow-up [40]. The health department also instituted enhanced statewide passive surveillance for inhalational anthrax and cutaneous anthrax by publishing case reporting criteria through press releases and on professional medical society and the health department Web sites. Similarly in Connecticut, after anthrax was identified in a 94-year-old female resident of a rural town, disease surveillance that had been initiated on September 11 and expanded after reports of the first US inhalational anthrax case was widened again. Retrospective reviews of death certificates, laboratory results data, medical examiner records, and postal worker absenteeism records were conducted. Intensive prospective surveillance began of hospital admissions, emergency room visits, and private physician reports. At each acute care hospital, a designated surveillance officer contacted the microbiology laboratory to look for any suspicious Gram stains or culture results. Suspect results were defined as any GPRs that had not been further identified or *Bacillus* species that had not yet been further typed. The surveillance officer also reviewed admissions of patients having any of five clinical syndromes (acute respiratory failure with pleural effusion; hemorrhagic enteritis with fever; a skin lesion characterized by vesicles, ulcer, or eschar; meningitis, encephalitis, or unexplained acute encephalopathy; or anthrax or suspected anthrax infection) and widened mediastinum on chest radiograph or consistent laboratory findings (gram-positive bacillus; *Bacillus* species from culture of a sterile site specimen; or hemorrhagic cerebrospinal fluid, pleural, or peritoneal fluid in patients without a traumatic lumbar puncture or event). Veterinarians were also queried by facsimile about deaths in animals with accompanying symptoms consistent with anthrax. Surveillance operated continuously around the clock for 3 weeks. No additional cases were found retrospectively or prospectively. Thus, the single Connecticut case was viewed as an isolated case [41].

During a multistate bioterrorism event, it would be helpful to rapidly develop a standardized data collection form and have a centralized repository of cases for epidemiological analysis purposes, as was done for the 2001 anthrax outbreak [36]. The CDC developed Web-based systems, such as that used during the SARS outbreak.

Rapid communication systems with clinicians, laboratorians, hospital emergency rooms, urgent care clinics, and hospital intensive care units should be developed. These would include both facsimile machines and electronic mail addresses, which can be collected in cooperation with professional societies and through joint preparedness activities. In pre-event situations these can be used to stimulate disease reporting by periodically sending out alerts of novel, but routine, infectious disease reports and outbreaks. In a postevent situation, the system can be used to announce case definitions, describe temporary reporting methods, provide crucial information on treatment and prophylaxis, and provide situational updates. Special telephone numbers and electronic mail addresses can be set up at the health department for receipt of reports and for questions from clinicians. Updates can be posted on public health agency Web sites, and news releases provided to the public media.

The potential for bioterrorism is not limited to the US; releases could occur anywhere. In addition, because of the rapid movement of people, a release in the US could result in cases occurring throughout the globe. The principles and methods discussed here can be modified as needed for local infrastructure and customs. Enhancing surveillance activities for the detection of bioterrorism will yield dividends in enhancing reporting for naturally occurring infectious diseases, including outbreaks and emerging infections. Collaboration with new surveillance partners, including veterinarians and law enforcement, will also enhance preparedness for natural public health threats like pandemic influenza.

Commenting on the anthrax events of 2001 and the role of public health and clinicians in bioterrorism preparedness and response, Gerberding, Hughes, and Koplan stated,

Knowledgeable clinicians, operating in the framework of a healthcare delivery system that is fully prepared to support the necessary diagnostic and treatment modalities to manage affected patients, and seamless linkages to local public health agencies will provide a strong foundation for detecting, responding to, and combating bioterrorism and other infectious disease threats to public health in the future [42].

This critical partnership between clinicians, laboratories, and public health is key to successful detection of bioterrorism that will hopefully lead to a healthier community outcome if bioterrorism were to strike at humans again.

References

1 Torok TJ, Tauxe RV, Wise RP, *et al*. A large community outbreak of salmonellosis caused by intentional contamination of restaurant salad bars. *JAMA* 1997;**278**:389–95.
2 Kolavic SA, Kimura A, Simons SL, Slutsker L, Barth S, Haley CE. An outbreak of *Shigella dysenteriae* type 2 among laboratory workers due to intentional food contamination. *JAMA* 1997;**278**:396–8.
3 Jernigan DB, Raghunathan PL, Bell BP, *et al*. and the National anthrax epidemiologic investigation team. Investigation of bioterrorism-related anthrax, United States, 2001: epidemiologic findings. *Emerg Infect Dis* 2002;**8**:1019–28.
4 Pavlin J. Epidemiology of bioterrorism. *Emerg Infect Dis* 1999;**5**:528–30.
5 Centers for Disease Control and Prevention. Biological and chemical terrorism: strategic plan for preparedness and response. Recommendations of the CDC strategic planning workgroup. *MMWR* 2000;**49**(RR-4):1–14.
6 Silk BJ, Berkelman RL. A review of strategies for enhancing the completeness of notifiable disease reporting. *J Public Health Manag Pract* 2005;**11**:191–200.

11

Surveillance for unexplained infectious disease-related deaths

Sarah Reagan, Ruth Lynfield, Kurt B. Nolte & Marc Fischer

Introduction

This chapter provides a framework for conducting surveillance for infectious disease related deaths, specifically in collaboration with medical examiners and coroners (MEs). This surveillance activity builds critical infrastructure to detect infections of public health importance, including reportable diseases, vaccine-preventable diseases, and emerging infections that may be missed by traditional public health surveillance. Topics covered in this chapter include:

1 Background and rationale for surveillance for potentially infectious disease related deaths
2 Infectious disease related death surveillance: Med-X system, Unexplained Death Project (UNEX)
3 Instituting infectious disease related surveillance
4 Challenges to implementing infectious disease related surveillance
5 Case studies

Background and rationale for surveillance

ME-based surveillance for infectious disease related deaths has the potential to identify public health threats, including bioterrorism, discover an emerging infection, recognize unique presentations of known pathogens, and detect reportable diseases that may be missed by more traditional public health reporting systems [1–8]. MEs have been involved in working on a number of infectious disease related public health issues. They were critical part-

ners in the identification of hantavirus pulmonary syndrome and West Nile viral encephalitis, in the investigation of bioterrorism-related anthrax, and in the recognition of pediatric influenza-associated mortality [9–14].

MEs investigate about 20% of all deaths in the US, including deaths that occur outside the hospital. ME jurisdictions are population-based and their investigations begin immediately after a death is reported. MEs have the legal authority to investigate sudden, unattended, and unexplained deaths. Clearly, some of these cases are due to infections of public health importance [4]; however, many MEs have not traditionally partnered with public health practitioners in evaluating these deaths because the MEs' practices generally focus on investigating intentional or accidental deaths.

Autopsies are inconsistently performed on possible infectious disease related deaths. When autopsies are performed, forensic pathologists are often satisfied with making general pathologic diagnoses (e.g., meningitis) and may not collect the appropriate specimens or pursue the laboratory evaluation needed to achieve an organism-specific diagnosis (e.g., meningitis due to *Neisseria meningitidis* or *Streptococcus pneumoniae*). This significantly limits their capacity to recognize and report infections to the appropriate public health agencies [4,15]. Because MEs are poorly integrated into the public health reporting system, they may not be aware of, or interested in, the implications that specific diagnoses may have for public health response (e.g., antimicrobial chemoprophylaxis, vaccination, contact tracing, or environmental investigations). Even if they are aware of these implications, they may not have sufficient resources or training to routinely pursue organism-specific diagnoses.

Collection of autopsy specimens for microbiologic evaluation is complicated by postmortem contamination of blood and tissues with intestinal, skin, oral, and environmental flora. However, by changing the timing of autopsies and improving sampling methods, the level of contamination can be reduced, allowing for more accurate microbiological diagnosis. Microbiological culture combined with immunohistochemical and molecular techniques are extremely useful for identifying organism-specific infectious diseases [2,8].

Infectious disease related death surveillance

Med-X system

The New Mexico Office of the Medical Investigator created a model pathology-based syndromic surveillance system, designed to recognize bioterrorism mortality and fatal infections of public health importance (Med-X). Med-X uses a set of antemortem signs/symptoms (e.g., fever) to identify cases that warrant an autopsy for infectious or toxin-related etiologies. Based on autopsy findings, a case is classified into a set of pathologic syndromes (e.g., community-acquired pneumonia). These syndromes provide an initial basis for reporting the case to the health department. The symptoms and syndromes are used to define a differential diagnosis and direct microbiologic testing. The pathologist attempts to achieve an organism-specific diagnosis in every infectious disease case [16].

In one year of surveillance, 150 cases in New Mexico were enrolled into Med-X and of these, 95 (63%) were classified as infectious disease deaths, 14 (9%) as toxin-related deaths, 31 (21%) as a non-infectious, non-toxin-related causes, and 10 (7%) as undetermined. An organism-specific diagnosis was made in 72 (76%) of the 95 infectious disease deaths. Thirty-four (47%) of the 72 Med-X cases with an organism-specific diagnosis were attributable to organisms that are notifiable by New Mexico public health standards, including invasive

Strep. pneumoniae (18 cases), *Strep. pyogenes* (7 cases), and *Haemophilus influenzae* (4 cases). Other reportable fatal infections identified included acquired immunodeficiency syndrome (1 case) and botulism (1 case) [16].

Unexplained death project

The Centers for Disease Control and Prevention's (CDC) Emerging Infections Program (EIP) began UNEX in 1994. This project established population-based surveillance for unexplained deaths and critical illnesses due to possible infectious etiologies in four EIP sites (i.e., California, Connecticut, Minnesota, and Oregon) [15,17]. UNEX was developed to address emerging infections that could present as a severe or fatal illness. Over the previous three decades, several new infectious diseases associated with life-threatening illness had been identified in the US, including Legionnaires' disease, toxic shock syndrome, acquired immunodeficiency syndrome, and hantavirus pulmonary syndrome. Each of these diseases was first identified following an outbreak investigation of unexplained severe illnesses. Subsequent studies found that each of these pathogens had been causing sporadic disease for years prior to their recognition. The delays in the recognition of new pathogens likely resulted from limitations in both surveillance methods and diagnostic techniques.

UNEX objectives were to (1) define the incidence and epidemiologic features of severe unexplained illness in selected populations in the US, (2) apply molecular diagnostic techniques to identify potential infectious etiologies for these illnesses, (3) develop and test a surveillance system for early detection of previously unrecognized life-threatening infectious agents, and (4) create a bank of clinical specimens for future testing as new pathogens and methods are identified.

A UNEX case patient was defined as a previously healthy resident of the surveillance area, 1–49 years old, who died or was admitted to an intensive care unit due to a possible infectious disease where no etiology was identified on initial testing. Hallmarks of an infectious disease included fever, leukocytosis, cerebrospinal fluid pleocytosis, or histopathologic evidence of an infection.

Exclusion criteria were extensive and included malignancy, diabetes, immunosuppressive therapy, HIV infection, or chronic cardiac, pulmonary, renal, hepatic, or rheumatologic conditions. Persons with toxic exposures, ingestions, trauma, or recent hospitalization were also excluded [15, 17].

Surveillance officers at participating EIP sites coordinated UNEX. Cases were detected through active (regular and frequent contact by the surveillance officer and the intensive care unit staff) and passive intensive care unit surveillance, and death certificate review. Epidemiologic and clinical data were obtained via chart abstraction and interviews with medical practitioners, patients, and their families. Previously collected clinical and pathologic specimens were obtained for additional diagnostic testing. Laboratory testing decisions were made based on the individual history of each case and the quality and quantity of available specimens. Over time, standard sets of syndrome-specific tests were developed and applied to all cases presenting with similar clinical features [15].

Beginning in 2000, the project decided that focusing on fatal cases and developing a more formal partnership with MEs would strengthen surveillance. The objectives were to (1) improve the identification of deaths potentially due to an infectious disease, (2) increase the proportion of potential cases submitted to autopsy, (3) obtain accurate and standardized data on all suspect cases in a timely manner, (4) collect adequate specimens for routine and reference testing for both toxins and infectious pathogens, and (5) implement state-of-the-art methods for autopsy-based microbiologic diagnosis. To accomplish this task, the program needed to (1) increase the pathologists' awareness of the importance of organism-specific diagnoses, (2) provide guidelines for the recognition of deaths that may be due to an infectious disease, (3) develop a standard approach to data collection, specimen retrieval, and diagnostic testing for cases of potential infectious etiology, and (4) provide adequate resources and training to allow forensic pathologists to safely and effectively perform autopsies on individuals with potentially transmissible infections.

A total of 227 fatal cases were submitted to UNEX between 1995 and 2003. Of 188 cases for which adequate specimens were available for evaluation, 53 (28%) had an etiology identified. *Strep. pneumoniae* and influenza viruses were the most frequent diagnoses. The change in surveillance methods affected the outcome of case evaluation. Only 15% of fatal cases identified before 2000 had an etiology identified, as compared to 34% of cases enrolled after that time ($p = 0.03$). A number of different factors led to this increase. One of the primary reasons has been a shift in laboratory methods. While immunohistochemical techniques contributed to the diagnosis of only 25% of cases identified prior to 2000, these contributed to the diagnosis of 64% of cases identified after that time. Reasons for this shift included an improvement in the adequacy of available autopsy specimens, a more systematic application of immunohistochemical assays to UNEX cases, and the optimization of key immunohistochemical assays, including *Strep. pneumoniae*, *Strep. pyogenes*, and *N. meningitidis*. In addition, the identification of an etiology had potential public health impact: 45% of explained cases were due to vaccine-preventable diseases, 30% were due to nationally notifiable infectious diseases, and 26% were initially reported as part of a cluster of unexplained illness and death [18].

In 2005–2006, UNEX initiated active "population-based" surveillance for all fatal infectious diseases in persons <50 years of age in selected EIP site ME jurisdictions. Specific activities included implementing guidelines for ME-based surveillance using the Med-X model and providing MEs with resources needed for specimen collection and laboratory evaluation of fatal infections. A protocol provides standardized methods for performing autopsies in the event of a potential infectious disease related death, and reporting cases to public health authorities.

Overall, this approach provides timely surveillance for deaths due to infections of public health importance (e.g., influenza) and increases the likelihood of recognizing bioterrorism-related deaths (e.g., anthrax). Furthermore, the system is designed to be exportable to multiple jurisdictions depending on existing infrastructure and available resources, and could be applied to multiple infectious disease syndromes based on public health priorities.

Instituting infectious disease related death surveillance

Objectives of population-based ME surveillance for infectious disease related deaths include the following:

1 Improve the identification of deaths potentially due to an infectious disease that fall under ME jurisdiction by:

a Establishing partnerships between public health agencies and MEs;

b Obtaining accurate and standardized data regarding infectious disease related deaths;

c Collecting a standardized set of specimens for routine and reference testing for both toxins and infectious pathogens;

d Implementing state-of-the-art methods for autopsy-based microbiologic evaluation to obtain an organism-specific diagnosis;

e Ensuring that infectious disease related deaths are reported to public health agencies in a timely manner.

2 Characterize the burden of infectious disease related deaths in a population by performing population-based surveillance for infectious disease related deaths that fall under ME jurisdiction.

Specific components of infectious disease related deaths surveillance

Case finding, categorization, and case definition

Cases should be identified through the routine death investigation, which may include death scene investigation, contact interviews, and/or medical record review. Fatal cases with antemortem signs/symptoms consistent with a possible infection should receive an autopsy (Box 11.1). At autopsy, cases should be categorized into selected pathologic syndromes associated with infectious disease related deaths as defined by the gross and histologic findings (Box 11.2). Cases autopsied for other reasons (e.g., unattended death with unknown symptom history) may still have pathologic syndromes suggestive of an infectious disease identified and should be brought into surveillance tracking. All cases with a defined pathologic syndrome should be enrolled into the surveillance activity. Pathologic syndromes should be used to classify the case for

> **Box 11.1 Antemortem signs/symptoms for identification of possible infectious disease related deaths.**
>
> • *Fever:* Documented antemortem fever ($\geq$38.0°C or $\geq$100.4°F) or the subjective perception of "fever" by the decedent or a caretaker.
> • *Acute encephalopathy or new onset seizures:* Acute mental status change (e.g., lethargy, confusion, disorientation, delirium, or coma) *or* acute onset of tonic-clonic seizure activity associated with the fatal illness.
> • *Acute flaccid paralysis or polyneuropathy:* Loss of voluntary power in muscles or symptoms involving many nerves associated with the fatal illness.
> • *New-onset jaundice:* Acute onset of yellow skin or sclerae.
> • *Acute diarrhea:* Recent history of acute watery diarrhea *or* grossly bloody stools without the presence of melena.
> • *New rash or soft tissue lesion:* Acute onset of any new rash (e.g., macular, papular, vesicular, pustular, petechial, hemorrhagic) *or* acute soft tissue lesion (e.g., eschar, cellulitis, necrotizing fasciitis, or abscess).
> • *Unexplained death:* Death of an individual <50 years of age where the past medical history, circumstances, and scene investigation provide inadequate diagnostic insight to establish the cause of death or to identify one of the signs/symptoms listed above. This category includes infants with a sudden infant death syndrome (SIDS) like presentation.

the initial report to the responsible public health agency.

Primary (minimum) specimen collection and laboratory evaluation

Results and specimens should be obtained from antemortem microbiologic and toxicologic sampling. Obtaining antemortem clinical samples for additional laboratory evaluation, if applicable, may be critical if the individual was hospitalized prior to death. In addition, a standardized set of autopsy specimens should be obtained and laboratory

Box 11.2 Pathologic syndromes associated with infectious disease related deaths.

Neurologic
- *Encephalitis:* Inflammation, necrosis, or hemorrhage in the brain parenchyma in a nonvascular, nontraumatic distribution.
- *Meningitis (including hemorrhagic):* Opacification, purulence, inflammation, or hemorrhage in the meninges without history of trauma or presence of traumatic injuries.

Respiratory
- *Pharyngitis, epiglottitis, or other upper airway infection:* Acute inflammation, edema, or membranes in the upper airways (i.e., between the pharynx and carina).
- *Bronchitis or bronchiolitis, acute:* Acute inflammation, edema, or membranes in the bronchi/bronchioles without a history or findings consistent with chronic obstructive pulmonary disease.
- *Pneumonia:* Interstitial or alveolar inflammation or consolidation that is community acquired (i.e., patient was not hospitalized within 2 weeks prior to onset of symptoms).
- *Diffuse alveolar damage:* Alveolar fibrin or hyaline membranes with reactive pneumocytes without a known noninfectious cause.
- *Mediastinitis, hemorrhagic:* Blood within the mediastinal soft tissues without history of trauma or presence of traumatic injuries.

Cardiac
- *Myocarditis:* Diffusely mottled myocardium *or* myocyte necrosis associated with acute inflammation in a nonvascular distribution.
- *Endocarditis:* Vegetation or significant thrombus on a cardiac valve.

Gastrointestinal
- *Acute hepatitis or fulminant hepatic necrosis:* Acute inflammation or necrosis in a pattern that is not characteristic of ethanol toxicity.
- *Enterocolitis:* Diffuse acute mucosal inflammation or ulcers of the colon not characteristic of inflammatory bowel disease *or* diffuse mucosal hemorrhage of the colon in a nonvascular distribution.

Dermatologic
- *Diffuse rash:* Any diffuse cutaneous lesions (e.g., macular, papular, vesicular, pustular, petechial, hemorrhagic).
- *Soft tissue lesion:* Discrete erythema, induration, purulence, necrosis, or acute inflammation of the soft tissues (e.g., ulcer, eschar, cellulitis, necrotizing fasciitis, or abscess).

Multisystem
- *Lymphadenitis:* Enlargement, acute inflammation, or necrosis of lymph nodes.
- *Sepsis syndrome:* Evidence of disseminated intravascular coagulation including cutaneous petechiae, adrenal hemorrhage, or fibrin thrombi in renal capillary loops.

evaluation should be pursued on all cases with a defined antemortem symptom or pathologic syndrome (Box 11.3) [19]. Initial testing should be performed through an established relationship between the MEs and local microbiology and toxicology laboratories. Additional specimens should be collected and applicable testing should be pursued at the discretion of the pathologist based on specific antemortem signs/symptoms and gross autopsy findings (Box 11.4). To encourage specimen collection and laboratory evaluation, public health agencies with adequate resources can develop and provide ME offices with a specimen collection kit, transport media, and an instructional quick ref-

erence guide to facilitate appropriate procedures. Public health laboratories can also provide diagnostic support that may not be readily available to MEs (e.g., viral culture, serologic assays) through other mechanisms.

Secondary laboratory evaluation

Secondary laboratory evaluation may be pursued at the discretion of the pathologist, together with public health staff and can be considered for cases (1) with a defined pathologic syndrome where no causative organism was identified by primary evaluation, (2) where the results of the primary

---

Box 11.3 Minimum specimen collection and testing to evaluate for infectious etiologies.

• Formalin-fixed tissues from all organs in stock jar
• Paraffin-embedded tissues/H&E stained slides from brain, heart, lung, liver, spleen, kidney, and organs that are thought to be diseased for routine histopathology
• Sterile percutaneous collection of femoral whole blood for bacterial culture (5 mL each inoculated into aerobic and anaerobic blood culture bottles)
• Additional femoral whole blood for toxicology (10 mL collected in a fluoridated tube; kept refrigerated).
• Serum for serologic assays (10 mL blood collected in a serum separator tube; centrifuged and separated in timely manner to minimize hemolysis)
• Nasopharyngeal swab for viral culture and/or PCR (1 swab placed into viral transport media; keep refrigerated).
• Urine for toxicology (20 mL; refrigerated in a toxicology container)
• Frozen tissue from primarily affected organ(s) for potential viral culture and/or PCR (1-cm cube(s) into small sterile containers)

Box 11.4 Additional specimen collection and testing to evaluate for infectious etiologies.

• *Fever (symptom) or respiratory syndrome (pathologic syndrome):* Sterile deep lung swabs for bacterial culture (1 swab from each lung placed into sterile culturette tubes)
• *Encephalopathy or new onset seizure (symptoms) or neurologic syndrome (pathologic syndrome):* Cerebrospinal fluid (10 mL in a sterile container) for bacterial culture/PCR
• *Rash/soft tissue lesion (symptom) or dermatologic syndrome (pathologic syndrome):* Excision of affected skin (full thickness) or soft tissue placed into formalin for routine histopathology *and/or* sterile deep swab of infected tissue or abscess for bacterial culture/PCR (1 swab placed into sterile culturette tube)
• *Acute diarrhea (symptom) or colitis (pathologic syndrome):* Stool for bacterial culture/toxin PCR (placed in a sterile container)
• Frozen tissue from brain, heart, lung, liver, spleen, and kidney for potential viral culture and/or PCR. (1-cm cubes into small sterile containers)

---

evaluation are ambiguous, or (3) where no primary microbiologic testing was performed. For some cases of specific public health importance, additional simultaneous microbiologic evaluation may also be warranted (e.g., unexplained clusters, suspected bioterrorism) [8,19]. Secondary testing may be performed through designated reference laboratories, including academic institutions, public health laboratories, and CDC and might include (1) immunohistochemistry on formalin-fixed, paraffin-embedded tissues, (2) viral culture of frozen tissues, (3) electron microscopy on tissues, (4) polymerase chain reaction (PCR) (including broad-range 16s rDNA PCR) on fixed tissues, frozen tissues, and/or normally sterile fluids (e.g., cerebrospinal fluid and pleural fluid), (5) serology (e.g., hepatitis B, hepatitis C, HIV), or (6) culture or PCR on antemortem-collected specimens.

Data flow, collection, and feedback

MEs should familiarize themselves with the list of notifiable diseases in their jurisdiction and report any such diagnoses to a public health agency. Any unusual clusters of potentially infectious deaths should also be reported. In addition, MEs and public health agencies should establish a dialogue to determine if cases with specific pathologic syndromes (e.g., diffuse rash, meningitis) and antemortem symptoms (e.g., fever and rash) or meeting other criteria should also be reported on a regular basis. Public health agencies should determine how they will respond to these case reports, and identify what additional data collection may be necessary. Suggested data flow includes timely feedback between involved agencies (Figure 11.1).

Public health agencies should work with MEs implementing this protocol to input the data

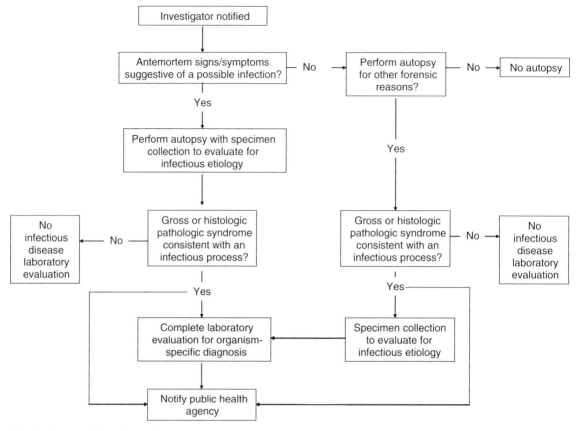

Fig 11.1 Suggested data flow and reporting.

recommended above (e.g., signs and symptoms, pathologic syndromes, laboratory testing performed, final diagnoses) into an electronic data management system in order to facilitate epidemiologic analysis and record-keeping [20]. MEs should be encouraged to adapt any existing electronic data management systems to collect these new variables. Public health agencies should advise MEs regarding additional data collection that may be necessary for any notifiable diseases or other types of cases identified.

In this vein, public health agencies may wish to establish a standardized set of additional epidemiologic, clinical, and laboratory data to collect on all infectious disease related deaths. The scope of data collected will likely vary considerably by case, depending on whether the individuals have been seen by the healthcare system for their illness and, if

hospitalized, the duration of their admission. These additional data will allow the public health agency to further characterize infectious disease related deaths, and guide any secondary laboratory evaluation. Public health agencies should work with their collaborating ME offices to determine which agency will be responsible for collecting supplemental data. Each agency involved should work together to establish standardized data-sharing policies, particularly for medical records, or reports from death scene investigations.

Biosafety

Implementation of appropriate biosafety precautions is critical for autopsy personnel who might handle human remains contaminated with infectious agents [1,21,22]. Infections can be transmitted at autopsies by percutaneous inoculation, splashes to unprotected mucosa, and inhalation of infectious aerosols. Basic protective measures should be maintained for all contact with potentially infectious materials. Additional precautions may be warranted for certain procedures that increase the risk for exposure. Specific recommendations for autopsy biosafety precautions are available in the published literature [1,22].

Analysis

Public health agencies should develop a routine data analysis strategy in partnership with participating ME offices. Regular periodic case reviews by a multidisciplinary infectious disease death review team can be valuable [4]. Detailed analyses of infectious disease related deaths by signs/symptoms, pathologic syndrome, final diagnosis, or other supplemental data (e.g., demographics, epidemiologic, or other clinical variables) should be performed on a regular basis to identify important characteristics of infectious disease related deaths and to uncover factors associated with identifying an organism-specific diagnosis. Overall numbers of cases can be used to calculate crude infectious disease related deaths mortality rates and specific mortality rates by age group, gender, and race/ethnicity or other demographic features. Additional analyses may include evaluating the contribution of infectious disease related deaths identified by MEs to the burden of reportable diseases in the public health jurisdiction.

Modifications to ME-based surveillance based on local resources

Depending on local resources and interest, public health agencies may opt to perform surveillance for a subset of pathologic syndromes that are felt to be of public health significance, or restrict the population under surveillance by age group (e.g., <50 years of age). These routine restrictions may help to optimize resources and not overburden staff. However, it is recommended that public health agencies partner with MEs to maintain the ability to be notified of specific cases of public health importance that may fall outside of the targeted age range or selected pathologic syndromes.

Challenges to implementing infectious disease related death surveillance

Public health agencies interested in implementing this surveillance activity should work to establish a close relationship with the ME offices in their jurisdiction. In order to assess the feasibility of surveillance for infectious disease related deaths, public health agencies should gather information regarding how candidate ME offices typically handle possible infectious disease related deaths. Important information might include what types of potential infectious deaths currently receive autopsies, what data are already routinely collected on possible infectious disease related deaths, including whether or not death scene investigators ask about antemortem signs/symptoms consistent with infection, and the extent of specimen collection and laboratory evaluation pursued for infectious disease related deaths. Next, public health agencies should clearly outline the expectations of this surveillance effort, identify what, if any, additional work would be required of the MEs beyond their current procedures, and identify funding resources that are available to offset the additional work and costs of MEs. Public health agencies should stress that these guidelines are not meant to recommend that MEs exceed their statutory scope and apply only to deaths that occur under ME jurisdiction.

Public health agencies should be aware of the obstacles to implementing ME-based surveillance. The quality and character of ME offices vary widely, and there may be vast differences in how evaluation of infectious disease related deaths are prioritized. Furthermore, ME offices may be challenged by having inadequate funding or staff for additional activities. ME office personnel will require training to implement recommendations for specimen collection and laboratory testing and data management. Death scene investigation procedures may also need to be modified to integrate obtaining information on antemortem signs/symptoms. Public health agencies may be able to offset these challenges by providing ME offices with support staff, supplies, and infrastructure. Selected ME jurisdictions

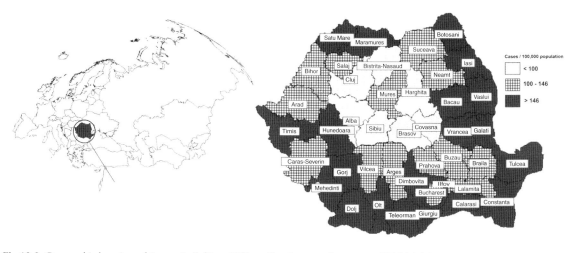

Fig 12.2 Geographic location of Romania (left) and TB notification rates by county, 2004 (right).

different cutoffs for defining success and failure [17].

TB mortality surveillance

Apart from reducing the burden of TB morbidity, global control also aims to reduce deaths associated with TB [18]. Mortality data are used to assess progress in this respect. TB mortality data are not the responsibility of disease surveillance bodies but are usually produced by the national vital registration authorities as part of the countries' mortality register. WHO collates these statistics from all countries into a database which is made available free of charge on the Internet [19]. An estimate of the completeness and the nationwide coverage is also given. TB mortality data allow the derivation of useful indicators such as proportional mortality due to TB and mortality rates, per total population or by age group, sex, and by site of disease (respiratory and nonrespiratory). For many countries, estimation of mortality trends is also possible. One limitation of these data is that TB deaths in HIV-infected patients may be classified as AIDS deaths. This results in an underestimation of TB deaths in areas of higher HIV prevalence.

The fact that these data do not derive from the national authority responsible for TB surveillance should be borne in mind when comparing notification and mortality rates. A relationship is nevertheless observed between mortality and notification rates. Outliers may be due to underreporting of TB deaths, undernotification of TB disease, or true differences in the mortality ratios due to underlying comorbidities and access to treatment.

Case study: Romania

Introduction

Romania is one of the largest Balkan countries of Europe, with an area of 237,500 km^2 and a population of 22 million (Figure 12.2). It comprises 42 administrative divisions or counties and has borders with five countries, of which two (Moldova Republic and Ukraine) once belonged to the Soviet Union. Romania became a democracy in the early 1990s in the wake of the dissolution of the Eastern socialist bloc. Radical economic reform followed, and today it is considered a lower middle-income country. Romania joined the EU in 2007.

TB epidemiology

In 2004, Romania reported 31,814 TB cases (rate: 146 cases per 100,000 population), an incidence much higher than other Balkan countries and similar to those observed in the FSU countries. Distal counties report higher rates of disease. TB notification rates and mortality rates increased until recently (Figure 12.3). Foreigners comprise a small fraction of TB cases and the proportion of TB cases seropositive for HIV is reportedly low (0.5% in

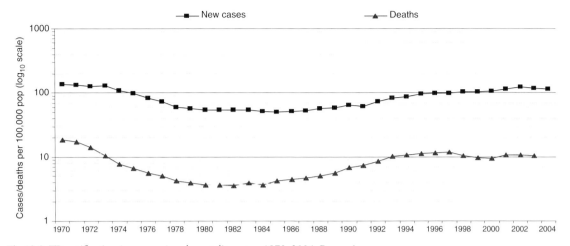

Fig 12.3 TB notification (new cases) and mortality rates, 1970–2004, Romania.

2003–2004). Despite the lack of reliable epidemiological data, it is widely believed that TB is highly prevalent among the Roma community as a result of lack of access to healthcare.

The frequency of drug resistance lies between the low levels observed in many western countries and higher ones in the FSU. In 2003–2004, primary MDR was 2.9% and secondary MDR was 10.7%. In 2003, 82% of previously untreated pulmonary culture positive cases were treated successfully, 4% died, 6% failed or had prolonged treatment, and 8% were lost to follow-up.

TB surveillance

For many years, the National TB Programme (NTP) of the Ministry of Health has been coordinated by a Central Unit located in the capital city. The Unit incorporates separate sections for surveillance, laboratory reference, and supervision and monitoring. A parallel TB program is operated through the penitentiary health system belonging to the Ministry of Justice. Cases in the penitentiary services are also notified to the NTP Central Unit (Figure 12.4).

In Romania, a network of over 200 TB dispensaries located at district and county level is responsible for both reporting and case management. District TB dispensaries diagnose and notify TB cases to the county health authorities which in turn report to the Central Unit by sending handwritten reports for each individual case. Until 2004, they also sent quarterly aggregate reports. Patient reports are entered on a case-based register maintained on computer at the Central Unit. This system is now

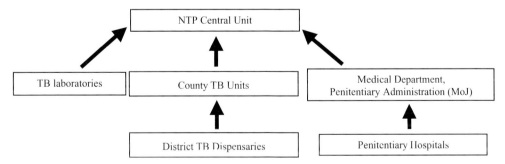

Fig 12.4 Simplified pathway for TB case reporting in the National TB Programme (NTP), Romania, 2006.

Table 12.4 Identified weaknesses in the TB surveillance system and recommended actions, Romania, 2005.

Points	Recommended actions	Situation by October 2006
Central Unit lacks technical staff for surveillance and is overwhelmed by routine work	Employ an epidemiologist to monitor implementation of the electronic surveillance system and other specialist tasks	Not in place
Electronic TB patient register in place but not validated	Conduct a user needs analysis and tailor system outputs at county and central level. Finalize, officially endorse TB surveillance manual, and use for training	Done
	Enter data on both old and new information systems to test consistency of system outputs ("parallel run")	Done
	Test the database module on treatment outcome using retrospective data for 2004 cases	Done (for 2005)
	Integrate reports from the penitentiary system in the electronic surveillance system	Done
Laboratory register is centered around examinations done rather than patients tested	Change to a patient-centered system, each row corresponding to a case, including all results for the tests done (smear microscopy and culture)	Done
Objectives of electronic laboratory reporting are not clear	Objectives of electronic laboratory reporting: decrease underreporting of bacteriological confirmed cases and improve completeness of information, avoiding delay in delivery of results to the patient's physician	Functioning
Treatment outcomes are assigned at 12 months	Only the first treatment outcome met by 12 months from start of treatment (or detection) should be reported. For MDR–TB, outcome also to be assessed at 24 months. All types of TB cases should be monitored	Done
Mortality data are underutilized	Obtain TB mortality data by age group, sex and country from the Institute of Statistics to verify and analyze regularly	Not done
Insufficient coordinated operational research; few publications in peer-reviewed journals	Retrospective data available at central level should be analyzed and published in scientific papers and used for public health action if possible. Priorities for operational research identified by consensus: (a) efficacy of observed treatment by general practitioners vs. by TB dispensaries (b) optimal length of hospital stay for noninfectious TB cases	Not yet started
Feedback of analyses to the peripheries is lacking	Publish progress reports on key program indicators on Internet yearly	Automated
External agencies make excessive demands for information	NTP should be considered the only official source of TB data, which can then be communicated as needed to other services and administrations	Not done

being phased out as a special program allowing Web-based notification from computer terminals situated in the dispensaries has been introduced. A parallel system of reporting from laboratories has been available for about 10 years but has only recently been computerized. In April 2005, a multidisciplinary team of experts reviewed all elements of the NTP, including the TB surveillance system [20]. The main findings and recommendations relating to surveillance are illustrative of the findings of an evaluation made on a system in the process of reform (Table 12.4).

Conclusion

The indicators of TB surveillance in Europe are more complete and reliable today than they were a decade ago. Nevertheless, there remains room for improvement in the uptake of European surveillance recommendations, particularly in the FSU and in the Balkan countries. Based on lessons learned from current TB surveillance in Europe, the following recommendations are made:

• Closer adherence to the European definitions for TB surveillance is necessary to provide a more accurate and comparable description of the TB situation between settings and over time.

• Data quality and utility can be improved through wider use of individual TB case reporting.

• Parallel TB case reporting from laboratories improves completeness of reporting.

• Special attention is needed to monitor problems in situations and population subgroups at increased risk of TB or of unfavorable outcome of TB disease.

• Surveillance of HIV serostatus among TB cases is important to assess the contribution of HIV to TB epidemiology and to advocate for joint case management of HIV/TB patients.

• The results of surveillance for drug resistance and treatment outcome monitoring should be used to ensure wider access to appropriate treatment, better patient management, and adherence to treatment; all are crucial elements for the interruption of TB transmission and in preventing the emergence of drug-resistant strains.

References

1 World Health Organization. Global tuberculosis control: surveillance, planning, financing. WHO Report. WHO/CDS/TB/2006.362. Geneva, Switzerland: WHO; 2006.

2 Raviglione MC, Sudre P, Rieder HL, Spinaci S, Kochi A. Secular trends of tuberculosis in western Europe. *Bull World Health Organ* 1993;**71**:297–306.

3 Coker RJ, Atun RA, McKee M. Health-care system frailties and public health control of communicable disease on the European Union's new eastern border. *Lancet* 2004;**363**:1389–92.

4 Raviglione M, Rieder HL, Styblo K, Khomenko AG, Esteves K, Kochi A. Tuberculosis trends in Eastern Europe and the former USSR. *Tuber Lung Dis* 1994;**6**:400–16.

5 Coninx R, Maher D, Reyes H, Grzemska M. Tuberculosis in prisons in countries with high prevalence. *BMJ* 2000;**320**:440–2.

6 Cox HS, Orozco JD, Male R, *et al.* Multidrug-resistant tuberculosis in Central Asia. *Emerg Infect Dis* 2004;**10**:865–72.

7 Ruddy M, Balabanova Y, Graham C, *et al.* Rates of drug resistance and risk factor analysis in civilian and prison patients with tuberculosis in Samara Region, Russia. *Thorax* 2005;**60**:130–5.

8 EuroTB. Surveillance of tuberculosis in Europe; 2006. Available from: www.eurotb.org. Accessed November 27, 2006.

9 Rieder HL, Watson J, Raviglione M, *et al.* Surveillance of tuberculosis in Europe. Recommendations of a Working Group of the World Health Organization (WHO) and the European Region of the International Union Against Tuberculosis and Lung Disease (IUATLD) for uniform reporting on tuberculosis cases. *Eur Respir J* 1996;**9**:1097–104.

10 Falzon D, Scholten J, Infuso A. Tuberculosis outcome monitoring—is it time to update European recommendations? *Euro Surveill* 2006;**11**(3):20–5.

11 EuroTB (CESES/KNCV) and the national coordinators for tuberculosis surveillance in the WHO European Region. Surveillance of tuberculosis in Europe. In: *Report on Tuberculosis Cases Notified in 1997.* Saint-Maurice, France: InVS; September 1999. Available from: www.eurotb.org. Accessed November 27, 2006.

12 Atun RA, Samyshkin YA, Drobniewski F, *et al.* Barriers to sustainable tuberculosis control in the Russian Federation health system. *Bull World Health Organ* 2005;**83**(3):217–23.

13 Coker R. Control of tuberculosis in Russia. *Lancet* 2001;**358**:434–5.

14 World Health Organization. Treatment of tuberculosis: guidelines for national programmes. Third edition. WHO/CDS/TB/2003.313. Geneva, Switzerland: WHO; 2003.

15 Schwoebel V, Lambregts-van Weezenbeek CSB, Moro ML, *et al.* Standardisation of anti-tuberculosis drug resistance surveillance in Europe. Recommendations of a WHO and IUATLD Working Group. *Eur Respir J* 2000;**16**:364–71.

16 Veen J, Raviglione MC, Rieder HL, *et al.* Standardized tuberculosis treatment outcome monitoring in Europe. Recommendations of a Working Group of the World Health Organization (WHO) and the European Region of the International Union Against Tuberculosis and Lung Disease (IUATLD) for uniform reporting by cohort analysis of treatment outcome in tuberculosis patients. *Eur Respir J* 1998;**12**:505–10.

17 World Health Organization. Guidelines for the programmatic management of drug-resistant tuberculosis. WHO/HTM/TB/2006.361. Geneva, Switzerland: WHO; 2006. Available from: http://whqlibdoc.who.int/publications/2006/9241546956_eng.pdf. Accessed September 13, 2006.

18 Dye C, Watt CJ, Bleed D, Hosseini SM, Raviglione M. Evolution of tuberculosis control and prospects for reducing tuberculosis incidence, prevalence, and deaths globally. *JAMA* 2005;**293**:2767–75.

19 World Health Organization. WHO mortality database. Available from: http://www.who.int/whosis/mort/en/index.html. Accessed October 10, 2006.

20 WHO Office for TB Control in the Balkans, Pneumology Institute "Marius Nasta" Romania. First review of the National Tuberculosis Programme in Romania. EUR/06/5068900. Copenhagen, Denmark: WHO; 2006.

13 Surveillance for healthcare-associated infections

Petra Gastmeier, Bruno Coignard & Teresa Horan

Healthcare-associated infections: epidemiology and impact

Epidemiology of healthcare-associated infections

Healthcare-associated infections (HAI) are those that are associated with hospital (nosocomial infections) or other medical treatment. They are by far the most common complication affecting hospitalized patients [1]. Currently, 5–10% of patients admitted to acute care hospitals acquire one or more infections; in special risk groups, the infection rate is even higher. Reasons why HAI are so common today include the following:

- Hospitals house large numbers of people who are severely ill and whose immune systems are often in a weakened state (e.g., stem cell or organ transplantation).
- The increasing use of outpatient treatment means that on average, people who are in the hospital are sicker.
- Many medical procedures (e.g., surgeries, catheter placement) bypass the body's natural protective barriers.
- Medical staff move from patient to patient, providing a way for pathogens to spread.

HAI are even more alarming in the twenty-first century as antimicrobial resistance spreads, and thus antimicrobial treatment becomes more difficult.

Four types of infections account for more than 80% of HAI: urinary tract, surgical site, respiratory tract, and bloodstream infections (BSI). The organisms causing HAI usually come from the patient's own flora (endogenous flora), but they can also come from contact with staff, contaminated instruments, and the environment. Therefore the proportion of HAI that could potentially be prevented by infection control measures applied under routine working conditions remains unclear. Experts estimate that at least 20–30% of all HAI are likely avoidable [2–4].

Impact of healthcare-associated infections

HAI add to functional disability, emotional stress, and in some cases, can lead to disabling conditions that reduce quality of life or cause death. Catheter-associated urinary tract infections are the most frequent HAI, but carry the lowest mortality and costs [5]. Surgical site infections (SSI) are second in frequency but are associated with substantial prolongation of length of stay. Pneumonia and BSI are less common, but are associated with much higher mortality and costs. Because of the morbidity, mortality, and economic consequences, measures to reduce HAI should have a high priority. Effective hospital infection control programs, guided by HAI surveillance, may be among the most cost-effective of all prevention programs in public health [6]. Hand hygiene is a critical tool in the prevention of HAI, and the use of standard and transmission-based precautions (airborne, droplet, contact) are important in reducing transmission of disease in a hospital setting (http://www.cdc.gov/ncidod/dhqp/gl_isolation_ptII.html).

Table 13.1 Advantages and disadvantages of various surveillance methods for healthcare-associated infections (HAI).

Method	Description	Advantage	Disadvantage	Example
Longitudinal survey (incidence)	Incidence rate: number of new HAI occurring during a given period divided by the number of patients at risk of acquiring HAI during the period	Provides a complete overview of the period from admission to discharge; also allows risk factor analyses	Requires substantial time and effort of trained personnel	Nosocomial MRSA cases per 100 patients admitted
Cross-sectional method (prevalence)	Prevalence rate: number of all currently active cases of disease within a specified population at risk during a specific period of time divided by the number of patients at risk during this period	Requires much less effort than a longitudinal survey and can be completed rapidly; primarily useful when a "quick and dirty" estimate is needed and there is insufficient time or resources to obtain a more useful measure of incidence	Because of the influence of the duration of infections, prevalence rates overestimate patients' risk of HAI. The number of patients included in point prevalence surveys is usually too small to obtain precise enough estimates of rates to detect important differences with statistical significance; repeated prevalence surveys may be informative	Prevalence of urinary tract infections in a given hospital on 1st of May
Prospective	Beginning from a starting point, patients are monitored, by repeated observations, for development of HAI	Uses all available resources of information for identifying HAI; if necessary, further investigations can be performed and interventions initiated	Requires substantial time and effort because the patients have to be evaluated repeatedly	Cases of BSI in a neonatal ICU
Retrospective	All newly occurring HAI are recorded for a specific observation period taking place sometime in the past (including risk factors)	Each patient chart has to be investigated only once, very useful in outbreak situations	The quality of the survey depends on the quality of clinical documentation; data may lack utility and timeliness if occurred too far in the past	Investigation of a cluster of SSI (outbreak analysis)
Active	Surveillance is performed by trained infection control personnel	Because of the more objective approach of the infection control personnel and their education in hospital epidemiology, a better surveillance quality can be expected	Requires infection control personnel	Surveillance of SSI by an infection control professional

Table 13.1 (*Continued*)

Method	Description	Advantage	Disadvantage	Example
Passive	Surveillance is performed by direct patient care staff	This allows consideration of information not documented in the patient's chart during case identification	For the direct patient care staff, surveillance is an additional task among many others, and cases are usually underreported. Inconsistent use or nonuse of standard case definitions is problematic	Surveillance of SSI following ambulatory surgery, as reported by the treating surgeon
Ongoing	Ongoing monitoring on a specific ward over many years	Provides a complete picture of the situation; stability of infection rates is likely to be achieved over time, and trends can be analyzed	Requires substantial time and effort	Cases of aspergillosis in a university hospital from year 2000 to present
Time-limited (rotating)	Limited or rotating surveillance periods on specific patient care areas (e.g., evaluation following an intervention or for periodic inspection for infection control problems)	Allows comprehensive surveillance activities even when limited infection control personnel are available	Random effects due to short surveillance periods may lead to mistaken conclusions, and infection control problems in other areas may be overlooked	Monitor urinary tract infections until reduction of an elevated infection rate is achieved

methods are widely used. Other investigators have developed methods for other patient groups, such as patients with bone marrow and stem cell transplantation, where days of neutropenia are used for adjustment [15].

In general, two major principles are used for adjustment of HAI data: Stratification (e.g., stratification of neonatal nosocomial infections rates according to birth-weight categories) and standardization (e.g., standardization of pneumonia rates according to ventilator utilization in ICU).

Feedback of surveillance data

One of the most important steps in surveillance is the dissemination of the data to those who will use them to prevent and control infections. A periodic reporting (e.g., at least twice a year) containing the calculated rates in comparison to data from former surveillance periods and a comparison to reference data is recommended. This information can be submitted to the head of the department surveyed. A presentation and interpretation of the data, to the department's staff, incorporating an interactive discussion can have a positive impact on improving infection control activities. Morbidity and mortality conferences of the departments may also be useful forums. Timeliness of these presentations is an important consideration, as outdated data tend to be less meaningful.

Surveillance of healthcare-associated infections in a facility

Selection of patient care areas

Hospital-wide surveillance is not recommended because the resources required to accurately monitor all HAI in the entire facility in an ongoing manner are generally not available [11]. Further, because many patient care areas house low-risk patients, this type of surveillance is inefficient. Therefore, surveillance personnel should concentrate their efforts on those patient groups at high risk for HAI (e.g., ICU patients, hematology–oncology patients, transplant patients, and postoperative patients) and on those areas with suspected or existing infection control problems. With certain infectious disease outbreaks, such as the severe acute respiratory syndrome (see Chapter 39, Part 1) or H5N1 avian influenza, surveillance for signs of infection should be performed among healthcare workers taking care of patients with those infections.

Selection of infection types

To perform surveillance cost-effectively, surveillance activities should concentrate on the most relevant types of HAI for the selected patient groups (e.g., SSI for postoperative patients, pneumonia and BSI for ICU patients). The frequency of these infections should be high enough to calculate meaningful infection rates, and morbidity, mortality, and related cost should be substantial.

Surveillance of healthcare-associated infections on a national level

The US system

NNIS was developed by CDC in 1970 to monitor the incidence of hospital-based HAI and their associated risk factors and pathogens. It was a voluntary, confidential reporting system that has guided infection-control efforts in hospitals across the US and around the world, and was also the only national source of systematically gathered data on hospital infections [1]. NNIS grew from about 60 hospitals at its inception to more than 300 at its peak at the turn of the century. Monthly reporting by this nonrandom sample of US hospitals allowed comparative infection rates to be established through the use of standardized case definitions and data collection methods, and computerized data entry and analysis.

In 2005, the NNIS system underwent a major redesign as a Web-based monitoring system. Renamed the National Healthcare Safety Network

(NHSN), it is available for use by all US hospitals, long-term care facilities, outpatient dialysis clinics, surgicenters, and other healthcare delivery organizations [16]. In addition to the traditional focus of the NNIS system, NHSN covers new areas of patient safety monitoring and evaluation, including adherence to infection prevention practices (process measures such as influenza vaccination rates of employees) and healthcare personnel safety. CDC's Division of Healthcare Quality Promotion manages NHSN and publications on the Division's Web site, including the protocols and definitions used in the system, descriptions of participating facilities, and current trends in the types of outcome and process measures that are monitored. For more information about NNIS and NHSN, refer to the Web site: www.cdc.gov/ncidod/dhqp/index.html.

The French system

In France, HAI surveillance activities were first developed at the regional level. Five regional infection control coordinating centers (Centre de Coordination de la Lutte contre les Infections Nosocomiales [CClin]) were created in 1992 and progressively five surveillance modules were developed: surgical site infections (SSI), intensive care units (ICU), blood and body fluids exposure (BBFE), bloodstream infections (BSI), and multiresistant bacteria (MRB). Participation is voluntary and modules are proposed each year to healthcare facilities.

The first two modules adapted the methods of the US NNIS system. Using CDC definitions for HAI, they produce standardized indicators (e.g., SSI rates adjusted by the NNIS index, pneumonia rates according to ventilator utilization). However, denominator data collection in France is patient-based and not aggregated by unit as in the NNIS system (e.g., risk factors for each ICU patient, such as type and duration of invasive device used, are documented). The third module adapted the methods of the US National Surveillance System for Healthcare Workers. The last two modules are laboratory-based and are targeted on MRB. For each module, data are collected, entered, and analyzed by participating healthcare facilities using dedicated software. They are sent to CClin, which validates and aggregates them into a regional database used for benchmarking purposes.

Beginning in 2001, HAI surveillance activities have been coordinated by the National Institute for Public Health Surveillance (Institut de Veille Sanitaire [InVS]) through the Nosocomial Infection Early Warning, Investigation, and Surveillance Network (Réseau d'Alerte, d'Investigation et de Surveillance des Infections Nosocomiales [RAISIN]). Regional surveillance methods have been harmonized and data are aggregated into a national database. In 2003, the SSI, ICU, BBFE, BSI, and MRB national networks included data from 272, 125, 263, 150, and 549 healthcare facilities, respectively [17]. Yearly national HAI surveillance reports are available on the RAISIN Web site (http://www.invs.sante.fr/raisin/). Current efforts focus on facilitating data collection and on developing new indicators such as the standardized incidence ratio [18].

In addition, three national prevalence surveys were conducted in 1990, 1996, and 2001 [19–21] in order to promote HAI surveillance A fourth national prevalence survey was underway in 2006. The 2001 survey included data from 1533 healthcare facilities and 305,656 patients. HAI prevalence was 7.5%. The most frequent infections were UTI (40%), skin and soft tissue infections (11%), pneumonia (10%), and SSI (10%).

Finally, as prevalence or incidence surveys do not cover all hospitals or HAI, a national nosocomial infections' notification system was implemented in August 2001. Its objectives are to detect unusual events, to promote outbreak investigation and control, and to reinforce recommendations. Healthcare facilities have to notify HAI to CClin, local health departments, and InVS if they are related to the following criteria: (1) rare or unusual infections, based on microorganism characteristics (including resistance), the infection site, a medical device/product, or medical malpractices; (2) infections leading to death; (3) airborne or waterborne infections (e.g., legionellosis); (4) otherwise reportable diseases (e.g., tuberculosis). The system is designed to detect the unusual events, and there is no restrictive list of events. The decision to notify is based on the knowledge of infection control practitioners. The notification form summarizes investigations and control measures and allows requests for assistance [22]. CClin and InVS provide support to hospitals for outbreak investigation when

necessary, and InVS analyzes national data in order to detect unusual trends. The system is now well accepted and has enabled the early detection and control of several regional and national outbreaks [23–25].

The German system

The field of hospital epidemiology and infection control in Germany has undergone changes in recent years. In addition to the traditional focus on disinfection and sterilization, epidemiological activities in the field of HAI have become important for many hospitals. In order to measure these infections, a surveillance system was established in Germany in 1997, which is known under the acronym KISS (Krankenhaus-Infektions-Surveillance-System) [26]. The system is based on the experiences and principles of the US NNIS system, but takes into account the local issues of participating hospitals in Germany. The hospitals can select among seven KISS components which focus on the following areas: ICU, neonatal intensive care patients with very low birth weight, hematology–oncology patients, surgical patients, non-ICU patients with vascular or urinary catheters, as well as outpatients with ambulatory operations. An additional module was developed for the surveillance of MRSA in hospitals.

KISS data may be used for quality management by individual hospitals and for benchmarking between hospitals. The time spent for surveillance in each hospital for one of the modules averages between 2 and 3 hours per week, depending on the size of the unit or department and the number of surgical procedures selected for surveillance. Data entry is Web-based. Cost-effectiveness is likely associated with activities within the KISS framework, as HAI reduction rates between 20 and 30% for individual surveillance components have been achieved [27].

International comparison of surveillance data

European networks of surveillance systems

During the 1990s, several European countries began to establish national or regional networks for

Table 13.2 List of European and US national surveillance systems.

Country	Acronym and name of the surveillance system	Web site
Belgium	NSIH, National Surveillance of Infections in Hospitals	www.nsih.be
Finland	Finnish Hospital Infection Program (SIRO)	www.ktl.fi/siro
France	RAISIN, Réseau d'Alerte, d'investigations et de Surveillance des Infectiones Nosocomiales	www.invs.sante.fr/raisin/
Germany	KISS, Krankenhaus-Infektions-Surveillance-System	www.nrz-hygiene.de
The Netherlands	PREZIES, Preventie Ziekenhusinfecties door surveillance	www.prezies.nl
UK-England	NINSS, Nosocomial Infection National Surveillance System	www.hpa.org.uk
US	NHSN (formerly NNIS), National Healthcare Safety Network	www.cdc.gov/ncidod/dhqp.index.html

surveillance of nosocomial infections. Most of these networks were based on the NNIS model. The European Union sponsored a project called Hospitals in Europe Link for Infection Control through Surveillance (HELICS). This was an international partnership of national and regional networks organized by the network coordinators, and started in 1994 [28]. The objectives of this project were:
• To standardize surveillance methods
• To promote and assist the development of new networks
• To improve the way results are used in feedback, prevention, and cost containment
• To promote the integration of surveillance of HAI with routine data collection

Subsequently, the HELICS project became part of the larger IPSE (Improving Patient Safety in Europe) project. A European database was established. Data for SSI for 2004 can be found at the IPSE Web site (http://ipse.univ-lyon1.fr).

Table 13.2 lists the European and US national surveillance systems and their Web sites.

The European Antimicrobial Resistance Surveillance System (EARSS; http://www. rivm.nl/earss) is a European network of national surveillance systems, providing data on antimicrobial resistance of selected pathogens (*Staphylococcus aureus*, *Enterococcus faecalis*, *E. faecium*, *Pseudomonas aeruginosa*, *Klebsiella pneumoniae*, *Escherichia coli*, *Streptococcus pneumoniae*). The data are useful for monitoring resistance trends within a country, but possibilities of international comparisons are limited, because the system does not feed back adjusted rates, and the number of participating laboratories varies greatly from one country to another.

Possibilities and limitations of international comparison of surveillance data

International comparisons yield interesting insights regarding quality and structure of care, reaching into the field of HAI prevention (e.g., the influence of different national approaches to prevent the spread of MRSA). Therefore, the exchange of experiences of national surveillance systems should be encouraged. However, the interpretation of differences of HAI rates should be done very carefully. Differences in healthcare systems, legal and cultural aspects, as well as differences in the methods of the surveillance systems may have an enormous influence on rates, for example, a comparison of SSI rates between Belgium and the Netherlands for herniorrhaphies [29]. The difference in SSI rates (0.4% in the Netherlands versus 1.2% in Belgium) is not explained by differences in the distribution of risk factors. The shorter hospital stay in the Netherlands (4 days) versus Belgium (6 days), the more effective postdischarge surveillance in Belgium, and the fact that more than two-thirds of the detected infections occurred after the first postoperative week may account for most of the observed difference.

Decrease of healthcare-associated infections by surveillance

Individual hospital success stories

Various studies have demonstrated that HAI can be significantly reduced by surveillance together with appropriate intervention methods in hospitals that are interested in quality management activities [2,3,30]. However, often these success stories

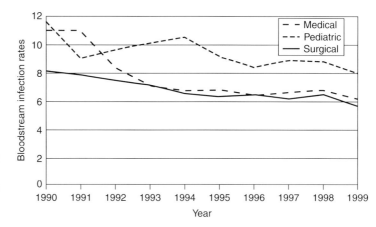

Fig 13.1 Trends in central line-associated bloodstream infection rates per 1000 central line-days by type of intensive care unit, National Nosocomial Infections Surveillance system, 1990–1999 [31].

emanate from hospital departments with very high initial infection rates, suggesting that a regression to the mean effect cannot be excluded.

National success stories

The NNIS system examined risk-adjusted HAI used by its participating hospitals and found that decreases in risk-adjusted infection rates occurred at all three body sites (respiratory tract, urinary tract, and bloodstream) monitored in ICUs [31] (Figure 13.1). The Dutch surveillance system (PREZIES) demonstrated a significant reduction of SSI rates from 50 hospitals [32]. Comparing the SSI rates from the first and the fourth year of participation, they showed a 31% reduction; between the first and

the fifth year, the reduction effect was even greater, at 57%.

Figure 13.2 shows the reduction of ventilator-associated pneumonia rates and central vascular catheter associated BSI rates in 150 ICUs participating for at least 36 months in Germany's KISS, and the reduction of SSI in 133 surgical departments participating in KISS for at least 36 months [27].

Cost-effectiveness of surveillance for healthcare-associated infections

Infection control professionals in hospitals usually perform HAI surveillance activities; the workload varies but in general is substantial. Several sources, including the microbiology laboratory, patient

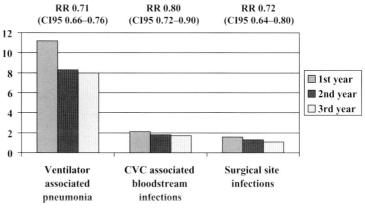

Fig 13.2 Reduction of ventilator associated pneumonia rates and central venous catheter associated bloodstream infection rates in 150 ICU participating for at least 36 months in KISS and reduction of surgical site infections in 133 surgical departments participating in KISS for at least 36 months [27].

167

care area information, and medical records, are searched. Beyond data collection, a major effort of infection control professionals should be timely data analysis and dissemination to support infection prevention collaborations with patient care areas. The cost-effectiveness of surveillance depends on the following factors:

• Initial infection rate (e.g., if the infection rate is above the 75th percentile, reduction will have important cost-saving implications)
• Economic importance of the type of infection selected for surveillance (e.g., 6 days prolongation of ICU stay in the case of ventilator-associated pneumonia, 3 days for central venous catheter associated BSI, and varying periods for SSI)
• Size of the patient care department and the hospital
• Intensity and frequency of data analysis and reporting
• Effectiveness of infection prevention programs
Assuming liberal costs, conservative benefits, and an infection control program capable of reducing infections by 12.5–25.0%, Wenzel was able to demonstrate cost-effectiveness for HAI surveillance [6].

Computer assistance

Computers are useful in many stages of surveillance. Usually, computerized data are used to identify a set of clinical factors or outcomes, signaling the possible presence of a HAI (e.g., use of antibiotics, isolation of unusual pathogens) that can be investigated further by human intervention. Although this approach typically involves going to the medical record to verify the event, it is much less costly because only a small proportion of charts needs to be reviewed. These types of warning signals may be derived from automated transfer of electronic microbiology data to the infection control office. Other investigators have used automated systems to facilitate surveillance by working with antibiotic prescriptions, ICD-9 codes, and other types of data available from various databases [33–37]. Denominator data may also be available electronically in existing databases, such as days of mechanical ventilation from a respiratory therapy database. In addition, Web-based systems for data entry allow an immediate feedback of infection rates to the individual hospitals, thus facilitating a prompt response to HAI problems.

Voluntary, confidential surveillance systems versus mandatory public reporting

In the US, state-based mandatory public reporting of HAI is a very controversial issue, but consumers, insurance companies, and other groups are demanding that such an effort be instituted to track healthcare facility performance. A systematic literature review was performed to determine whether public reporting systems improve healthcare performance and whether there was evidence of the effectiveness of private reporting systems to reduce HAI [38]. The investigators reported that published studies do not provide strong support for the effectiveness of public reporting of HAI as a means to improve HAI prevention and control practices or to prevent the occurrence of HAI. The key questions for mandatory public reporting of HAI remain: Will the information mislead or confuse, rather than empower consumers? Will there be an increased motivation for clinicians and hospital administrators to address HAI reduction that leads to safer care and fewer HAI? In France, public reporting began in 2006 with a composite indicator of infection control organizations, resources, and actions. Two further indicators were added in 2007: alcohol-based handrub solution consumption and existence of SSI surveillance. Information on the French public reporting Web site is at: http://www.sante.gouv.fr/htm/dossiers/nosoco/tab_bord/accueil.htm.

Future

New and sophisticated analytical tools are needed in both public health and hospital infection control programs to improve how surveillance is conducted and results are disseminated. Alternative approaches include adopting simpler methods and more objective definitions, using sampling and estimation, substituting information in computer databases for manually collected data, and increasing surveillance for process measures with known prevention efficacy [16]. The ideal system will include analysis tools that automatically identify, on different time and geographical scales, unusual and interesting patterns from time slices of raw data. Data-mining systems represent the first generation of these tools [39], although they currently suffer from the lack of available standardized data systems from which all pertinent data can be readily extracted. However, as the electronic medical record becomes more robust, such approaches will greatly assist HAI surveillance efforts.

References

1 Burke J. Infection control—a problem for patient safety. *N Engl J Med* 2003;**348**:651–6.

2 Haley RW, Culver DH, White JW, *et al.* The efficacy of infection control programs in preventing nosocomial infections in US hospitals. *Am J Epidemiol* 1985;**212**:182–205.

3 Harbarth S, Sax H, Gastmeier P. What proportion of nosocomial infections is preventable? A tentative evaluation of published reports. *J Hosp Infect* 2003;**54**:258–66.

4 Grundmann H-J, Bärwolff S, Schwab F, *et al.* How many infections are caused by transmission in intensive care units? *Crit Care Med* 2005;**33**:946–51.

5 Gastmeier P, Kampf G, Wischnewski N, *et al.* Prevalence of nosocomial infections in representatively selected German hospitals. *J Hosp Infect* 1998;**38**:37–49.

6 Wenzel RP. The Lowbury Lecture: the economics of nosocomial infections. *J Hosp Infect* 1995;**31**:79–87.

7 Deming WE. *Out of the Crisis.* Cambridge, MA: Center for Advanced Engineering Study; 1986.

8 Horan T, Gaynes R. Surveillance of nosocomial infections. In: Mayhall C (ed.), *Hospital Epidemiology and Infection Control.* Atlanta, GA: Lippincott Williams & Wilkins; 2004:1659–89.

9 Miller P, Johnson J, Karchmer T, Hoth J, Meredith J, Chang M. National nosocomial infection surveillance system: from benchmark to bedside in trauma patients. *J Trauma* 2006;**60**:98–103.

10 Horan T, Emori T. Definitions of nosocomial infections. In: Abrutyn E (ed.), *Saunders Infection Control Reference Service.* Philadelphia: WB Saunders Company; 1998:17–21.

11 McKibben L, Horan T, Tokars J, *et al.* Guidance on public reporting of healthcare-associated infections: recommendations of the Healthcare Infection Control Practices Advisory Committee. *Infect Control Hosp Epidemiol* 2005;**26**:580–7.

12 McGeer A, Campbell B, Emori T, *et al.* Definitions of infection for surveillance in long-term care facilities. *Am J Infect Control* 1991;**19**:1–7.

13 Freeman J, McGowan JJ. Day-specific incidence of nosocomial infection estimated from a prevalence survey. *Am J Epidemiol* 1981;**114**:888–901.

14 Gastmeier P, Bräuer H, Sohr D, *et al.* Converting incidence and prevalence data of nosocomial infections: results from eight hospitals. *Infect Control Hosp Epidemiol* 2001;**22**:31–4.

15 Dettenkofer M, Ebner W, Bertz H, *et al.* Surveillance of nosocomial infections in adult recipients of allogeneic and autologous bone marrow and peripheral blood stem-cell transplantation. *Bone Marrow Transplant* 2003;**31**:795–801.

16 Tokars J, Richards C, Andrus M, *et al.* The changing face of surveillance for healthcare-associated infections. *Clin Infect Dis* 2004;**39**:1347–52.

17 Poirier Bègue E, Chaib A, Georges S, Coignard B. pour le Réseau d'Alerte d'Investigation et de Surveillance des Infections Nosocomiales (RAISIN). Caractéristiques des établissements de santé participants aux réseaux de surveillance des infections nosocomiales du Raisin en 2003 [Poster]. *Journées de veille sanitaire, Paris* November 29–30, 2005. Available from: http://www.invs.sante.fr/publications/2005/jvs_2005/poster_16.pdf. Accessed April 23, 2007.

18 Rioux C, Grandbastien B, Astagneau P. The standardized incidence ratio as a reliable tool for surgical site infection surveillance. *Infect Control Hosp Epidemiol* 2006;**27**:817–24.

19 Anonymous. Enquête nationale de prévalence des infections nosocomiales en France : Hôpital Propre. BEH no. 39/1993; 1993.

20 Anonymous. Enquête nationale de prévalence des infections nosocomiales, 1996. BEH no. 36/1997; 1997. Available from: http://www.invs.sante.fr/beh/1997/9736/beh_36_1997.pdf. Accessed April 23, 2007.

21 Anonymous. Deuxième enquête nationale de prévalence des infections nosocomiales, France, 2001. Surveillance nationale des maladies infectieuses, 2001–2003. Institut de veille sanitaire; 2005. Available from: http://www.invs.sante.fr/publications/2005/snmi/infections_noso_enquete.html.

22 Coignard B, Poujol I, Carbonne A, *et al.* Le signalement des infections nosocomiales, France, 2001–2005 [Nosocomial infection mandatory notification, France, 2001–2005]. BEH no. 51-52/2006; December 26, 2006. Available from: http://www.invs.sante.fr/beh/2006/51_52/index.htm.

23 Coignard B, Vaillant V, Vincent J, *et al.* Infections sévères à Enterobacter sakazakii chez des nouveau-nés ayant consommé une préparation en poudre pour nourrissons,

France, octobre à décembre 2004. BEH no. 2-3/2006; January 17, 2006. Available from: http://www.invs.sante .fr/beh/2006/02_03/index.htm.

24 Naas T, Coignard B, Carbonne A, *et al.* VEB-1 extended-spectrum ß-lactamase-producing *Acinetobacter baumannii*, France. *Emerg Infect Dis* 2006;**12**:1214–22.

25 Tachon M, Cattoen C, Blanckaert K, *et al.* First cluster of *C. difficile* toxinotype III, PCR-ribotype 027 associated disease in France: preliminary report; 2006. Available from: http://www.eurosurveillance.org/ew/2006/060504 .asp#1.

26 Gastmeier P, Geffers C, Sohr D, Dettenkofer M, Daschner F, Rüden H. Five years working with the German Nosocomial Infection Surveillance System KISS. *Am J Infect Control* 2003;**31**:316–21.

27 Gastmeier P, Geffers C, Brandt C, *et al.* Effectiveness of a nationwide nosocomial infection surveillance system for reducing nosocomial infections. *J Hosp Infect* 2006;**64**:16–22.

28 Mertens R, van den Berg J, Fabry J, Jepsen O. HELICS: a European project to standardise the surveillance of hospital acquired infection 1994–1995. *Euro Surveill* 1996;**1**:28–30.

29 Mertens R, Van den Berg JM, Veerman-Brenzikofer MLV, Kurz X, Jans B, Klazinga N. International comparison of results of infection surveillance: The Netherlands versus Belgium. *Infect Control Hosp Epidemiol* 1994;**15**:574–80.

30 Gastmeier P. Nosocomial infection surveillance and control policies. *Curr Opin Infect Dis* 2004;**17**:295–301.

31 Gaynes R, Richards C, Edwards J, *et al.* Feeding back surveillance data to prevent hospital acquired infection rates. *Emerg Infect Dis* 2001;**7**:295–8.

32 Geubbels E, Nagelkerke N, Mintjes-de Groot A, Vandenbroucke-Grauls C, Grobbee D, de Boer A. Reduced risk of surgical site infections through surveillance in a network. *Int J Qual Health Care* 2006;**18**:127–33.

33 Evans RS, Burke JP, Classen DC, *et al.* Computerized identification of patients at high risk for hospital—acquired infection. *Am J Infect Control* 1992;**20**:4–10.

34 Hirschhorn L, Currier J, Platt R. Electronic surveillance of antibiotic exposure and coded discharge diagnoses as indicators of postoperative infection and other quality assurance measures. *Infect Control Hosp Epidemiol* 1993;**14**:21–8.

35 Bouam S, Girou E, Brun-Buisson C, Karadimas H, Lepage E. An intranet-based automated system for the surveillance of nosocomial infections: prospective validation compared with physicians' self-reports. *Infect Control Hosp Epidemiol* 2003;**24**:51–5.

36 Pokorny L, Rovira A, Baranera M, Gimeno C, Alonso-Tarres C, Vilarasau J. Automatic detection of patients with nosocomial infection by a computer-based surveillance system: a validation study in a general hospital. *Infect Control Hosp Epidemiol* 2006;**27**:500–3.

37 Leth R, Moller J. Surveillance of hospital-acquired infections based on electronic hospital registries. *J Hosp Infect* 2006;**62**:71–6.

38 McKibben L, Fowler G, Horan T, Brennen P. Ensuring rational public reporting systems for healthcare—associated infections: systematic literature review and evaluation recommendations. *Am J Infect Control* 2006; **34**:142–9.

39 Brosette S, Sprague A, Jones W, Moser S. A data mining system for infection control surveillance. *Methods Inf Med* 2000;**39**:303–10.

14 Surveillance for methicillin-resistant *Staphylococcus aureus* (MRSA) in the community

R. Monina Klevens, Kathleen Harriman & Melissa A. Morrison

Introduction

Staphylococcus aureus is a formidable human pathogen; it has caused infections throughout history (e.g., there are references to boils in the Bible) and developed mechanisms to evade specific therapy. Penicillin-resistant strains of *S. aureus* were reported in hospitalized patients in 1942 [1], just one year after penicillin was used in clinical care. Methicillin-resistant *S. aureus* (MRSA) was first identified in the United Kingdom in 1961, just one year after this antibiotic was introduced [2,3]. In 1968, a healthcare-associated (HA) MRSA outbreak was reported in the United States (US) [4], and since then the prevalence of HA-MRSA in the US and many other countries has rapidly increased. Surveillance for nosocomial infections, including MRSA, is discussed in Chapter 13.

US reports of MRSA in the community first appeared among injection drug users in the early 1980s [5]. During the mid- to late-1990s, MRSA outbreaks were reported among diverse populations, including Native Americans [6], sports teams [7], prison inmates [8], and child care attendees [9], typically with little or no previous contact with the healthcare system. In 1999, four children in Minnesota and North Dakota died from community-associated (CA) MRSA [10]. Subsequently, numerous cases of MRSA occurring in the community, in previously healthy individuals have been reported. Although about 80% of these infections are skin and soft tissue disease [11], some cases have been severe, including necrotizing pneumonia, osteomyelitis, septic thrombophlebitis, necrotizing fasciitis,

and other syndromes [12–14]. By 2005, MRSA strains of community origin were being seen in infections associated with healthcare settings [15].

Surveillance projects in a variety of geographic areas using a variety of methods have been initiated to understand the epidemiology of CA-MRSA, including disease incidence, prevalence, risk factors, and trends. These data are being used to develop prevention and control activities. This chapter will discuss how surveillance activities were initiated in the US and the advantages and disadvantages of different types of surveillance. Lessons learned from the development of surveillance systems for a rapidly emerging infection like CA-MRSA can be applied to other emerging diseases.

Components of CA-MRSA surveillance

Case definition

A standardized case definition ensures that cases reported are comparable. The development of a case definition for MRSA in the community starts with a determination of the data needs, and then is adjusted based on resources available for conducting surveillance (see Table 14.1). Epidemiologic case definitions for MRSA in the community have differentiated MRSA cases from those in healthcare settings by ruling out exposures to healthcare. The case definition used by the US Centers for Disease Control and Prevention (CDC) and collaborators since 2000, begins with identifying patients with a positive culture for MRSA. Among those patients the presence of any of the

Table 14.1 Comparison of methods used in surveillance for methicillin-resistant *Staphylococcus aureus* (MRSA) in the community.

	Population-based	Time-limited	Sentinel site	Antibiogram
Case definition	A resident of the catchment area from whom MRSA has been isolated	Patient with MRSA infection of specified severity during a specified period of time	An individual from whom MRSA has been isolated, identified by a participating site	A positive MRSA culture
Case ascertainment	Surveillance personnel contact laboratories and or healthcare providers to identify cases	Laboratory personnel or healthcare providers report cases to the health department	Facility personnel report cases to the health department	Laboratory personnel report to the health department
Denominator	Population of the catchment area	Population of the catchment area included in the reporting requirement	Varies; examples: number of individuals seen at a facility; number of cultures collected at that facility; number of all *S. aureus* infections at that facility	Number of cultures; for example, the number of MRSA isolates out of all *S. aureus* isolates
Numerator	MRSA or CA-MRSA cases identified in a defined period	Number of CA-MRSA cases identified in the defined period	Number of CA-MRSA cases	Number of MRSA cultures
Analysis	Incidence rate: number of MRSA or CA-MRSA infections/100,000 population per year. Can adjust for age and race	Incidence rate: number of CA-MRSA (or MRSA) infections/100,000 population per time period	Prevalence of CA-MRSA (or MRSA) among individuals receiving medical care at specific facilities	Prevalence of methicillin resistance among isolates tested
Resources required	Significant	Moderate	Moderate	Minimal
Strengths	Able to calculate incidence rates (by age, sex, etc.) among low-risk population, monitor trends in a population over time; identify special populations, scope of disease, and targets for intervention; may identify unusual strain or new epidemiologic trend	Able to calculate incidence rate among population selected; identify special populations at risk; identify scope and spectrum of disease in the selected population; identify targets for intervention	Allows monitoring of intra-facility trends over time	Provides local resistance; patterns to guide empiric treatment; can be used to track resistance trends
Weaknesses	Often difficult to sustain due to personnel time required	Relying upon persons outside of health department to report; cannot describe trends; might be biased by seasonal infections	Identifies infections only in persons receiving care at participating facilities; limited interfacility comparisons and generalization; meaningful denominator difficult to define	Variability in practices across laboratories, including deduplication of isolates, susceptibility testing methods, and stratification of data (e.g., by age, inpatient/outpatient, body site source of isolate)

following healthcare-related risk factors is determined: (1) a history of MRSA infection or colonization; (2) a positive culture for MRSA infection obtained greater than 48 hours of admission to a healthcare facility; (3) a history of hospitalization, surgery, residence in long-term care, or dialysis in the prior year; or (4) an indwelling percutaneous device or catheter. Patients with one or more healthcare-related risk factors are classified as HA-MRSA, and those without are classified as CA-MRSA. HA-MRSA cases can be classified further as of hospital-onset (>48 hours) or community-onset.

Partners

Successful surveillance systems require the collaboration of healthcare providers, infection control professionals (ICPs), laboratorians, and public health professionals. Partners should be involved in developing methods for MRSA surveillance to ensure that these methods are feasible and sustainable. When involvement of partners in the planning stages of surveillance is not possible, advance notification and a description of surveillance activities can help create awareness and allow partners to prepare for the activities.

Role of the laboratory in surveillance

The microbiology laboratory is crucial to MRSA surveillance in the following ways:

Case finding

Both active and passive reporting systems depend on laboratory identification of MRSA cases. To ensure completeness of cases ascertained by laboratory-initiated reporting of MRSA, periodic audits of laboratory results are helpful (see section on *Quality assurance*). In addition, antibiogram-based surveillance for MRSA cannot be conducted without laboratory participation.

Characterization of MRSA

The microbiologic and genetic characterization of case isolates can inform the epidemiology of MRSA. MRSA strains in different geographic regions can vary. Characteristics of interest include (1) *in vitro* antimicrobial susceptibility patterns; (2) SCC*mec* type, the genetic element containing the gene that confers methicillin resistance, which is different in CA-MRSA versus HA-MRSA strains; (3) pulsed-field gel electrophoresis subtyping (Figure 14.1) [16]; and (4) the presence of staphylococcal virulence factors. Testing methods for each of these characteristics are described elsewhere [17].

Surveillance methods

Various methods can be used for surveillance of CA-MRSA (see Table 14.1). These methods differ with respect to method of case ascertainment, strengths and weaknesses of the surveillance system, resources required, and potential data analysis. Each

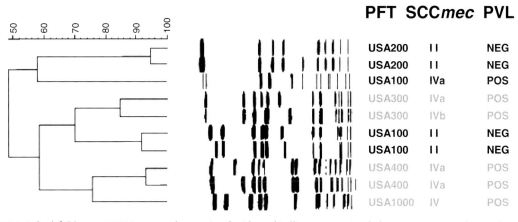

Fig 14.1 Pulsed-field types (PFTs) commonly associated with methicillin-resistant *Staphylococcus aureus* in the US, their staphylococcal chromosomal cassette (SCC)*mec* type, and the presence of the gene encoding for Panton-Valentine leukocidin (PVL). Types in bold represent strains of healthcare origin. Types in light print are of community origin. (Courtesy of Sigrid McAllister, CDC.)

option can be used as part of a combination of methods or as the sole surveillance activity. For example, the state of Tennessee uses passive reporting of all MRSA infections from a normally sterile body site for surveillance. However, one county within the state conducts active surveillance for infections among its residents and investigates cases to classify them as CA or HA.

Antibiogram surveillance

Antibiograms show the proportion of isolates from a particular bacterial species that are susceptible to a panel of antibiotics. Most hospitals routinely develop and disseminate antibiograms annually. The primary goal of antibiogram surveillance is to monitor antimicrobial resistance at the local level and disseminate this information to clinicians to guide empiric prescribing. Antibiograms from multiple hospitals can be aggregated to estimate the level of MRSA in a community. Because these data already exist, this type of surveillance can be easily implemented. However, most CA-MRSA infections occur among outpatients, and antibiograms for outpatient isolates are uncommon. Therefore, susceptibilities from noninvasive CA-MRSA isolates may be underrepresented in hospital antibiograms.

Susceptibility data obtained from antibiograms may be aggregated by subgroups, for example: patient location (e.g., outpatient); clinical service; source of specimen (e.g., blood, wound); organism subgroups (e.g., MRSA); and patient subpopulation (e.g., pediatric). Clinical and Laboratory Standards Institute (CLSI, formerly NCCLS) [18] guidelines indicate that stratification, if undertaken, should be based on local needs. Before results are stratified, adequate numbers of isolates should be included (usually >10 isolates) in each stratum.

One example of antibiogram development comes from a network of laboratories and an interdisciplinary team in Jacksonville, FL, that included microbiologists, clinical pharmacists, infection control professionals (ICPs), and infectious disease specialists [19]. The network provided training on antibiogram development, including antimicrobial resistance and laboratory methods and facilitated communication during conferences.

In Jacksonville, the first step in data collection was a survey to determine hospital susceptibility testing methods, compliance with CLSI [18] guidelines, and how antibiogram results were reported. Compliance with CLSI guidelines requires the selection of the first isolate of any species per patient per period of the report (at least annually is recommended). Furthermore, isolates should be selected from those causing clinically relevant infections and should not include surveillance cultures.

Laboratories can submit their results by mail, fax, or increasingly, electronically for aggregation, which may be done at the state or regional level. Many laboratories use automated systems for testing isolates. To facilitate surveillance, mechanisms for using electronic data generated by these systems are in development. Although antibiograms are widely available, few stratify and report MRSA separately from *S. aureus*. Approaches to approximate CA-MRSA isolates include selecting isolates from cultures obtained within 48 hours of admission, isolates from outpatient locations, or those from skin and soft tissue infections.

Aggregate antibiogram reports should consist of tables that include the organisms, numbers of isolates tested, and percentage susceptible to each antimicrobial tested (see example in Chapter 4). To allow stratification of results by a particular subgroup, information on the patient location, specimen source, and patient population should be displayed as well as the date of the report noting the culture dates of included isolates. An example of this type of antibiogram is at http://www.dhh.louisiana.gov/reports.asp?ID=1&Detail=330.

An alternative to pooling data from multiple area laboratories is to report susceptibilities from isolates tested at a central laboratory (e.g., the state public health reference laboratory). However, these isolates may not be representative of isolates from all clinical infections in the community because isolates selected for submission to the central laboratory may be more frequently resistant or from more serious infections.

The major advantages of antibiogram surveillance are that relatively minimal resources are required to develop and disseminate the information, and that information regarding local antimicrobial susceptibilities can enable clinicians to make judicious empiric treatment choices. Weaknesses include (1) the variability in susceptibility testing, resulting in aggregation of data that are not comparable [20]; (2) the possible inclusion of more than one isolate per patient, resulting in an overestimate of MRSA[21]; (3) an overestimate of resistance due to culturing bias (i.e., infections more likely to be resistant may be cultured more frequently and submitted for testing); and (4) the frequent pooling of data from various age groups, clinical settings, and body source of isolates, yielding less useful data.

Sentinel site surveillance
Sentinel site surveillance, whereby a group of individual facilities participate in a surveillance system, is a feasible option for health departments that desire clinical descriptions of CA-MRSA infections and trend data. Sentinel site surveillance can be active or passive. Selection of sites to conduct sentinel surveillance may be based on a site's willingness and capacity to participate, and whether the site can provide representative data for the population of interest.

The application of a standardized surveillance protocol, case definition, and case report form (see example in Figure 14.2) is essential across all sites. A surveillance coordinator is required to ensure that the protocol is implemented consistently across all sites and that data collection is standardized. A mechanism for case report form submission must be identified for centralized data management and analysis.

The population under sentinel site surveillance typically consists of the individuals seeking care at a sentinel site or of those whose providers send cultures to a sentinel site laboratory. The numerator and denominator vary but generally, the numerator is the number of MRSA infections and the denominator is the number of individuals seeking care, number of admissions, number of emergency room visits, or the total number of *S. aureus* infections. Therefore, the rates that can be calculated will not reflect the frequency of the event in the resident population.

The ability of a sentinel system to be representative of the larger population depends upon the types and catchment areas of facilities included in the surveillance model [22].Because sentinel surveillance networks are not randomly selected, findings are not representative of the larger population. However, trends over time in the same sites can provide insights into antimicrobial resistance trends. State public health professionals need to be aware of potential biases as they draw conclusions or implement new programs based on these data.

An advantage of a sentinel system is the ability to collect information on individual cases and link epidemiologic and microbiologic information at the individual level. For example, sentinel surveillance can allow for comparison of trends in resistance among pediatric cases, adult cases, or between age groups or culture-positive clinical syndromes. In addition, reports have suggested that sentinel networks may provide a more accurate profile of antimicrobial resistance patterns in the community compared with antibiograms, because data from antibiograms may include duplicate isolates [21].

Sentinel networks may also provide value to states beyond the data collected. These include (1) partnerships built between participating facilities and the state; (2) awareness of antimicrobial resistance trends; (3) opportunities for clinical laboratory evaluations and feedback; and (4) coordination and communication between historically separate institutions.

Sentinel surveillance systems, depending upon design, can require a substantial investment in financial and human resources, laboratory personnel, training, and logistical coordination, although typically less than that required for population-based surveillance. In addition, collection, transport and testing of isolates, if included, may require a large amount of laboratory personnel time.

An example of sentinel surveillance is the prospective surveillance for CA-MRSA at 12 sentinel sites conducted in Minnesota since 2000 [23]. A yearly antibiogram produced by the Minnesota Department of Health includes CA-MRSA isolates from the sentinel sites: http://www.health. state.mn.us/divs/idepc/dtopics/antibioticresistance/ antibiogram.html.

Time-limited surveillance
Conducting CA-MRSA surveillance for a specified time period is an approach that balances resources with the need to provide answers to epidemiologic questions. Successful implementation of such an option is exemplified by work from Los Angeles County.

Los Angeles County, CA, is the second largest metropolitan area in the US, and had an estimated population of almost 10 million people in 2004.

After investigating a large MRSA outbreak in the Los Angeles County Jail and receiving numerous reports of previously healthy children with MRSA infections, the Los Angeles County Health Department conducted a targeted surveillance project to describe the epidemiology of MRSA in the community. During May through November 2003, pediatric MRSA infections requiring hospitalization were reportable to public health authorities. Reported cases were investigated by medical record review and, if possible, parent interview. In addition, available isolates were collected and tested in the public health laboratory. Findings from this highly targeted surveillance project were used to measure the frequency of disease in this population during this time period. However, the resources necessary to conduct this surveillance led public health authorities to question whether repeating this effort would be feasible. For more information on CA-MRSA in Los Angeles, see http://search .lapublichealth.org/acd/mrsa_0ld_51105.htm.

Population-based surveillance
Population-based surveillance refers to surveillance that covers all residents in a selected geographic area. Population-based surveillance is considered the "gold standard" and enables calculation of incidence rates and the monitoring of trends within a population. An important consideration of population-based surveillance is the catchment area. The population must be well defined and of an adequate size so that epidemiologic follow-up is feasible. The denominator is the population of the defined catchment area and the numerator is the number of infections identified in residents of the catchment area. Population-based surveillance may be active or passive, laboratory or provider-based, and may be limited to a small area, such as a city, or include a larger population such as an entire state. Population-based surveillance can be used to detect the emergence of infection in low-risk populations, monitor trends over time, identify geographic differences, and identify changes in epidemiology. Population-based surveillance is resource-intensive, so feasibility and sustainability are often limited. Also, if surveillance is conducted in a smaller area, it may not be generalizable to the larger population. The follow-ing provide examples of population-based surveillance systems adapted to address MRSA in the community.

Surveillance for MRSA-positive cultures from all body sites Active, laboratory-based surveillance for CA-MRSA was conducted in Georgia and Maryland from 2001 to 2002 through the Active Bacterial Core surveillance (ABCs) program of the CDC's Emerging Infections Program [11]. The objectives of the ABCs CA-MRSA surveillance were to determine the incidence of CA-MRSA and to describe the epidemiologic characteristics of CA-MRSA infections. The Georgia catchment area was defined as the eight-county Atlanta metropolitan area, population 3.3 million. The Maryland catchment area was defined as Baltimore City, population 700,000. CA-MRSA surveillance included all MRSA positive cultures in order to identify all cases.

ABCs surveillance officers regularly contacted laboratories serving residents of the catchment areas to identify cases. Laboratories with the capability to produce computerized reports sent a printout of all MRSA positive cultures monthly and surveillance officers reviewed laboratory records in those without this capacity. Surveillance officers determined whether the individuals were residents of the catchment area. Medical records of cases were then reviewed to identify any established healthcare-related risk factors. If risk factors were identified, the case was determined to be HA-MRSA and no further information was collected. If no risk factors were identified in the medical record, the cases were determined to be probable CA cases. Interviews of probable CA cases were attempted in an effort to identify any risk factors not recorded in the medical record and to obtain additional case characteristics and outcome information.

Findings from this surveillance indicated a CA-MRSA incidence ranging from 18 to 26 per 100,000 population in the two US communities. The incidence was greatest in children under 2 years of age, and was significantly higher in African–American children in Atlanta. Most patients presented with skin and soft tissue infection; 6% of disease was invasive, and 23% of patients required hospitalization [11].

In preparation for surveillance, laboratory surveys were conducted to estimate the number of cases that would need to be investigated. The actual number of cases exceeded the estimated number and the resources required to conduct population-based surveillance for all culture sites were too burdensome to be sustainable. The objective of the initial surveillance had been met; therefore, the lessons learned were used to develop a more feasible protocol that could be ongoing and expanded to other geographic areas.

Surveillance limited to invasive infections The new ABCs MRSA surveillance methods had the following objectives: (1) determine the incidence and epidemiologic characteristics of invasive disease due to MRSA in diverse geographic areas; and (2) categorize MRSA infections as HA or CA-MRSA. The case report form is shown in Figure 14.3.

Surveillance is active, laboratory-based, and population-based, but the case definition was a resident of the surveillance area from whom MRSA has been isolated from a normally sterile site. All cases were investigated through medical record review to determine the presence of HA risk factors and case characteristics. During 2004–2006, population-based surveillance in nine ABCs sites found that the incidence of invasive CA-MRSA was approximately 5 per 100,000 (range 2–30 per 100,000) and the projected number of annual cases in the US was approximately 94,000 [24]. While estimates from invasive infections are limited compared to all infections, they represent the most severe disease and have relatively high mortality.

Mandatory reporting
An alternative to active population-based surveillance is passive surveillance through regulation or law. Passive surveillance relies on reports from clinicians, ICPs, or microbiology laboratories and thus depends on voluntary collaboration of personnel outside the health department. Because data from passive reporting systems tend to underestimate the event, periodic evaluation of reporting practices and case ascertainment may be performed to determine the completeness and validity of the data [25].

Tennessee began mandatory reporting for MRSA in 2004. Only invasive infections were reported.

Active surveillance was conducted in Davidson County through ABCs, and passive surveillance was conducted statewide. Under the state reporting law, all providers and laboratories are required to report invasive MRSA infections to the state health department. The report form collects basic demographic information as well as hospital admission and outcome (for more details, see http://www2 .state.tn.us/health/CEDS/notifiable.htm). Although the healthcare risk factors are not reported, a proxy of community- or hospital-onset of infection may be determined from the hospital admission and specimen collection dates provided on the report form. The strength of this approach is that the health department can estimate a minimum incidence of invasive MRSA in the population and monitor trends over time with a minimal burden on the state health department.

Feedback of surveillance data

Surveillance data are meant to effect action, and MRSA surveillance data should be reported to surveillance partners, clinicians, public health decision makers, and policymakers. The data and format in which feedback is presented should be targeted for the intended audience. Successful tools for communicating surveillance data include newsletters, publications in the scientific literature, and oral presentations at local meetings. Surveillance partners may value facility-specific reports that can be developed with their input. Clinicians may appreciate data on incidence rates, antimicrobial susceptibilities, clinical presentations, and characteristics of the populations at risk. Data may also be used to evaluate prevention and control measures.

The prioritization of limited resources is critical to any public health program; likewise it is important that individuals allocating resources are informed of public health issues. Perceptions of the prevalence of CA-MRSA are frequently inaccurate. Data elements of interest for public health officials might include estimates of the local incidence of MRSA in the community, and data evaluating the impact of prevention activities. Aggregated data from sentinel site surveillance, and resistance patterns of *S. aureus* isolates from antibiograms can also be helpful.

179

The findings from CA-MRSA surveillance in the community can impact public policy, from funding to legislation. While policymakers are typically not involved in the development and implementation of surveillance, they are often responsible for allocating funds for public health activities. A regular report on the burden of MRSA in the community may support continued allocation of funds, an expansion of funds, or the development of interventions. Surveillance data can support evaluations of legislation on public reporting, mandatory patient screening, and other measures.

The status of CA-MRSA surveillance in the US

In a CDC survey initially conducted in 2005, and updated in 2006, 37 (73%) of states and the District of Columbia reported conducting surveillance activities for MRSA in the community (see Figure 14.4). In 2006, MRSA in the community is a reportable condition in 24 (47%) states; however, case definitions and surveillance methods vary by state and in some places, within the state. For example, some states require that only clusters of cases be reported. Thirty percent of survey respondents described their surveillance activities as population-based, 20% as antibiogram-based, 20% as sentinel site, and 14% conducted surveillance for invasive MRSA (MRSA isolated from blood, cerebrospinal fluid, or other normally sterile site). The source of reports was more frequently a laboratory than healthcare providers. About 30% of states conducting surveillance reported publishing a Web-based report summarizing surveillance data.

As of 2006, at least two states have discussed legislation requiring hospitals to screen patients at admission for MRSA and report results to public health authorities; however, this practice has not yet been mandated in any state. Many hospitals currently screen patients for MRSA for infection control purposes. Because the purpose of screening is to ensure that patients colonized or infected with MRSA are appropriately managed, determining whether the MRSA is community-acquired is less relevant.

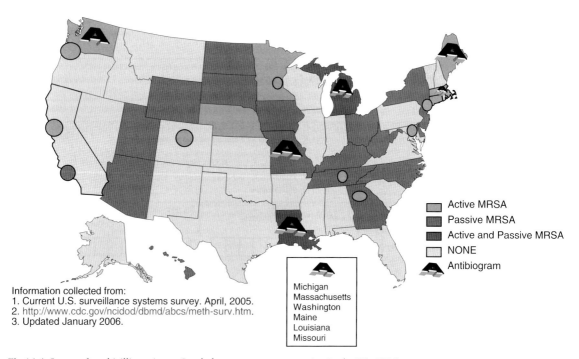

Information collected from:
1. Current U.S. surveillance systems survey. April, 2005.
2. http://www.cdc.gov/ncidod/dbmd/abcs/meth-surv.htm.
3. Updated January 2006.

Active MRSA
Passive MRSA
Active and Passive MRSA
NONE
Antibiogram

Michigan
Massachusetts
Washington
Maine
Louisiana
Missouri

Fig 14.4 Status of methicillin-resistant *Staphylococcus aureus* reporting in the US, 2005.

Surveillance for MRSA in both the hospital and the community is important because of concern about the emergence of vancomycin-resistant *S. aureus* (VRSA). Coexistence of vancomycin-resistant enterococci and MRSA in the same individual has facilitated the development of VRSA [26]. As of 2006, six clinical cases of VRSA have been reported in the US. In contrast to MRSA, VRSA is a notifiable condition throughout the US. Reporting is frequently the responsibility of the testing laboratories, however, the provider and hospital are also required to report in many states (see http://www.cste.org/nndssmainmenu2005.htm for details). CDC has developed guidance for investigating and reporting vancomycin-intermediate *S. aureus* (VISA) and VRSA (see http://www.cdc.gov/ncidod/dhqp/ar_visavrsa_ prevention.html).

Opportunities and challenges

Surveillance of MRSA in the community requires selection of the appropriate method to provide useful information and careful consideration of logistical issues. Some key considerations in the development of surveillance protocols and data collection instruments are the volume of cases that will require investigation, the availability of information, and local needs. After a protocol and data collection instruments have been developed, the surveillance system should be piloted to identify logistical problems that were or could not be anticipated so that revisions can be made before full implementation. Similarly, opportunities for expansion or the collection of additional information may be identified during piloting and implementation.

Perhaps the main challenge of surveillance for MRSA in the community is the number of cases that require investigation. For example, to document the 1590 cases of CA-MRSA reported during the initial Atlanta surveillance effort, 7819 cases had to be investigated [11]. The investigation of all MRSA cases should be anticipated since the patient information available from the laboratory reports is typically insufficient to determine whether or not a case is CA-MRSA. A survey of area laboratories to estimate the number of cultures processed per month can be used to estimate the resources that

will be required. The scope of surveillance may be limited if the burden of case investigation would be greater than the resources available. Information typically available from the laboratory, such as culture site and location of collection, can be used to restrict the volume of cases in a manner that will address the surveillance questions efficiently. For example, surveillance could be limited only to sterile site cultures or to cultures obtained in the emergency department. Likewise, all culture sites may be included from a smaller geographic area or from target populations, such as children or patients receiving dialysis.

Differences in the availability of information complicate the standardization of methods for CA-MRSA. As discussed previously in this chapter, reporting requirements for MRSA vary by state and within some states. The legal status of reporting and concerns about confidentiality can have significant impact on the performance of a surveillance system. Where MRSA is not reportable, case identification may be difficult. Medical record review is often required to collect information on health-care risk factors; therefore determination if a case is epidemiologically CA-MRSA, may be challenging if access to this information is difficult. At some facilities, hospital staff may not be able to assist in obtaining additional information because of a lack of resources. The information available directly from the laboratory also varies; some laboratories may be able to provide detailed information on reports that will reduce the number of cases that have to be investigated, such as patient demographics and hospital admission dates. Communication with partners about the type of information that will be needed and what information is available is essential in the development of effective data collection instruments.

A time period should be defined for pilot testing the data collection instruments and methods. During the pilot phase, the surveillance system may be implemented in the entire surveillance population or in selected facilities. The purpose of piloting a surveillance system is to identify difficulties in methods and instruments. While some issues may arise that are unanticipated, there are specific issues that should be evaluated during a pilot. The number of cases investigated should be compared to the expected number to assess the completeness of reporting and to determine if the available resources are adequate for surveillance. The availability of the information needed should also be assessed; if the majority of values are missing for a particular item, revision of the data collection instrument may be necessary or other sources of information may need to be identified.

Monitoring and quality assurance activities

Ideally, after surveillance has been implemented, the quality of the data should be evaluated and monitored. Results should translate into actions to improve or eliminate the system. Several surveillance system performance indicators can be applied. For example, completeness and timeliness of reporting should be assessed [25]. A comparison of the cases identified through surveillance to the baseline information on isolates processed annually per laboratory and between-laboratory variability can be used to evaluate how well the system is performing. If the number of cases is significantly lower than that expected or the interlaboratory variability is high, case ascertainment methods should be closely examined. For example, if a laboratory is reporting fewer cases than was estimated from previous annual isolates processed, it is possible that the estimates included duplicate isolates while the cases currently identified represent only the initial culture for an individual. The standardization of methods across laboratories and surveillance personnel is essential and should be periodically assessed through surveys, training, and validation analyses.

Data entry errors are common and can result in inaccurate findings, therefore, reports should be regularly reviewed and items that appear inconsistent or missing should be returned for clarification. Many data entry errors can be avoided by incorporating checks into the data entry application, and simple data editing programs can be developed and run periodically to capture potentially invalid entries. Dates, especially those related to date of culture and date of hospital admission, can lead to errors in classification of whether the case is CA- or HA-MRSA.

Lessons learned and recommendations to the reader

As with all surveillance systems, building relationships with surveillance partners is crucial and requires frequent contact and ongoing communication. If participation in surveillance is voluntary, partners should be queried at least annually about their willingness to continue participation and their recommendations for improvements in surveillance protocols. Revisions based on feedback should be made. Changes in protocol should be made as some surveillance questions are answered and new questions arise. Flexibility in reporting (e.g., electronic mail, fax, electronic submission) is extremely important and batched reporting and batched isolate submission may be helpful. Providing partners with regular feedback on surveillance data, both in aggregate and for their own facility, is very important. It is also important to provide partners with any published reports using surveillance data so that partners can see the value of their work. For example, in addition to publishing a statewide antibiogram and providing laboratory support to healthcare facilities, the Minnesota Department of Health (MDH) has found that hosting an annual "MRSA Appreciation Day" for participating site ICPs and laboratorians is beneficial. Surveillance partners are invited to MDH for a program in which surveillance results and reports are presented and issues are discussed.

Future directions

It is difficult to predict future MRSA surveillance needs. Mandatory reporting of all or a selected subset of MRSA infections has been implemented in many geographic areas. However, long-term experience with this approach will determine its usefulness and feasibility to maintain. Electronic reporting will likely have a more prominent role in the future. Currently, systems used to manage information in laboratories and hospitals are not compatible across facilities and do not use standardized definitions and protocols; hopefully, these issues will be addressed. Objectives of MRSA surveillance may change; surveillance data might help direct resources toward prevention and control of

MRSA and result in a decline in the rate of MRSA infections. More likely, the future will bring more cases of MRSA with increasing resistance to other antimicrobial classes, including VRSA. Surveillance will be important not only to detect and describe, but also to help implement and monitor the effectiveness of public health measures.

Summary

• Surveillance for CA-MRSA has provided important information on prevalence and incidence, characteristics of populations at greatest risk for severe infection, and local susceptibility patterns. However, the resources necessary to conduct surveillance are significant, and questions to be addressed by surveillance should be balanced with availability of resources.
• There are multiple options for conducting surveillance depending on local needs and resources. A surveillance strategy can consist of one or a combination of methods to maximize resources.
• The needs of stakeholders and partners should be considered early in the process, and feedback of data to these groups is an important incentive to continued collaboration and success.

Acknowledgments

The authors are grateful for the contributions of Ms Pei Jean Chang, Dr Elizabeth Bancroft, and Dr Marion Kainer to this chapter.

References

1 1 Rammelkamp C MT. Resistance of *Staphylococcus aureus* to the action of penicillin. *Proc. Soc Exp Biol Med* 1942;**51**:386–9.

2 Jevons MP. Celbenin-resistant staphylococci. *BMJ* 1961;**1**:124–5.

3 Barber M. Methicillin-resistant staphylococci. *J Clin Path* 1961;**14**:385–93.

4 Barrett F RMJ, Finland, M. Methicillin-resistant *Staphylococcus aureus* at Boston City Hospital. *N Engl J Med* 1968;**279**(9):441–8.

5 Saravolatz LD, Markowitz N, Arking L, Pohlod D, Fisher E. Methicillin-resistant *Staphylococcus aureus*: epidemiologic observations during a community-acquired outbreak. *Ann Intern Med* 1982;**96**(1):11–6.

6 Baggett HC, Hennessy TW, Rudolph K, *et al.* Community-onset methicillin-resistant *Staphylococcus aureus* associated with antibiotic use and the cytotoxin Panton-Valentine leukocidin during a furunculosis outbreak in rural Alaska. *J Infect Dis* 2004;**189**(9): 1565–73.

7 CDC. Methicillin-resistant *Staphylococcus aureus* infections among competitive sports participants–Colorado, Indiana, Pennsylvania, and Los Angeles County, 2000–2003. *MMWR Morb Mortal Wkly Rep* August 22, 2003; **52**(33):793–5.

8 CDC. Methicillin-resistant *Staphylococcus aureus* infections in correctional facilities—Georgia, California, and Texas, 2001–2003. *MMWR Morb Mortal Wkly Rep* October 17, 2003;**52**(41):992–6.

9 Adcock PM, Pastor P, Medley F, Patterson JE, Murphy TV. Methicillin-resistant *Staphylococcus aureus* in two child care centers. *J Infect Dis* 1998;**178**(2):577–80.

10 CDC. Four pediatric deaths from community-acquired methicillin-resistant *Staphylococcus aureus*—Minnesota and North Dakota, 1997–1999. *MMWR Morb Mortal Wkly Rep* 1999;**48**(32):707–10.

11 Fridkin SK, Hageman JC, Morrison M, *et al.* Methicillin-resistant *Staphylococcus aureus* disease in three communities. *N Engl J Med* 2005;**352**(14):1436–44.

12 Crum NF. The emergence of severe, community-acquired methicillin-resistant *Staphylococcus aureus* infections. *Scand J Infect Dis* 2005;**37**(9):651–6.

13 Francis JS, Doherty M, Lopatin U, *et al.* Severe community-onset pneumonia in healthy adults caused by methicillin-resistant *Staphylococcus aureus* carrying the Panton-Valentine Leukocidin genes. *Clin Infect Dis* 2005;**40**:100–7.

14 Miller LG, Perdreau-Remington F, Rieg G, *et al.* Necrotizing fasciitis caused by community-associated methicillin-resistant *Staphylococcus aureus* in Los Angeles. *N Engl J Med* 2005;**352**(14):1445–53.

15 Klevens RM, Morrison MA, Fridkin SK, *et al.* Spread of community-associated methicillin-resistant *Staphylococcus aureus* (MRSA) strains in healthcare settings. *Emerg Infect Dis* 2006;**12**(12):1991–3. Available from: http://www.cdc.gov/ncidod/EID/vol12no12/06-0505.htm. Accessed April 24, 2007.

16 McDougal LK, Steward CD, Killgore GE, Chaitram JM, McAllister SK, Tenover FC. Pulsed-field gel electrophoresis typing of oxacillin-resistant *Staphylococcus aureus* isolates from the United States: establishing a national database. *J Clin Microbiol* 2003;**41**(11):5113–20.

17 Tenover FC, McDougal LK, Goering RV, *et al*. Characterization of a strain of community-associated methicillin-resistant *Staphylococcus aureus* widely disseminated in the United States. *J Clin Microbiol* 2006;**44**(1):108–18.

18 NCCLS. Analysis and presentation of cumulative susceptibility test data; approved guideline. *NCCLS document M39-A* 2002;**22**(8):1–8.

19 Halstead DC, Gomez N, McCarter YS. Reality of developing a community-wide antibiogram. *J Clin Microbiol* 2004;**42**(1):1–6.

20 Zapantis A, Lacy MK, Horvat RT, *et al*. Nationwide antibiogram analysis using NCCLS M39-A guidelines. *J Clin Microbiol* 2005;**43**(6):2629–34.

21 Horvat RT, Klutman NE, Lacy MK, Grauer D, Wilson M. Effect of duplicate isolates of methicillin-susceptible and methicillin-resistant *Staphylococcus aureus* on antibiogram data. *J Clin Microbiol* 2003;**41**(10): 4611–6.

22 Charlebois ED, Bangsberg DR, Moss NJ, *et al*. Population-based community prevalence of methicillin-resistant *Staphylococcus aureus* in the urban poor of San Francisco. *Clin Infect Dis* 2002;**34**(4):425–33.

23 Naimi TS, LeDell KH, Como-Sabetti KM, *et al*. Comparison of community-and health care—associated methicillin-resistant *Staphylococcus aureus* infection. *JAMA* 2003;**290**(22):2976–84.

24 Klevens RM, Morrison MA, Fridkin SK, *et al*. Epidemiology of invasive methicillin-resistant *Staphylococcus aureus* infections in the United States, 2004–2005. CDC unpublished data.

25 CDC. Updated guidelines for evaluating public health surveillance systems. *MMWR Morb Mortal Wkly Rep* July 27, 2001;**50**(RR-13):1–35.

26 Chang S, Sievert DM, Hageman JC, *et al*. Infection with vancomycin-resistant *Staphylococcus aureus* containing the vanA resistance gene. *N Engl J Med* 2003;**348**(14):1342–7.

15 Surveillance for viral hepatitis

Mary Ramsay, Koye Balogun & Catherine Quigley

Introduction and background

Hepatitis is caused by several viruses that differ in clinical presentation, risk of chronicity, transmission, and means of prevention. The most common are hepatitis A (HAV), hepatitis B (HBV), hepatitis C (HCV), and hepatitis E. Clinical hepatitis occurs rarely due to hepatitis A or B infection acquired in childhood but is more common in adults; acute symptomatic hepatitis occurs infrequently with hepatitis C at any age. Although most hepatitis A and E infections are acute, self-limiting conditions, chronic infection is a common consequence of hepatitis B and C infection; hepatitis B leads to chronic infection in less than 10% of adults, but up to 90% of infants infected at birth, and hepatitis C leads to chronic infection in approximately 75–80% of those infected. The World Health Organization (WHO) estimates that globally 350 million and 180 million individuals are chronically infected with hepatitis B and C, respectively.

Hepatitis A and E are mainly transmitted via the faecal-oral route—spread from person to person or from contaminated food and water. Hepatitis B and C can be transmitted by sexual or parenteral exposure to blood or body fluids from an infected individual, leading to major differences in disease prevalence globally. In countries with limited economic and medical resources, most people become infected with hepatitis B virus during childhood and more than 8% of the general population are chronically infected. Hepatitis C prevalence is high (>2%) in many countries in Africa, Latin America,

and Central and Southeast Asia; prevalence figures above 5% are frequently reported.

The principal control measures for each infection also vary. Hepatitis A and E can be controlled by good sanitation and hygiene. Effective vaccines also exist for prevention of both hepatitis A and B infections. Sexual transmission of hepatitis B can be reduced through the use of condoms and by limiting the numbers of sexual partners. Hepatitis B and C can be prevented by reducing blood exposure in the medical setting, for example, through the use of clean needles, and by instituting blood donor screening and avoiding sharing of needles and syringes amongst drug users.

Because of these key differences in exposure routes, clinical complications, and control measures, the objectives, appropriate methods, and relative priorities for the surveillance of each cause of viral hepatitis requires different approaches. In this chapter, we concentrate on surveillance of hepatitis A, B, and C, using surveillance in Europe as a model. We describe case definitions, routine and supplementary data sources, their strengths and weaknesses, and the analysis and use of data for public health at both local and national levels.

Aims of hepatitis surveillance

The general objectives of the surveillance of viral hepatitis are to:
• determine incidence, prevalence, burden, and trends of disease

187

- select and monitor prevention and control strategies
- identify and control outbreaks
- assist in planning appropriate healthcare for those infected

Case definition

Case definitions used in European countries differ in the specific clinical or laboratory criteria included. Surveillance may be based only on a clinical diagnosis, although in many countries laboratory confirmation is required. The definition advised by the European Center for Disease Control (ECDC) is a case with a clinical picture compatible with acute hepatitis, combined with specific laboratory criteria (Table 15.1).

Laboratory tests can distinguish between the various causes of acute hepatitis and therefore are increasingly included in case definitions. For example, in England and Wales, notifications (Box 15.1) of viral hepatitis (infective jaundice) were further classified into hepatitis A, hepatitis B, non-A, non-B, and "other" in 1987; from 1998 non-A, non-B was reclassified as hepatitis C. As laboratory diagnosis has become more common, the number of cases of "other hepatitis" has declined dramatically (Figure 15.1).

Challenges to hepatitis surveillance

All reporting systems are subject to underreporting. The extent of underreporting can be established using techniques such as capture–recapture [1], or by auditing against complete data extracted from exhaustive systems (such as laboratory or hospital databases) [2]. Acute infections are particularly susceptible to under-ascertainment due to undiagnosed, mild, or asymptomatic infection. Hepatitis A, for example, is usually mild or asymptomatic in childhood, and most surveillance systems underestimate the true incidence of infection by several fold [3]. Similarly, hepatitis E testing is often not routinely performed in individuals with symptoms of hepatitis who have negative tests for hepatitis A, B, and C. Testing is often only performed in individuals who have traveled to an endemic country, therefore indigenous cases are not recognised [4].

Table 15.1 Proposed case definitions for reporting communicable diseases to the European community network, 2006.

	Clinical criteria
Hepatitis A, B, and C	Discrete onset of symptoms and at least one of the following: • Jaundice • Elevated serum aminotransferase levels
	Laboratory criteria
Hepatitis A*	One of the following three laboratory tests: • Detection of hepatitis A IgM antibody in serum • Detection of hepatitis A virus nucleic acid in serum or stool • Detection of hepatitis A antigen in stool
Acute hepatitis B*	• Detection of IgM antibody to the hepatitis B virus core antigen
Hepatitis C*	One of the following three laboratory tests: • Detection of hepatitis C IgG antibody in serum • Detection of hepatitis C virus nucleic acid in serum • Detection of hepatitis C virus antigen in serum
Chronic hepatitis B	One of the following two sets of laboratory tests: • Detection of hepatitis B surface antigen (HBsAg) in serum on two occasions at least 6 months apart • Detection of HBsAg in serum that is negative for IgM antibody to the hepatitis B virus core antigen

*Adapted from European Center for Disease Control draft document.

Another challenge to hepatitis surveillance is the specificity of the diagnosis. In most developed countries, laboratory tests to distinguish between the hepatitides are routinely used in medical practice; laboratory-based surveillance will therefore be the preferred option. As clinical criteria are not required to confirm the diagnosis, direct laboratory reporting may be preferable. In this type of surveillance the timeliness of laboratory confirmation and reporting is important; delaying a laboratory diagnosis can delay any local public health action [5]. In many countries, however, clinical and laboratory

Box 15.1 Case study: routine hepatitis surveillance in England.

Routine surveillance of hepatitis in England relies on clinician notification and laboratory reporting to the Health Protection Agency (HPA) (Figure 15.2). Physicians in England and Wales are statutorily obliged to notify cases of viral hepatitis to the proper public health officer of the local authority where the patient is resident. Although no microbiological confirmation is required, the physician can specify whether the case is due to hepatitis A, B, C, or "other" virus. The data reported at a local level include name, date of birth, address, diagnosis, date of onset, and where the infection was acquired. Notified cases are then reported to the national centre (HPA Centre for Infection) on a weekly basis (Figure 15.2), but only age, sex, and local authority of residence are included.

Diagnostic samples submitted to local National Health Service (NHS) or HPA laboratories are tested for hepatitis markers; results are returned to the requesting clinician. Approximately, 250 NHS and HPA laboratories voluntarily report laboratory-confirmed cases to local units and to the national centre of the HPA using the following case definitions:

Acute hepatitis B: HBsAg *and* anti-HBc IgM positive with liver function tests consistent with acute viral hepatitis

Chronic hepatitis B: Two HBsAg positive tests taken 6 months apart *or* HBsAg positive *and* anti-HBc IgM negative *and* anti-HBc positive

Acute hepatitis A: anti-HAV IgM positive

Confirmed hepatitis C: anti-HCV positive or HCV RNA positive

Reports include a patient identifier (used to avoid duplicates), age, sex, specimen date, type of specimen, and method of confirmation. Reporting to regional and national centers is usually electronic or on paper using the case form in the Appendix. Local HPA teams contact the reporting physician to obtain further information and institute control measures.

Analysis, interpretation, and feedback of surveillance data to local laboratories and clinicians occur. At the national level, quarterly reports appear in the national surveillance bulletin—*The Health Protection Report*—and on the Web site (www.hpa.org.uk).

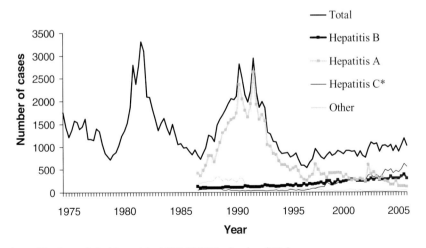

Fig 15.1 Quarterly notifications of viral hepatitis, 1975–2000 England and Wales.
*Classified as non-A, non-B hepatitis until 1998.

systems operate separately and are not easily linked. The use of case definitions that include both clinical and laboratory criteria, such as the ECDC case definition (Table 15.1), is therefore often problematic for routine surveillance.

Because hepatitis B and C may lead to chronic infection, laboratory reporting of all infected individuals cannot be used to infer trends in incidence. Laboratory markers of acute infection, such as serum IgM antibody, do not exist for hepatitis C and are not perfect for hepatitis B. Surveillance of chronic infection is complicated by the fact that most individuals are only aware of their status if tested as part of medical care. Numbers reported therefore reflect medical practice and access to healthcare in that country. Better information is available from routine screening, and information can be improved by linking the numerator of infections diagnosed to the denominator of tests performed. This allows interpretation of trends in diagnoses and can be used to infer prevalence in certain groups [6].

Routine surveillance data sources

In many European countries, clinical notification, laboratory reporting, and death registrations are the major sources of data for hepatitis surveillance. An example of routine surveillance data flows in England is shown in Figure 15.2.

Clinical notification of viral hepatitis

In many European countries, healthcare providers are required by statute to notify cases of hepatitis to local public health authorities. Such infections are normally reported on a weekly or monthly basis to regional or national levels to allow for the collation and feedback of data and the national monitoring and analysis of disease trends. Information collected at a local level includes the individual's name and address, date of birth, sex, the clinical condition, and date of onset. Usually, only limited data are reported at a national level (e.g., age, sex, week/month of notification, and local area).

In some countries (e.g., Austria) all newly identified cases are notifiable, and therefore hepatitis surveillance systems contain both acute and chronic infections [7]. In England and Wales, the number of notified cases of hepatitis B and C has increased in recent years, suggesting that increased identification of chronically infected individuals is obscuring trends in acute infections (Figure 15.1). The Netherlands has established a notification system

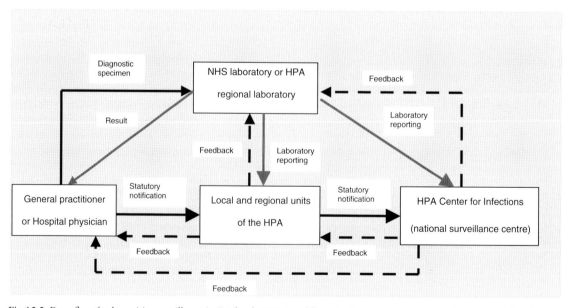

Fig 15.2 Data flow for hepatitis surveillance in England. HPA, Health Protection Agency; NHS, National Health Service.

that allows for the differentiation between acute and chronic hepatitis C infection [8].

Laboratory reporting of confirmed cases of viral hepatitis

Laboratory reporting of confirmed infection is the preferred method for hepatitis surveillance in many countries. Laboratories may report to a national center, to the local public health departments, or to both. In a number of European countries, laboratory surveillance is performed as part of a generic reporting system for all infections confirmed by laboratories. Alternative models of laboratory surveillance include collation of data in a single reference laboratory where specimens are referred for confirmation or reporting from a small group of sentinel laboratories [9]. Laboratory-based case definitions tend to be more consistent between countries, with most countries using the detection of hepatitis A- and B-specific IgM antibody in serum to define an acute infection, with or without additional clinical criteria. Secondary and confirmatory testing can be carried out at national or regional reference laboratory if the facilities for carrying out certain tests are not present in the primary testing laboratory. Newer techniques, based upon detection of nucleic acid in serum, are becoming more commonly used and have been incorporated into recent ECDC case definitions (Table 15.1).

Death certification

In most countries, a physician completes a death certificate for each patient who dies in his or her care, outlining the likely cause of death. The death certificates are then registered and both the immediate and the underlying causes of death coded, normally using the International Classification of Diseases (ICD) codes. Deaths due to acute hepatitis or to cirrhosis and primary liver cancer caused by hepatitis B and C should be coded with viral hepatitis as the underlying cause of death. The ICD system is revised periodically and is currently in its tenth edition (ICD-10) [10], the first to include a specific code for hepatitis C (previously recorded as non-A, non-B hepatitis) and to differentiate between deaths from acute and chronic complications of hepatitis B and C. These data are often collated nationally to provide mortality statistics. Trends in mortality as a result of both acute and chronic viral hepatitis infection can therefore be monitored over time.

Enhanced surveillance

Because of the weaknesses of the routine surveillance systems described above and the relatively heterogeneous risk of hepatitis across the population, enhanced and active surveillance for hepatitis are often used in addition to routine reporting systems. Enhanced surveillance involves the collection of additional clinical, epidemiological, or laboratory information on some or all cases. Where resources are limited, or compliance with follow-up of routine reports is poor, enhanced information can be collected more easily through sentinel schemes. Such schemes use a group of motivated practitioners or microbiologists who agree to report on a regular basis. These reporters can be chosen geographically (e.g., by conducting surveillance in one area), from selected centers (e.g., hospitals or laboratories), or from established professional networks. Enhanced surveillance can also be targeted at particular risk groups, such as injecting drug users (IDUs), or at vulnerable populations, such as children.

Active surveillance can improve ascertainment of hepatitis cases. This may be achieved using automated exhaustive data extraction (e.g., from laboratory or hospital computers) or by conducting manual searches through medical records on a regular basis. Ascertainment can also be improved by prompting the practitioner to report on a regular basis and by requiring a response in each period even if no case has been seen.

Supplementary information collected as part of enhanced surveillance

Risk factor information

Collection of risk factor information can help identify the main exposure routes for infection. Additional information may be obtained by contacting reporting clinicians or the patients themselves. Linking of clinical reporting systems for acute hepatitis to laboratory results and risk factor data was found to be particularly valuable in Italy [11]. Because this is resource-intensive, however, some countries may survey only a limited population.

Molecular typing

Molecular typing can further enhance laboratory-based reporting. For example, sequence-based typing of viral nucleic acid was used in Norway to define links between cases [12] of hepatitis A. Establishment of international databases as repositories of sequence information (http://www.hpa-bioinfodatabases.org.uk/hepatitis/main.php) will provide a background of virus diversity, allowing tracking of strains between countries and identification of clusters.

Hepatitis testing

Collecting information on testing for hepatitis can be useful in interpreting trends in diagnoses, can provide prevalence estimates for groups undergoing testing, and may help in planning services. Because the number of tests performed in some countries is likely to be large, sentinel surveillance may be used to monitor screening for chronic hepatitis B and C infections [13]. Because different providers may test infected patients for markers of hepatitis, duplicate tests for a single individual should be removed to avoid overestimating hepatitis prevalence.

Hospital admission data

Statistics on hospitalizations for hepatitis are becoming increasingly available and a minimum data set is often available in a computerised format. Hospitalized cases reflect only the more severe, symptomatic infections but the associated data sources are usually fairly complete. Hospital admissions are typically coded for the cause of admission using established coding schemes such as ICD10 [10]. As coding is often made using clinical notes, specific codes may be missing or inaccurate, and misclassification between acute and chronic hepatitis is common [2]. In England, hospital data have been used to look for admissions due to end stage liver disease where the underlying cause is chronic viral hepatitis (http://www.hpa.org.uk/hpa/ publications/hepC_2005/default.htm).

Seroprevalence studies

Seroprevalence studies can be performed on a regular or intermittent basis as part of a formal survey or by using anonymized residual serum samples submitted to laboratories for other tests. These serum samples can be tested for markers of acute and chronic infection or for vaccine-derived and natural immunity. Studies of the prevalence of markers of past or current hepatitis infection can be used to estimate past cumulative incidence. These data can be used to help validate information from disease surveillance and to assess the extent of under-ascertainment in routine systems.

Age-specific seroprevalence of IgG antibody to hepatitis A indicates that the childhood incidence has been declining in most industrialized countries [14]. This not only tells us about past incidence, but also identifies a pool of susceptible adults. This change has been accompanied by increased recognition of hepatitis A in adult risk groups such as IDUs and gay men [15]. Because adults may develop severe infection if exposed [16] and disease is preventable by vaccine, identification of risk factors for hepatitis A infection in adults has become a major priority.

Repeated cross-sectional prevalence studies can also be used to estimate incidence and follow disease trends. In a low incidence country, however, a large number of samples are needed to show any change. Such surveys may be more useful in high-risk groups such as IDUs attending clinics. In England, assays have been developed to detect evidence of past exposure to hepatitis B virus (the presence of anti-hepatitis B core antigen or anti-HBc) in saliva specimens and have been used to infer a decline in the incidence between 1990 and 1995, and subsequent increase in the early part of the twenty-first century (http://www.hpa.org.uk/ infections/topics_az/injectingdrugusers/Shooting_Up_2004_data. pdf).

Seroprevalence studies can also be used to determine the prevalence of chronic infection with hepatitis B and C. Data on the seroprevalence of chronic hepatitis B are often routinely available from blood donors and from antenatal women who are screened for hepatitis B surface antigen (HBsAg) (http://www.hpa.org.uk/infections/topics_az/BIBD/menu.htm). However, blood donors are a highly

Table 15.2 Advantages and disadvantages of supplementary data sources for hepatitis surveillance.

Data source or type	Advantages	Disadvantages
Patient risk factor information	Identify preventable exposures	Resource intensive
Molecular typing	May identify imported strains and links between cases	Requires specialized laboratory capacity
Hepatitis testing requests	Identify prevalence among those tested; predict future workload for health services	Large amount of data handling required
Hospital admissions	More complete data on severe disease	Coding of acute and chronic infection often not clear; only tracks severe disease
Seroprevalence	Complete data on past exposure and current infection	Difficult to obtain representative samples; resource intensive

selected group and antenatal populations exclude males, who may be at greater risk of hepatitis infection. Seroprevalence studies for hepatitis B and C are often carried out in high-risk populations, such as IDUs. Estimation of overall prevalence requires knowledge of the size of the group being studied and the extent of overlap between populations. Seroprevalence studies in general populations are more difficult to conduct, but residual sera have been used in Australia [17] and from individuals undergoing social security checks in France [18]. The strengths and weaknesses of various types of supplementary information are summarized in Table 15.2.

Surveillance as part of public health intelligence

Public health intelligence is based on the integration of routine surveillance data, available supplementary data, and informal reports. The product resulting from the analysis, integration, and interpretation of all available information is used in the formulation of health strategy and policy across that population.

Knowing the denominator for the population under surveillance is essential for appropriate use of surveillance. For national surveillance, population data, broken down by age and sex, are usually available from the census. If data from sentinel schemes can be linked to the correct denominator for the population under surveillance, and if the sentinel sites are representative of a larger population, then

extrapolations can be made to a national level, avoiding the need to collect detailed information on all cases. More commonly, defining populations for sentinel schemes is problematic, as individuals from one region may attend providers in neighboring regions. In some health services, it is possible to define a catchment population for certain providers; this occurs when individuals are registered with a single practitioner or receive all their healthcare in certain units as part of their health insurance plan.

Other sources of data can help describe the epidemiology of hepatitis. Monitoring risk factors for infection in a community may be helpful. For example, data on local prevalence of injecting drug use can guide targeted harm reduction measures and data on needle sharing amongst IDUs may indicate a potential problem before increasing rates of infection are recognized (http://www.hpa.org.uk/infections/topics_az/injectingdrugusers/Shooting_Up_2004_data.pdf). Monitoring of the likely sources of infection may also be useful. For example, hepatitis E infections acquired in western Europe are thought to be due to transmission from animals; therefore, seroprevalence studies in animal populations in Sweden [19] and typing of veterinary and human isolates in Spain [20] have been conducted.

Monitoring control measures can help identify potential reasons for changes in hepatitis incidence. Interventions that can be monitored include vaccination coverage [21], screening programs (http://www.hpa.org.uk/infections/topics_az/BIBD/menu.htm), and access to drug treatment programs (http://www.nta.nhs.uk/areas/ndtms/default.aspx).

193

Uses of public health intelligence (Box 15.2)

Estimating incidence, prevalence, and burden of disease

Routine reporting by providers, laboratory reports, and death certificates may be used to assess the burden of viral hepatitis infection. Reports from providers and laboratories can be used to estimate age-specific incidence although adjustments should be made for underdiagnosis and for underreporting [22]. Incidence can also be inferred from seroprevalence studies of the markers of past or current infection (anti-HAV, anti-HBc, and anti-HCV) but in older populations these markers will reflect cumulative exposure over many years, and may include

---

Box 15.2 Uses of public health intelligence at a local and national level and examples of important public health questions.

Estimating incidence, prevalence, and burden
• What are the trends in the rate of acute hepatitis A and B?
• What is the estimated prevalence of chronic hepatitis B and C?
Assessing the contribution of relevant exposures
• What are the risk factors for acute hepatitis A and B?
• Which groups/communities are affected by chronic hepatitis B and C?
Evaluating prevention and control programmes
• What is the uptake for antenatal screening women for hepatitis B?
• What is the immunisation coverage in the target groups?
Healthcare planning for treatment of chronic liver disease
• What resources are required to care for those with chronic hepatitis B and C in the future?
Prevention of secondary disease
• Who requires postexposure vaccination and how will they get it?
Identification and investigation of clusters/ outbreaks
• Is this a true increase?
• Is the increase due to an avoidable exposure?

---

exposure in other countries prior to immigration [23].

Knowing the rate of complications from acute disease and the proportion of acute hepatitis B and C infections that become chronic is useful and necessary to plan appropriate healthcare. This rate may vary between populations or among populations (e.g., by age groups) [22]. It can be combined with data on the rate of progression from chronic infection to liver disease to estimate the potentially preventable burden.

Assessing the contribution of relevant exposures

Local surveillance data on acute hepatitis A and B infections can help ascertain patterns of disease transmission, identify local populations at risk, and guide disease prevention. Although acute hepatitis C infection is rarely recognized, identification of recent infections (e.g., seroconverters) may identify nosocomial transmissions. In this situation, a retrospective cohort study may identify other exposed patients who may benefit from early diagnosis and treatment. Because asymptomatic infection is common and because of the relatively long incubation period for hepatitis, collation of risk factor data at a national level may identify the emergence of infections in specific populations before local outbreaks are recognized. This can be used to guide national policy and guidance on prevention.

Routine collection of local risk factor data for cases of chronic hepatitis B and C is resource-intensive and of lower benefit because transmission may have occurred many years earlier or in other countries. Alternatively, sentinel surveillance to identify local patterns of transmission and populations at risk of infection may be worthwhile. Such surveillance may be coordinated regionally or nationally. For areas not undertaking such surveillance, data from sentinel sites with similar sociodemographic profiles may help to guide local public health action.

Evaluating prevention and control programs

Surveillance can be used to develop and evaluate prevention and control activities. For example, national or local, selective or universal vaccination programs have the potential to reduce the burden of hepatitis A and B infections. The decision on whether to introduce universal vaccination should be based upon an economic analysis that estimates the potential benefits and costs of that option. Such analyses require accurate disease surveillance data [24]. Once hepatitis A or B vaccines have been implemented, surveillance of the preventable infection in the target group is essential. This will require a reporting system that includes laboratory investigation of almost all cases. Vaccine coverage information and vaccination status of reported cases is also needed to interpret any changes in incidence. Local scrutiny of hepatitis A and B cases can be used to identify those who should have been vaccinated and assess other missed opportunities for prevention (e.g., transmission from an infected household contact, perinatal transmission). Local monitoring of hepatitis B testing among antenatal women and provision of harm reduction services among drug users (e.g., needle exchange) will also guide prevention policies.

The impact of mass vaccination on herd immunity can be modeled using surveillance data. In England, models were used to predict the coverage that could be achieved and the impact of transmission of hepatitis B amongst IDUs in the community by the introduction of a program to immunize prisoners with hepatitis B vaccine [25].

In the absence of an effective vaccine, one of the primary means for preventing hepatitis C infection is by blood donor selection and screening policies. Surveillance of the prevalence of hepatitis in blood donors and monitoring of transfusion-transmitted infections can be used to evaluate these policies (http://www.hpa.org.uk/infections/topics_az/BIBD/menu.htm). In most industrialized countries, injecting drug use is the most important route of hepatitis C acquisition and should be the target of prevention strategies. Surveillance data can be used to provide an impetus for educational initiatives, for drug treatment services, and for needle exchange schemes.

Healthcare planning for treatment of chronic liver disease

Individuals with chronic hepatitis B and C infection are at risk of developing cirrhosis, liver failure, and primary liver cancer. The treatment and care for these conditions may be expensive [26]. The recent availability of effective treatment for both infections, therefore, requires cost–benefit analyses and planning for the provision of such treatment. Such planning of service provision may be guided by surveillance data. The estimated number of individuals likely to require treatment and further care can be used to establish care pathways to ensure access to services. By using data on a disease endpoint and information on the period of time from infection to that endpoint, modeling can also be used to estimate the past incidence and to predict the future burden of an infection. In France, deaths from hepatocellular carcinoma (HCC) due to hepatitis C have been used to investigate the past incidence of infection and predict an increase in future HCC cases [27].

Prevention of secondary disease

When acute hepatitis A and B cases are identified it is important to determine (where possible) the source of infection and potential for prevention of secondary cases. Public health staff or healthcare providers should contact the patient to provide information and advice on how to prevent transmission of infection. Contacts should be identified, advised, tested, and offered vaccine or other interventions as appropriate.

Similarly, cases of newly diagnosed chronic hepatitis B need information and advice and contacts should be identified, advised, tested, and vaccinated as appropriate. Barriers to using local surveillance for such case management include resource constraints, difficulties distinguishing acute from chronic cases, and privacy concerns [28]. The priority for local surveillance should be the identification of HBsAg-positive pregnant women so that babies born to such mothers receive hepatitis B vaccination and hepatitis B-specific immunoglobulin as appropriate.

As transmission of hepatitis C to sexual and household contacts of cases is uncommon (although such individuals may share other risk factors for infection), use of local surveillance to identify cases and contacts is of lower public health benefit and is likely to be very resource-intensive. Public health departments can work with healthcare providers to

territories) that have implemented confidential name-based HIV infection surveillance are eligible to report both HIV and AIDS cases to the national HIV/AIDS surveillance system and combined reported 92% of persons diagnosed with AIDS in 2004 [4,9]. HIV/AIDS surveillance in the US has evolved as advances in treatment transformed HIV from an apparently acute and fatal disease (i.e., AIDS) to one that can be chronic and medically managed for decades. Because treatment is dependent on HIV diagnosis, only persons who are tested for HIV and access appropriate care can maximally benefit.

The Ryan White Comprehensive AIDS Resources Emergency Act (RWCA), the large emergency financial assistance program overseen by the Health Resources Services Administration (HRSA) and authorized by Congress, is intended to serve as the provider of last resort for comprehensive HIV care. Allocation of federal funds under the RWCA has been based on the reporting of AIDS cases to CDC, causing states to prioritize AIDS reporting over HIV reporting. Starting in 2007, RWCA funds were to be allocated based on all cases of HIV disease (HIV and AIDS) [10]. The key effect on surveillance has been to tie the award of federal funds to case surveillance data.

Case definitions

Case definitions for HIV and AIDS surveillance have evolved over time and are defined according to age and disease status. Cases are defined as HIV infection (without AIDS) or as AIDS. For purposes of public health surveillance, progression from HIV to AIDS is unidirectional. Once a case has met the criteria to be classified as AIDS, it cannot be reclassified as HIV/not AIDS even if the patient clinically improves and achieves a less immunocompromised state.

Adolescent/adult AIDS case definition
Effective July 2006, AIDS diagnosed in a person at least 13 years of age is defined as HIV infection with any variant of HIV (e.g., HIV-1 and HIV-2) accompanied by a CD4+ T-lymphocyte count of <200 cells/µL (or less than 14% of total lymphocytes) and/or at least 1 of 26 AIDS defining conditions [11]. Three preceding AIDS case definitions

were established between 1981 and 1993, each of which affected trend analyses. The most dramatic case definition change came in 1993, when low CD4 count was added as an AIDS criterion [12]. This addition resulted in a perturbation of AIDS incidence trends due to the immediate addition of reported "immunologic" AIDS cases, an enhanced role for laboratory-based reporting, and the virtual disappearance of AIDS cases that met the case definition based solely on clinical criteria.

HIV case definition for adolescents/adults
The HIV case definition has undergone less change. Since the initial definition in 1986, changes have reflected advances in the sensitivity and specificity of antibody tests, and improvements in HIV detection tests. The current HIV case definition for adolescents and adults, introduced in 1999 and having undergone minor revisions in 2005, defines a case based on either confirmed HIV antibodies or detection of virus or viral antigens [13].

Pediatric AIDS case definition
HIV affects younger individuals differently; hence, a separate case definition exists for children [14]. In 1987 and 1994 the main case definition modifications were made and combined comprise the current case definition for surveillance [15]. This case definition includes 24 AIDS-defining conditions but, unlike the adolescent/adult case definition, does not include any immunologic criterion (i.e., CD4 count) for case defining purposes. In 2006, for children aged 18 months through 12 years of age at diagnosis, an AIDS diagnosis became contingent upon laboratory confirmation of HIV infection [16].

Perinatal and pediatric HIV case definitions
Pediatric cases are divided into those diagnosed in children 18 months through 12 years of age and infants <18 months of age. Virtually all children diagnosed with HIV at <18 months of age are born to HIV-infected mothers therefore, HIV antibodies detected at <18 months may be maternal and may not indicate infection in the child. Perinatal case definitions, therefore, cover HIV infection (subcategorized as definitive or presumptive) and HIV noninfection in the HIV-exposed infant (also subcategorized as presumptive or definitive).

Table 16.1 Minimum performance standards for critical attributes and activities to achieve maximum performance established by the CDC and CSTE.

Attribute	Minimum performance measure	Examples of activities to achieve acceptable performance
Accuracy		
Interstate	≤5% duplicate case reports	Participate in routine interstate duplication review
		Conduct interstate reciprocal case notification
Intrastate	≤5% duplicate case reports	Verify accuracy of key patient identifiers
	≤5% incorrect matched surveillance reports	Assess accuracy of matching algorithms
Completeness of case ascertainment	≥85% of diagnosed cases reported to public health for a given diagnostic year	Include reporting from multiple sources (e.g., healthcare provider, laboratory, vital statistics)
Timeliness of case reporting	≥66% of cases reported to public health within 6 mo of diagnosis	Electronic reporting Active surveillance driven by laboratory reporting
Risk factor ascertainment	≥85% of cases (or representative sample with identified HIV exposure risk factor	Healthcare provider education Patient and provider risk assessment tools Matching to other public health databases with risk factor information

These definitions rely on results of HIV viral detection tests such as PCR, p24 antigen, or viral culture and are dependent on the age of the infant when the tests are performed. Determining HIV infection status of HIV-exposed infants is complicated and requires multiple tests over time. Incomplete testing leads to an indeterminate HIV infection status. For children ≥18 months of age, confirmed HIV antibody tests are indicative of HIV infection. For these older pediatric cases, the HIV infection case definition is identical to that for adolescents and adults.

National HIV/AIDS surveillance and the Michigan State perspective

Guidelines for surveillance

Although HIV/AIDS case reporting uses established case reporting forms, some states have made modifications to these forms for local needs. All states use standardized surveillance software for electronic reporting. To be eligible for reporting to CDC, a case must have a minimum set of data elements: soundex code of the last name (a nonunique four-digit alphanumeric code), date of birth, sex, race/ethnicity, and date of diagnosis. If the patient is reported as dead, the date of death is required. Data are checked for omissions or inconsistencies as they are reported

to CDC; critical data inconsistencies result in exclusion of the case report from national data. At least quarterly, areas should assess cases with missing required data elements to improve completeness and accuracy of case reporting.

In 1999, CDC established key performance standards that define a well-functioning HIV/AIDS surveillance system as follows: (1) provide accurate case counts with complete case ascertainment, (2) maximize ascertainment of HIV transmission risk factors, and (3) provide timely case reporting. The required attributes, measures, and minimum performance standards for HIV/AIDS surveillance systems are listed in Table 16.1 [13]. To assist surveillance programs in measuring and achieving these minimum standards and provide a framework for improving performance, in 2005, CDC and the Council of State and Territorial Epidemiologists (CSTE) developed technical guidance for local and state health departments and conducted regional trainings for surveillance staff. These guidance documents focus on (1) outlining structural requirements needed to achieve success in specific areas, (2) process requirements—or steps to be taken to achieve success, and (3) outcomes to be measured to evaluate success. An example of such technical guidance relates to mortality ascertainment. A structural requirement is that the surveillance program has access to death certificates and vital

203

registry data sets to identify deaths in persons with HIV or AIDS. A process requirement would be that each program annually matches with their state death registry to determine vital status of known HIV/AIDS cases and to identify new cases. An outcome measure would be that fewer than 5% of cases reported annually are initially identified through death registry matching.

Risk factor ascertainment

Individual risk factors for HIV acquisition should be collected for all newly diagnosed cases. The risk factors include sexual behaviors (e.g., male–male sexual contact or male–female sex with a known HIV-infected person), injection drug use, transfusion or transplantation of blood/tissues known to be from an HIV-infected donor, or being born to an HIV-infected mother. Based on the historic probability of likely route of infection, risk factors are hierarchically classified into assigned HIV transmission categories. Unfortunately, ascertainment of risk factors has become difficult [17]. However, demand for this information remains high because it helps focus prevention programs.

Consequently, Michigan (and many other states) has developed a variety of techniques for obtaining risk factor information. The most prominent is prioritizing cases without mode of transmission for investigation. For example, a person who is HIV-infected and has not had sex in the prior decade and does not inject drugs would be a higher priority for follow-up investigation than a sexually active adult.

Risk ascertainment is higher for persons with AIDS than with HIV alone. Seventeen percent of AIDS cases and 24% of HIV cases had an undetermined mode of transmission among cases in Michigan in July 2006. Among major race/ethnic groups in Michigan, African-American women have the highest rate of no identified risk—31% of those living with AIDS and 43% of those with HIV/not AIDS. For women, these higher rates are likely due to their lack of knowledge of their male sex partners' HIV status and/or behaviors.

CDC and CSTE have established national guidance to assist in ascertainment of risk factors including examples of risk factor assessment tools for use by patients and providers. Methods for maximiz-ing risk information in Michigan include ongoing training of surveillance staff and providers on why risk factors are important and how the information is used. To maximize collection of risk factors, surveillance staff take a list of cases without identified risk to facility/provider site visits to talk to site staff about whether they have identified risk behaviors for HIV transmission since the initial case report form was completed. Because risk factor documentation in medical records varies, it can be more efficient to have a specific contact person at the site who provides updates. In the medical record, risk factor information is most commonly found in the social worker notes and "history and physical" sections. Sexually transmitted disease records may also reveal information on mode of transmission, but the effort it takes to access these records must be weighed against the fruitfulness of the search.

Laboratory reporting/surveillance

Reporting of individual HIV-related laboratory results (e.g., positive confirmatory HIV antibody tests, viral detection results, CD4 counts) directly from laboratories to surveillance programs can support key surveillance objectives and facilitate timely case ascertainment [18]. Using laboratory results to identify new cases can facilitate more focused field investigations (medical chart abstractions) or serve as a trigger to request that a healthcare provider report a case.

Collection of all CD4 counts and viral load results allows better characterization of the stage of disease at the time of initial HIV diagnosis and provides population-based measures of the number of patients who could benefit from antiretroviral treatment. Where allowed by local laws, surveillance staff can work with other HIV/AIDS program areas to link newly identified or progressing individual patients to appropriate healthcare services. Requiring laboratories to report only those CD4 counts <200 cells/μL (i.e., restricted to levels defining an AIDS case), as was done by approximately half of states in the US by 2005, limits the ability to measure the overall number of HIV-infected persons who might benefit from HAART.

Complete collection of laboratory results, including any preceding negative HIV tests found upon medical record review, can allow identification of newly diagnosed cases as truly incident, or even a case in the primary stage of HIV infection. New infections, particularly in persons with high viral loads, are thought to account for a large number of new HIV transmissions, especially when the infected person is not aware of his or her HIV infection [19].

Because CD4 and viral load monitoring are a part of routine HIV care in the US, their reporting can indicate when patients are "in care" [20]. The minimum indication of "receiving adequate care" is defined by HRSA as having a viral load, a CD4 count, or prescription of antiretroviral therapy during a 1-year period. The absence of such results in surveillance registries would suggest that these patients are not in care or are now receiving care in another jurisdiction. Area measures of 'in-care" and "not-in-care" can be used to assess the effectiveness of programs intended to link patients to care, and provide an overall estimate of unmet need necessary for planning purposes.

Record linkage

HIV/AIDS data should be linked to other public health databases for evaluation, checking the validity of individual data elements, and for overall case ascertainment completeness. The frequency of such linkages depends on both program resources as well as morbidity level and yield from the matches. At a minimum, all HIV/AIDS registries should be linked to the state death registry annually. Other databases to be linked include birth certificates (which may reveal children with perinatal exposure), tuberculosis, and cancer case registries. If laboratory data are not a routine data source for the surveillance program, matching with laboratory databases at least annually will allow the addition of CD4 counts and viral loads.

Most birth, death, tuberculosis, and cancer registries are part of state health departments, making them relatively accessible to a state HIV/AIDS surveillance program. The confidentiality standards used by these programs need to be reviewed to assure that their security and confidentiality standards are at least as high as those that the HIV/AIDS surveillance program maintains. If they are not, then the names should come to the HIV/AIDS surveillance program for linking and should not

be provided to the program with the lower standards. It helps to set up an agreement in writing that addresses the responsibilities of each program involved in the match, specifies what is done with the data, and prohibits the placement of named data on laptops or removable devices (e.g., flash drives, CDs).

Case residency

Geographic assignment for a case is given to the city and state of residence at time of HIV diagnosis and/or at time of AIDS diagnosis. This method of measurement is intended to best represent where the infection (transmission) occurred. However, because HIV infection is now a chronic disease, current residence is increasingly important. It gives a measure of the burden of disease prevalence in a given area and can be used to assess the need for HIV-related services. Accurate current residence data are difficult to obtain in practice, because a surveillance program would need to track both who moves in and who moves out of the jurisdiction. Recent CDC initiatives that assist states in conducting interstate duplicate review will improve this tracking, but evaluation will still be needed to establish how accurately this can be performed.

Security and confidentiality

Security and confidentiality are central to the work of HIV/AIDS surveillance due to several features, some of which are unique to HIV/AIDS data: (1) identifying information may be maintained for decades; (2) the registry includes personal and sensitive information about sexual practices and potentially illegal behaviors; (3) society still stigmatizes some of these behaviors; (4) all of the above factors, if not addressed carefully, could result in providers not reporting cases of HIV or AIDS or reporting false names. CDC and CSTE have completed guidelines that jurisdictions must follow to maintain funding for HIV/AIDS surveillance: *Technical Guidance for HIV/AIDS Surveillance Programs, Volume III: Security and Confidentiality Guidelines* [21]. These guidelines include a Security and Confidentiality Program Requirement Checklist that contains five guiding principles and 35 requirements used to evaluate program compliance. Integrating security and confidentiality into daily work and attendance at mandatory annual trainings should become a part of standard operating procedures. Michigan finds that collecting anecdotes of "real-life" situations and using them as scenarios for discussion makes the trainings more meaningful.

Use of HIV/AIDS surveillance data

HIV/AIDS surveillance data have a variety of uses including (1) monitoring the incidence and prevalence of HIV infection and AIDS, and HIV-related morbidity and mortality in the population, (2) measuring levels of viral resistance in newly diagnosed persons, and (3) identifying changes in trends of HIV transmission and identifying populations at risk. These data can also be utilized to target prevention interventions and evaluate their effectiveness, allocate funds for social and medical services and facilitate access to health, social, and prevention services, including medical treatment. In addition, there is a legislatively mandated link between nationally reported HIV/AIDS cases and the allocation of more than $2 billion of RWCA funds for care. All of these uses of surveillance data require an ongoing need to ensure the highest accuracy possible.

Development of HIV/AIDS surveillance in Michigan

Michigan's active AIDS surveillance system began in 1986 in Detroit. This location placed staff within a 10-minute drive of the hospitals that were seeing the majority of AIDS cases at that time. Regular contact with Infection Control Practitioners at hospitals was established. Keeping files on each site and analyzing patterns in reports helped determine site visit frequency. Examples of variables monitored included timeliness of reporting from that site, level of risk factor ascertainment, and willingness to report cases without prompting by the health department. Change in staff either at the site or the health department necessitated a site visit. Other case-finding methods included death certificate review for AIDS, HIV, or the more common AIDS-defining conditions. Hospitals with many AIDS cases initially identified via death certificate were targeted for increased attention.

More recently, medical care for HIV-infected persons has shifted to the outpatient setting but similar surveillance techniques apply: (1) identifying contacts who report cases, (2) reviewing methods to identify HIV-infected persons, (3) setting up a regular schedule of phone calls and site visits, and (4) deciding who will complete case report forms. It is not uncommon for patients to be tested in one place (e.g., community-based organizations, hospital emergency departments, physicians' offices) and enter care elsewhere. We recommend that reporting be pursued anywhere that tests and/or care are administered for HIV-infected persons, because building redundancy into the program improves completeness of reporting. It is best to pursue sources of reports that are able to give the information required to complete the case report form; however, because surveillance is shifting toward a focus on new infections, this needs to be balanced with the goal of obtaining the first positive HIV test.

In the outpatient setting there is usually not a particular person who routinely reports diseases. Consequently, "provider-buy-in," including giving useful information back to clinicians, is important. At a minimum, reporting sources should receive regular statistical summaries. This can be efficiently accomplished using a listserve which also includes data users.

Surveillance staff must earn the trust of providers by knowing the confidentiality laws in their jurisdiction. This includes understanding how the Health Insurance Portability and Accountability Act (HIPAA) applies to surveillance. HIPAA applies to health information created or maintained by healthcare providers who engage in certain electronic transactions, health plans, and healthcare clearing houses. It requires consent for the release of "protected health information," including names and other identifying information. However, HIPAA has a specific exemption for reporting cases to the health department for purposes of surveillance. Many health departments have found it useful to discuss the surveillance exemption in a standard letter. It may be beneficial to include such a letter in a packet of information sent out to new providers.

Developing relationships with those who both report cases and use the data as well as affected communities increases the strength of an active

HIV/AIDS surveillance systems. For example, as the epidemic increased in the African-American community, MDCH built relationships with key African-American health leaders and physicians. To complete the circle of organizations, we met with leaders of key gay organizations. These relationships helped create trust and kept surveillance staff aware of ongoing community issues that might impact surveillance.

Role of local (city or county) health departments

The Michigan Communicable Disease Rules state that reporting of notifiable diseases goes from the provider to the local health department (LHD) and then to the state. The LHDs are mostly county-specific, but also include the City of Detroit Health Department and multicounty district health departments in the more rural northern parts of the state. At the state level, surveillance staff needed the approval of the LHDs to request providers to send HIV/AIDS case reports directly to the state health department. In Michigan, in the 1980s we met with representatives of the LHDs to set up policies and practices that would aid surveillance and give LHDs the information they needed. Seeking the advice of the LHDs on surveillance challenges and producing routine statistical summaries of HIV/AIDS in their jurisdiction have helped maintain these relationships.

Pediatric case ascertainment

Distinguishing infants who are HIV-infected from those who are perinatally HIV-exposed but not infected is resource-intensive. A potential barrier to conducting surveillance among perinatally HIV-exposed children can be the language of reporting regulations, because surveillance is being conducted for persons not yet identified as infected with HIV. CSTE passed a position statement in 2002 to support reporting of these children before their serostatus can be definitively determined [22]. Many states have added HIV-exposure among newborns as a reportable event. In Michigan, the Communicable Disease Rules allow "reporting of suspect illness" and reporting of conditions not listed. These sections allow Michigan physicans to report perinatally HIV-exposed children since such exposure is

considered to be a "suspect illness". New cases of HIV identified among children with uninfected mothers are unusual and may be due to sexual or other abuse or early initiation of sexual behaviors and/or injection drug use. As such, they are individually investigated as cases of public health importance.

Laboratory reporting

Regulatory changes requiring HIV case reporting and later, reporting of HIV test results by laboratories, have enhanced Michigan's HIV/AIDS surveillance over time. HIV was added to the list of notifiable diseases by the state legislature in December 1988. However, this law exempted clinical laboratories from the reporting requirement and led to an HIV reporting system that, like the AIDS reporting system that preceded it, was clinically based. As medical care became more decentralized, the system's dependence on conducting surveillance with a manageable number of key physicians became less reliable. MDCH requested a law change that would require laboratories to report positive HIV laboratory results to the health department. In December 2004, Public Act 514 was signed into law and required clinical laboratories to report positive HIV antibody test results and all CD4 counts/percents and all HIV viral load results (including undetectable results) among HIV-infected persons.

Laboratory reporting has become the most frequent mechanism for learning of new cases. However, case report forms must still be obtained from providers, because laboratory data are insufficient for completing case report forms. Lab results can also be used to update a case from HIV to AIDS if a CD4 count <200 or 14% is reported. MDCH interprets Michigan disease reporting rules to mean that any clinician who cares for an HIV-infected person is responsible to report that case. This helps insure that reporting is complete and that we have current care information on individuals.

Data management

A critical part of collecting HIV/AIDS data is maintaining the database. Regularly scheduled data cleaning should be part of ongoing work routines.

In Michigan, statistics are produced on a quarterly basis. In preparation for producing those reports, standard cleaning programs are run. To identify potential duplicates, a list of cases that match on soundex code and date of birth is generated. An error-checking component involves running a standard analytic program that prints information on cases with suspect vital status, state identification number, death information, or other questionable diagnostic and demographic information. For both steps, original paper case report forms are pulled and compared, and duplicates or errors are reconciled. A site cleaning procedure involves running a SAS program that compares all facilities of diagnosis and sites of care to the legal list of facilities updated during the previous quarter's cleaning. Additional data cleaning projects are also developed based on errors that are revealed when responding to data requests.

The Michigan surveillance system manages duplicate reports for a case (e.g., case reports from different providers who provide HIV-related care for a patient, multiple CD4 and viral load tests results from laboratories, and/or interstate reciprocal case notifications) by having multiple methods for searching for persons in the registry in addition to maintaining fields for multiple names, multiple dates of birth (DOB) and, if needed, multiple social security numbers. We suggest that, if local laws allow, a "noncase file" should be maintained. This file folder has paper case report forms that have been completed on someone later discovered to be uninfected. Rather than shred these case report forms, these files are maintained, using the same security and confidentiality procedures as for cases, in case the person presents for care again with questionable diagnostic status.

Evaluation of surveillance

Having high quality data is critical for targeting of prevention programs and for designing programs for persons in care. The national guidance on evaluation recommends that reabstractions be conducted at least annually and that they target demographic, risk factors, laboratory, and clinical data from a representative sample of records.

Timeliness and completion are assessed according to the CSTE/CDC guidelines (Table 16.1). Timeliness calculations suggest which sites may benefit from visits by surveillance staff. Improving completeness can cause timeliness to decrease. For example, in Michigan, a clinically based HIV case reporting system existed for 15 years. When laboratory reporting began, reports were received on old cases that had been missed, resulting in a long delay between date of diagnosis and date of report, but increasing completeness.

Data quality is also evaluated through validation of key analytic variables, determined by the frequency with which the variable is analyzed. For example, date of HIV and AIDS diagnoses, race, sex, age at diagnosis, HIV transmission category, and residence at diagnosis are used in many, if not, most analyses, and are therefore important to prioritize for accuracy. Patient name is also an important variable because it is used to rule out duplicate reports. For example, names are reviewed for potential misspellings, use of nicknames (which are recorded as aliases), correct assignment of "Jr." and addition of a middle name or initial.

Routine analyses

As shown in Figure 16.1, HIV/AIDS can be diagnosed at varying amounts of time after initial infection, and the time between infection and diagnosis and the time between diagnosis and report can vary substantially. Consequently, trends in reported cases may not represent either trends in new diagnoses or trends in new infections. At the national level, both HIV and AIDS cases are presented both by date of report (which will include reporting delay artifact, but accurately represents the burden of reporting on a surveillance program) and by estimated date of diagnosis. The diagnoses are estimates that have been adjusted for reporting delays [23]. In Michigan, adjustments for reporting delay are made and trends by year of diagnosis are provided annually [24].

Routine analyses should be conducted to evaluate both the state of the epidemic and the surveillance system, including analyzing current prevalence and trends in (1) new HIV diagnoses, (2) new AIDS diagnoses, and (3) the number and proportion of persons diagnosed with AIDS within a month of their initial HIV diagnosis. States can use CDC-provided software programs to adjust their data for reporting

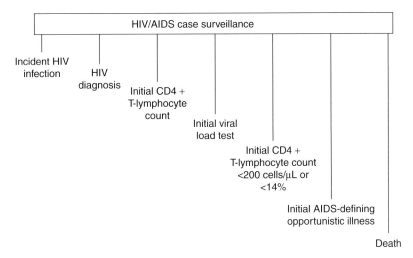

Fig 16.1 Sentinel events in HIV/AIDS case surveillance.

delays. Trends in new HIV diagnoses indicate who is being tested. Although HIV incidence should ideally represent new HIV infections, new diagnoses are a surrogate measure for incidence. New infections are not the same as new diagnoses, and only a subset of those persons recently diagnosed were recently infected. Trends in new AIDS diagnoses will evaluate both successes at early HIV diagnosis as well as keeping HIV-infected persons from progressing to severe immune suppression. If analysis reveals that a large proportion (more than a quarter) of persons newly diagnosed with HIV were diagnosed with AIDS at the same time or shortly thereafter, this may show a lack of success in getting infected persons diagnosed early and should fuel efforts to increase routine testing [24,25].

An analysis of Detroit area data indicated that about half of persons who had a first CD4 count reported within 6 months of their HIV diagnosis had a count under 200 cells/µL. Pregnant women were diagnosed with HIV at higher CD4 counts than nonpregnant women or men. Evidence points to routine testing of pregnant women as a major contributing factor in this earlier diagnosis [26]. There are several scenarios that influence the proportion of people reported with an AIDS diagnosis at the time of their initial HIV diagnosis. The most obvious is testing long after initial infection when testing is motivated by the onset of symptoms. However, it is possible that persons may have tested anonymously and either not received their test results or not gone into care. Another possibility is that some persons tested confidentially, but in another state. Without interstate communication, an original earlier HIV test date in the other state would not be linked to what appears to be the initial case report in a jurisdiction. Routine interstate deduplication can evaluate the accuracy of HIV diagnosis date and improve the accuracy of the national surveillance system. For further discussion, please see Chapter 29.

Data dissemination

Creatively thinking about how to best disseminate data and make them useful for reporting sources will strengthen the surveillance program's relationship with the reporters and dramatically increase its relevance. Examples include making state, city, or metropolitan area slide sets available. It is helpful to track data requests and incorporate recurring requests into routine data dissemination. This will assist with responding rapidly to data requests, which will, in turn, assist with creating a reciprocal relationship with reporting sources. Surveillance programs should be prepared to respond rapidly to grant-related data requests from healthcare facilities, local health departments, community-based organizations, AIDS service organizations, and academics. Because it is important

209

to build and maintain relationships with affected communities and providers, directed and ongoing data dissemination to key partners is critical. CDC and HRSA have developed guidance for developing an integrated epidemiologic profile to address planning needs for prevention and care [27]. However, these profiles should be tailored to fit the needs of prevention and care programs in the state or city and respond to local requests. They are very time-consuming to create, but when done properly are an enormous source of data on the epidemic and can be used to respond to many other data requests.

If adequate staff are available, it works well to have staff assigned to groups that routinely use the data that your program collects, such as HIV Prevention Community Planning Groups, and planning councils that advise on how RWCA funding should be distributed and used. Surveillance staff can play a role in training on data interpretation so that informed decisions can be made. These staff can keep planning groups focused on what the epidemic looks like in the particular state, county, or city, rather than the demographic or risk group that is receiving national attention at the time or is of personal interest to influential group members.

Current and future directions for HIV/AIDS surveillance

Until recently, biomedical technology did not allow discrimination between recent and chronic HIV infection; as a result, HIV surveillance predominantly monitors prevalence. New serologic testing methods, particularly the Serologic Testing Algorithm for Recent HIV Seroconversion (STARHS) [28], make it possible to establish a system to differentiate between recent and long-standing HIV-1 infection on a population level. In conjunction with information collected through standard case surveillance and statistical estimation procedures, data from these laboratory methods provide the means to estimate national population-based HIV incidence from the number of recent infections among persons newly diagnosed with HIV [29].

HIV case surveillance faces opportunities and potential challenges introduced by increasingly improved laboratory diagnostics. Highly sensitive and specific rapid HIV antibody tests, some of which can be performed on saliva, are increasing access to HIV testing. The perception that these tests can function as confirmatory tests may mean that a decreasing proportion of screening test results are confirmed. For example, a provider may combine positive results of a rapid HIV test with a low CD4 count and initiate HAART. Depending on the health jurisdiction's reporting regulations, this combination of test results may not meet the case definition for surveillance. The high specificity of rapid HIV tests may allow implementation of alternate confirmatory algorithms for a preliminary positive HIV rapid test that do not require confirmation in a laboratory, allowing easier and rapid, yet accurate confirmation (or determination of negative serostatus) even in low prevalence settings. Surveillance systems that are dependent on laboratory reporting will need to change to meet this challenge.

Case surveillance is designed to monitor the spectrum of HIV infection (Figure 16.1). Historically, AIDS surveillance started at the far right end of this spectrum because death and AIDS were the initial presentation of this epidemic. As the epidemic has evolved, the need to monitor earlier clinical events, corresponding to the left side of the figure, has been increasingly emphasized. This is essential for the two main activities that are informed by surveillance data—prevention and care. Prevention programs are best designed by knowing the "leading edge" of the epidemic. Care is most successful when people enter care with an intact immune system. Continued surveillance of immunologic status (i.e., CD4 cells) will allow documentation of success with early testing and treatment. State and city surveillance programs must continue to work together with each other, CSTE and CDC to increase and maintain the high levels of accuracy needed for the data that are pivotal to the work needed to end this epidemic.

References

1 Gallo RC, Sallahudin S, Popovic M, *et al*. Frequent detection and isolation of cytopathic retroviruses (HTLV-III) from patients with AIDS and at risk for AIDS. *Science* 1984;**224**:500–3.
2 Barre-Sinoussi F, Chermann JC, Rey F, *et al*. Isolation of a T-lympho- tropic retrovirus from a patient at risk

for acquired immune deficiency syndrome (AIDS). *Science* 1983;**220**:868–71.

3 Centers for Disease Control and Prevention. Update: Public Health Service Workshop on Human T-Lymphotropic Virus Type III Antibody Testing—United States. *MMWR Morb Mortal Wkly Rep* 1985;**34**:477–8.

4 Centers for Disease Control and Prevention. Cases of HIV infection and AIDS in the United States, 2004. *HIV/AIDS Surveill Rep* 2005;**16**:1 16.

5 Fraser DW, Tsai TR, Orenstein W, *et al.* Legionnaires' disease: description of an epidemic of pneumonia. *N Engl J Med* 1977;**297**:1189–97.

6 Fairchild AL, Bayer R, Colgrove J, Wolfe D. Searching Eyes: Privacy, the State, and disease surveillance in America (Berkeley: University of California Press, 2007).

7 Burris S. Surveillance, social risk, and symbolism: framing the analysis for research and policy. *J Acquire Immune Defic Syndr* 2000;**25**:S120–7.

8 Morin SF. Early Detection of HIV: Assessing the legislative context. *J Acquir Immune Defic Syndr* 2000;**25**:S144–50.

9 Glynn MK, Lee LM, McKenna MT. The status of national HIV case surveillance, United States 2006. *Public Health Rep* 2007;**122**(suppl 1): 63–71.

10 Ryan White HIV/AIDS Treatment Modernization Act: 2006 Health Resources Services Administration; 2006. Available from: http://hab.hrsa.gov/treatmentmodernization/. Accessed April 25, 2007.

11 Council of State and Territorial Epidemiologists. CSTE Position Statement 05-ID-04: revision of surveillance case definition for AIDS among adults and adolescents ≥13 years of age. Council of State and Territorial Epidemiologists; 2005. Available from: http://www.cste.org/PS/2005pdf/final2005/05-ID-04final.pdf. Accessed July 25, 2006.

12 Centers for Disease Control and Prevention. 1993 Revised classification system for HIV infection and expanded surveillance case definition for AIDS among adolescents and adults. *MMWR Recommend Rep* 1992;**41**:1–19.

13 Centers for Disease Control and Prevention. CDC guidelines for national human immunodeficiency virus case surveillance, including monitoring for human immunodeficiency virus infection and acquired immunodeficiency syndrome. *MMWR Recommend Rep* 1999;**48**:1–27.

14 Lindegren ML, Steinberg S, Byers RH, Jr. Epidemiology of HIV/AIDS in children. *Pediatr Clin North Am* 2000;**47**:1–20.

15 Centers for Disease Control and Prevention. 1994 Revised classification system for human immunodeficiency virus infection in children less than 13 years of age. *MMWR Recommend Rep* 1994;**43**:1–10.

16 Council of State and Territorial Epidemiologists. CSTE Position Statement 06-ID-02: revision of the surveillance case definition for HIV infection and AIDS among children age >18 months but <13 years. Council of State and Territorial Epidemiologists; 2006. Available from: http://www.cste.org/PS/2006pdfs/PSFINAL2006/06-ID-02FINAL.pdf. Accessed August 5, 2006.

17 McDavid K, McKenna MT. HIV/AIDS risk factor ascertainment: a critical challenge. *AIDS Patient Care and STDs* 2006;**20**:285–92.

18 Klevens RM, Fleming PL, Li J, Karon J. Impact of laboratory-initiated reporting of CD4$^+$ T lymphocytes on U.S. AIDS surveillance. *J Acquire Immune Defic Syndr* 1997;**14**:56–60.

19 Marks G, Crepaz N, Janssen RS. Estimating sexual transmission of HIV from persons aware and unaware that they are infected with the virus in the USA. *AIDS* 2006;**20**:1447–50.

20 Council of State and Territorial Epidemiologists. Position Statement 04-ID-07: Laboratory Reporting of Clinical Test Results Indicative of HIV Infection: New Standards for a New Era of Surveillance and Prevention. Council of State and Territorial Epidemiologists; 2004. Available from: http://www.cste.org/ps/2004pdf/04-ID-07-final.pdf. Accessed April 25, 2007.

21 Centers for Disease Control and Prevention. *Technical Guidance for HIV/AIDS Surveillance Programs, Volume III: Security and Confidentiality Guidelines*. Centers for Disease Control and Prevention; 2006. Available from: http://www.cdc.gov/hiv/topics/surveillance/resources/guidelines/guidance/index.htm. Accessed October 1, 2006.

22 Council of State and Territorial Epidemiologists. Position Statement 02-ID-04: surveillance for perinatal HIV exposure. Council of State and Territorial Epidemiologists; 2004. Available from: http://www.cste.org/position%20statements/02-ID-04.pdf. Accessed October 1, 2006.

23 Green TA. Using surveillance data to monitor trends in the AIDS epidemic. *Stat Med* 1998;**17**:143–54.

24 Michigan Department of Community Health. Annual Review of HIV Trends in Michigan 2001–2005. Michigan Department of Community Health; 2007. Available from: http://www.michigan.gov/documents/mdch/MIReport07_195579_7.pdf. Accessed May 7, 2007.

25 Branson BM, Handsfield HH, Lampe MA, Janssen RS, Lyss SB, Clark JE. Revised Recommendations for HIV testing of adults, adolescents, and pregnant women in health-care settings. *MMWR Recommend Rep* 2006;**55**:1–17.

26 Wotring LL, Montgomery JP, Mokotoff ED, Inungu JN, Markowitz N, Crane LR. Pregnancy and other factors associated with higher CD4+ T-cell

counts at HIV diagnosis in Southeast Michigan, 1992–2002. *Medscape Gen Med* 2005. Available from: http://www.medscape.com/viewarticle/498351. Accessed March 16, 2005.

27 Centers for Disease Control and Prevention and Health Resources Services Administration. *Integrated Guidelines for Developing Epidemiologic Profiles: HIV Prevention and Ryan White CARE Act Community Planning*. Centers for Disease Control and Prevention; 2004. Available from: http://www.cdc.gov/hiv/epi_guidelines.htm. Accessed October 1, 2006.

28 Janssen RS, Satten GA, Stramer SL, *et al.* New testing strategy to detect early HIV-1 infection for use in incidence estimates and for clinical and prevention purposes. *JAMA* 1998;**280**:42–8.

29 Lee LM, McKenna MT. Monitoring the incidence of HIV infection in the United States. *Public Health Rep* 2007;**122**(suppl 1):72–9.

17 Surveillance for sexually transmitted diseases

Samuel L. Groseclose, Michael C. Samuel & Hillard Weinstock

Introduction

Sexually transmitted disease (STD) surveillance is a complex endeavor because of the large variety of STD pathogens and associated syndromes and the simultaneous ubiquity of, variability in, and human sensitivity around the behaviors that facilitate transmission of these infections [1]. Fortunately, recently developed laboratory technologies allow more affordable detection and characterization of these agents. This chapter will describe the STD surveillance methods that have furthered our understanding of the distribution of STDs in the community and have informed prevention efforts. This chapter focuses on STD surveillance approaches that have been used in the United States (US); however, most of the principles apply to STD surveillance in other countries with established medical, diagnostic laboratory, and public health infrastructure. Surveillance for HIV/AIDS is discussed in Chapter 16.

Background

Prior to 1900, "venereal diseases" were considered a moral rather than a public health problem in the US, so initiation of STD surveillance lagged behind surveillance for other communicable conditions [2]. As the medical profession began to recognize venereology as a medical specialty, the diagnosis and treatment of STDs in patients and their partners was adopted as the approach to STD control. Surveillance for STDs began in California in 1911, in New York in 1912, and subsequently in other states. In the late 1930s, a number of states began to require premarital blood testing and antenatal screening for syphilis and reporting of syphilis and gonorrhea cases. Federal grants to support STD control initiatives in local and state health departments began in 1939. Since 1941, state health departments have reported cases of all stages of syphilis and gonorrhea annually to the Centers for Disease Control and Prevention (CDC).

In 1972, a national gonorrhea control program was initiated with federal funds appropriated to establish screening programs to identify asymptomatic women with gonococcal infection. In the 1980s, the increased availability of diagnostic tests for chlamydia made large-scale screening programs feasible. During the 1990s, regional infertility prevention programs focused on chlamydia screening and treatment of women were established throughout the US in public family planning clinics and other settings. Chlamydia became a nationally notifiable condition in 1995. In addition to syphilis, gonorrhea, and chlamydia, many local and state health departments conduct surveillance for other bacterial and viral STDs and their sequelae. The continued strong practical disease control focus of most STD programs (i.e., screening, treatment, and partner management) has led to an inextricable linkage of case and partner management, screening, and STD surveillance.

STD surveillance purposes

STD surveillance supports public health efforts by providing a framework for detecting and describing the emergence of an STD (e.g., lymphogranuloma venereum outbreak in Europe in 2003) or changes in an endemic disease (e.g., syphilis outbreaks among men who have sex with men [MSM], 2000 to present), for developing and implementing interventions to address health disparities, and for evaluating the effectiveness of STD prevention interventions [3]. Within this framework, STD surveillance can include monitoring the incidence and prevalence of STDs or their sequelae, pathogen-specific antimicrobial resistance, sexual behaviors, and STD screening and care coverage and quality. Table 17.1 presents a number of surveillance purposes relevant to STD prevention and control and recommends surveillance methods (described below) that can be used to achieve that purpose. Changes in STD prevalence or distribution, the pathogen's biology, diagnostic technologies, or clinical or behavioral interventions may necessitate a change in or reprioritization of surveillance purposes. The progressive elimination of syphilis from many jurisdictions in the US emphasized the need to reorient syphilis prevention and, therefore, surveillance toward early detection and control of outbreaks arising from newly imported infections. Identification of penicillinase-producing *Neisseria gonorrhoeae* and chromosomally mediated penicillin- and tetracycline-resistant *N. gonorrhoeae* in the 1970's led to implementation of sentinel surveillance for gonococcal antimicrobial susceptibility to guide the selection of gonococcal therapies.

STD surveillance approaches

There are several main types of STD surveillance activities: case reporting, prevalence monitoring, sentinel surveillance, behavioral surveillance, population-based surveys, and health services and administrative data-based surveillance.

Case reporting

Currently, syphilis, gonorrhea, and chlamydia are designated as reportable conditions in all 50 states. Other STDs, including chancroid, granuloma inguinale, and lymphogranuloma venereum are reportable in many states. Still others, including genital warts, neonatal herpes, mucopurulent cervicitis, nongonococcal urethritis, and pelvic inflammatory disease are reportable in a few states. At a national level, the only nationally notifiable STDs (other than HIV infection, AIDS, and other conditions that have both sexual and nonsexual modes of transmission, like hepatitis B) are chancroid, chlamydia, gonorrhea, and all stages of syphilis. CDC receives provisional STD morbidity data weekly from state health departments and the District of Columbia. These data are reviewed each week and disseminated in the *Morbidity and Mortality Weekly Report (MMWR)*. In 2005, there were more than 1.3 million case reports of syphilis, gonorrhea, and chlamydia, accounting for >80% of all infectious disease notifications to the CDC; these case reports are considered to substantially undercount the true burden of disease.

Syphilis case reports

After reaching a nadir in 2000, the rate of primary and secondary syphilis increased from 2001 to 2005. Some states and cities that collect information on the sex of sex partners documented an increase in syphilis that was almost entirely among MSM. Information on the sex of partners of persons with syphilis was not available at the national level until 2005. In the absence of national sexual behavior information, trends in the syphilis male to female incidence rate ratio, which are assumed to reflect syphilis trends among MSM, have been increasing in the US in recent years [4]. Such information has been used to refocus STD prevention efforts [5].

Gonorrhea case reports

Gonorrhea remains the second most commonly reported condition to CDC. Over 330,000 cases were reported in both 2004 and 2005 with rates greater than 2 per 100 population in some age and racial/ethnic groups. Gonorrhea rates were 18 times higher in African-Americans than in whites in 2005; this reflects a health disparity that is greater for many STDs than for most other reportable conditions in the US [6]. Incidence rate ratios by demographic subgroup (e.g., race/ethnicity) can be useful

Table 17.1 STD surveillance purposes by surveillance method(s).

Surveillance purpose	Surveillance method(s) to consider
Monitor rates, trends, and geographic distribution of STDs and their sequelae	Case reporting Prevalence monitoring Sentinel provider or laboratory surveillance Assessment of administrative or financial data derived from health information systems Hospital discharge or outpatient clinic records
Early outbreak detection	Case reporting Sentinel provider surveillance
Identify population subgroups and communities at high risk	Case reporting Enhanced case-based surveillance Prevalence monitoring Sentinel provider or laboratory surveillance Special surveillance-related study or survey
Develop operational definition of core group membership for application to program activities and research	Case reporting Enhanced case-based surveillance Sentinel provider surveillance Special surveillance-related study or survey (e.g., social network analysis)
Monitor population-level risk behaviors and social factors that contribute to disease acquisition and transmission	General population-based behavioral surveys +/− biomarkers Special surveillance-related study or survey (e.g., behavioral survey)
Identify persons at increased risk of HIV infection	Case reporting Enhanced case-based surveillance Prevalence monitoring Sentinel provider or laboratory surveillance
Monitor frequency and distribution of antimicrobial susceptibility of STD etiologic agents	Sentinel surveillance for antimicrobial resistance
Assess effectiveness of prevention and control measures	Case reporting Enhanced case-based surveillance Prevalence monitoring Sentinel provider or laboratory surveillance Special surveillance-related study or survey
Develop, evaluate, and modify screening criteria	Prevalence monitoring Sentinel provider surveillance Special surveillance-related study or survey
Monitor screening coverage in defined populations	Prevalence monitoring Sentinel provider surveillance Special surveillance-related study or survey (e.g., administrative data linkage)
Develop, evaluate, and modify case investigation criteria	Case reporting Enhanced case-based surveillance Prevalence monitoring Provider visitation for case management evaluation

Table 17.1 (*Continued*)

Surveillance purpose	Surveillance method(s) to consider
Identify gaps in healthcare and missed opportunities for interventions	Case reporting Enhanced case-based surveillance Prevalence monitoring Provider visitation for case management evaluation Assessment of administrative or financial data derived from healthcare records (e.g., insurance claims) Healthcare provider medical record review
Identify providers and laboratories not testing or reporting	Case reporting Prevalence monitoring Provider or laboratory reporting evaluation visits
Ensure proper treatment and partner management	Case reporting Enhanced case-based surveillance Prevalence monitoring Provider visitation for case management evaluation
Stimulate epidemiologic research and program evaluation	Case reporting Enhanced case-based surveillance Prevalence monitoring Sentinel provider or laboratory surveillance Assessment of administrative or financial data derived from health information systems
Demonstrate need for funding of control programs	Case reporting Enhanced case-based surveillance Prevalence monitoring Sentinel provider or laboratory surveillance

to illustrate the magnitude of health disparities for intervention and planning purposes. Race and ethnicity in the US are risk markers that correlate with other more fundamental determinants of health status such as poverty, access to quality healthcare, healthcare seeking behavior, illicit drug use, and living in communities with high prevalence of STDs.

Chlamydia case reports
The number of chlamydia cases has increased each year for the last 10 years in men and women. This has been attributed to expansion of chlamydia screening activities, use of increasingly sensitive diagnostic tests, increased emphasis on case reporting from providers and laboratories, and improvements in the information systems for reporting. Over 900,000 cases of chlamydia were reported to CDC in both 2004 and 2005 making it the

most commonly reported notifiable disease. These numbers probably underestimate the true incidence of disease. Using prevalence data, the incidence of chlamydial infections in the US was estimated to be about 2.8 million new infections per year in 2000, more than three times the number of reported cases [7].

Enhanced surveillance to supplement case reports of STDs
In response to divergent or emerging trends in STD incidence in different population subgroups, local and state health departments often collect additional data about cases reported via routine morbidity surveillance. Key behavioral data collected during enhanced surveillance may include sex of partner(s), number of sexual partners and sexual network connections, condom use, substance use,

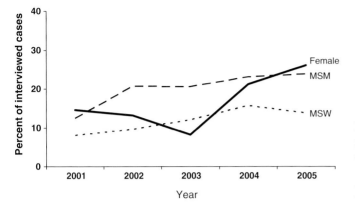

Fig 17.1 Enhanced case-based surveillance: percent of interviewed primary and secondary syphilis cases reporting methamphetamine use by sexual orientation, California, 2001–2005. MSM, men who have sex with men; MSW, men who have sex with women only.

history of incarceration, exchange of sex for money or drugs, and venues used for meeting new or anonymous sex partners. California conducts enhanced surveillance in some areas and has documented increases in methamphetamine use among MSM and heterosexual men and women with syphilis in recent years (Figure 17.1). Similarly, knowledge of venues where persons with STDs meet new or anonymous partners is key to understanding where and how new infections are being acquired, as well as for determining which venues to target for intervention. The Internet has been identified as a venue used by MSM for meeting new sex partners and, therefore, a new venue for education, outreach, and innovative control efforts [8]. Enhanced surveillance data can be collected on a sample of reported STD cases or via sentinel clinics or healthcare providers [9].

Syndromic surveillance for STDs
Notifiable STD surveillance in the US utilizes case definitions that require laboratory confirmation. In countries where clinical and laboratory resources are scarce, syndromic case reporting, which does not require confirmatory diagnostic testing, is often conducted instead. The World Health Organization provides STD-associated syndromic case definitions and recommends that, in the absence of routinely available, high-quality laboratory diagnostic testing, case reporting should be based on syndromes [10]. However, because STDs are often asymptomatic among women and men, and since many clinical characteristics of STDs are not

pathogen-specific, the only syndromes useful for meaningful assessment of STD incidence patterns are urethral discharge and nonvesicular genital ulcer disease [10]. For case management and health services planning, periodic limited prevalence monitoring should be conducted in selected healthcare settings to identify the pathogens associated with STD-associated syndromes.

Prevalence monitoring

Prevalence monitoring is the assessment of STD prevalence among persons in defined populations that are routinely screened. In this context, prevalence refers to the number of persons with positive test results divided by the number of persons screened for the first time in a defined time interval. In situations where repeat tests cannot be excluded, positivity (the number of positive tests/number of adequate test results, ignoring repeat tests) can be used as a surrogate for prevalence. In most clinic settings, chlamydia positivity differs little from prevalence [11].

In the US, the federally funded Regional Infertility Prevention Projects, in each of the 10 public health service regions, monitor chlamydia positivity among approximately 3 million women annually who are screened for chlamydial infection in selected family planning clinics, prenatal care clinics, STD clinics, and corrections facilities [12]. Other sources of STD prevalence include STD screening of persons entering jails and juvenile detention facilities, MSM attending STD clinics and other

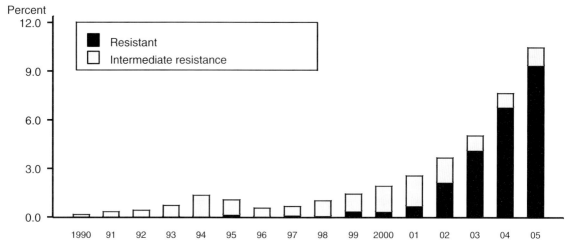

Fig 17.2 Sentinel surveillance: percent of *Neisseria gonorrhoeae* isolates with resistance or intermediate resistance to ciprofloxacin, Gonococcal Isolate Surveillance Project, United States, 1990–2005. Resistant isolates have ciprofloxacin mean inhibitory concentrations (MICs) of ≥1 µg/mL. Isolates with intermediate resistance have ciprofloxacin MICs of 0.125–0.5 µg/mL. Susceptibility to ciprofloxacin was first measured in GISP in 1990.

primary care settings, and adolescent and young adult women and men entering the National Job Training Program [12]. These data augment case reporting data but can be difficult to interpret because both screening policies and the populations screened may change over time. Little behavioral information is available about persons with STDs identified through prevalence monitoring.

Sentinel surveillance

The sentinel surveillance approach can also be used to monitor a variety of STDs or their sequelae when ongoing, detailed surveillance of the entire population is not feasible. Sentinel surveillance typically involves the collection of data from a representative sample of the population of interest. Sentinel STD surveillance systems may be useful in identifying the burden of disease for conditions that are not notifiable, for special populations, or for obtaining information that is not routinely collected (e.g., behavioral or laboratory data). When resources are limited, intermittent sentinel surveillance may be useful.

In 25–30 cities in the US, antimicrobial resistance to *Neisseria gonorroheae* has been monitored since 1986 through the Gonococcal Isolate Surveillance Project (GISP) [13]. The first 25 isolates per month from male patients with gonococcal urethritis in each of these cities are submitted for antimicrobial susceptibility testing at regional laboratories. Demographic, clinical, and behavioral data are also collected from participating patients. With the increased use of nucleic acid amplification tests for the detection of gonorrhea and chlamydia, culture capacity that enables gonococcal susceptibility testing has decreased over time, and GISP data have become increasingly important. GISP data have been used in developing state and national treatment recommendations. In 2007, on the basis of GISP findings, fluoroquinolones were no longer recommended for the treatment of gonococcal infections. (Figure 17.2).

Behavioral surveillance

Typically, information included in STD case reports and prevalence monitoring systems is limited to patients' demographic characteristics. The periodic collection and interpretation of behavioral risk factor information (e.g., describing the general or specific at-risk populations' risk behaviors or linking behavioral risk information with other case patient information) provides critical contextual information to explain changes in STD rates over time and to inform prevention efforts. Behavioral surveillance information from national and state-specific representative samples of the general population is a key source of population-level data on STD-related behaviors, knowledge, and attitudes.

National surveys of the US population that collect useful STD-related behavioral data include the Youth Risk Behavior Survey (YRBS) and the National Survey of Family Growth (NSFG). The YRBS measures the prevalence of health-risk behaviors among high school students through national, state, and local self-administered surveys conducted biennially. Analysis of YRBS data indicates that from 1991 to 1997 the percentage of US high school students who have had sexual intercourse decreased and the prevalence of condom use among sexually active students increased [14]. The NSFG sample represents women and men 15–44 years of age in the US household population and is designed to produce national data. NSFG provides estimates of statistics on sexual behaviors (e.g., anal, vaginal, or oral sex), sexual orientation and attraction (e.g., same- or opposite-sex sexual behavior) [15]. Data from YRBS and NSFG can be used by STD prevention programs to estimate the size and location of at-risk groups in their jurisdictions, to aid interpretation of STD trends, and to tailor prevention messages and other interventions.

Some states collect additional population-based behavioral surveillance data to generate local and state-specific information. Data from two California-specific surveys, the California Women's Health Survey (CWHS) and the California Health Interview Survey (CHIS) have been used to assess STD program needs, evaluate program effectiveness, and interpret STD morbidity trends. CWHS data indicating gaps in chlamydia awareness were used to secure state funds to support a regional health educator network and build local capacity for chlamydia outreach and prevention activities [16]. Similarly, CHIS data from adolescents informed the development of culturally appropriate school-based curricula for STD education [17].

Although these data have been very useful for targeting prevention program activities, behavioral surveillance data can be difficult to interpret because of lack of question validation and standardization and lack of inclusion of compre-

hensive sexual health- and behavior-related questions due to perceived respondent sensitivities. To address questions of validity, local and state programs interested in conducting behavioral surveillance should consider using previously validated questions from other surveys to allow greater comparability.

Population-based surveys

Some local and national surveys incorporate the assessment of STD biomarkers and self-reported behavioral information among a sample of persons representing a larger population. The largest national survey that includes collection of both biologic samples and information on healthcare seeking and behavioral risk factors is the National Health and Nutrition Examination Survey. This nationally representative probability sample survey of the noninstitutionalized US population has examined the prevalence of human papillomavirus [18], herpes simplex virus types 1 and 2 antibodies [19], reactive syphilis serologies, chlamydia, gonorrhea, trichomoniasis, and bacterial vaginosis.

Health services and administrative data-based surveillance

Other sources of national STD surveillance data include health services databases. The National Hospital Discharge Survey (NHDS) is a continuous probability sample of medical records of patients discharged from acute care hospitals in the US. The National Ambulatory Medical Care Survey (NAMCS), a survey of private physicians' office practices, the NHAMCS-ED, an emergency room discharge survey, and the NHAMCS-OPD, a hospital outpatient clinic survey are performed through abstraction of information from medical records. The National Disease and Therapeutic Index (NDTI) is a probability sample survey of private physicians' clinical management practices and provides estimates of the number of initial visits to private physicians' offices for many conditions, including STDs. Despite limitations, NDTI is the only source of national data on office visits for genital herpes, genital warts, and trichomoniasis [12]. Data from four surveys—NAMCS, NHAMCS-ED, NHAMCS-OPD, NDTI—were used to estimate

219

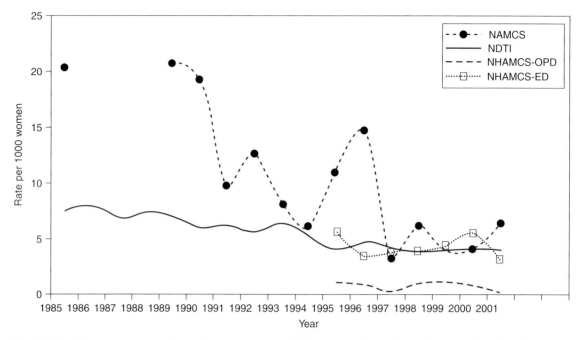

Fig 17.3 Health services data-based surveillance: rates of pelvic inflammatory disease in ambulatory settings, based on NAMCS, NHAMCS-OPD, NHAMCS-ED, and NDTI data, United States, 1985–2001.

rates of pelvic inflammatory disease (PID), a severe complication of chlamydia and gonorrhea infections (Figure 17.3) [20]. Analyses of state-specific health services data sets like the California hospital discharge and vital statistics data have also been used to estimate rates of neonatal herpes, to assess deaths from neonatal herpes, and to assess trends in cesarean section rates associated with herpes [21,22].

Administrative data sources (e.g., billing, pharmacy, or laboratory records from managed care organizations or government-funded healthcare programs) have been used to assess STD-related morbidity or quality of care and provider's compliance with testing and treatment guidelines, including monitoring the percentage of sexually active women under 26 years of age screened annually for chlamydia, a Health Plan Employer Data and Information Set (HEDIS) measure [23,24]. California has used administrative data to assess the chlamydia screening rates in a large-scale entitlement program and compliance with screening guidelines. Administrative data that are most useful for surveillance purposes consist of electronically managed health-

care service and outcome data on large numbers of individuals that allow linkage of multiple observations (e.g., laboratory tests and procedures performed, reported diagnoses) [25]. However, administrative data are typically limited to data needed to bill for care received. The assignment of diagnosis codes (e.g., International Classification of Diseases, Ninth Revision, Clinical Modification (ICD-9-CM)) may be based on local practice or policy and are often difficult to validate. The characteristics and data quality of administrative data sources must be assessed prior to using them for surveillance purposes.

Other surveillance approaches

Laboratory surveys of test usage
Periodic laboratory surveys that monitor STD test volume by test type provide data to assist in interpretation of both case-based surveillance and prevalence monitoring data [26]. Findings from state and national surveys of public health laboratories indicate the increasing use of nucleic acid amplification tests (NAATS) for chlamydia and

gonorrhea testing and declining use of culture for detection of gonorrhea [27].

Combining data from multiple sources
Behavioral surveillance data, population-based survey data, and other secondary data can be used to validate STD incidence and prevalence data. This analysis method is referred to as data synthesis or triangulation—the purpose is to determine if findings from one or more data sources support or differ from information derived from other data sources [28]. If differences are observed, the data analyst is required to account for information discrepancies. Figure 17.3 illustrates synthesis of data from sample surveys that monitor the same outcome, PID, in different types of healthcare settings. In this case, the incidence estimate from each survey has different reliability (based on event frequency), but the declining PID trend observed in data from each source provides stronger evidence for declining PID incidence in the general population than the findings from a single survey.

Another adjunct to basic STD surveillance is the linkage of STD-related surveillance data sets to other data sets to gain information and insight into STD epidemiology or the planning of comprehensive public health interventions. STD data can be matched to other disease registries to assess comorbidity patterns. Data linkage may also be performed to improve demographic, laboratory test result, or clinical data quality and completeness by borrowing information that may be available in one data set but not another. STD-related data matching projects can also link hospital discharge data, substance abuse treatment program data, birth and death statistics, and a range of other data sources to add value to surveillance system data [29].

Surveillance for STD reinfection
Several investigators have defined a repeat chlamydia or gonorrhea infection as an infection detected in the same individual more than 30 days from the initially reported infection [30,31]. Several STD programs have assessed repeat infections in order to target resources to the highest risk cases and to develop and evaluate guidelines for retesting of persons previously infected with an STD [30,32].

Incorporation of Geographic Information Systems into STD surveillance
Mapping and spatial analyses of STD incidence, prevalence, and their correlates allows visualization and monitoring of the spatiotemporal distribution of STDs in the community, detection of disease clusters, and focusing of case management and intervention resources. When behavioral, socioeconomic, or social network data are not available, geographic location may be used as a surrogate in ecological analyses by associating geographically referenced STD surveillance data with data derived from the US Census or population-based surveys [33]. Several investigators have used geographic clustering of repeat STD infections rather than high prevalence regions as an indicator for geographically and socially defined sexual networks or STD high-risk groups [34–37].

STD surveillance case definitions

In the US, the Council of State and Territorial Epidemiologists and the CDC collaboratively develop and maintain the surveillance case definitions used for case reporting of nationally notifiable STDs [38]. The STD surveillance case definitions typically specify clinical and laboratory criteria. For some reportable STDs, the case definitions are fairly clear and simple. For example, for gonorrhea and chlamydial infections, a confirmed case is based on a positive laboratory test for the organism. For other STDs, particularly syphilis, congenital syphilis, and PID, the case definitions are not straightforward. Because of the complex and variable manifestations of syphilis, epidemiologic (e.g., history of sexual exposure to a partner who had confirmed or probable primary or secondary syphilis), clinical (e.g., presence of rash or chancre), and laboratory (e.g., prior serologic test results) criteria must be reviewed to allow staging of syphilis. For surveillance and disease control purposes, "primary" and "secondary" syphilis case data are often combined since they represent infectious stages of syphilis, are typically uniformly classified across jurisdictions, and are most relevant for directing new intervention or prevention efforts.

Specifying case definitions allows similar STD outcomes to be monitored in different data sources, a practice that can improve the interpretation of surveillance information from any single source. ICD-9-CM and Current Procedural Terminology (CPT) codes have been used for STD surveillance purposes [20–23,39]. ICD-9-CM and CPT codes represent both clinical diagnoses and disease-associated procedures, respectively, for selected STDs and their sequelae and are routinely used by health services and administrative data sources.

STD surveillance case definitions are not intended to be used for establishing clinical diagnoses, determining the standard of care necessary for a particular patient, setting guidelines for quality assurance, or providing standards for reimbursement. Use of additional clinical, epidemiologic, and laboratory data may enable a physician to diagnose an STD even though the formal surveillance case definition may not be met. Conversely, the STD surveillance case definition may be quite sensitive but lack specificity and be met under certain conditions even though the clinician does not make the clinical diagnosis. Even though the processes are related, proper clinical management of an STD must often be dissociated from the public health surveillance reporting process.

STD surveillance evaluation

Completeness
Completeness of STD reporting is affected by both underdetection and underreporting. Chlamydial infections and, to a lesser extent, gonorrhea are often underdetected due to their asymptomatic nature (i.e., approximately 70% of chlamydial infections and 50% of gonorrhea infections in women are asymptomatic). As chlamydia screening programs have expanded in the US since the 1990s, case detection and reporting has increased. The US chlamydia male/female incidence rate ratio of approximately 0.3 during 2002–2005 suggests that a greater number of women are screened for chlamydia and that many sex partners of women with chlamydia are not diagnosed or reported.

Monitoring STD test positivity or prevalence of clinic-based populations over time should provide less biased trend data than reported morbidity data. However, in the absence of publicly funded screening programs, there may be a financial disincentive for diagnostic laboratory testing in some healthcare settings. Empiric treatment of STDs can also limit the completeness of surveillance. Strategies for improving completeness of reporting include conducting active surveillance, implementing electronic laboratory-based reporting, strengthening ties with clinicians and other key partners to encourage reporting and case management consultation, and facilitating increased use of laboratory diagnostic tests to identify new cases [40].

Numerous evaluations of the completeness of STD reporting since the 1980s suggest that completeness ranges between 64 and 95% for gonorrhea, between 55 and 98% for chlamydia, and is 79% for syphilis [41–43]. Use of capture–recapture methods to assess the degree of underreporting may improve the interpretation of STD surveillance data [44]; however, the underlying assumptions of the capture–recapture method (i.e., independence of data sources, equal probability of individuals being identified in the data source, and constant probability of individuals being included in a data source for the period of observation) are often not met. When using capture–recapture methods, increasing the number of data sources and using analytic methods like log-linear models can limit the risk of bias [45].

Timeliness
Timeliness of STD surveillance data is critical for outbreak detection and effective public health intervention, such as case and partner management. Assessing STD incidence based on date of disease onset, date of specimen collection, or date of first report to the public health system illustrates how specific steps in the surveillance process impact assessments of overall surveillance timeliness. In one study comparing temporal line graphs of early syphilis by date of report and estimated infection date, syphilis reports underestimated infections during the growth period of the outbreak and overestimated infections during the period of highest reported incidence [46].

Standardized use of surveillance case definitions
The interpretation and use of STD surveillance case definitions should be assessed periodically. Are standardized surveillance case definitions being used? Are cases classified as probable or confirmed

based upon the reported information? A recent evaluation of syphilis case classification in six US jurisdictions indicated that information for staging syphilis according to the current case definition is often not available—that is, case classification was occurring in the absence of information regarding case definition criteria [47]. Such misclassification results in poor data quality.

STD surveillance challenges

The wide range of bacterial and viral STDs and their sequelae that can be considered for surveillance complicates monitoring and evaluation efforts. The asymptomatic nature of chlamydia, gonorrhea, latent syphilis, and some viral STDs results in substantial underdetection. Additionally,

---

Box 17.1 Syphilis reactor grid evaluation.

Surveillance for new syphilis cases depends primarily on case identification via laboratory reporting of serologic tests for syphilis (STSs— e.g., RPR (rapid plasma reagin)), and, secondarily, on healthcare provider reporting and health department investigations of case patients and their partners. Because STSs are not specific for new, untreated syphilis and health departments do not have resources to investigate every person with a reported reactive STS (reactors); they use syphilis reactor registries (containing information on previously treated persons), medical records, provider input, and a table algorithm known as the syphilis reactor grid (SRG) to determine which reactors to investigate further [48] (Figure 17.4). SRGs vary by locality and are used to assign reactors to be investigated based on results of a quan-

titative (titer) nontreponemal-specific STS (e.g., RPR), age, sex, and other factors (e.g., test from a HIV clinic). In general, SRGs assign higher priority for investigation to younger persons with higher titers compared to older persons with lower titers. Evaluation of SRGs in several communities indicates that the percentage of cases missed by a SRG is influenced by the SRG design and the prevalence of syphilis among reactors [48]. Because syphilis prevalence changes over time, to maximize case identification and use of local resources, periodic SRG evaluation is recommended [49]. When STD investigation resources are scarce, one can imagine that syphilis case investigation and the associated surveillance outcomes would be restricted to only those cases considered to be at greatest risk.

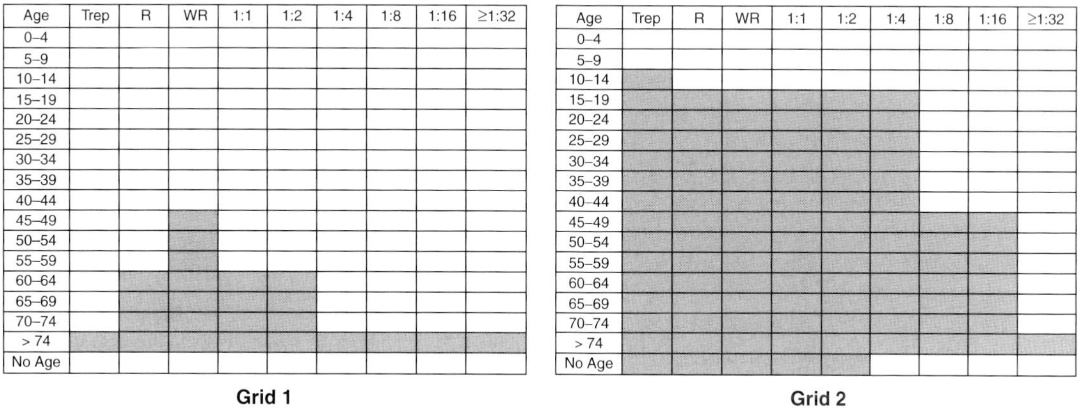

Age	Trep	R	WR	1:1	1:2	1:4	1:8	1:16	≥1:32
0–4									
5–9									
10–14									
15–19									
20–24									
25–29									
30–34									
35–39									
40–44									
45–49			▓						
50–54			▓						
55–59		▓	▓						
60–64		▓	▓						
65–69		▓	▓						
70–74		▓	▓	▓					
> 74	▓	▓	▓	▓	▓	▓	▓	▓	▓
No Age									

Grid 1

Age	Trep	R	WR	1:1	1:2	1:4	1:8	1:16	≥1:32
0–4									
5–9									
10–14	▓								
15–19	▓	▓	▓	▓	▓	▓			
20–24	▓	▓	▓	▓	▓	▓			
25–29	▓	▓	▓	▓	▓	▓			
30–34	▓	▓	▓	▓	▓	▓			
35–39	▓	▓	▓	▓	▓	▓			
40–44	▓	▓	▓	▓	▓	▓			
45–49	▓	▓	▓	▓	▓	▓			
50–54	▓	▓	▓	▓	▓	▓			
55–59	▓	▓	▓	▓	▓	▓			
60–64	▓	▓	▓	▓	▓	▓			
65–69	▓	▓	▓	▓	▓	▓			
70–74	▓	▓	▓	▓	▓	▓			
> 74	▓	▓	▓	▓	▓	▓			
No Age							▓	▓	▓

Grid 2

Fig 17.4 Syphilis reactor grids (SRGs). This grid assigns reactors with younger ages and higher titers to investigation (unshaded cells) and not reactors with older ages and lower titers (shaded cells). Investigation of reactors with an intermediate age and/or titer varies between health departments. Two representative SRGs currently in use are presented: very inclusive (Grid 1) and very exclusive (Grid 2). Trep = positive treponemal test result; R = reactive; WR — weakly reactive.

different STDs may be distributed differently in the same population. Therefore, analysis of surveillance data for different STDs should be conducted separately for each STD and also in an integrated fashion to identify similar and different epidemiological, spatial, or temporal patterns.

The inextricable linkage between STD prevention and control program activities and STD surveillance occasionally confounds accurate surveillance data interpretation. For example, variability in screening practices over time directly impacts case detection and morbidity trends [26]. Partner notification activities conducted as an intervention for early syphilis may also result in increased case detection. Accurate information on method (e.g., screening testing of an asymptomatic person) and venue of case detection (e.g., STD clinic, correctional facility) should be monitored to improve the ability to interpret disease trends. Similarly, STD diagnostic technologies and protocols modify surveillance data in a number of ways and should be routinely monitored. Prevention program activities may also affect surveillance data interpretation and delay public health action by introducing additional steps such as elicitation and treatment of partners prior to case reporting. Such reporting delays can lead to late recognition of outbreaks or common epidemiologic or behavioral features amenable to intervention.

Changing clinical care practice, such as the shift from inpatient to outpatient management of ectopic pregnancy and PID since the 1990s, may also impact the interpretation of STD surveillance data. Similarly, changes in access to STD care in the US—reductions in public STD clinic hours and clinic closings—have resulted in reporting of more gonorrhea cases since 1998 and more syphilis cases since 2002 from clinical settings other than public STD clinics [12]. Periodic evaluations of surveillance data sources are required to reveal changing clinical practices and patterns of health care.

Finally, STD surveillance and prevention efforts are impacted by the stigma associated with STDs and human sexuality in some communities. Secrecy and stigma may limit patients from seeking healthcare and result in underdetection of STDs. Clinicians uncomfortable with discussing sexual health issues with their patients may not offer STD risk assessment or test patients for STDs, further limiting diagnosis and reporting of STDs. These clinicians may also be reluctant to report diagnosed STDs.

Conclusion

Surveillance for STDs is challenging due to the varied nature of the infections themselves: they are viral, bacterial, and parasitic. Some are symptomatic whereas others are mostly asymptomatic. A clinical syndrome defines some and others are defined by the identification of an organism. The epidemiology of these infections varies as well. For these reasons, STD surveillance must be as multifaceted as the biologic and clinical characteristics. Most state and local programs focus surveillance efforts on case reporting of the bacterial STDs—syphilis, gonorrhea, and chlamydia—for which prevention and control programs have been established. In addition, many health departments also have access to prevalence monitoring data, behavioral surveillance information, and administrative databases. It is only through multiple approaches that the burden of these complex infections may be truly understood and prevention interventions be appropriately targeted.

References

1 Cates W Jr, Holmes KK. Sexually transmitted diseases. In: Wallace RB, Doebbeling BN, Last JM (eds.), *Public Health and Preventive Medicine*, 14th ed. Stamford, CT: Appleton & Lange; 1998.

2 Brandt AM. *No Magic Bullet: A Social History of Venereal Disease in the United States Since 1880*. New York: Oxford University Press; 1987:42–3.

3 Centers for Disease Control and Prevention. *Program Operations Guidelines for STD Prevention*. Atlanta, GA: US Department of Health and Human Services; July 2001. Available from: http://www.cdc.gov/std/program/. Accessed April 25, 2007.

4 Beltrami JF, Shouse RL, Blake PA. Trends in infectious diseases and the male to female ratio: possible clues to changes in behavior among men who have sex with men. *AIDS Educ Prev* 2005;**17**:S49–59.

5 Centers for Disease Control and Prevention. Together we can. *The National Plan to Eliminate Syphilis from the United States*. Atlanta, GA: US Department

of Health and Human Services; May 2006. Available from: http://www.cdc.gov/stopsyphilis/plan.htm. Accessed April 25, 2007.

6 Centers for Disease Control and Prevention. Racial disparities in nationally notifiable diseases—United States, 2002. *MMWR* 2005;**54**:9–11.

7 Weinstock H, Berman S, Cates W Jr. Sexually transmitted diseases among American youth: incidence and prevalence estimates, 2000. *Perspect Sex Reprod Health* 2004;**36**:6–10.

8 Mcfarlane M, Kachur R, Klausner JD, Roland E, Cohen M. Internet-based health promotion and disease control in the 8 cities: successes, barriers, and future plans. *Sex Transm Dis* 2005;**32**(10, suppl):S60–4.

9 Mark KE, Gunn RA. Gonorrhea surveillance: estimating epidemiologic and clinical characteristics of reported cases using a sample survey methodology. *Sex Transm Dis* 2004;**31**:215–20.

10 World Health Organization and Joint United Nations Programme on HIV/AIDS. *Guidelines for Sexually Transmitted Infections Surveillance*. UNAIDS/WHO Working Group on Global HIV/AIDS/STI Surveillance; 1999. WHO/CDS/CSR/EDS/99.3. Available from: http://www.who.int/hiv/pub/sti/pubstiguidelines/en/. Accessed April 25, 2007.

11 Dicker LW, Mosure DJ, Levine WC. Chlamydia positivity versus prevalence. What's the difference? *Sex Transm Dis* 1998;**25**:251–3.

12 Centers for Disease Control and Prevention. *Sexually Transmitted Disease Surveillance, 2005*. Atlanta, GA: US Department of Health and Human Services; October 2006. Available from: http://www.cdc.gov/nchstp/dstd/Stats_Trends/Stats_and_Trends.htm. Accessed April 25, 2007.

13 Centers for Disease Control and Prevention. *Sexually Transmitted Disease Surveillance 2005 Supplement: Gonococcal Isolate Surveillance Project (GISP) Annual Report—2005*. Atlanta, GA: US Department of Health and Human Services; January 2007. Available from: http://www.cdc.gov/nchstp/dstd/Stats_Trends/Stats_and_Trends.htm. Accessed April 25, 2007.

14 Centers for Disease Control and Prevention. Trends in sexual risk behaviors among high school students—United States, 1991–1997. *MMWR* 1998;**47**:749–52.

15 Mosher WD, Chandra A, Jones J. Sexual behavior and selected health measures: men and women 15–44 years of age, United States, 2002. Advance data from vital and health statistics. No. 362. Hyattsville, MD: National Center for Health Statistics; 2005.

16 Chase J, Chow JM, Lifshay J, Bolan G. STD/HIV knowledge, care-related behaviors, and morbidity. In: *Women's Health: Findings from the California Women's Health Survey, 1997–2003*. California: Office of Women's

Health, California Department of Health Services; Chap. 6. Available from: http://www.dhs.ca.gov/director/owh/owh_main/cwhs/wmns_hlth_survey/survey.htm. Accessed April 25, 2007.

17 Brindis C, Ozer E, Adams S, *et al. Health Profile of California's Adolescents: Findings from the 2001 California Health Interview Survey*. Los Angeles, CA: UCLA Center for Health Policy Research; 2005. Available from: http://www.chis.ucla.edu/pubs/publication.asp?publD=124. Accessed April 25, 2007.

18 Dunne EF, Unger ER, Sternberg M, *et al.* Prevalence of HPV infection among females in the United States. *JAMA* 2007;**297**:813–9.

19 Xu F, Sternberg MR, Kottiri BJ, *et al.* Trends in herpes simplex virus type 1 and type 2 seroprevalence in the United States. *JAMA* 2006;**296**:964–73.

20 Sutton MY, Sternberg M, Zaidi A, St. Louis ME, Markowitz LE. Trends in pelvic inflammatory disease hospital discharges and ambulatory visits, United States, 1985–2001. *Sex Transm Dis* 2005;**32**:778–84.

21 Morris SR, Bauer HM, Samuel MC, Johnston D, Bolan G. Surveillance of neonatal herpes in California using hospital discharge data: an alternative to mandatory case-based reporting. Abstract No 274. In: *Proceedings from the 2006 National STD Prevention Conference*, Jacksonville, FL, May 8–11, 2006.

22 Gutierrez KM, Halpern MSF, Maldonado Y, Arvin AM. The epidemiology of neonatal herpes simplex virus infections in California from 1985–1995. *JID* 1999;**180**:199–202.

23 Centers for Disease Control and Prevention. Chlamydia screening among sexually active young female enrollees of health plans, United States, 1999–2001. *MMWR* 2004;**53**:983–5.

24 Chow JM, Guo J, Bradsberry M, Thiel de Bocanegra H, Steinberg S, Bolan G. Impact of a targeted provider intervention to improve Chlamydia screening practices in a large California family planning program. Abstract No. 338. In: *Proceedings from the 2006 National STD Prevention Conference*, Jacksonville, FL, May 8–11, 2006.

25 Virnig GA, McBean M. Administrative data for public health surveillance and planning. *Annu Rev Public Health* 2001;**22**:213–30.

26 Gotz H, Lindback J, Ripa T, Arenborn M, Ranstedt K, Ekdahl K. Is the increase in notifications of *Chlamydia trachomatis* infections in Sweden the result of changes in prevalence, sampling frequency or diagnostic methods? *Scand J Infect Dis* 2002;**34**:28–34.

27 Dicker LW, Mosure DJ, Steece R, Stone KM. Laboratory tests used in US public health laboratories for sexually transmitted diseases, 2000. *Sex Transm Dis* 2004;**31**:259–64.

28 Guion LA. Triangulation: establishing the validity of qualitative studies. Publication No. FCS6014. Florida: Florida Cooperative Extension Service, Institute of Food and Agricultural Sciences, University of Florida; September 2002.

29 Newman LM, Samuel M, Stover J, Stenger M, Ellen J. Outcomes for Assessment through Systems of Integrated Surveillance (OASIS). Turning STD surveillance data into action. Abstract No. B03. In: *Proceedings from the 2005 National STD Prevention Conference*, Philadelphia, PA, March 8–10, 2005.

30 Gunn RA, Maroufi A, Fox KK, Berman SM. Surveillance for repeat gonorrhea infection, San Diego, California, 1995–2001: establishing definitions and methods. *Sex Transm Dis* 2004;**31**:373–9.

31 Bernstein KT, Zenilman J, Olthoff G, Marsiglia VC, Erbelding EJ. Gonorrhea reinfection among sexually transmitted disease clinic attendees in Baltimore, MD. *Sex Transm Dis* 2006;**33**:80–6.

32 Bernstein KT, Curriero FC, Jennings JM, Olthoff G, Erbelding EJ, Zenilman J. Defining core gonorrhea transmission utilizing spatial data. *Am J Epidemiol* 2004;**160**:51–8.

33 Kilmarx PH, Zaidi AA, Thomas JC, *et al.* Sociodemographic factors and the variation in syphilis rates among US counties, 1984 through 1993: an ecological analysis. *Am J Public Health* 1997;**87**:1937–43.

34 Elliott LJ, Blanchard JF, Beaudoin CM. Geographical variations in the epidemiology of bacterial sexually transmitted infections in Manitoba, Canada. *STI* 2002;**78**:139–44.

35 Zenilman JM, Glass G, Shields T, Jenkins PR, Gaydos JC, McKee KT, Jr. Geographic epidemiology of gonorrhoea and Chlamydia on a large military installation: application of a GIS system. *STI* 2002;**78**:40–4.

36 Law DCG, Serre ML, Christakos G, Leone PA, Miller WC. Spatial analysis and mapping of sexually transmitted diseases to optimize intervention and prevention strategies. *STI* 2004;**80**:294–9.

37 Blanchard JF. Populations, pathogens, and epidemic phases: closing the gap between theory and practice in the prevention of sexually transmitted diseases. *STI* 2002;**78**(suppl I):i183–8.

38 Centers for Disease Control and Prevention. Case definitions for infectious conditions under public health surveillance. Available from: http://www.cdc.gov/epo/dphsi/casedef/index.htm. Accessed April 25, 2007.

39 Chorba T, Tao G, Irwin KL. Sexually transmitted diseases. In: Litwin MS, Saigal CS (eds.), *Urologic Diseases in America*. Washington, DC: US Government Publishing Office, US Department of Health and Human Services; 2004:233–79. NIH Publication No. 04-5512.

40 Silk BJ, Berkelman RL. A review of strategies for enhancing the completeness of notifiable disease reporting. *J Public Health Manag Pract* 2005;**11**:191–200.

41 Centers for Disease Control and Prevention. Reporting of laboratory-confirmed Chlamydia infection and gonorrhea by provider affiliated with three large managed care organizations—United States, 1995–1999. *MMWR* 2002;**51**:256–9.

42 Tao G, Carr P, Stiffman M, Defor TA. Incompleteness of reporting of laboratory-confirmed chlamydial infection by providers affiliated with a managed care organization, 1997–1999. *Sex Transm Dis* 2004;**31**:139–42.

43 Doyle TJ, Glynn MK, Groseclose SL. Completeness of notifiable infectious disease reporting in the United States: an analytical literature review. *Am J Epidemiol* 2002;**155**:866–74.

44 Reintjes R, Termorshuizen F, van de Laar MJW. Assessing the sensitivity of STD surveillance in the Netherlands: an application of the capture–recapture method. *Epidemiol Infect* 1999;**122**:97–102.

45 Papoz L, Balkau B, Lellouch J. Case counting in epidemiology: limitations of methods based on multiple data sources. *Int J Epidemiol* 1996;**25**:474–8.

46 Schumacher CM, Bernstein KT, Zenilman JM, Rompalo AM. Reassessing a large-scale syphilis epidemic using an estimated infection date. *Sex Transm Dis* 2005;**32**:659–64.

47 Peterman TA, Kahn RH, Ciesielski CA, *et al.* Misclassification of the stages of syphilis: implications for surveillance. *Sex Transm Dis* 2005;**32**:144–9.

48 Schaffzin JK, Koumans EH, Kahn RH, Markowitz LE. Evaluation of syphilis reactor grids: optimizing impact. *Sex Transm Dis* 2003;**30**:700–6.

49 Centers for Disease Control and Prevention. *Recommendations for Public Health Surveillance of Syphilis in the United States*. Atlanta, GA: US Department of Health and Human Services; March 2003. Available from http://www.cdc.gov/std/SyphSurvReco.pdf. Accessed April 25, 2007.

Appendix: ICD-9-CM and CPT codes used for STD surveillance

International Classification of Diseases, Ninth Revision, Clinical Modification (ICD-9-CM) codes were developed to allow assignment of codes to diagnoses and procedures associated with hospital utilization in the US and are often used for third-party insurance reimbursement purposes. Current Procedural Terminology (CPT) is a listing of descriptive terms and identifying codes for reporting

Table A.1 Selected STD-associated diseases and conditions and their corresponding International Classification of Diseases, Ninth Revision, Clinical Modification (ICD-9-CM) codes

STD-associated disease or condition	ICD-9-CM Codes
Chancroid	Chancroid 099.0
Chlamydia	Unspecified diseases of conjunctiva due to Chlamydiae 077.98
	Other diseases due to Chlamydiae 078.88
	Other specified chlamydial infection 079.88
	Unspecified chlamydial infection 079.98
	Urethritis due to *Chlamydia trachomatis* 099.41
	Other venereal diseases due to *Chlamydia trachomatis* 099.50-099.59
	Other VD in pregnancy 647.2
	Special screening for other chlamydial diseases V73.88
	Special screening for unspecified chlamydial diseases V73.98
Genital herpes	Genital herpes 054.10-054.19
Genital warts	Viral warts, unspecified 078.10
	Condyloma acuminatum 078.11
	Other viral warts 078.19
	Genital warts due to HPV 079.4
Gonorrhea	Gonoccocal infections 098.0-098.89
	Gonorrhea in pregnancy 647.1
Granuloma inguinale	Granuloma inguinale 099.2
Lymphogranuloma venereum	Lymphogranuloma venereum 099.1
Pelvic inflammatory disease	Salpingitis and oophoritis 614.0-614.2, 098.17, 098.37
	Parametritis and pelvic peritonitis 614.3-614.5, 098.86
	Pelvic inflammatory disease 614.7-614.9, 098.10, 098.30, 098.39
	Inflammatory disease of the uterus, except cervix 615.0, 615.1, 615.9, 098.16, 098.36
Syphilis, adult, all stages	Early syphilis, symptomatic (P&S) 091.0-091.9
	Early syphilis, latent 092.0-092.9
	Neurosyphilis 094.0-094.9
	Other forms of late syphilis, with symptoms 095.0-095.9
	Late syphilis, latent 096
	Syphilis, unknown latency 097.0-097.9
	Syphilis in pregnancy 647.0
Syphilis, congenital	Congenital syphilis 090.0-090.9

medical services and procedures under insurance programs and for administrative management purposes, such as claims processing and developing guidelines for medical care review. ICD-9-CM and CPT codes have been monitored in several settings to support public health surveillance.

STD surveillance using ICD-9-CM- or CPT-coded health information may be considered because the codes are readily available for use by healthcare systems, are used in multiple clinical settings (e.g., outpatient, inpatient, emergency departments), are often available electronically, and can be shared easily among different information systems. However, prior to implementing surveillance for STD-associated health outcomes based on the use of ICD-9-CM- or CPT-coded health information, public health agencies should evaluate the usefulness of the codes with regard to the goals of the surveillance system. Nonspecific ICD-9-CM codes (e.g., Other VD in pregnancy [647.2] in the

Table A.2 Medical procedures and services' Current Procedural Terminology (CPT) codes corresponding to Chlamydia, gonorrhea, and syphilis

STD	Current Procedural Terminology
Chlamydia	Chlamydia 86631
	Chlamydia, IgM 86632
	Chlamydia, culture 87110
	Chlamydia trachomatis 97270
	Infectious agent antigen detection by enzyme immunoassay technique, *Chlamydia trachomatis* 87320
	Infectious agent detection by nucleic acid (DNA or RNA); *Chlamydia trachomatis*, direct probe technique 87490
	Infectious agent detection by nucleic acid (DNA or RNA); *Chlamydia trachomatis*, amplified probe technique 87491
	Infectious agent detection by nucleic acid (DNA or RNA); *Chlamydia trachomatis*, quantification 87492
	Infectious agent detection by immunoassay with direct optical observation; *Chlamydia trachomatis* 87810
Gonorrhea	*Neisseria gonorrhoeae*, direct probe technique 87590
	N. gonorrhoeae, amplified probe technique 87591
	N. gonorrhoeae, quantification 87592
	Infectious agent detection by immunoassay with direct optical observation; *N. gonorrhoeae* 87850
Syphilis	Obstetric panel (including syphilis test) 80055
	Treponema pallidum, confirmatory test 86781
	Syphilis test; qualitative (e.g., VDRL*, RPR*, ART*) 86592
	Syphilis test; quantitative 86593
	Treponema pallidum 87285

*VDRL: Venereal Disease Research Laboratory; RPR: Rapid plasma reagin; ART: Automated reagin test.

Chlamydia category) may yield low specificity for the outcome of interest. There may be bias in the use of the codes by some data providers (e.g., using codes for greater severity of illness to justify patient treatment or claims reimbursement). Use of a limited number of ICD-9-CM or CPT codes to describe a clinical encounter may further limit appropriate interpretation. However, given the widespread availability and use of ICD-9-CM codes, it is prudent to consider their use and to encourage the evaluation of their use for STD surveillance. Tables A.1 and A.2 present ICD-9-CM codes and CPT codes, respectively, that have been used to monitor STD-associated diseases and conditions using health services and administrative data (20, 39).

18 Vaccine preventable diseases

PART 1: Vaccine preventable disease surveillance

Hanna Nohynek & Elizabeth Miller

Introduction

Vaccines are one of the most cost-effective health intervention tools. The objectives of surveillance for vaccine preventable diseases (VPD) depend on the phase of the vaccination program. Preintroduction data are required to estimate the burden of disease, to identify risk groups, and to decide on the appropriate vaccination or vaccine development strategy. Postintroduction data are required to monitor vaccine program performance and to identify remaining pockets of susceptible individuals, as well as to provide alert signals to identify and control outbreaks. Data sources used for surveillance for VPD include both clinical and laboratory reporting. Special studies can be performed if VPD surveillance data are not available via routine systems. In most countries, most VPD are notifiable by law.

Vaccine program related surveillance has three components: coordinated monitoring of vaccine coverage, VPD incidence, and vaccine-related adverse events. This chapter will concentrate on the methods and resources required to monitor universal vaccination program performance and discuss these in the light of VPD surveillance. VPD related methodology in the context of new vaccine development will also be discussed. Table 18(1).1 lists the most commonly used vaccines. Vaccine related adverse events are addressed in Chapter 18, Part 2.

Vaccine program related surveillance

In order for vaccines to work effectively, they need to be safe, immunogenic, and reach their intended target group in a timely manner. The strict good manufacturing practice and quality control requirements to which the producers need to adhere are implemented to make sure that vaccines sold and delivered are both as efficacious and as harmless as possible. Supranational control agencies like the European Medical Agency (EMEA) in Europe and national control authorities like the Food and Drug Administration (FDA) in the United States (US) assure that vaccines licensed for use in these countries all meet high quality standards (see additional resources at the end of this chapter).

Depending on the pathology and immunology of the disease to be prevented, vaccine program performance is measured with different indicators. These include vaccine coverage, immunological markers of vaccine protection (such as concentration of antibodies indicating humoral immunity or concentration of different T cells as indicators of cell mediated immunity), and estimates of vaccine efficacy or effectiveness that can be direct (i.e., reduction of incidence of VPD in vaccine target group) or indirect (i.e., reduction of incidence of VPD in other groups, the so-called herd immunity effect).

Measuring vaccine coverage

Vaccines can prevent disease only if they reach the intended target populations. Measures of vaccine coverage are used to address the question of what proportion of the population has been reached with the vaccine. Several different epidemiological methods can be used to measure vaccine coverage. The

Table 18(1).1 Most commonly used vaccines in universal immunization programs of rich and middle-income countries to prevent communicable diseases and surrogate methods used to measure protection against the disease elicited by the vaccine.

Disease	Vaccine preventing from disease (Acronym used)	Type of vaccine	Surrogate methods used to measure vaccine protection	Comment
Tuberculosis; meningitis and military forms	Bacillus Calmette-Guérin (BCG)	Live	Tuberculin test	Vaccine efficacy reported against other forms of tuberculosis contradictory [1]
Diphtheria	Diphtheria toxoid D or d	Inactivated	Antibodies against diphtheria toxin	
Tetanus	Tetanus toxoid T or t	Inactivated	Antibodies against tetanus toxoid	
Pertussis	Acellular pertussis (aP); whole cell pertussis (wcP)	Inactivated or component	Antibodies against whole cell or toxin components	Most rich countries are using aP, whereas middle-income and poor countries continue to use wcP
Polio	Oral polio vaccine or Sabin (OPV); injectable polio vaccine or Salk (IPV)	Live Inactivated	Antibodies against different polio serotypes	
Hepatitis B	Hepatitis B vaccine (HBV)	Yeast-derived component vaccine	Antibodies against hepatitis B surface antigen	
Haemophilus influenzae type b (Hib)	Hib vaccine	Polysaccharide conjugated to carrier protein	Antibodies against polysaccharide, functionality of antibodies (killing assay)	
Pneumococcal invasive and noninvasive disease	Pneumococcal polysaccharide (23PPS) and conjugated vaccine (7PCV)	Plain polysaccharide; polysaccharide conjugated to carrier protein	Antibodies against polysaccharide or functionality of antibodies (killing assay)	
Measles	Measles vaccine (M)	Live	Neutralizing antibodies	
Mumps	Mumps vaccine (M)	Live	Neutralizing antibodies	
Rubella	Rubella vaccine (R)	Live	Neutralizing antibodies	

simplest is to calculate *vaccine distribution*. This is, however, a crude and inaccurate method because it does not take into consideration doses gone to waste. Nor does it give accurate information on the target groups reached because no denominator is available at the time vaccine is given.

Population assessment is usually the preferred method. In *total population assessment* information is gathered on the vaccination status of each eligible individual (numerator) and the denominator (total eligible population) is obtained from census count or demographic registries on permanent and migrating populations. Population assessment can provide accurate data on coverage but is laborious if done manually. The electronic vaccine registries presently being established in several resource rich countries allow the remote entry of vaccination data at the vaccination site, thus, in principle, providing both simplified and timely measures of coverage. In practice, due to missing information, vaccine registries have seldom been able to replace the more traditional means [2], even though they are mostly seen as a positive development [3]. Electronic vaccine registries also enable linkage of vaccine specific information to information collected in disease or other specific registries. This can be very useful for causality assessment of short- and long-term associations claimed to be vaccine-related adverse events (see Chapter 18, Part 2).

If total population assessment is not a practical approach, *sample population assessment* is an alternative that is less resource intensive. The sample can be drawn as a cluster representing the chosen population or as randomly chosen individuals. The World Health Organization (WHO) promotes the so-called *EPI cluster surveys* that are easy to perform and mostly used in resource poor country settings [4]. In the EPI cluster survey, 30 communities (clusters) are selected with probability proportional to the most recent census estimate of the community population size, by systematic selection from a list of cumulative population sizes. In each selected cluster, the study team starts at a central point, selects a random direction from that point and chooses a dwelling at random among those along the line from the center to the edge of the community. Information on vaccination of the individuals in the chosen age range of the target group of interest living in the first household is then collected. Starting from this household, the next nearest household is visited in turn until at least seven children have been found. The sample size allows vaccine coverage to be estimated with a 95% confidence interval (CI) of ±10 percentage points on the assumption of a design effect (increase in variance due to clustering) of two. Recently, WHO has recommended enhanced precision with ±5, or even ±3 percentage points [5]. If the region to be surveyed is very large, or heterogeneous, it may be split into strata and 30 clusters selected from each stratum, allowing estimates to be made on subregional levels.

In countries with ample resources, the EPI cluster survey has also been used successfully [6], but due to the inherent problems (i.e., difficulties in ensuring objectivity of household selection, problems in appropriately dealing with nonresponse, and in estimating total numbers of those vaccinated, which is needed for program planning purposes), *individual random sampling* methods are preferred. Depending on the research and programmatic questions of interest, the sample of randomly selected individuals needs to be large and representative. Bias is entered in the estimates if the sampled individuals do not arise from the total population but rather from an easily available target group (like all families with telephones or all children attending well-baby clinics delivering vaccines), leaving unattended those minority groups with vaccine coverage that is lower than in the general population [7].

The method chosen depends on the main public health and/or scientific aim of the coverage survey, type of vaccination program (i.e., whether it is universal or selective for certain risk groups), the methods of vaccine delivery (i.e., centralized or decentralized), and the general organization of vaccination services, as well as the availability of recorded information, mainly vaccination status and denominator data. When comparing vaccine coverage rates in different countries, careful note needs to be taken of the sampling method used. The official coverage and coverage rates reported by WHO and/or UNICEF often differ (Figure 18(1).1). In Table 18(1).2, a summary is given of the methods used to measure vaccine coverage in the European Nordic countries, demonstrating the prevailing variability even in a rather homogenous group of countries.

Immunological markers of protection

When the incidence of VPD is low, it may be difficult to estimate the prevailing vaccine-related protection in the population via surveillance of clinical cases of VPD. For those VPDs with established serological surrogate of protection (i.e., protection from infection or from clinical disease) as is the case, for example, with polio, rubella, diphtheria, and hepatitis B, the measurement of concentrations or titers of antibodies via targeted serosurveys is an important additional tool for VPD surveillance [8,9].

The survey can be done as a one-time seroprevalence study. For this, only one serum sample from the selected target group individuals is required. Age-specific seroprevalence surveys can be used to measure the duration of humoral immunity, but not immunological memory. An example of a seroprevalence study providing useful information for program design comes from Finland. Both the general public and vaccine program officers were concerned about the level of protection against diphtheria in the population [10]

(disease burden). Based on this encouraging example, similar systems have been set up elsewhere. In 1998, the International Network of Paediatric Surveillance Units (INoPSU, http://www.inopsu.com/) was established, and it now involves 10,000 pediatricians covering a population of 50 million children in 14 countries [21].

Instead of relying on regular passive surveillance, active sentinel surveillance systems, such as surveillance at several sites for acute respiratory infections to monitor baseline acute respiratory incidence rates, have been established to give alert signs of advancing influenza epidemics and to monitor the prevalent circulating influenza strains, which then can be used to predict the expected vaccine efficacy of the yearly seasonal influenza vaccine (see Chapter 19).

Passive surveillance provides the baseline trends of most common VPDs. When interpreting trends and time series, one needs to critically appraise whether the case definition has changed overtime and whether diagnosis and treatment practices have changed. This was the case for pertussis in Finland; along with a true increase in incidence, there was an artificial increase caused by the introduction of a specific and sensitive polymerase chain reaction test to detect pertussis in very young children, in whom serological tests perform poorly [22].

Even if passive surveillance is problematic, it is important to have country-specific incidence data to be able to formulate local vaccination policies. For example, the Nordic countries and the UK maintain a policy of immunizing risk groups only for hepatitis B, rather than complying with the WHO recommendation of universal hepatitis B vaccination for infants (Plate 18(1).1). This policy is based on carefully collected local incidence data and cost-effectiveness calculations of the universal vs. the risk group vaccination approach—for all these countries it is more cost-effective to continue vaccinating risk groups only.

When unexpected observations of increases in VPD occur, there are several explanations that need to be explored and tested to be able to take measures to control the outbreak. There are several reasons why sudden increases in VPD might occur. Increases can result from loss of vaccine potency because of having been frozen (e.g., hepatitis B vaccine is vulnerable to low temperatures) or having been exposed to high temperatures for too long (e.g., oral polio vaccine looses potency at high temperature) [23]. A vaccine can lose its potency in relation to the pathogenic agent it was supposed to prevent (e.g., escape mutants such as reported with *Bordetella pertussis* or antigenic drifts such as those seen with influenza). It may also be that vaccine coverage is not optimal; pockets of unimmunized populations or pools of susceptible individuals have been accumulating and the setting is ripe for an outbreak. Very few official reports document the mean ages when the intended coverage was reached. In Sweden, it was shown that the design of the national surveillance system overestimated coverage at 2 years and failed to record delayed vaccination [24]. The pool of measles susceptible population silently grew due to delayed vaccinations, presumably as a result of the impact of increased public concern over the alleged potential harmful effects of measles vaccination and resulted in a measles outbreak [25].

Vaccine efficacy and effectiveness

Observational methods to detect vaccine effectiveness

There are several observational methods that can be employed to study vaccine effectiveness. These include rapid screening, retrospective or prospective cohort studies, household contact studies, case-control studies, and the EPI cluster sampling method.

Rapid screening method
The rapid screening method gives an idea of how vaccine coverage and vaccine effectiveness are associated during an outbreak. It is used to determine if another more detailed study is necessary. In short, the rapid screening method compares the number of cases who had been vaccinated who fell ill with the VPD (percent cases vaccinated or PCV) with population vaccine uptake (percent population vaccinated or PPV). The effectiveness of the vaccine (VE) is calculated using the following formula, VE = 1 − [PCV(1 − PPV)]/[(1 − PCV)PPV]. The rapid screening method gives a very rough estimate of vaccine effectiveness. There are no controls for confounding variables and the estimates are poor

at the limits of the curve. It has been used, however, in combination with other methods to rapidly generate hypotheses for reduced vaccine effectiveness. Ramsay *et al.* used the rapid screening method as an adjunct to regular passive surveillance of VPD to generate hypotheses on possible reasons for the lower than expected effectiveness of Hib vaccine in the UK [26]. The researchers concluded that during the study period the effectiveness of Hib vaccine was only 58–72%, considerably lower than expected. The effectiveness was lower in children vaccinated during infancy, compared with those who were vaccinated during the catch-up campaign, declined with time since vaccination, and was lower in children born during years 2000–2002, compared with other children scheduled for infant vaccination.

Cohort study

Cohort studies can give much more accurate information on vaccine effectiveness than rapid screening. These studies are used during or after an outbreak of VPD and can be analyzed either prospectively or retrospectively. The population at risk is defined as accurately as possible. Vaccination status at the start of outbreak is preferably verified from existing records rather than by personal recall. Random mixing is assumed (i.e., both vaccinated and unvaccinated should have equal chance of exposure to pathogen). If the vaccination status of the population under study changes during the outbreak, as is often the case when the outbreak is being controlled by vaccination, the person-time approach can be used and analysis can be restricted to cases before vaccination. Disease status can be ascertained either clinically or by using direct laboratory confirmation, as was the case in the Italian hepatitis A outbreak, which was studied as a prospective cohort study to provide evidence on the feasibility of stopping the outbreak by vaccinating secondary household contacts [27]. This was a special case of a cohort study—a household contact study. In households, random mixing occurs more readily than in the general population. Exposure to the index case is similar regardless of vaccination status. In the analysis, past cases and the index case are excluded from the at risk population.

Case-control study

Case-control studies are more frequently used and often less laborious than cohort studies. Cases of illness are detected as they arise and are compared to controls who are identified using matching variables such as age, gender, access to vaccination and care, location of dwelling, and season of illness. Vaccine history is obtained from both cases and controls. There is considerable potential for bias and confounding; controls need to be representative of the population from which cases arose. Bias and confounders can be controlled for by matching, although care has to be given not to overmatch.

A recent example of the excellent use of the case-control method to estimate vaccine effectiveness was reported from the US on invasive pneumococcal disease [28]. Due to an unexpected manufacturing shortage, the seven-valent pneumococcal conjugate vaccine was given not according to the recommended four-dose schedule starting at 2 months of age, but with different schedules and at different ages. Effectiveness against vaccine serotypes for one or more doses was 96% (95% CI 93–98) in healthy children under 5 years of age and 81% (95% CI 57–92) in children with coexisting conditions. These results provided further evidence to support suggestions from phase II immunological studies that a three-dose schedule with two doses given in the first year of life, followed by a third dose in second year of life, yields antibody concentrations postbooster comparable to those offered by the official four-dose schedule [29]. The design of the matched case-control study carefully addressed potential bias and confounding variables. Control children were matched by age and zip code. Bias was minimized by rigorous methods in locating and enrolling control children. Many possible confounding variables were controlled for, such as known risk for disease and access to vaccines. This study demonstrated that case-control studies can be a useful and economical means to test vaccine efficacy in situations where randomized controlled trials would not be possible, or would be too lengthy, or costly.

For vaccines such as pneumococcal vaccines which only offer protection against a **proportion** of all the pneumococci that can cause disease, the Broome method can be used to measure efficacy [30]. This simply requires information on the vaccination status of cases of pneumococcal infection that are caused by vaccine and non-vaccine serotypes, the latter acting as controls that are already matched for potential confounding factors relating to risk of disease. Clearly the extent to which the vaccine is effective will be reflected in the lower proportion of vaccinated cases with a vaccine serotype than unvaccinated cases.

EPI cluster sampling
If the disease is very common, the EPI cluster sampling, a cross-sectional survey generally for studying vaccine coverage (see p. 231), can also be used to gather data on vaccine effectiveness. At the same time as the informant is asked about vaccination, he or she can be asked about history of illness. Data thus obtained can then be analyzed as retrospective cohort data. The value of this method, however, is limited by biases, including the recognition and recall of illness and the recall of the sequence between illness and vaccination.

Indirect vaccine effectiveness

It is important to measure and analyze trends in VPD incidence in age groups other than those targeted in the universal vaccination programs. Unexpectedly high indirect public health benefits have been demonstrated for rubella, Hib, pneumococcus, varicella, hepatitis A, and influenza vaccines. This so-called herd effect means that the vaccine, by reducing or interfering with the transmission of the infective pathogen, extends its preventive effect to those not vaccinated. This phenomenon is seldom seen in the prelicensure phase III efficacy studies due to their short duration, limited sample size, and study design, which for the licensure purposes mostly uses individual rather than cluster randomization [31]. For example, immunization of school-aged children with influenza vaccine reduced influenza rates not only in the vaccinated school children but also in their parents and others family members in Japan [32]. Similarly, Hib-conjugate vaccination reduced Hib disease in older age groups. Recently, use of pneumococcal conjugate vaccine in children, via a similar mechanism of reducing upper respiratory tract carriage of vaccine specific serotypes, has resulted in major reductions in invasive pneumococcal disease among adults and the elderly in the US [33]. These indirect effects have clear implications to cost-effectiveness calculations, which, if failing to include indirect effects in the model [34,35], lead to a gross underestimate of the overall impact of the vaccine on a population level [36,37].

Surveillance related to new vaccine development

The breakthrough discovery in the pathogenesis of a disease and identification of a potentially protective vaccine epitope may not be enough to start clinical development of a new vaccine. Both the pharmaceutical industry and decision makers call for evidence of a significant disease burden. This emphasizes the need to establish nationwide surveillance systems that are sensitive enough to measure the overall disease burden that could be prevented by a new vaccine. If the disease is rare, active surveillance may be the preferred method.

In a phase III trial to test the efficacy of a new vaccine, surveillance systems need to be comprehensive enough to capture the majority of the clinical endpoint cases (i.e., those episodes where the vaccinated study subjects fall ill with the clinical disease the vaccine is supposed to be preventing). In order not to bias vaccine efficacy toward zero, the efficacy endpoint case detection needs to emphasize specificity over sensitivity. In allocation of the intervention, the gold standard method uses randomization to allocate participants to receive the vaccine antigen or control (ideally placebo) in order to minimize bias and confounding, which is easily introduced when using observational methods. The randomized controlled trial under carefully standardized and controlled circumstances is the ultimate method of choice to study vaccine efficacy. This is the method regulatory authorities usually require to demonstrate efficacy of new products prior to licensure and large-scale use.

Vaccine probe method

When the direct detection of the pathogen is difficult, as is the case with common bacteria causing the majority of serious childhood pneumonia globally [38], the vaccine probe method may be the only means to provide understanding of the true disease burden caused by these pathogens. This was first demonstrated in the large-scale randomized controlled trial for efficacy of the Hib conjugate vaccine in the Gambia [39], in which the vaccine had an expected 95% efficacy against invasive Hib disease. At the same time, and unexpectedly, 21% of radiologically proven pneumonia [40] was prevented indirectly, indicating that at least 21% of this type of pneumonia was caused by Hib. Recently, the vaccine probe method has also been used for measuring the global disease burden caused by pneumococcus [41].

Program development

Vaccination schedules need to be adjusted to the changing epidemiology of VPD and to better respond to new information on how vaccines work. Schedules also need to be revisited when new vaccines become available. Pressures from industry and nongovernmental interest groups can be strong. National and regional decision makers need accurate data and reliable tools with which to make evidence based decisions. There are four key elements to decision making: (1) existing or predicted disease burden preventable by vaccination, (2) safety of the vaccine on an individual level, (3) safety of the vaccine on a population level, and (4) cost-effectiveness of the intervention.

The existing disease burden can be used as a starting point in modeling the impacts of different vaccination schedules. In the US, a recent modeling exercise taking into consideration both herd impact and hepatitis A importation predicted that nationwide routine immunization with hepatitis A vaccine at 1 year of age with 70% coverage would prevent 57% of additional cases during the period 1995–2029, compared with the continuation of the regional strategy of vaccinating children at 2 years of age, as recommended by the US Advisory Committee for Immunization Practices in 1999 [42].

The emphasis and visibility of speculations on potential adverse events has substantially increased during the past decade. Countries are increasingly concerned about possible population level adverse events that the universal use of a vaccine may cause. The disease could move to older age groups when vaccine coverage remains below optimal levels or when the possibility to natural boosting diminishes with increasing vaccine uptake. An example of the former comes from Greece, where congenital rubella cases increased to epidemic levels as a result of rubella vaccination coverage constantly remaining below 50% [43]. Since 1986 in the UK, a mathematical modeling tool utilizing disease-specific surveillance data and seroepidemiological data has been used to analyze the extent to which the measles, mumps, and rubella diseases can be controlled and when it is most timely to adjust the current strategies to avoid outbreaks [44,45]. Many countries have not wanted to introduce varicella vaccine because of the concern that it may lead to increases of zoster in older age groups [46,47] despite rather favorable costing calculations made from societal perspective for chickenpox cases averted [48].

The fourth, and increasingly the decisive element of decision making especially in middle-income countries, is the cost of the vaccine and its introduction. Any change in schedule is bound to have economic consequences, which usually are not one-time changes (except in cases where only the cold chain needs to be extended), but are increases that need to be sustained for the vaccine and vaccination budgets for years after the introduction. Mathematical modeling is an important tool to address cost concerns. Cost–benefit and cost-effectiveness calculations are becoming routine steps in national decision making before introduction of new vaccines. In order for calculations to be reliable, carefully collected locally available data are needed. Extrapolating from nearby countries can give an idea of the magnitude of disability-adjusted life years (DALYs) and lives saved, but the differences in care-seeking behavior, access to care, diagnostic and treatment practices, and social security systems (both for illness and health events) can make such extrapolations difficult to interpret. An example of the intelligent use of extensive sensitivity analyses to capture direct and indirect vaccine effects is given by Melegaro *et al.* [49]. These estimations were used to make decisions on the introduction of the seven-valent pneumococcal conjugate vaccine into the national program in the UK with a three-dose schedule (i.e., at 2, 4, and 13 mo with a catch-up program for children under 2 yr) [50]. Similarly in Finland, cost-effectiveness analyses based on comprehensive clinical data on virologically confirmed influenza infections, hospital medical records, and national registers demonstrated that introduction of influenza vaccine to children ≤ 13 years of age would be cost-saving from the healthcare providers perspective. According to Salo *et al.*, investing € 1.7 million in vaccination of children <5 years of age yielded savings of € 2.7 million in healthcare costs [51] and Finland is now considering introducing influenza vaccine to this age group.

In summary, surveillance of VPDs is essential for monitoring the performance of national vaccination programs and thus control of VPDs. Despite reduction and even elimination of VPDs, the significance of VPD surveillance will not diminish as increasingly both vaccinees and decision makers are requesting best available evidence to support the decision of whether or not to vaccinate individuals, risk groups, or larger populations. Clinical research and product development will make new vaccines available; in order to support this development and enhance introduction of new vaccines into national programs, data arising from surveillance of VPD needs to be sensitive, timely, and readily available for different stakeholders.

References

1 Fine PE. Variation in protection by BCG: implications of and for heterologous immunity. *Lancet* 1995;**346**:1339–45.

2 Khare M, Piccinino L, Barker LE, Linkins RW. Assessment of immunization registry databases as supplemental sources of data to improve ascertainment of vaccination coverage estimates in the national immunization survey. *Arch Pediatr Adolesc Med* 2006;**160**:838–42.

3 Linkins RW, Salmon DA, Omer SB, Pan WK, Stokley S, Halsey NA. Support for immunization registries among parents of vaccinated and unvaccinated school-aged children: a case control study. *BMC Public Health* 2006;**6**:236.

4 World Health Organization. *Training for Mid-Level Managers: The EPI Coverage Survey*. Expanded Programme on Immunization. WHO/EPI/MLM/91.10. Geneva: World Health Organization; 1999.

5 World Health Organization. Immunization coverage cluster survey. Reference Manual. Expanded Programme on Immunization. WHO/VB/04.23. Geneva: World Health Organization; 2005.

6 Ellinga A, Depoorter AM, Van Damme P. Vaccination coverage estimates by EPI cluster sampling survey of children (18–24 months) in Flanders, Belgium. *Acta Paediatr* 2002;**91**:599–603.

7 Durrheim DN, Ogunbanjo GA. Measles elimination—is it achievable? Lessons from an immunisation coverage survey. *S Afr Med J* 2000;**90**:130–5.

8 Edmunds WJ, Pebody RG, Aggerback H, *et al*. The seroepidemiology of diphtheria in Western Europe. ESEN Project. European Sero-Epidemiology Network. *Epidemiol Infect* 2000;**125**:113–25.

9 Pebody RG, Gay NJ, Giammanco A, *et al*. The seroepidemiology of *Bordetella pertussis* infection in Western Europe. *Epidemiol Infect* 2005;**133**:159–71.

10 Lumio J, Olander RM, Groundstroem K, Suomalainen P, Honkanen T, Vuopio-Varkila J. Epidemiology of three cases of severe diphtheria in Finnish patients with low antitoxin antibody levels. *Eur J Clin Microbiol Infect Dis* 2001;**20**:705–10.

11 Galazka AM, Robertson SE, Oblapenko GP. Resurgence of diphtheria. *Eur J Epidemiol* 1995;**11**:95–105.

12 Eskola J, Olander RM, Kuronen T. Reasons for diphtheria vaccination campaign. *Duodecim* 1994;**110**:449.

13 Herremans T, Kimman TG, Conyn-Van Spaendonck MA, *et al*. Immunoglobulin a as a serological marker for the (silent) circulation of poliovirus in an inactivated poliovirus-vaccinated population. *Clin Infect Dis* 2002;**34**:1067–75.

14 Vyse AJ, Gay NJ, Hesketh LM, Pebody R, Morgan-Capner P, Miller E. Interpreting serological surveys using mixture models: the seroepidemiology of measles, mumps and rubella in England and Wales at the beginning of the 21st century. *Epidemiol Infect* 2006;**2**:1–10.

15 Giammanco A, Chiarini A, Maple PA, *et al*. European Sero-Epidemiology Network: standardisation of the assay results for pertussis. *Vaccine* 2003;**22**:112–20.

16 von Hunolstein C, Aggerbeck H, Andrews N, *et al*. European sero-epidemiology network: standardisation of the results of diphtheria antitoxin assays. *Vaccine* 2000;**18**:3287–96.

17 Sagliocca L, Bianco E, Amoroso P, Quarto M, Richichi I, Tosti ME. Feasibility of vaccination in preventing secondary cases of hepatitis A virus infection. *Vaccine* 2005;**23**:910–4.

18 World Health Organization Programme for the Control of Acute Respiratory Infections. Acute respiratory infections in children: case management in small hospitals in developing countries. WHO/ARI/90.5. Geneva: World Health Organization; 1990.

19 Ladhani S, Slack MP, Heath PT, Ramsay ME. Changes in ascertainment of Hib and its influence on the estimation

of disease incidence in the United Kingdom. *Epidemiol Infect* November 9, 2006;1–7. [Epub ahead of print]

20 Lynn RM, Pebody R, Knowles R. Twenty years of active paediatric surveillance in the UK and Republic of Ireland. *Euro Surveill* 2006;**11**(7):E060720.4.

21 Eliott EJ, Nicoll A, Lynn R, Marchessault V, Hirasing R, Ridley G. Rare disease surveillance: an international perspective. *Paediatr Child Health* 2001;**6**:251–60.

22 He Q, Schmidt-Schlapfer G, Just M, *et al.* Impact of polymerase chain reaction on clinical pertussis research: Finnish and Swiss experiences. *J Infect Dis* 1996;**174**:1288–95.

23 World Health Organization. Temperature sensitivity of vaccines. WHO/IVB/06.10. Geneva: World Health Organization; 2006.

24 Dannetun E, Tegnell A, Hermansson G, Torner A, Giesecke J. Timeliness of MMR vaccination—influence on vaccination coverage. *Vaccine* 2004;**22**:4228–32.

25 Muscat M, Christiansen AH, Persson K, *et al.* Measles outbreak in the Oresund region of Denmark and Sweden. *Euro Surveill* March 30, 2006;**11**(3):E060330.4.

26 Ramsay ME, McVernon J, Andrews NJ, Heath PT, Slack MP. Estimating *Haemophilus influenzae* type b vaccine effectiveness in England and Wales by use of the screening method. *J Infect Dis* 2003;**188**:481–5.

27 Sagliocca L, Bianco E, Amoroso P, *et al.* Feasibility of vaccination in preventing secondary cases of hepatitis A virus infection. *Vaccine* 2005;**23**:910–4.

28 Whitney CG, Pilishvili T, Farley MM, *et al.* Effectiveness of seven-valent pneumococcal conjugate vaccine against invasive pneumococcal disease: a matched case-control study. *Lancet* 2006;**368**:1495–502.

29 Käyhty H, Åhman H, Eriksson K, Sorberg M, Nilsson L. Immunogenicity and tolerability of a heptavalent pneumococcal conjugate vaccine administered at 3, 5 and 12 months of age. *Pediatr Infect Dis J* 2005;**24**:108–14.

30 Broome CV, Facklam RR, Fraser DW. Pneumococcal disease after pneumococcal vaccination: an alternative method to estimate efficacy of pneumococcal vaccination. *N Engl J Med* 1980;**303**:549–52.

31 Moulton LH, O'Brien KL, Kohberger R, *et al.* Design of a group-randomized *Streptococcus pneumoniae* vaccine trial. *Control Clin Trials* 2001;**22**:438–52.

32 Reichert TA, Sugaya N, Fedson DS, Glezen WP, Simonsen L, Tashiro M. The Japanese experience with vaccinating schoolchildren against influenza. *N Engl J Med* 2001;**344**:889–96.

33 Centers for Disease Control and Prevention (CDC). Direct and indirect effects of routine vaccination of children with 7-valent pneumococcal conjugate vaccine on incidence of invasive pneumococcal disease—United

States, 1998-2003. *MMWR Morb Mortal Wkly Rep* 2005;**54**:893–7.

34 Lieu TA, Ray GT, Black SB, *et al.* Projected cost-effectiveness of pneumococcal conjugate vaccination of healthy infants and young children. *JAMA* 2000; **283**:1460–8.

35 Salo H, Sintonen H, Pekka Nuorti J, *et al.* Economic evaluation of pneumococcal conjugate vaccination in Finland. *Scand J Infect Dis* 2005;**37**:821–32.

36 Melegaro A, Edmunds WJ. Cost-effectiveness analysis of pneumococcal conjugate vaccination in England and Wales. *Vaccine* 2004;**22**:4203–14.

37 Ray GT, Whitney CG, Fireman BH, Ciuryla V, Black SB. Cost-effectiveness of pneumococcal conjugate vaccine: evidence from the first 5 years of use in the United States incorporating herd effects. *Pediatr Infect Dis J* 2006;**25**:494–501.

38 Williams BG, Gouws E, Boschi-Pinto C, Bryce J, Dye C. Estimates of world-wide distribution of child deaths from acute respiratory infections. *Lancet Infect Dis* 2002;**2**:25–32.

39 Mulholland K, Hilton S, Adegbola R, Usen S, *et al.* Randomised trial of *Haemophilus influenzae* type-b tetanus protein conjugate vaccine [corrected] for prevention of pneumonia and meningitis in Gambian infants. *Lancet* 1997;**349**:1191–7. [Erratum in: *Lancet* 1997;**350**:524.]

40 World Health Organization Pneumonia Vaccine Trial Investigators' Group. Standardization of interpretation of chest radiographs for the diagnosis of pneumonia in children. WHO/V&B/01.35. Geneva: World Health Organization; 2001.

41 Madhi SA, Kuwanda L, Cutland C, Klugman KP. The impact of a 9-valent pneumococcal conjugate vaccine on the public health burden of pneumonia in HIV-infected and -uninfected children. *Clin Infect Dis* May 15, 2005;**40**(10):1511–8.

42 Van Effelterre TP, Zink TK, Hoet BJ, Hausdorff WP, Rosenthal P. A mathematical model of hepatitis a transmission in the United States indicates value of universal childhood immunization. *Clin Infect Dis* 2006;**43**:158–64.

43 Panagiotopoulos T, Antoniadou I, Valassi-Adam E. Increase in congenital rubella occurrence after immunisation in Greece: retrospective survey and systematic review. *BMJ* 1999;**319**:1462–7. [Erratum in: *BMJ* 2000;**320**:361.]

44 Jansen VA, Stollenwerk N, Jensen HJ, Ramsay ME, Edmunds WJ, Rhodes CJ. Measles outbreaks in a population with declining vaccine uptake. *Science* 2003;**301**:804.

45 Vyse AJ, Gay NJ, White JM, *et al.* Evolution of surveillance of measles, mumps, and rubella in England and Wales: providing the platform for evidence-based vaccination policy. *Epidemiol Rev* 2002;**24**:125–36.

46 Brisson M, Edmunds WJ, Gay NJ, Law B, De Serres G. Modelling the impact of immunization on the epidemiology of varicella zoster virus. *Epidemiol Infect* 2000;**125**:651–69.

47 Brisson M, Gay NJ, Edmunds WJ, Andrews NJ. Exposure to varicella boosts immunity to herpes-zoster: implications for mass vaccination against chickenpox. *Vaccine* 2002;**20**:2500–7.

48 Lieu TA, Cochi SL, Black SB, *et al.* Cost-effectiveness of a routine varicella vaccination program for US children. *JAMA* 1994;271:375–81.

49 Melegaro A, Edmunds WJ. Cost-effectiveness analysis of pneumococcal conjugate vaccination in England and Wales. *Vaccine* 2004;**22**:4203–14.

50 Cameron C, Pebody R. Introduction of pneumococcal conjugate vaccine to the UK childhood immunisation programme, and changes to the meningitis C and Hib schedules. *Euro Surveill* 2006;**11**(3):E060302.4.

51 Salo H, Kilpi T, Sintonen H, Linna M, Peltola V, Heikkinen T. Cost-effectiveness of influenza vaccination of healthy children. *Vaccine* 2006;**24**:4934–41.

Additional Web resources

National Immunization Program, Center for Diseases Control (CDC): www.cdc.gov/nip.

Vaccines and immunizations division of European Center for Disease Control: http://www.ecdc.eu.int/Health_topics/VI/VI.html.

Supranational Regulatory Authority of the European Commission, European Agency for the Evaluation of Medicinal Products (EMEA): www.emea.eu.int.

The vaccine section of the US Food and Drug Agency (FDA) Web site: http://www.fda.gov/cber/vaccines.htm.

GAVI Alliance, a public-private partnership focused on increasing children's access to vaccines in poor countries: www.gavialliance.org.

Technet 21, a technical network for strengthening immunization services in developing countries: www.technet21.org.

Immunization Action Coalition, newsletter on vaccination and VPD related issues from the US: www.immunize.org.

The immunization section of the World Health Organization Web site: http://www.who.int/topics/immunization/en/.

18 Vaccine preventable diseases

PART 2: Public health surveillance for vaccine adverse events

John K. Iskander & Robert T. Chen

Introduction

Surveillance of the safety of vaccines and immunizations is an integral and vital part of vaccine preventable disease (VPD) surveillance [1]. Because of the importance of immunization and its widespread use as a preventive intervention, public health officials and scientists should possess a working knowledge of vaccine safety. For the purposes of this text, vaccine safety surveillance is considered separately primarily because of the distinct methodologies involved. Vaccine safety monitoring exists as a specialized discipline within pharmacoepidemiology. Pharmacovigilance refers primarily to early detection of medical product safety concerns via passive surveillance; this may be further specified as vaccine vigilance or vaccinovigilance.

This chapter will describe the primary reasons for undertaking systematic vaccine safety surveillance, including the historical context in which such activities have become increasingly important in both the developed and developing world with maturing of immunization programs [2]. Regulatory and programmatic aspects of vaccine safety systems will be outlined briefly. Key methodological concepts and definitions, including the distinctions between active and passive surveillance systems, will be summarized. Finally, a series of case studies will be presented which integrate key scientific and public health concepts.

The primary scientific rationale for postlicensure monitoring of vaccine safety is detection of rare or novel adverse reactions not detected in prelicensure trials [3]. Such trials are rarely large enough to be able to detect reactions with incidence of 1 in 10,000 or rarer. The tolerance for serious reactions is much lower for vaccines than for drugs as the former are primarily given to healthy persons for prevention of disease; vaccines differ also in that they are used in infants, often universally. In contrast, most drugs are given to ill persons for therapeutic or curative purposes. While side effects commonly occur with drugs, serious reactions as rare as 1/100,000 doses (e.g., Guillain–Barré syndrome after Swine influenza vaccine) [4] or even 1 per million doses (e.g., paralysis after oral polio vaccine) [5] have resulted in withdrawal of vaccines or changes in immunization policy. Even rare side effects may result in a considerable numbers of affected individuals; more than 100 reported intussusceptions occurred following licensure of the first rotavirus vaccine, despite the product's limited distribution [6].

Postlicensure monitoring is also necessary to assess the safety of new vaccines among at-risk groups. Vaccine trials may deliberately exclude special populations, such as the elderly, those with chronic medical conditions, or pregnant women. Safety monitoring may uncover risk factors for adverse events among these groups once vaccine licensure permits broader use of a new vaccine [7,8]. Postlicensure study can also help to calm vaccine safety controversies. Concerns that tetanus toxoid was causing spontaneous abortions among vaccinated pregnant women in the Philippines hampered efforts to control neonatal tetanus, until epidemiologic study refuted the association [9].

Programmatically, surveillance of an immunization program can be conceived of as a "three-legged stool," with coordinated monitoring of VPD levels, vaccine coverage, and risks from vaccines. Monitoring vaccine safety plays an important role in maintaining public confidence needed to keep vaccination levels above disease prevention thresholds [10]. Concerns about combined measles, mumps, and rubella (MMR) vaccine's alleged link to autism led to decreased vaccine uptake in the United Kingdom (UK) and a brief upsurge in reported measles cases. In order to maximize scientific credibility, primary responsibility for vaccine safety surveillance may be organizationally separate from the national immunization program.

Concerns about the safety of vaccines date back to Jenner's initial use of cowpox as a vaccine against smallpox [11]. The 1955 "Cutter incident," in which several inadequately inactivated lots of the newly developed Salk polio vaccine caused disabling or fatal polio in 174 persons [12], was one of the first modern field investigations of vaccine safety (Figure 18(2).1). With the near elimination of the target VPD's due to high vaccine

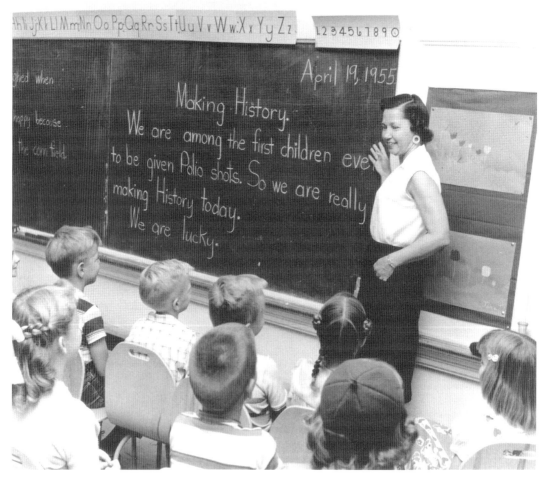

Fig 18(2).1 The children in this class were among the first to receive the newly developed Salk polio vaccine in 1955. The investigation of the "Cutter incident," in which several inadequately inactivated lots of this new vaccine caused disabling or fatal polio, highlighted the importance of vaccine safety [12]. Used with permission from March of Dimes.

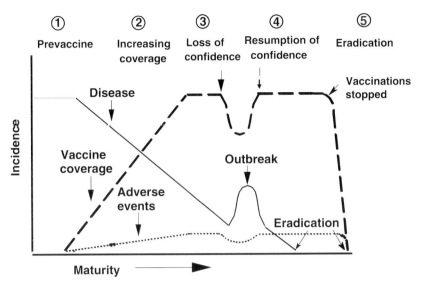

Fig 18(2).2 Evolution of immunization program and prominence of vaccine safety. (From Ref. [2].)

coverage in many countries with well-developed immunization programs, vaccine safety issues paradoxically became more prominent (Figure 18(2).2). This new paradigm was last seen with smallpox vaccine. When pivotal studies undertaken by Lane *et al.* during the late 1960s documented the burden of adverse reactions to smallpox (vaccinia) vaccine, the ultimate result was a policy decision to discontinue its routine use in some countries prior to smallpox eradication [13,14]. The rare association of Guillain–Barré syndrome (GBS) with the 1976–1977 "Swine flu" vaccine mass campaign in the United States (US) has had far ranging scientific and policy consequences [4,15]. Concerns about the safety of the whole cell pertussis vaccine globally led to the rise of vaccine consumer groups, lawsuits, loss of vaccine manufacturers, vaccine injury compensation programs, and finally a safer acellular vaccine [10]. The late 1980s and early 1990s saw the initiation and development of many current vaccine safety surveillance systems in the US to meet the needs of the mature immunization program [16,17]. During the late 1990s, this paradigm appeared to spread to other countries; high-profile vaccine safety issues included the hypothesized (but so far scientifically unsupported) link between MMR and autism [18], concern about the mercury containing preservative

thimerosal [19], the proven association between the first licensed rotavirus vaccine and intussusception [20,21], and rumors about contamination of oral polio vaccine (OPV) used as part of polio eradication campaigns [22].

Unlike traditional communicable disease surveillance which operates primarily at subnational levels, some aspects of vaccine safety monitoring are governed by national regulatory requirements. General roles of national regulatory authorities (NRAs), such as the US Food and Drug Administration (FDA) and the European Medicines Agency (EMEA), include requiring "phase IV" postlicensure studies as a condition of new vaccine licensure [23], mandating manufacturer reporting of spontaneously received adverse event reports [24], and initiating label changes or other regulatory actions, including product withdrawal, based on review of safety surveillance data [25]. NRAs are also involved in monitoring the purity, efficacy, and safety of individual vaccine lots, both prior to their release and during their general use [3]. Any apparent clustering of similar events by lot is investigated in detail. Governmental agencies in more than one dozen countries also oversee compensation schemes for individuals presumed to have been harmed by vaccine; one such system is the US Vaccine Injury Compensation Program (VICP) [26].

Table 18(2).1 Classification of AEFI by clinical characteristics and relationship to vaccination, with illustrative examples.

	Local	Systemic	Allergic
Program error	Administration of incorrect vaccine or injectable product	Administration of nonvaccine product with systemic effects	Rare allergic reactions in persons with known hypersensitivity to vaccine component (e.g., yeast in hepatitis B vaccine)
Adverse reaction	Injection site reactions	Fever	Anaphylaxis
Coincidental adverse event	Not applicable	Upper respiratory infection following inactivated influenza vaccine	Allergic reaction related to nonvaccine exposure (e.g., infant formula)

Unlike vaccine efficacy and effectiveness, vaccine safety cannot be directly measured. Instead, it is inferred from the relative absence of adverse events when a functional monitoring system is in place. An adverse event following immunization (AEFI) or vaccine adverse event (VAE) is "... a medical incident that takes place after an immunization ... and is believed to be caused by the immunization" [27]. AEFIs may include (1) true adverse reactions, (2) coincidental events that would have occurred even if the person had not been vaccinated, (3) program errors related to mistakes in vaccine preparation, handling, or administration (e.g., injection site abscesses), and (4) unknown events that cannot be directly related to the vaccine or its administration [28]. The term "adverse reaction" or side effect refers to untoward effects of vaccination caused by the vaccination [29].

Vaccine adverse reactions may be grouped into three general categories: local, systemic, and allergic. Local reactions such as pain, swelling, or redness at the site of injection are usually the least severe and most frequent; they are brief, self-limited, and rarely result in complications. Systemic reactions (e.g., fever) occur less frequently than local reactions; they may be similar to a mild form of the natural disease but only infrequently pose a serious health risk. These reactions occur more commonly after live attenuated vaccines such as MMR. Data from some prelicensure trials suggest that some minor systemic events may not be vaccine attributable [30]. Rarely, systemic reactions may be severe or even life-threatening. Thrombocytopenia (TP) occurs following MMR with an approximate incidence of 1 in 30–40,000 vaccinations; however, this is less than the occurrence of TP following either wild measles or rubella [1,31]. Serious allergic reactions, although the most severe, are the least frequent. The most serious type of allergic reaction, anaphylaxis, occurs approximately once per million vaccinations [32].

AEFI may be classified according to the clinical characteristics of the event and/or the known or suspected relationship to vaccination [28,29]. Table 18(2).1 presents examples of adverse events categorized according to both clinical manifestations and relationship to vaccination.

Formal epidemiologic study is usually required to distinguish between coincidental adverse events and adverse reactions [33]. Although methods for case-based adverse event causality assessment have been selectively employed in the US and Canada [34,35], the scientific merit of these approaches is controversial [36] primarily because of the inherent limitations of case reports. Most reported adverse events do not have features permitting easy conclusions on causality [37]. Except for injection site reactions, some immediate-type allergic reactions, recurrence of unique symptoms following subsequent vaccinations [38], or the finding of a unique clinical syndrome or laboratory result that would not occur in the absence of vaccination (e.g., the rare occurrence of vaccine-associated paralytic polio with isolation of vaccine virus strain derived from OPV), it is usually not possible to state definitively whether a vaccine caused the reported event [33]. Because case reports usually do not contain all the information needed for epidemiologic assessments

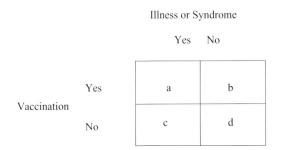

Fig 18(2).3 Establishing causality for vaccine adverse events. Rate in vaccinated persons = a/(a + b); rate in unvaccinated persons = c/(c + d); SRS only receive data on an unknown proportion of box a.

(Figure 18(2).3), elevated risks of specific adverse events following immunization are best demonstrated epidemiologically through controlled study.

Almost all national immunization programs have some type of passive surveillance or spontaneous reporting systems (SRS) for AEFIs. Reviews of case reports are most useful for identifying adverse events of concern that should be evaluated in future studies or inquiries. The US Vaccine Adverse Event Reporting System (VAERS) and the Canadian Adverse Event Following Immunization Surveillance System (CAEFISS) are examples of vaccine-specific SRS. Alternatively, SRS can be part of broader medication safety systems (e.g., the Yellow Card program used in the UK and other countries) [39]. Vaccine manufacturers also maintain internal safety reporting systems for their products, which are then forwarded to appropriate NRAs.

The US VAERS, operational since 1990 [16], serves as an "early warning" system for potential vaccine safety concerns and is typical of passive surveillance systems. It is jointly operated by the US Centers for Disease Control and Prevention (CDC) and the FDA. Reports may be submitted by healthcare providers, patients, state and local health departments, or by anyone else who wishes to report an AEFI. Manufacturers are required to report all adverse events of which they become aware [24]. In many other countries reporting to SRS is limited to healthcare professionals; the Yellow Card system recently changed its policies to permit other individuals to report as well [40].

VAERS, like other SRS, has well-described strengths and limitations. The system collects reports on a national scale and has been able to rapidly detect rare events in a cost-effective manner. Because VAERS is centralized, isolated rare events that would ordinarily escape attention may become apparent more readily, especially when larger numbers of doses are administered over a short period of time. It is also simple: healthcare providers or patients only have to fill out a one-page form and mail or fax in the report to a central location. Secure electronic reporting via the Internet is also available (www.vaers.hhs.gov). VAERS allows the rapid generation of hypotheses that can be further tested in controlled studies. For example, VAERS has successfully alerted public health authorities about safety concerns involving rotavirus (intussusception), yellow fever (viscero- and neurotropic disease), and smallpox (myo/pericarditis) vaccines [41–43]. When concerns have arisen about the need to monitor specific lots of vaccine, VAERS data have proved useful, for example, in monitoring how long specific lots were in use in practice Figure 18(2).4, which summarizes temporal trends in reporting to VAERS since its inception, indicates that while overall reporting has increased, the number of reports meeting FDA criteria for seriousness has remained relatively constant.

VAERS is subject to underreporting, reporting biases that may be related to media coverage of vaccine adverse events, and reporting of events that are unconfirmed or incompletely described [45]. The term "reporting efficiency" describes the proportion of occurrences of a specific type of event after administration of a particular vaccine that is actually reported to VAERS. Reporting efficiency may have been as high as 72% for OPV-associated poliomyelitis and as low as 1% for rashes occurring after MMR. Serious events and events occurring sooner after vaccination are more likely to be reported [46]. A capture–recapture study found that reporting efficiency of intussusception following rotavirus vaccine approached 50%, though reports in both the medical literature and the media undoubtedly stimulated reporting [47]. The effects of publicity on reporting should be taken into account when analyzing any spontaneously reported vaccine safety data [48,49].

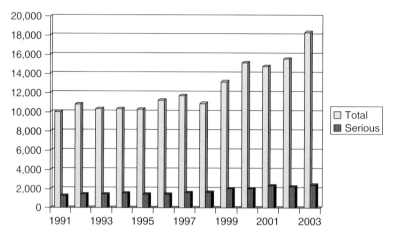

Fig 18(2).4 Reports to the US Vaccine Adverse Event Reporting System, 1991–2003. (*Source*: www.vaers.hhs.gov.)

Other limitations of passive surveillance systems include variability in quality and completeness of reports and reporter bias [45,49]. In its current configuration, VAERS and most similar nationally based systems do not permit calculation of population-based incidence rates of adverse events. This is due to both incomplete reporting of adverse events, and lack of knowledge of the total number of persons receiving a given vaccine or vaccine combination. Case definitions developed by the Brighton Collaboration, an international voluntary collective of subject matter experts, provide a means to classify adverse events in a standardized manner [50].

Reporters to VAERS and CAEFISS are asked to denote whether the adverse event led to hospitalization, life-threatening illness, disability, death, or closely related outcomes. These events are classified as "serious" according to regulatory definitions and international criteria [24]. Reports of special interest, including all deaths and hospitalizations, are often subject to further study. Follow-up often yields important information. For example, investigation of deaths reported to VAERS determined that the cause of death was significantly different from what originally was stated on the original report in nearly one-quarter of the cases [51].

SRS data have been evaluated using descriptive epidemiological approaches combined with medical judgment [36]. Case series analysis combined with case level review and application of case definitions or classification criteria is one typical methodology. Advanced signal detection or "data mining" techniques which trace their origins to drug safety research [52] seem promising as methods for identifying vaccine safety signals in need of further evaluation, although they require cautious interpretation due to inherent system biases. Bias is very difficult to quantify or control in nonexperimental studies [53], and is likely to be a far greater source of uncertainty than the effect of chance. The application of statistical significance tests or calculation of confidence intervals for vaccine safety data reported through SRS should therefore not be undertaken routinely [45].

Other national vaccine safety systems have successfully detected early signals which were validated in subsequent studies. Reports to CAEFISS identified oculorespiratory syndrome among influenza vaccinees from one Canadian manufacturer in one season [54]. Bell's palsy was also detected in recipients of a new Swiss intranasal influenza vaccine [55]. The Brazilian SRS detected higher rates of allergic adverse events with one brand of MMR after a mass campaign, with subsequent confirmation by the Italian system leading to the product's withdrawal [56]. Equally important, such systems have provided reassurance of safety of new vaccines such as the new meningococcal B and C vaccines in New Zealand and the UK [57]. As expected, some signals were not validated by follow-up studies, such as initial concerns about the safety of the infant hexavalent vaccine in Germany [58].

Regardless of the method used, vaccine-adverse event combinations that are identified as safety concerns should be subjected to further clinical and epidemiological analysis. Confirmation using data from a controlled study is usually required. This requires unbiased collection of data regarding incidence of the AEFI in question in both vaccine exposed and unexposed persons.

The primary mechanism used for vaccine safety hypothesis testing in the US is the Vaccine Safety Datalink (VSD). The VSD project is a collaboration between CDC and several geographically diverse health maintenance organizations (HMOs); it utilizes the HMO databases to collect information on enrollees' vaccination status, health outcomes, and demographic characteristics. The VSD covers about 3% of the US population [17,59]. This general approach, referred to as a large-linked database (LLDB), allows assessment of the rate with which medical events occur in both vaccinated and unvaccinated persons. Verification of diagnoses coded in automated data can be accomplished through chart review, and the VSD has been successfully used for studies needed to answer urgent public health questions, most notably when it confirmed the association of intussusception with the first US licensed rotavirus vaccine [20]. However, even LLDBs such as the VSD may not be sufficiently powerful for detection of extremely rare events such as GBS, whose incidence or vaccine attributable risk may range from 1/100,000 to 1/1,000,000 [4,60],

Although LLDB studies are typically used for hypothesis testing [20,59], they may also be conducted for purposes of hypothesis generation or safety screening [61]. Applicable study designs include cohort or case-control studies and so-called self-controlled case series analyses. Active surveillance studies have typically been conducted retrospectively, but newer technologies allow the possibility of conducting prospective vaccine safety inquiries in near real time [62]. Other LLDBs that have been used to conduct vaccine safety studies include the UK's General Practice Research Database (GPRD) [63], and the US Department of Defense's Defense Medical Surveillance System (DMSS) [64]. The UK, Denmark, Canada, and Vietnam have also used LLDBs for vaccine safety studies [65].

Other types of active surveillance used to conduct vaccine safety studies include hospital-based networks, such as the Canadian IMPACT system [66] which is used to monitor AEFI, vaccine failures, and selected infectious diseases in children. Ad hoc case-control studies can also be conducted to address vaccine safety issues with important public health implications [4,9,21,55,60] especially when LLDBs are unavailable, although such studies are both labor and resource intensive.

In developing countries, the World Health Organization (WHO) has encouraged the establishment of functional routine AEFI surveillance systems and support for NRAs as part of the Expanded Programme on Immunization (EPI) [67]. The primary focus is on detection of correctable programmatic errors like injection site abscesses (suggestive of inadequate sterilization), and development of a rapid response/assessment team for clusters of more serious events (e.g., toxic shock syndrome from contamination of vaccine vials or deaths from confusing other medications for vaccines). Both polio and measles elimination programs have provided opportunities to pilot AEFI surveillance, but much work remains. As of 2004, only 67 of 192 national EPIs (35%) have a functioning program for monitoring AEFIs (A. Bentsi-Enchill, Personal communication, World Health Organization, 2004).

Case studies

Intussusception after rotavirus vaccine

Among participants of prelicensing trials of several candidate rotavirus vaccines, intussusception was noted in five of 10,054 recipients of any reassortant rhesus vaccine compared with 1 of 4633 placebo recipients. The difference between the rates of intussusception in these groups was not statistically significant, and the rates observed among vaccinated children were similar to those seen in comparison populations. A reassortant rhesus vaccine (RRV-TV) was licensed for use in the US in August 1998 and recommendations for its use were published in March 1999 by the Advisory Committee on Immunization Practices (ACIP) [68]. As a precaution, intussusception was listed in the package insert of the vaccine as a possible side effect, and physicians were encouraged to report all adverse reactions to VAERS. Before RRV-TV was licensed and marketed in the US, VAERS had received a total of only three reports of intussusception after all other vaccinations [69].

The first intussusception case following RRV-TV was reported to VAERS in December 1998. During the first half of 1999, a total of 14 additional cases were reported. CDC announced this finding in July 1999 and recommended that healthcare providers postpone use of RRV-TV at least until November 1999, pending results of a national case-control study [41]. The manufacturer, in consultation with FDA, voluntarily ceased further distribution of the vaccine in mid-July 1999.

From September 1998 through December 1999, VAERS received 121 reports of intussusception among infants who received RRV-TV. The majority of cases were reported during July–August 1999, with a peak occurring soon after the *MMWR* publication [6]. On October 22, 1999, after a review of scientific data from multiple sources [20,21], ACIP concluded that intussusception occurred with substantially increased frequency in the first 1–2 weeks after vaccination with RRV-TV, particularly after the first dose. ACIP withdrew its recommendation for vaccination of infants in the US with RRV-TV [70], and the manufacturer subsequently withdrew the vaccine.

Influenza vaccine and GBS

Vaccination with swine influenza vaccine (used in 1976–1977) is known to increase the risk for GBS [5]. Studies of influenza vaccines used in the US in subsequent years did not find evidence of a causal link with GBS [71]. Reports of GBS after any vaccination are followed up by VAERS to confirm the diagnosis. The number of reports to VAERS of influenza vaccine-associated GBS doubled between 1992–1993 and 1993–1994, arousing concern about a possible increase in vaccine-associated risk. ACIP recommended that a special study be initiated to investigate the VAERS signal.

Patients given a diagnosis of GBS in the 1992–1993 and 1993–1994 influenza vaccination seasons were identified in the hospital-discharge databases of four states. Vaccination histories were obtained

and were confirmed by the vaccine providers. Disease with an onset within 6 weeks after vaccination was defined as vaccine-associated. In 9 of the 19 vaccine-associated cases, the onset was in the second week after vaccination. The relative risk of GBS associated with vaccination, adjusted for age, sex, and vaccine season, was 1.7 for the two seasons combined (95% confidence interval, 1.0–2.8, $p = 0.04$). However, there was no increase in the risk of vaccine-associated GBS from 1992–1993 to 1993–1994. The adjusted relative risk of 1.7 suggests slightly more than one additional case of Guillain–Barré per million persons vaccinated [60]. Because of its apparent rarity, a prior history of GBS is now considered a relative precaution, rather than an absolute contraindication, to receipt of influenza vaccine [72].

This example indicates that spontaneously reported data are useful in preliminary evaluation of rare adverse events when the relation to vaccination is uncertain. Recent data from VAERS have documented decreased reporting of post influenza vaccine GBS across age groups, despite overall increased adverse event reporting for influenza vaccine [73]. Studies to investigate the pathophysiology of swine-flu-associated GBS have been undertaken [71], using banked frozen vaccine.

Hepatitis B vaccination and multiple sclerosis (MS) in France

Beginning in the 1994, over 20 million French were vaccinated against hepatitis B in the largest mass vaccination campaign conducted in France in the modern era [74]. Within months of the start of the campaign in 1994, neurologists reported to French pharmacovigilance centers that they were seeing patients with MS who had recently received hepatitis B vaccine. In response, several investigations were initiated in France and elsewhere. In a controversial move which was opposed by many public health and immunization experts, the French Ministry of Health also temporarily suspended the school adolescent hepatitis B vaccination program in 1998 due to these safety concerns.

The age and gender distribution of the reported vaccine-associated cases was similar to the known epidemiologic profile of MS, with most cases occurring among females. No cases were reported among children <25 months of age despite recommendations for routine childhood hepatitis B vaccination. At least 10 epidemiologic studies have been completed examining this possible association [75]. Nine studies, including one using the VSD, failed to show statistically significant positive associations. A recent study using the GPRD in the UK did find a significant association, with an odds ratio of 3.1 (95% CI 1.5–6.3) [63]. However, even these researchers concluded that the proven benefits of hepatitis B vaccination outweigh the potential risks.

Influenza vaccines and Bell's palsy

Bell's palsy (BP) is a paralysis of the nerves of the face from which people typically recover fully. In 2000–2001, BP was strongly associated with a Swiss-licensed inactivated intranasal influenza vaccine [55]. The vaccine contained *Escherichia coli* heat-labile toxin as a mucosal adjuvant, which may have been responsible for the development of BP [76]. When a follow-up study in VAERS indicated the possibility of an association between inactivated injectable influenza vaccines and BP [77], a population-based VSD study was launched to assess the validity of this hypothesized link. This example illustrates the potential for conducting vaccine safety studies in an internationally coordinated manner, using both active and passive surveillance methods.

Conclusion

The importance of public health surveillance for vaccine safety is likely to continue to increase in consequence of ongoing licensure of new vaccines, implementation of expanded vaccine recommendations [72], and new global immunization initiatives including the Global Alliance for Vaccine and Immunization [78]. Vaccines will continue to be held to very high standards of safety. Although recent prelicensure trials for second-generation rotavirus vaccine shave involved nearly 70,000 subjects [79,80], it is unlikely that studies of this size will become routine because of attendant increased cost and logistic difficulties. The burden of monitoring rare, serious, and/or unexpected adverse events will continue to fall to postlicensure surveillance systems, both active and passive. The twenty-first century public health practitioner needs to understand the objectives and relative strengths and weaknesses of both types of systems. These are summarized in Table 18(2).2.

Vaccination policy decisions and reviews, as well as communications with healthcare providers or the public related to vaccine safety issues, should take into account available scientific surveillance data from all sources [81]. Clear communication of rare but potentially serious risks to an increasingly risk-adverse public may pose substantial challenges [82], but can be addressed through scientific principles of risk communication [83].

Table 18(2).2 Characteristics of vaccine safety surveillance systems.

General type of surveillance	Active	Passive
Examples	VSD, GPRD, IMPACT	VAERS, CAEFISS, Yellow Card
Is population based	Yes	No
Primary objective	Hypothesis testing	Hypothesis generation
Can be used to calculate incidence of AEFI	Yes	No
Can be used to calculate vaccine attributable risk of AEFI	Yes	No
Sensitivity for rare event detection	Relatively low	Relatively high
Cost	Relatively high	Relatively low
Study designs	Cohort, case-control, self-controlled case series	Case series, advanced signal detection, or "data mining"

References

1 Atkinson W, Hamborsky J, McIntyre L, Wolfe S (eds.). *Epidemiology and Prevention of Vaccine-Preventable Diseases*, 8th edn. Washington, DC: Public Health Foundation; 2005.

2 Chen RT. Evaluation of vaccine safety after the events of 11 September 2001: role of cohort and case-control studies. *Vaccine* May 7, 2004;**22**(15–16):2047–53.

3 Ellenberg SS, Chen RT. The complicated task of monitoring vaccine safety. *Public Health Rep* January–February1997;**112**(1):10–20.

4 Schonberger LB, Bregman DJ, Sullivan-Bolyai JZ. Guillain–Barré syndrome following vaccination in the National Influenza Immunization Program, United States, 1976–1977. *Am J Epidemiol* August 1979; **110**(2):105–23.

5 Alexander LN, Seward JF, Santibanez TA, *et al.* Vaccine policy changes and epidemiology of poliomyelitis in the United States. *JAMA* October 13, 2004;**292**(14):1696–701.

6 Zanardi LR, Haber P, Mootrey GT, *et al.* Intussusception among recipients of rotavirus vaccine—reports to the Vaccine Adverse Event Reporting System. *Pediatrics* 2001;**107**(6):E97. Available from http://www.pediatrics.org/cgi/content/full/107/6/e97.

7 Martin M, Weld LH, Tsai TF, *et al.* Advanced age a risk factor for illness temporally associated with yellow fever vaccination. Emerg Infect Dis 2001;7:945–51.

8 Barwick R; Eidex for the Yellow Fever Vaccine Safety Working Group. History of thymoma and yellow fever vaccination. *Lancet* September 11–17, 2004;**364**(9438):936.

9 Catindig N, Abad-Viola G, Magboo F, *et al.* Tetanus toxoid and spontaneous abortions: is there epidemiological evidence of an association? *Lancet* October 19, 1996;**348**(9034):1098–9.

10 Gangarosa EJ, Galzka AM, Wolfe CR, *et al.* Impact of anti-vaccine movements on pertussis control: the untold story. *Lancet* January 31, 1998;**351**(9099): 356–61.

11 Plotkin SA, Orenstein W. *Vaccines*, 4th edn. Philadelphia: WB Saunders; 2003.

12 Nathanson N, Langmuir AD. The Cutter incident. Poliomyelitis following formaldehyde-inactivated poliovirus vaccination in the United States during the spring of 1955. II: Relationship of poliomyelitis to Cutter Vaccine. *Am J Hyg* 1963;**78**:29–60.

13 Lane JM, Ruben FL, Neff JM, *et al.* Complications of smallpox vaccination, 1968: results of ten statewide surveys. *J Infect Dis* 1970;**122**:303–9.

14 Lane JM, Ruben FL, Neff JM, *et al.* Complications of smallpox vaccination: national surveillance in the United States, 1968.*N Engl J Med* 1969;**281**: 1201–7.

15 US Department of Health and Human Services. *Pandemic Influenza Preparedness and Response Plan. Annex 11: Lessons Learned from 1976 Swine Influenza Program.* Washington, DC: US Department of Health and Human Services; August 2004.

16 Chen RT, Rastogi SC, Mullen JR, Hayes SW, Cochi SL, Donlon JA. The Vaccine Adverse Event Reporting System (VAERS). *Vaccine* 1994;**12**:542–50.

17 Chen RT, Glasser JW, Rhodes PH, *et al.* The Vaccine Safety Datalink Project: a new tool for improving vaccine safety monitoring in the United States. *Pediatrics* 1997;**99**:765–73.

18 Wakefield AJ, Murch SH, Anthony A, *et al.* Ileal-lymphoid-nodular hyperplasia, non-specific colitis, and pervasive developmental disorder in children. *Lancet* February 28, 1998;**351**(9103):637–41.

19 Centers for Disease Control and Prevention. Thimerosal in vaccines: a joint statement of the American Academy of Pediatrics and the Public Health Service. *MMWR Morb Mortal Wkly Rep* 1999;**48**:563–5.

20 Kramarz P, France EK, Destefano F, *et al.* Population-based study of rotavirus vaccination and intussusception. *Pediatr Infect Dis J* April 2001;**20**(4):410–6.

21 Murphy TV, Gargiullo PM, Massoudi MS, *et al.* Intussusception among infants given an oral rotavirus vaccine. *N Engl J Med* 2001;**344**:564–72.

22 Chen C. Rebellion against the polio vaccine in Nigeria: implications for humanitarian policy. *Afr Health Sci* 2004;**4**(3):205–7.

23 Baylor NW, Midthun K. Regulation and testing of vaccines. In: Plotkin SA, Orenstein WA (eds.), *Vaccines*. Philadelphia: WB Saunders; 2004:1539–56.

24 Postmarketing reporting of adverse experiences, 21 C.F.R. Sect. 600.80 (1999).

25 Centers for Disease Control and Prevention. Guillain–Barre syndrome among recipients of Menactra meningococcal conjugate vaccine—United States, June–July 2005. *MMWR Morb Mortal Wkly Rep* October 14, 2005;**54**(40):1023–5.

26 Evans G. Vaccine injury compensation programs worldwide. *Vaccine* October 29, 1999;**17**(suppl 3):S25–35.

27 World Health Organization. *Immunization Safety Surveillance*. Manila: Immunization Focus, Western Pacific Regional Office; 1999. Available from: http://www.who.int/immunization_safety/publications/aefi/en/AEFI_WPRO.pdf. Accessed May 30, 2006.

28 United States Agency for International Development; Office of Health, Infectious Diseases, and Nutrition, Bureau for Global Health. *Immunization Essentials*. Washington, DC: United States Agency for International Development; 2003.

29 Centers for Disease Control and Prevention. General recommendations on immunization: recommendations of the Advisory Committee on Immunization Practices and the American Academy of Family Physicians. *MMWR Morb Mortal Wkly Rep* 2002;**51**(RR-2).

30 Peltola H, Heinonen OP. Frequency of true adverse reactions to measles-mumps-rubella vaccine: a double-blind placebo-controlled trial in twins. *Lancet* April 26, 1986;**1**(8487):939–42.

31 Jefferson T, EUSAFEVAC project. Unintended events following immunization with MMR: a systematic review. *Vaccine* September 8, 2003;**21**(25–26):3954–60.

32 Bohlke K, Davis RL, Marcy SM, *et al*. Risk of anaphylaxis after vaccination of children and adolescents. *Pediatrics* October 2003;**112**(4):815–20.

33 Halsey N. The science of evaluation of adverse events associated with vaccination. *Semin Pediatr Infect Dis* 2002;**13**:205–14.

34 Sever JL, Brenner AI, Gale AD, *et al*. Safety of anthrax vaccine: a review by the Anthrax Vaccine Expert committee (AVEC) of adverse events reported to the Vaccine Adverse Event Reporting System (VAERS). *Pharmacoepidemiol Drug Saf* 2002;**11**:189–202.

35 Collet J-P, MacDonald N, Cashman N, *et al*. Monitoring for signals for vaccine safety: the assessment of individual adverse event reports by an expert advisory committee. The Advisory Committee on Causality Assessment. *Bull World Health Organ* 2000;**78**:178–85.

36 Ball R. Methods for ensuring vaccine safety. *Expert Rev Vaccines* 2002;**1**:161–8.

37 Iskander Jk, Miller ER, Chen RT. The role of the Vaccine Adverse Event Reporting system (VAERS) in monitoring vaccine safety. *Pediatr Ann* September 2004;**33**(9):599–606.

38 Wise R, Kiminyo K, Salive M. Hair loss after routine immunizations. *JAMA* 1997;**278**(14):1176–8.

39 Morales-Olivas FJ, Martinez-Mir I, Ferrer JM, *et al*. Adverse drug reactions in children reported by means of the yellow card in Spain. *J Clin Epidemiol* October 2000;**53**(10):1076–80.

40 Patient Reporting Working Group. London: Medicines and Healthcare Products Regulatory Agency; c2004–2006. Available from: www.mhra.gov.uk/home/idcplg?IdcService=SS_GET_PAGE&nodeId=620. Accessed May 26, 2006.

41 Centers for Disease Control and Prevention. Intussusception among recipients of rotavirus vaccine—United States, 1998–1999. *MMWR Morb Mortal Wkly Rep* 1999;**48**:577–81.

42 Centers for Disease Control and Prevention. Adverse events associated with 17d-derived yellow fever vaccination—United States, 2001–2002. *MMWR Morb Mortal Wkly Rep* 2002;**51**:989–93.

43 Centers for Disease Control and Prevention. Cardiac adverse events following smallpox vaccination—United States, 2003. *MMWR Morb Mortal Wkly Rep* 2003;**52**:248–50.

44 Dayan G, Iskander J, Glasser J, *et al*. Tracking vaccine lot lifecycles using reports to the Vaccine Adverse Event Reporting System (VAERS). *Pharmacoepidemiol Drug Saf* January 20, 2005.

45 Varricchio F, Iskander J, Destefano F, *et al*. Understanding vaccine safety information from the Vaccine Adverse Event Reporting System. *Pediatr Infect Dis J* 2004;**23**:287–94.

46 Rosenthal S, Chen RT. Reporting sensitivities of two passive surveillance systems for vaccine adverse events. *Am J Public Health* 1995;**85**:1706–9.

47 Verstraeten T, Baughman AL, Cadwell B, *et al*. Enhancing vaccine safety surveillance: a capture–recapture analysis of intussusception after rotavirus vaccination. *Am J Epidemiol* 2001;**154**(11):1006–12.

48 Goodman MJ, Nordin J. Vaccine adverse event reporting system reporting source: a possible source of bias in longitudinal studies. *Pediatrics* February 2006;**117**(2):387–90.

49 Woo EJ, Ball R, Bostrom A, *et al*. Vaccine risk perception among reporters of autism after vaccination: vaccine adverse event reporting system 1990–2001. *Am J Public Health* June 2004;**94**(6):990–5.

50 Bonhoeffer J, Kohl K, Chen R, *et al*. The Brighton Collaboration-enhancing vaccine safety. *Vaccine* May 7, 2004;**22**(15–16):2046.

51 Silvers LE, Varricchio FE, Ellenberg SS, *et al*. Pediatric deaths reported after vaccination: the utility of information obtained from parents. *Am J Prev Med* April 2002;**22**(3):170–6.

52 Niu MT, Erwin DE, Braun MM. Data mining in the US Vaccine Adverse Event Reporting System (VAERS): early detection of intussusception and other events after rotavirus vaccination. *Vaccine* 2001;**19**:4627–34.

53 Sparrow JM, Thompson JR. Bias: adding to the uncertainty. *Br J Opthalmol* 1999;**83**:637–8.

54 Skowronski DM, Strauss B, De Serres G, *et al*. Oculo-respiratory syndrome: a new influenza vaccine-associated adverse event? *Clin Infect Dis* 2003;**36**:705–13.

55 Mutsch M, Zhou W, Rhodes P, *et al*. Use of the inactivated intranasal influenza vaccine and the risk of Bell's palsy in Switzerland. *N Engl J Med* February 26, 2004;**350**(9):896–903.

56 Chiron Vaccines. Chiron recalls and withdraws MORU-PAR(R) MMR vaccine from Italian and developing

world markets. Marburg: Chiron Vaccines; c2006. Available from: http://www.chironvaccines.com/company/vaccines_Press_Area_16_March_2006_2.php. Accessed May 1, 2006.

57 Ruggeberg J, Heath PT. Safety and efficacy of meningococcal group C conjugate vaccines. *Expert Opin Drug Saf* January 2003;**2**(1):7–19.

58 Lackmann GM. Comparative investigation of the safety of hexavalent vaccines for primary scheduled infant immunizations in Germany over a time period of 2 years. *Med Sci Monit* September 2004;**10**(9):PI96–8.

59 DeStefano F; Vaccine Safety Datalink Research Group. The Vaccine Safety Datalink project. *Pharmacoepidemiol Drug Saf* August–September 2001;**10**(5):403–6.

60 Lasky T, Terracciano GJ, Magder L, *et al.* The Guillain–Barre syndrome and the 1992–1993 and 1993–1994 influenza vaccines. *N Engl J Med* 1998;**339**:1797–802.

61 France EK, Glanz JM, Xu S, *et al.* Safety of the trivalent inactivated influenza vaccine among children: a population-based study. *Arch Pediatr Adolesc Med* November 2004;**158**(11):1031–6.

62 Davis RL, Kolczak M, Lewis E, *et al.* Active Surveillance of Vaccine Safety: a system to detect early signs of adverse events. *Epidemiology* May 2005;**16**(3):336–41.

63 Hernan MA, Jick SS, Olek MJ, *et al.* Recombinant hepatitis B vaccine and the risk of multiple sclerosis: a prospective study. *Neurology* September 14, 2004;**63**(5):838–42.

64 Rubertone MV, Brundage JF. The Defense Medical Surveillance System and the Department of Defense serum repository: glimpses of the future of public health surveillance. *Am J Public Health* December 2002;**92**(12):1900–4.

65 Verstraeten T, DeStefano F, Chen RT, *et al.* Vaccine safety surveillance using large linked databases: opportunities, hazards and proposed guidelines. *Expert Rev Vaccines* February 2003;**2**(1):21–9.

66 Moore DL, Le Saux N, Scheifele D, *et al.* Lack of evidence of encephalopathy related to pertussis vaccine: active surveillance by IMPACT, Canada, 1993–2002. *Pediatr Infect Dis J* 2004;**23**:568–71.

67 Duclos P, Delo A, Aguado T, *et al.* Immunization safety priority project at the World Health Organization. *Semin Pediatr Infect Dis* July 2003;**14**(3):233–9.

68 Centers for Disease Control and Prevention. Rotavirus vaccine for the prevention of rotavirus gastroenteritis among children: recommendations of the Advisory Committee on Immunization Practices. *MMWR Morb Mortal Wkly Rep* 1999;**48**(RR-2).

69 Zhou W, Pool V, Iskander J, *et al.* Surveillance for safety after immunization: Vaccine Adverse Event Reporting System (VAERS)—United States, 1991–2001. In: CDC surveillance summaries (January 24). *Morb Mortal Wkly Rep* 2003;**52**(SS-1).

70 CDC. Withdrawal of rotavirus vaccine recommendation. *MMWR Morb Mortal Wkly Rep* 1999;**48**:1007.

71 Institute of Medicine. *Immunization Safety Review: Influenza Vaccines and Neurological Complications.* Washington, DC: National Academies Press; 2003.

72 Prevention and Control of Influenza. Recommendations of the Advisory Committee on Immunization Practices (ACIP). *Morb Mortal Wkly Rep Recomm Rep* July 29, 2005;**54**(RR-8):1–40.

73 Haber P, DeStefano F, Angulo F, *et al.* Guillain–Barré syndrome following influenza vaccination. *JAMA* November 24, 2004;**292**(20):2478–81.

74 Balinska MA. L'affaire hepatite B en France. *Espirit* 2001;**276**:34–48.

75 Zuckerman JN. Protective efficacy, immunotherapeutic potential, and safety of hepatitis B vaccines. *J Med Virol* February 2006;**78**(2):169–77.

76 Couch RB. Nasal vaccination, Escherichia coli enterotoxin, and Bell's palsy. *N Engl J Med* February 26, 2004;**350**(9):860–1.

77 Zhou W, Pool V, DeStefano F, *et al.* A potential signal of Bell's palsy after parenteral inactivated influenza vaccines: reports to the Vaccine Adverse Event Reporting System (VAERS)—United States, 1991–2001. *Pharmacoepidemiol Drug Saf* August 2004;**13**(8):505–10.

78 Balaji KA. GAVI and the Vaccine Fund—a boon for immunization in the developing world. *Indian J Public Health* April–June 2004;**48**(2):45–8.

79 Vesikari T, Matson DO, Dennehy P, *et al.* Safety and efficacy of a pentavalent human-bovine (WC3) reassortant rotavirus vaccine. *N Engl J Med* January 5, 2006;**354**(1):23–33.

80 Ruiz-Palacios GM, Perez-Schael I, Velazquez FR, *et al.* Safety and efficacy of an attenuated vaccine against severe rotavirus gastroenteritis. *N Engl J Med* January 5, 2006;**354**(1):11–22.

81 Giffin R, Stratton K, Chalk R. Childhood vaccine finance and safety issues. *Health Aff (Millwood)* September–October 2004;**23**(5):98–111.

82 Breiman RF, Zanca JA. Of floors and ceilings—defining, assuring, and communicating vaccine safety. *Am J Public Health* December 1997;**87**(12):1919–20.

83 Gust DA, Woodruff R, Kennedy A, *et al.* Parental perceptions surrounding risks and benefits of immunization. *Semin Pediatr Infect Dis* July 2003;**14**(3):207–12.

Appendix: List of abbreviations

ACIP: US Advisory Committee on Immunization Practices

AEFI: Adverse Event Following Immunization

BP: Bell's palsy

CAEFISS: Canadian Adverse Event Following Immunization Surveillance System

CDC: US Centers for Disease Control and Prevention

DMSS: Defense Medical Surveillance System

EMEA: European Medicines Agency

EPI: Expanded Programme on Immunization

FDA: US Food and Drug Administration

GBS: Guillain–Barré syndrome

GPRD: General Practice Research Database

HMO: Health Maintenance Organization

IMPACT: Immunization Monitoring Program-Active

LLDB: Large-linked database

MMR: Measles, mumps, and rubella vaccine

MS: Multiple sclerosis

NRA: National Regulatory Authority

OPV: Oral polio vaccine

RRV-TV: Tetravalent rhesus-based rotavirus vaccine

SRS: Spontaneous reporting system

TP: Thrombocytopenia

VAE: Vaccine adverse event

VAERS: US Vaccine Adverse Event Reporting System

VICP: US Vaccine Injury Compensation System

VPD: Vaccine-preventable disease

VSD: US Vaccine Safety Datalink

WHO: World Health Organization

19 Seasonal and pandemic influenza surveillance

Lynnette Brammer, Alicia Postema & Nancy Cox

Introduction

Influenza viruses belong to the Orthomyxoviridae family and are divided into types A, B, and C. Influenza type A and B viruses are responsible for epidemics of respiratory illness that occur every winter in temperate climates and year-round in the tropics. Influenza type C virus produces a milder infection, does not cause epidemics, and will not be discussed further in this chapter. Influenza type A viruses are divided into subtypes based on surface proteins called hemagglutinin (HA) and neuraminidase (NA). To date, 16 HA subtypes and nine NA subtypes have been identified. However, in the twentieth century, influenza viruses bearing only three HA (H1, H2, and H3) and two NA subtypes (N1 and N2) have circulated widely in humans. Influenza viruses are notable for their ability to change through two different mechanisms: antigenic drift and antigenic shift. Antigenic drift is the slow, continuous change affecting both influenza type A and B viruses that allows for multiple infections of an individual over their lifetime and requires frequent updating of the viral components of trivalent influenza vaccine. Antigenic shift is an infrequent but dramatic change, occurring only among influenza type A viruses, that results in a new influenza A subtype to which most or all of the population has no immunity. If the new virus can infect humans and transmit easily from person to person, a pandemic may occur.

The burden of influenza in nonindustrialized countries is not well defined. However, during annual epidemics in industrialized nations, between 5% and 20% of the population may be infected [1]. Influenza illness can range in severity from asymptomatic infection to mild respiratory illness to primary viral pneumonia and death [1–7]. More than 90% of influenza-related deaths occur in persons 65 years of age and older, but school-age children generally have the highest infection rates [2–7]. Although influenza virus infection may result in more severe illness than that caused by other respiratory viruses and have a greater impact on the population as a whole, individual cases of influenza cannot be diagnosed based on clinical information alone. Laboratory testing is required to differentiate influenza from other respiratory virus infections. Surveillance for influenza must take into account a constantly changing virus, the pervasiveness of infection, and the nonspecificity and range of clinical illness. Laboratory surveillance serves as the foundation of influenza surveillance and is necessary for the selection of appropriate vaccine strains. However, additional components that provide morbidity and mortality information are needed to provide a complete picture of the impact of influenza necessary to guide prevention, control, and mitigation policies. Descriptions of laboratory-based surveillance and systems to monitor outpatient illness, hospitalizations, and deaths due to influenza will be discussed. Specific examples from the United States (US) are used.

Components of influenza surveillance

Worldwide influenza surveillance is conducted through the World Health Organization (WHO)

Global Influenza Program that was conceived in 1947 and the WHO Global Influenza Surveillance Network that was established in 1952. The network currently consists of four international WHO Collaborating Centers for Reference and Research on Influenza and 116 laboratories in 87 countries recognized by WHO as National Influenza Centers (NIC). The NICs collect specimens from patients within their country with influenza-like-illness (ILI; defined as fever >38°C and either cough or sore throat [8]), either directly from physicians, clinics, and hospitals, or through a network of laboratories, for viral isolation. NICs perform preliminary analysis of influenza isolates, including virus typing and subtyping. Results are reported to WHO and made publicly available through a Web-based reporting system, called FluNet (http://gamapserver.who.int/GlobalAtlas/home.asp). A subset of the routine seasonal influenza isolates and all isolates for which the subtype cannot be determined are sent from the NICs to one or more of the four WHO Collaborating Centers for more detailed antigenic and genetic characterization and antiviral resistance testing. Seed viruses for vaccine production are obtained through this surveillance network.

The design of an influenza surveillance system should be based on the goals and objectives of surveillance. The goals of influenza surveillance at the international level may differ from those at the national, state, or local level. The primary goals of the international influenza surveillance network are to provide virologic data to inform twice-yearly trivalent vaccine strain selection and to rapidly detect and respond to human infections with novel influenza A subtypes that may have pandemic potential. Other goals of WHO's Global Influenza Program are detailed at http://www.who.int/csr/disease/influenza/en/index.html. National level goals may focus on measuring disease burden and impact to inform prevention and control policy development. Local jurisdictions may need information to inform patient treatment decisions and outbreak response. Additionally, whereas interpandemic influenza surveillance forms the foundation for pandemic surveillance, it is unlikely that those systems alone will be sufficient for detecting the initial introduction and spread of pandemic influenza or be able to fulfill all the information needs during a pandemic. Further

information on interpandemic surveillance as part of pandemic preparedness can be accessed at http://www.who.int/csr/resources/publications/influenza/FluCheck6web.pdf.

Regardless of the surveillance goals or objectives, a combination of virologic data and influenza-related morbidity and/or mortality components is typically needed. Several considerations should guide the selection of the clinical outcomes to be monitored and the sources of data to be used. Emphasis should be placed on collection of the minimum amount of data required in order to make public health decisions, collection of data that can be used by local, state, and national level public health officials, use of existing electronic data when available, and use of all the data that are collected. Sources of data frequently used for influenza surveillance include:

• Laboratory records
• Vital statistics records
• Emergency room or outpatient clinic visits
• Sentinel physician or clinic records
• Hospital admissions or discharge records
• School or workplace records
• Notifiable disease records
• Long-term care facility or other institution surveys and records
• Healthcare worker surveys

Laboratory surveillance

Laboratory surveillance is the foundation of influenza surveillance. In addition to providing basic information on the geographic distribution and temporal patterns of circulating viruses, the goals of influenza virologic surveillance include monitoring for antigenic changes in the viruses for vaccine strain selection, monitoring for antiviral resistance, and detecting novel influenza subtypes that pose a pandemic threat. Virologic data can be used in combination with morbidity or mortality data to provide estimates of the burden of influenza. Although influenza infection generally leads to more severe illness among adults than other respiratory viruses, individual cases of influenza infection cannot be distinguished with certainty from other respiratory virus infections based on clinical information alone. Laboratory testing is necessary to confirm the diagnosis but testing of all ill persons is neither feasible nor necessary. Methods available for the diagnosis of influenza include virus isolation (standard methods and rapid culture assays), molecular detection (reverse transcriptase polymerase chain reaction, RT-PCR, and real-time RT-PCR), detection of viral antigens (enzyme immunoassays, EIA, and direct or indirect immunofluorescent antibody [DFA or IFA] testing), commercially available rapid diagnostic kits, and less frequently, electron microscopy, and serologic testing.

Appropriate clinical specimens for influenza virus testing include nasal washes, nasopharyngeal aspirates, nasal and throat swabs, transtracheal aspirates, and bronchoalveolar lavage. For commercially available rapid diagnostic kits, the optimal specimen varies depending upon the kit used. Specimens may come from multiple sources: physician's offices, outpatient clinics, institutional outbreaks, emergency departments, and hospitals. Respiratory specimens collected and tested as a part of routine patient care rather than purely for surveillance purposes may contribute a large proportion of samples reported for influenza surveillance. Optimally, samples should be collected from both severely ill cases, such as those requiring hospitalization, and those with milder illness requiring only outpatient care, as the predominant virus type or subtype may differ with disease severity. Systematic sampling of ill or hospitalized persons within a defined population can allow for calculation of rates of disease. Laboratory surveillance may be enhanced during pandemic alert phases by targeted sampling of persons who, based on the epidemiology of the virus of interest as it is known at the time, are at increased risk for infection with a virus with pandemic potential.

Commercially available, rapid diagnostic tests and laboratory methods such as RT-PCR, real-time RT-PCR, EIA, DFA, or IFA can provide results quickly and are useful for patient management. However, viral isolates are necessary for antigenic characterization and susceptibility testing to antiviral agents. These tests have little immediate impact on the treatment of an individual, but provide data necessary for the selection of influenza vaccine strains and recommendations for antiviral drug use.

Although it is a rare event, detection of human infections with a novel influenza A virus is one of the most important functions of the WHO Global Influenza Surveillance Network. Detection of a novel virus may occur as a result of increased surveillance among persons, such as swine or poultry workers or cullers, exposed to influenza-infected animals. Human infections with influenza A (H7N7) in the Netherlands [9], influenza A (H7N2) in the US [10], and influenza A (H7N3) in Canada [11] were detected as a result of increased surveillance of occupationally exposed persons during recognized poultry outbreaks. Other cases, such as the initial case of influenza A (H5N1) infection of a child in Hong Kong in 1997 [12] and influenza A (H9N2) in two children in Hong Kong in 1999 [13] were recognized during the course of the routine virologic surveillance performed as part of the WHO Global Surveillance Network. These viruses were initially identified as influenza A viruses that could not be subtyped with the standard reagents for identification of human H1 or H3 subtypes and were sent to one or more of the WHO Collaborating Centers for further identification. Once a new subtype is identified, reagents for detection of that subtype can be produced and distributed, if necessary. Because of the increased biosafety requirements posed by influenza A (H5N1) viruses [14], diagnostic testing has focused on methods such as RT-PCR that can be performed under biosafety level 2 conditions and can provide results in a timely manner. Commercially available rapid diagnostic tests to diagnose influenza A appear to be less sensitive for influenza A (H5N1) viruses [15,16]; testing with more sensitive and specific methods should be performed on patients suspected to have influenza A (H5N1) infection.

The US influenza virologic surveillance system provides an example of an in-country network of laboratories. A group of approximately 140 US WHO collaborating laboratories and National Respiratory and Enteric Virus Surveillance System (NREVSS) (http://www.cdc.gov/ncidod/dvrd/revb/nrevss/index.htm) laboratories report to Centers for Disease Control and Prevention (CDC) the number of respiratory specimens tested for influenza and the number that were positive by influenza virus type or subtype. The US WHO collaborating laboratories report the data by age group. The US WHO collaborating laboratories consist of all state public health laboratories, some local public health laboratories, and some hospital or academic center laboratories. NREVSS laboratories that are not also

WHO laboratories are primarily hospital laboratories. CDC compiles and analyzes data from the US WHO collaborating laboratories and NREVSS laboratories on a national and regional level each week. The data are included in a weekly national influenza activity summary posted on the CDC Web site www.cdc.gov/flu, and are reported to WHO via FluNet.

The US WHO collaborating laboratories also submit a subset of viruses they have isolated to CDC for antigenic and genetic characterization and antiviral resistance testing. Each laboratory is asked to submit a few isolates from early in the season, a few from peak influenza activity, some late season isolates, summer isolates, and any unusual isolates. Unusual isolates may include those that do not react as expected in testing, isolates that may be the result of animal to human transmission, isolates from unusually severe cases, or any influenza A isolate that the laboratory is unable to subtype.

Enhanced surveillance for influenza A (H5N1) virus provides an example of how laboratory surveillance can be focused to increase the probability of detecting the introduction of a novel influenza virus subtype into human populations. Influenza A (H5N1) viruses were first detected in humans in 1997; and again in early 2003 in Hong Kong; in January 2004 H5N1 human infections were reported in Vietnam and Thailand. By November 2006, the virus had been detected in more than 250 humans in 10 countries in Asia and Africa and hundreds of millions of birds were infected in numerous countries including some in Europe. The majority of human cases were associated with direct contact with sick or dead birds or their excretions. Most patients were severely ill and more than 50% of the cases were fatal. This information was used in the US to focus surveillance on severely ill patients with a recent travel history to an H5N1-affected country and direct contact with either birds or suspected or confirmed human cases. State public health laboratories were provided with protocols and training for real-time RT-PCR testing methods that allow for rapid (within 4 hours) detection and subtyping of influenza viruses including influenza A (H5) virus. Recommendations for enhanced surveillance will remain in place until the epidemiology of the virus changes, requiring adjustment in the case definition, or the threat of H5N1 diminishes.

Virologic surveillance frequently leads to changes in the seasonal trivalent vaccine composition, but in January 2006 virologic surveillance also led to a change in recommendations for influenza antiviral use. There are two classes of antiviral drugs effective against influenza viruses, the adamantanes (amantadine and rimatadine) and the neuraminidase inhibitors (oseltamivir and zanamivir). Resistance against adamantanes can emerge rapidly during treatment, but during 1995–2002 global surveillance showed less than 2% of influenza A isolates tested were resistant to this class of drugs. Resistance increased to 13.3% during 2003, driven primarily by increased resistance of viruses isolated in Asia [17]. In the US, 1.9% of influenza A viruses were resistant to the adamantanes during the 2003–2004 season, 11% were resistant during the 2004–2005 season [18], and 91% were resistant between October 2005 and January 14, 2006. In response, CDC issued an alert in January 2006 that recommended that adamantanes not be used for treatment or chemoprophylaxis of influenza A in the US until there are data that indicate that circulating influenza A strains are susceptible to these agents [19].

Morbidity surveillance

Disease surveillance for influenza presents many challenges. Most persons infected with influenza do not seek medical care and remain unidentified; cases of influenza usually are not confirmed by laboratory tests, and in most areas, reporting of influenza is not mandated. Therefore, influenza disease activity must be measured or monitored indirectly. Since the impact of influenza on morbidity and mortality can differ and may not follow a parallel course depending on the circulating viruses and the population under surveillance (e.g., mortality may be low in some years in which there still are substantial numbers of visits to clinicians), monitoring more than one clinical outcome is necessary to obtain an understanding of the impact of influenza during a given influenza season.

The selection of the clinical outcomes to be monitored and the data sources to be used should take into account the availability of existing data sources, the healthcare structure, the ease of collecting and reporting the data, the potential for sustainable reporting, and the potential for collecting data that are reasonably representative of the groups of interest.

Sentinel outpatient surveillance

In its most simple form, sentinel surveillance for ILI among outpatients can provide early evidence of increases in influenza virus circulation and information on where influenza activity is occurring, track the course of influenza activity during the season, and serve as a source of samples for virus isolation. In situations where the population under surveillance is known, population-based rates of ILI can be calculated. If, in addition, samples are collected in the sentinel sites in a systematic manner, the proportion of ILI due to influenza can be determined, rates of influenza infection requiring medical care can be calculated, and the burden of influenza in terms of outpatient visits can be estimated.

In Europe, the countries reporting to the European Influenza Surveillance System (EISS) have national sentinel surveillance systems for collecting and reporting information on ILI, acute respiratory infection (ARI), or both; most countries collect this information by age group. The case definitions used for ILI or ARI differ slightly from country to country. Many of the European countries have a centralized and government funded system of medical care, and therefore the population under surveillance can be more accurately defined than in countries like the US with a largely private-sector healthcare delivery system. For the countries where the population under surveillance is known, population-based rates can be calculated and reported. This allows for better assessment of the differences in impact between age groups and between influenza seasons.

In the US, outpatient ILI data are collected through the US Influenza Sentinel Provider Surveillance Network, a collaborative effort between CDC, state and local health departments, and healthcare providers. In this system, states are responsible for identifying an influenza surveillance coordinator, recruiting and retaining sentinel providers, maintaining data quality, and providing testing of specimens from sentinel providers. CDC is responsible for coordinating and managing the network, maintaining the reporting systems, serving as a data repository, and analyzing and disseminating the data.

The system has grown more than fivefold from approximately 500 providers enrolled in 29 states reporting 1.8 million patient visits during the 1997–1998 season to approximately 2400 providers enrolled in 50 states reporting 12 million patient visits during the 2005–2006 season. The purpose of the sentinel provider system is to monitor ILI activity in the general population as a surrogate for influenza. Therefore, states recruit sentinel providers who will, in aggregate, see a broad mix of patients that are representative of the state population particularly with regards to age and geographic distribution. Any primary care provider is eligible to participate, including practitioners in family practice, internal medicine, pediatrics, infectious disease, obstetrics and gynecology, and emergency medicine. Participation is open to private providers, emergency departments, urgent care centers, college/university student health centers, and health maintenance organizations. Sentinel providers report weekly summary data including the total number of patient visits for any reason and the number of patient visits for ILI (fever $\geq 100°$F and cough or sore throat in the absence of a known cause other than influenza) by age group (0–4 yr, 5–24 yr, 25–64 yr, >65 yr).

Sentinel providers are encouraged to submit throat or nasopharyngeal swab specimens from a subset of ILI cases for virologic testing at the participating state laboratory. Providers are asked to limit specimen collection to 2–3 swabs taken during each of the following times/types of cases: (1) ILI cases at the beginning of the season, peak of the season, toward the season's end, and during the summer; (2) unusual clinical cases or unusually severe cases, and (3) outbreak-related cases. The virus isolation data are entered into the virus surveillance system. Due to the time lag in obtaining results (approximately a week for viral culture), the information obtained from viral culture results usually will not be useful to the provider for confirming individual cases of influenza but does provide information about influenza virus circulation in the community.

Data reported by sentinel providers are used to calculate the percentage of all patient visits due to ILI. These data are analyzed weekly on the national and regional level and are reported in the weekly influenza surveillance report. Because the strength of ILI surveillance and the proportion of the population covered by the participating providers can vary widely from state to state, the national and regional percentages of patient visits for ILI are weighted relative to the population of the contributing states. The national and regional percent of visits for ILI is compared to national or regional baselines, respectively, and values above the baseline usually correlate with increased influenza activity. The baseline is obtained by (1) calculating a 3-week moving average of the laboratory surveillance data (the percent of specimens testing positive for influenza) for each week during the influenza surveillance season, (2) calculating the average percent of visits for ILI during the weeks in which <10% of specimens tested positive for influenza, and (3) adding two standard deviations to this mean. Weeks during which the percent of visits for ILI rises above the baseline can be interpreted as weeks during which there were excess visits to healthcare providers most likely attributable to influenza.

The US sentinel provider system is a very labor-intensive system and in many states it does not provide enough data to adequately represent influenza activity at the state or local level. CDC and state health departments are exploring the utility of various electronic data sources as adjuncts to sentinel provider data. Such data sources might include emergency departments or other syndromic surveillance systems or large managed care organizations.

Hospital surveillance
Hospital-based surveillance for influenza can be useful in tracking levels of severe illness related to influenza. As discussed earlier, it is helpful to collect viruses from hospitalized patients because they may differ from outpatient case isolates in the proportion of viruses from one subtype. Other hospital data that can be collected include discharge diagnosis, admission diagnosis, chief complaint, admissions defined using both clinical and/or laboratory criteria, total number of admissions regardless of diagnoses, or bed census (including information about cancellation of elective procedures).

Collection of hospital discharge diagnoses is useful in documenting the impact of influenza but lacks timeliness and is therefore more appropriate for studies. As an alternative, some surveillance systems have monitored hospital admission diagnosis or chief complaint data, which can be available sooner than discharge data. However, admission data may not be coded or available in computerized files. Additionally, admission data and discharge data are prone to coding biases and errors.

The Emerging Infections Program (EIP) and the New Vaccine Surveillance Network (NVSN) in the US are examples of population-based surveillance for laboratory-confirmed influenza-associated hospitalizations. These systems involve collaborations between CDC, state health departments, and universities. EIP began influenza surveillance during the 2003–2004 season and focused on pediatric populations until the 2005–2006 season, during which surveillance was expanded to include all age groups. This system seeks to capture information from 60 counties in 12 metropolitan areas on hospitalizations of individuals with a positive influenza test conducted as part of routine patient care [20]. The NVSN began surveillance for influenza among children aged <5 years in three counties in 2000. Respiratory swab specimens are obtained from a systematically established sample of children hospitalized with fever or acute respiratory illness and does not rely on physician ordering of influenza testing [21]. Regardless of the system, once a case is identified additional information is obtained via laboratory and medical record review and in some cases parental and provider interview.

Every other week pediatric surveillance data from each system are analyzed, preliminary hospitalization rates are calculated, and a graph of the current and previous seasons' data is presented in the weekly influenza surveillance report. Additional analyses on complete data are performed at the end of the season and provide valuable information about the type of individuals with severe outcomes associated with laboratory confirmed influenza. Data from these systems were recently used by the Advisory Committee on Immunization Practices, the advisory committee to CDC that makes recommendations on vaccine use, to expand vaccination recommendations for persons with a broader group of underlying medical conditions and to children aged <5 years.

Another example of hospitalization surveillance in the US is BioSense, a system newly developed by CDC that focuses on capturing information contained in electronic hospital records systems.

The initial focus is on obtaining chief complaint and diagnosis information from a small number of hospitals with plans to increase the number of participating hospitals and data elements to include laboratory, radiology, pharmacy, bed census, and emergency department clinical data. More information about BioSense is available at http://www.cdc.gov/biosense/.

Influenza activity level assessment
The WHO, the European Influenza Surveillance Scheme (EISS), and US Influenza Surveillance System each include reports of estimated levels of overall influenza activity. In the WHO and EISS systems, estimated levels of activity are reported for countries or regions of a country and in the US system estimated levels of activity are reported for each state. Standard definitions are used within each of these systems but the definitions vary from system to system, and within a single system the surveillance methods used to make the activity level determination may vary from country to country and state to state. Although these assessments are not strictly standardized, they do provide a level of local interpretation of influenza activity and surveillance data that may be lacking otherwise.

Participating countries can report their influenza activity level each week through WHO's internet reporting system, FluNet (http://rhone.b3e.jussieu.fr/flunet/www/).

Activity level definitions in the WHO/FluNet system are:
• *No activity*—no influenza viral isolates or clinical signs of influenza activity
• *Sporadic*—an isolated case of ILI or laboratory/culture confirmed cases in a limited area
• *Local outbreak*—ILI activity above baseline values with laboratory confirmed cases in a limited area
• *Regional activity*—outbreaks of ILI or laboratory confirmed influenza in one or more regions with a population comprising less than 50% of the country's total population
• *Widespread activity*—outbreaks of ILI or laboratory confirmed influenza in one or more regions with a population comprising 50% or more of the country's population

The EISS system activity levels are similar to those used by WHO. However, EISS incorporates a sec-ond variable to describe the intensity of influenza activity in addition to the geographic distribution of influenza viruses. The intensity of influenza activity is described as low, medium, high, or very high.

The system in the US for reporting statewide activity is the State and Territorial Epidemiologist's Report. The state or territorial epidemiologists (or their designee) from each state, New York City, Washington, DC, and Puerto Rico report the overall level of influenza activity in the state or territory each week. The activity level definitions that have been in place since the 2003–2004 season are summarized in Table 19.1.

Each week the states' reports are displayed in a color-coded map of the US. The weekly maps provide information on spread of influenza across the country at a glance. At the end of each season, the number of states reporting regional or widespread influenza activity in a given week are graphed and compared to previous seasons to estimate timing of peak influenza activity in the country. The state data are the most widely disseminated and quoted component of the national influenza system. The system has minimal resources and operational requirements since it draws on data already collected for other purposes. Modifications to activity level definitions adopted in 2003 appear to have strengthened the correlation with virologic and sentinel provider surveillance data.

Other sources of morbidity data
Other events that may reflect levels of influenza activity include school or workplace absenteeism, including healthcare worker absenteeism, sales of over-the-counter or prescription medicines used to treat influenza or the secondary complications of influenza, increases in ambulance calls, and institutional outbreaks. Each of these systems has strengths and weaknesses. In particular, outcomes such as absenteeism are highly nonspecific, and should be interpreted with caution. However, absenteeism can be useful on a local level to spur further investigation and to monitor the community burden of disease. Over-the-counter drug sales and to a lesser degree prescription drug sales are also nonspecific and the cause of increases may be difficult and time consuming to determine. Nonetheless, these outcomes can complement other surveillance methods if the data are readily available.

Table 19.1 Influenza activity level definitions in the State and Territorial Epidemiologist's Report, United States.

Activity level	ILI activity* or outbreaks		Laboratory data
No activity	Low	AND	No laboratory confirmed cases[†]
Sporadic	Not increased	AND	Isolated laboratory-confirmed cases
			OR
	Not increased	AND	Laboratory-confirmed outbreak in one institution[‡]
Local	Increased ILI in 1 region*[§]; ILI activity in other regions is not increased	AND	Recent (within the past 3 weeks) laboratory evidence of influenza in region with increased ILI
			OR
	2 or more institutional outbreaks (ILI or laboratory confirmed) in 1 region; ILI activity in other regions is not increased	AND	Recent (within the past 3 weeks) laboratory evidence of influenza in region with the outbreaks; virus activity is no greater than sporadic in other regions
Regional (does not apply to states with ≤4 regions)	Increased ILI in ≥2 but less than half of the regions	AND	Recent (within the past 3 weeks) laboratory-confirmed influenza in the affected regions
			OR
	Institutional outbreaks (ILI or laboratory confirmed) in ≥2 and less than half of the regions	AND	Recent (within the past 3 weeks) laboratory-confirmed influenza in the affected regions
Widespread	Increased ILI and/or institutional outbreaks (ILI or laboratory confirmed) in at least half of the regions	AND	Recent (within the past 3 weeks) laboratory-confirmed influenza in the state.

* ILI activity can be assessed using a variety of data sources including sentinel providers, school or workplace absenteeism, and other syndromic surveillance systems that monitor influenza-like illness.

[†] Laboratory-confirmed case: case confirmed by rapid diagnostic test, antigen detection, culture, or PCR.

[‡] Institution includes nursing home, hospital, prison, school, etc.

[§] Region: population under surveillance in a defined geographical subdivision of a state.

Surveillance for influenza and ILI in institutions helps the facility identify influenza outbreaks early and limit spread of influenza to patients/residents and staff. Institutional outbreak surveillance is another marker of influenza activity in the community.

Mortality surveillance

Mortality surveillance provides a marker for severity of disease. This information can help policy makers, the healthcare community, and the general public understand the serious consequences of influenza and both justify implementation of preventive measures such as vaccination and determine high-risk groups likely to benefit most from these interventions. However, most influenza-related deaths are not due directly to the primary viral infection but are from complications such as secondary bacterial pneumonia or worsening of chronic health conditions such as congestive heart failure or pulmonary disease. As a result, most persons for whom influenza initiated the chain of events leading to death will not be tested for influenza at the time of death or even at the time of hospitalization and will no longer be shedding virus by the time they are brought to medical attention.

Most measures of influenza-related mortality are estimates based on calculating the number of deaths occurring above, or in excess of, the number expected for that time of year if influenza viruses were not circulating. Data are typically collected from death certificates and the outcomes most frequently used are pneumonia and influenza deaths, respiratory and circulatory deaths, or all cause deaths [2]. Counting only pneumonia and influenza deaths produces a very conservative estimate of influenza-associated mortality that likely underestimates the true impact of influenza, while using increases in deaths due to all causes attributes any seasonal increase in the number of deaths to influenza and likely overestimates the impact of influenza. Using respiratory and circulatory deaths as proposed by Thompson *et al.* includes pneumonia and influenza deaths and deaths from other causes such as congestive heart failure known to increase during influenza season and produces estimates of the impact of influenza between those obtained using other outcomes [2]. Estimates can be calculated using a variety of mathematical models, one of the more straightforward being rate difference models [22]. In rate difference models, the numbers of deaths during periods of influenza virus circulation are compared to those seen during periods of low influenza virus circulation and the difference is said to be the influenza-associated excess mortality. Some investigators use the summer months as the comparison period and others use the weeks in the fall and spring where little or no influenza virus is detected but other respiratory viruses are expected to be circulating. This period is referred to as the "peri-season" period [23]. As expected, models using a summer baseline produce higher rates of influenza-associated mortality than those using the peri-season as a baseline for comparison.

In the US, three systems are used to monitor influenza-related mortality. The 122 Cities Mortality Reporting System provides a rapid assessment of influenza mortality. Each week throughout the year the vital statistics offices of 122 US cities report the total number of death certificates filed for that week and the number of deaths for which pneumonia or influenza was listed as an underlying or contributing cause of death on the certificate. The number of deaths reported through this system represents approximately 25% of all deaths in the US. A robust regression procedure is used to calculate a seasonal baseline. If the proportion of pneumonia and influenza deaths for a given week exceeds the baseline value for that week by a statistically significant amount, then influenza-related deaths are said to be above the epidemic threshold.

The US mortality data are also available from the National Vital Statistics System (NVSS) of the National Center for Health Statistics (NCHS) at CDC. Data from the NVSS differs from that received through the 122 Cities Mortality Reporting System in several important ways. First, the NVSS data set contains information for >99% of all deaths occurring in the US. There is a separate record in the NVSS data set for each death. In contrast, a record in the 122 Cities System contains a weekly summary of the number deaths from a city. Basic demographic data, the date of death, and the underlying and contributing causes of death are included in the NVSS data allowing for a more detailed analysis and more accurate assessment of the timing of P&I deaths. The cause of death is classified using International Classification of Diseases (ICD) coding. The largest drawback of these data is the lack of timeliness; the data for a given year are not available until approximately 2 years later.

During the 2003–2004 influenza season, following the reports of several deaths in children associated with influenza infection, CDC requested voluntary reporting of influenza associated deaths in children <18 years of age from state health departments. In 2004, laboratory confirmed, influenza-associated deaths in children was added to the US list of nationally notifiable diseases. This is the only mortality reporting system in the US that uses a laboratory confirmed outcome and can directly produce population-based rates. The data are collected via a Web-based case report form that feeds into the National Notifiable Disease Surveillance System. Basic demographic information is collected along with information on preexisting health conditions and complications, including secondary bacterial infections, vaccination status, and laboratory testing methods. The informally collected information from the 2003–2004 season showed that 67% of the children that died did not have medical conditions that placed them in one of the existing high-risk groups for whom influenza vaccination is recommended, but 20% had other chronic health conditions [24]. The most common of these were neuromuscular problems and developmental delays. This information led to the expansion of influenza vaccine recommendations by adding as a high-risk group adults and children who have any condition (e.g., cognitive dysfunction, spinal cord injuries, seizure disorders, or other neuromuscular disorders) that can compromise respiratory function or the handling of respiratory secretions or that can increase the risk for aspiration.

Conclusion

Influenza surveillance is a collection of surveillance components rather than a single system. Laboratory surveillance should form the foundation for any influenza surveillance system but selection of other components should be driven by the goals and objectives set for the system and the anticipated uses of the data. The challenges of influenza surveillance are numerous: the viruses are constantly changing and the vaccine requires annual updates, both the number of people affected and the severity of disease can vary substantially, the symptoms of influenza are nonspecific and testing is necessary to confirm diagnoses, electronic data sources for surveillance are often not available, and the possibility of the emergence of a novel influenza subtype and pandemic disease requires constant vigilance. However, data collected through surveillance can inform outbreak response and patient treatment decisions and rapidly lead to changes in vaccination and antiviral drug use policy. Demands for timely influenza surveillance data will likely increase as influenza vaccination programs expand and will certainly increase in the event of a pandemic. Systems should be designed with enough flexibility to meet changing needs and to be robust enough to be sustainable in both interpandemic and pandemic periods.

Acknowledgments

We acknowledge with gratitude Dr Andrea Forde, New Zealand Ministry of Health, for her timely, rigorous, and insightful comments.

References

1 Monto AS, Kioumehr F. The Tecumseh Study of Respiratory Illness. IX: Occurrence of influenza in the community, 1966–1971. *Am J Epidemiol* 1975;**102**(6):553–63.

2 Thompson WW, Shay DK, Weintraub E, *et al.* Mortality associated with influenza and respiratory syncytial virus in the United States [see comment]. *JAMA* 2003;**289**(2):179–86.

3 Barker WH. Excess pneumonia and influenza associated hospitalization during influenza epidemics in the United States, 1970–78. *Am J Public Health* 1986;**76**(7):761–5.

4 Barker WH, Mullooly JP. Impact of epidemic type A influenza in a defined adult population. *Am J Epidemiol* 1980;**112**(6):798–811.

5 Glezen WP. Serious morbidity and mortality associated with influenza epidemics. *Epidemiol Rev* 1982;**4**:25–44.

6 Glezen WP, Couch RB. Interpandemic influenza in the Houston area, 1974–76. *N Engl J Med* 1978;**298**(11):587–92.

7 Glezen WP, Greenberg SB, Atmar RL, Piedra PA, Couch RB. Impact of respiratory virus infections on persons with chronic underlying conditions. *JAMA* 2000;**283**(4):499–505.

8 WHO. *WHO Recommended Surveillance Standards*, 2nd edn. Available from: http://www.who.int/csr/ resources/ publications/surveillance/WHO_CDS_CSR_ISR_99_2_EN/ en/. Accessed December 1, 2006.

9 Koopmans M, Wilbrink B, Conyn M, *et al.* Transmission of H7N7 avian influenza A virus to human beings during a large outbreak in commercial poultry farms in the Netherlands [see comment]. *Lancet* 2004;**363**(9409):587–93.

10 Centers for Disease Control and Prevention. Avian influenza infection in humans. Available from: http://www.cdc.gov/flu/avian/gen-info/avian-flu-humans. htm. Accessed December 1, 2006.

11 Tweed SA, Skowronski DM, David ST, *et al.* Human illness from avian influenza H7N3, British Columbia. *Emerg Infect Dis* 2004;**10**(12):2196–9.

12 Centers for Disease Control and Prevention. Isolation of avian influenza A(H5N1) viruses from humans—Hong Kong, May–December 1997. *MMWR Morb Mortal Wkly Rep* 1997;**46**(50):1204–7.

13 Uyeki TM, Chong YH, Katz JM, *et al.* Lack of evidence for human-to-human transmission of avian influenza A (H9N2) viruses in Hong Kong, China 1999. *Emerg Infect Dis* 2002;**8**(2):154–9.

14 Interim CDC-NIH Recommendation for Raising the Biosafety Level for Laboratory Work Involving Noncontemporary Human Influenza Viruses Excerpted from the draft Biosafety in Microbiological and Biomedical Laboratories, 5th edn. Available from: http://0-www.cdc. gov.mill1.sjlibrary.org/flu/h2n2bsl3.htm. Accessed December 1, 2006.

15 Fedorko DP, Nelson NA, McAuliffe JM, Subbarao K. Performance of rapid tests for detection of avian influenza

A virus types H5N1 and H9N2. *J Clin Microbiol* 2006;**44**(4):1596–7.

16 Oner AF, Bay A, Arslan S, Akdeniz H, Sahin HA, *et al.* Avian Influenza A (H5N1) Infection in Eastern Turkey in 2006. *N Engl J Med* 2006; **355**:2179–85.

17 Bright RA, Medina MJ, Xu X, *et al.* Incidence of adamantane resistance among influenza A (H3N2) viruses isolated worldwide from 1994 to 2005: a cause for concern [see comment]. *Lancet* 2005;**366**(9492):1175–81.

18 Bright RA, Shay DK, Shu B, Cox NJ, Klimov AI. Adamantane resistance among influenza A viruses isolated early during the 2005–2006 influenza season in the United States [see comment]. *JAMA* 2006;**295**(8):891–4.

19 Centers for Disease Control and Prevention. High levels of adamantane resistance among influenza A (H3N2) viruses and interim guidelines for use of antiviral agents—United States, 2005–06 influenza season. *MMWR Morb Mortal Wkly Rep* 2006;**55**(2):44–6.

20 Schrag SJ, Shay DK, Gershman K, *et al.* Multistate surveillance for laboratory-confirmed, influenza-associated hospitalizations in children: 2003–2004. *Pediatr Infect Dis J* 2006;**25**(5):395–400.

21 Poehling KA, Edwards KM, Weinberg GA, *et al.* The underrecognized burden of influenza in young children [see comment]. *N Engl J Med* 2006;**355**(1):31–40.

22 Thompson WW, Comanor, Lorraine, Shay, David K. Epidemiology of seasonal influenza: use of surveillance data and statistical models to estimate the burden of disease. *J Infect Dis* 2006;**194**(suppl 2):S82–91.

23 Izurieta HS, Thompson WW, Kramarz P, *et al.* Influenza and the rates of hospitalization for respiratory disease among infants and young children [see comment]. *N Engl J Med* 2000;**342**(4):232–9.

24 Bhat N, Wright JG, Broder KR, *et al.* Influenza-associated deaths among children in the United States, 2003–2004 [see comment]. *N Engl J Med* 2005;**353**(24):2559–67.

20 Communicable disease surveillance in complex emergencies

Marta Valenciano & Alain Moren

Introduction

The goal of this chapter is to present practical aspects of communicable diseases (CD) surveillance in complex emergency (CE) situations. We will define complex emergencies and discuss the underlying constraints that influence the design of a surveillance system useful in CE situations. Finally, we describe the systems developed for three different CE situations: refugees in a hosting country integrated in the local population (Albania, 1999), population in the aftermath of a war (Iraq, 2003), and a population displaced in its own country (Darfur, 2004). This chapter focuses on the surveillance systems for epidemic-prone diseases. Other important public health problems that are part of CE public health surveillance systems such as malnutrition, injuries and violence, and post-traumatic disorders are not addressed. The chapter does not include mortality surveys that are important tools needed to complement CD surveillance systems in CE [1].

Complex emergencies

Definition

Complex emergencies are defined as "situations of war or civil strife affecting large civilian populations with food shortages and population displacement, resulting in excess mortality and morbidity" [2]. During these situations, the capacity to sustain livelihood and life may be threatened by political factors and, in particular, by high levels of violence [3].

Rationale for communicable disease surveillance in CE

Complex emergencies result in a dramatic increase in morbidity and mortality in the affected population. It is estimated that more than 70% of the victims are civilians [3]. CDs are major contributors to the high mortality and morbidity [4,5]. In the first phases of the emergency, infectious diseases like diarrhea (including cholera and shigellosis), measles, acute respiratory infections, and malaria occur in the areas where the disease is endemic. [6]. Other diseases such as meningitis, tuberculosis, and hepatitis E [7] can also cause outbreaks. Most complex emergency situations occur in countries or regions with limited capacity to detect and to respond effectively to CD outbreaks. Therefore, one of the public health priorities during initial interventions is to set up or to strengthen the existing surveillance system to promptly detect and respond to outbreaks of epidemic-prone diseases [4,8].

Characteristics of CE influencing the surveillance system

Ideally, the CD surveillance system in CE should have the same characteristics as a surveillance system in a stable situation. However, when developing the system during a crisis, some context-specific features, including the target population, presence of multiple partners in the field, the political context, and poor infrastructure should be taken into account.

Population under surveillance

Populations affected by complex emergencies have often escaped from violence, undertaken a long exodus, and lost members of their families. People are exhausted, in poor nutritional states, and highly stressed. They are more susceptible to epidemic-prone diseases.

In many crises, part of the population is difficult to access due to poor infrastructure or lack of security in the area. Obtaining information on the diseases affecting inaccessible groups is a challenge. Information on the situation of the isolated groups can sometimes be obtained through radio contact, contact with nongovernmental organizations (NGOs) working in the area, and exploratory missions. Under crisis situations, the population is not stable. There are new arrivals and departures every day. It is difficult to estimate the size of the population and difficult to determine valid denominators for the calculation of surveillance indicators. Methods for obtaining timely and precise estimates of population size are one of the current CE research areas [9].

Partners

During a crisis, there are often many organizations in the field, each with different priorities, resources, and background: local authorities, national and international NGOs from various disciplines and ideologies, United Nations (UN) agencies, military groups (e.g., Coalition Forces in Iraq, NATO in Albania), representatives of donor agencies, diplomatic missions, journalists, etc. Consequently, actions are difficult to coordinate and the communication among the various organizations is generally poor. In most CEs it is impossible to define precisely which organizations and health staff can contribute to surveillance as there is no central listing of staff, competencies, planned activities, resources, locations, or expected duration of work.

Political context

The political context, the attitude of the local government, the relations between international organizations and national structures often represent a barrier to access the affected population. The political context can also hinder dissemination of surveillance results and implementation of activities. Issues of who should have the mandate to coordinate activities may create tensions and hamper the implementation of interventions.

Infrastructures, resources

Most complex emergencies take place in poor countries, with poor infrastructures and lack of resources. The crisis further deteriorates the situation. The design of the surveillance system, especially the terms of data flow, should take into account these limitations in order to develop an adaptable and flexible system. Resources available locally or brought by international organizations should be assessed to identify which could be available to support the surveillance system (e.g., fax, phone, radio, cars, satellite Internet connections).

Objective of CD surveillance in CE

The general objective is to reduce mortality and morbidity related to CDs. All information collected through the surveillance system should serve that purpose. Any information collected that is not action-oriented is useless and detrimental to other priority tasks conducted by those who collect surveillance data.

In the first phase of the emergency, the primary objective is to detect cases of epidemic-prone diseases, implement rapid responses, and minimize mortality. Diseases with potential for outbreaks should be targeted.

Secondary objectives include providing health indicators for monitoring and evaluating the impact of humanitarian action and evaluating the activity of health structures in order to optimize resource allocation.

Main attributes of CD surveillance in CE

Sensitivity

In order to detect cases of diseases with outbreak potential as soon as possible, the system should be sensitive. Any suspicion of outbreak should be reported to a level where action can be taken. Systems based on rumors of epidemic cases have frequently been set up for cholera, shigellosis, meningitis, jaundice, hemorrhagic fevers, etc. A rapid verification of rumors is necessary. Case definitions must be sensitive (suspect cases reported,

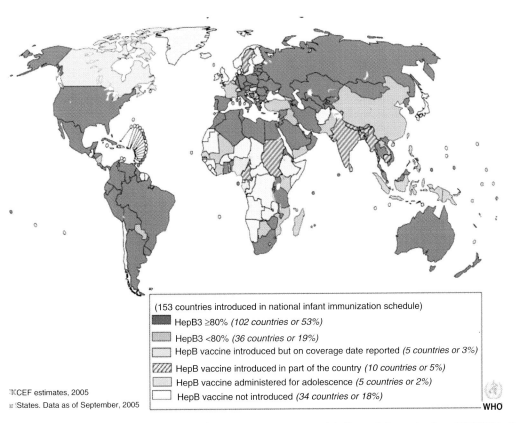

(153 countries introduced in national infant immunization schedule)
HepB3 ≥80% *(102 countries or 53%)*
HepB3 <80% *(36 countries or 19%)*
HepB vaccine introduced but on coverage date reported *(5 countries or 3%)*
HepB vaccine introduced in part of the country *(10 countries or 5%)*
HepB vaccine administered for adolescence *(5 countries or 2%)*
HepB vaccine not introduced *(34 countries or 18%)*

WHO

Plate 18(1).1 HBV vaccination as part of universal immunization programs globally per information from UNICEF in 2005.

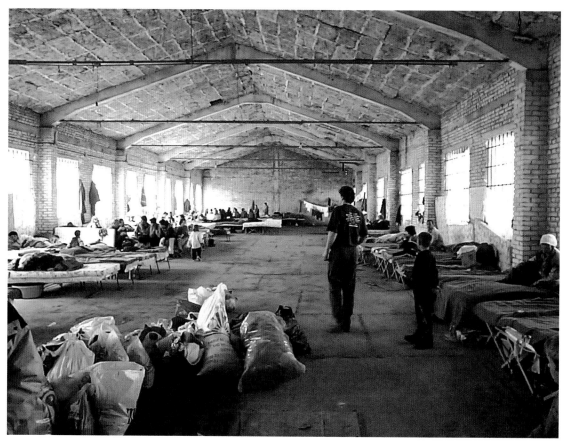

Plate 20(1).1 Collective center for Kosovar Refugees, Tirana (Albania), 1999. (Courtesy of Marta Valenciano.)

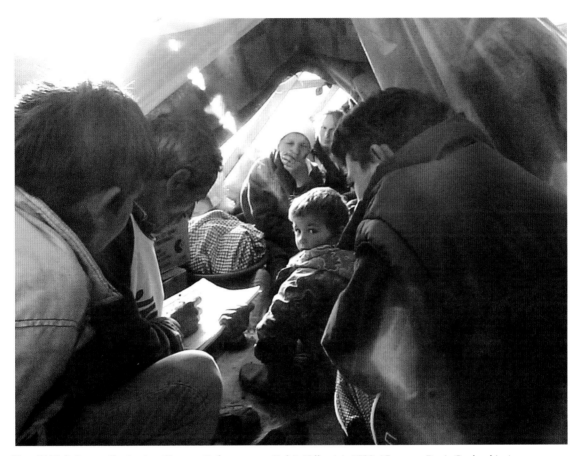

Plate 20(1).2 Data collection in a Kosovar Refugee camp, Kukës (Albania), 1999. (Courtesy Denis Coulombier.)

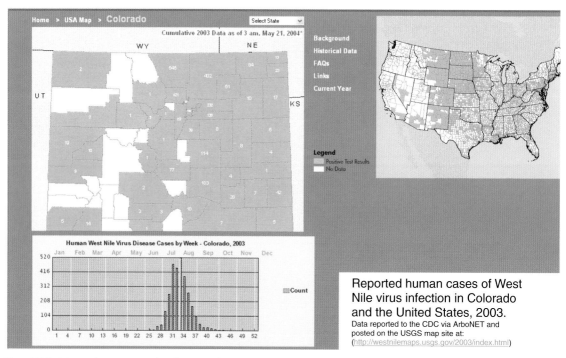

Plate 31(1).1 Map showing spatial and temporal pattern of arbovirus activity (West Nile virus) in humans in Colorado, USA, 2003, from the ArboNET surveillance system. (Courtesy of US Geological Survey.)

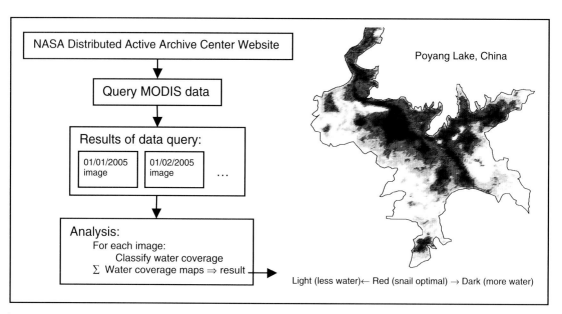

Plate 31(1).2 Poyang Lake schistosomiasis warning system. A disease warning system based on identification of probable snail habitats from water coverage maps.

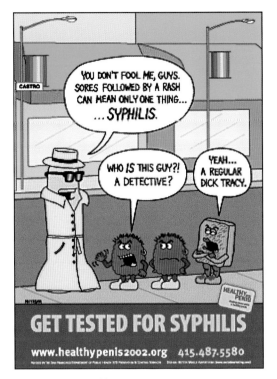

Plate 32(2).1 One of the comic strips used in the Healthy Penis campaign. Cartoon images and humor were used to impart key messages regarding syphilis symptoms and transmission. Web site address and telephone number where more information could be obtained were also displayed.

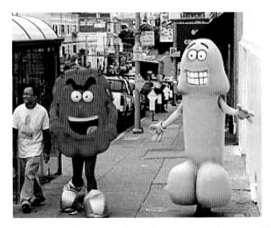

Plate 32(2).2 Healthy Penis costumes were worn by outreach workers at places frequented by the target population.

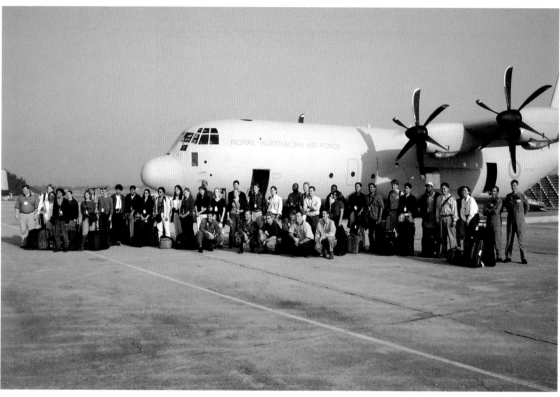

Plate 36.1 A team of Epidemic Intelligence Service (EIS) officers preparing to depart for New York City 3 days after the September 11, 2001, terrorists' attack. EIS officers assisted local public health officials with implementation of an emergency disease surveillance system to monitor for bioterrorist-related events. At the time only military aircrafts were allowed in US airspace. (*Source*: DH Hamilton, Centers for Disease Control and Prevention.)

syndromes reported) and all reporting units should know how to immediately report.

Simplicity

In complex emergencies, local healthcare structures are overwhelmed by patients. Often there is lack of public health staff and the infrastructures are damaged. Therefore, the surveillance system should be simple so that it does not add too much to the workload of health staff. New and complicated forms, different reporting mechanisms, and sophisticated analysis should be avoided. Feedback should be as simple as possible while meeting the surveillance objective. A limited amount of information can be collected; often the total number of cases by day or week and by two age groups are reported.

Acceptability

All partners—national and international staff, affected population, and local authorities—should accept the system. To achieve acceptability, the system should be simple and useful to all partners.

Timeliness

The ultimate objective of CD surveillance is outbreak control, and, therefore, the delay between onset of symptoms and action has to be as short as possible. Surveillance data should trigger action at the level of the response (and should be as decentralized as possible). There should be the capacity to interpret data and take action accordingly at the local level.

Flexibility

In unstable situations, the system should be flexible and able to adapt to changes in the population (new arrivals, new settlements, new health priorities, new partners).

Steps in the implementation of CD surveillance during CE

Preparation phase

Documentation
To organize a surveillance system focusing on major epidemic-prone diseases and adapted to CE,

it is essential to gather all preexisting information concerning the affected population, the hosting country/region, and the availability of resources. Information should be collected from country health status reports (Ministry of Health), international organizations reports (United Nations Children's Fund (UNICEF), World Health Organization (WHO), United Nations High Commissioner for Refugees (UNHCR)), and from local and international NGOs working in the area (rapid assessments, surveys).

Key issues to be considered include:

a Health status of the affected population before the crisis:
• Diseases affecting the population in the country of origin
• Most recent outbreaks
• Disease specific vaccination coverage in this specific population
• Age structure

b Health status in the host country/region: The same information as above should be gathered with regards to the population of the host country. In addition, the environment in which the affected population is settled should be taken into account to identify potential sources of outbreaks: presence of vectors (population moving from noninfected to malaria-infected areas), access to and type of water, sanitation (possibility to dig latrines).

c History from the beginning of the crisis:
• Cause of displacement (war, attack during displacement, famine, natural disaster)
• If the population is displaced, how long was the displacement?
• How did the affected population arrive in the area?

d Surveillance system in hosting country/region: Ideally, the surveillance system implemented for the affected population should be integrated into the host country surveillance system. The following information on the existing surveillance system has to be taken into account:
• Is the existing system adaptable to the emergency?
• Is it sensitive and timely enough?
• Is it focused on the priority epidemic-prone diseases?
• Which parts of the system can be used?
• Which components need to be adapted or reinforced?

e Infrastructure, resources: Any existing surveillance system has to be adapted to the situation. For its design, the logistical, financial, and human resources should be taken into account. Relevant questions include:
• How accessible is the affected population?
• Is there a communication network (telephone lines, fax, Internet connections, satellite connections, radio network)?
• Which resources exist to carry out the surveillance system activities?
• What are the human resources and competencies at all surveillance levels?
• What is the diagnosis capacity at healthcare delivery level?
• What is the quality of the laboratory support (if any)?
• What are the financial resources available?

f Identification of stakeholders, consensus building: As mentioned before, one of the challenges in complex emergencies is to coordinate actions among all organizations and groups involved in the crisis. The surveillance system is based on a human network of motivated people and institutions working together. Therefore, a preliminary step in the implementation phase is to identify all stakeholders and build consensus among all of them. They should be convinced that surveillance is one of the priorities for the health sector, and need to have a sense of ownership. It is essential to involve all stakeholders in the design of the system so that it can answer to their needs.

Usually stakeholders include:
• National authorities (Ministry of Health)
• Representative of all surveillance levels (central, intermediate, peripheral)
• Healthcare providers
• National Public Health Laboratory
• International organizations, including WHO, Office for the Coordination of Humanitarian Affairs (OCHA), UNHCR, UNICEF
• National and international medical NGOs

Protocol development

A working group may be organized to develop a surveillance protocol that has to include and rapidly specify the following items:

1 Events to be included   To keep the system as simple as possible, the list of health events to be reported should be limited (<10 health events). Only diseases with high epidemic potential should be reported. In addition, any suspicion of outbreak has to be immediately reported.

The agreement among all partners is sometimes difficult to achieve due to different priorities. A short prioritization exercise to define events to be reported may be needed. Criteria to incorporate an event in the list of priority diseases include, among others, its potential for outbreak in the specific complex emergency context (population susceptibility, environment), the case fatality, the need for immediate control measures.

Deaths from CD represent a key indicator in CE. Sources of information on death and causes of death include among others: political and religious leaders, graveyards' watch, hospital and dispensary death registers, and community health workers [8].

2 Case definitions   For each category of the health events included, a standard case definition should be agreed upon. The case definition should be:
• Sensitive
• Simple
• Adapted to the local situation (local expertise, diagnosis capacity at peripheral level, local knowledge, cultural perception of the disease)

Syndromic case definitions are used to target some events (e.g., jaundice for hepatitis or yellow fever, rash with fever for measles). When possible, WHO has developed standard case definitions that should be adapted to the local context [2]. If deaths and causes of death are reported, simple algorithms for verbal autopsy can be used by community health workers to estimate, with the help of families, the most likely cause of death [10]. Because of lack of diagnosis capacity at peripheral level, suspect cases are frequently reported. In addition, case definitions for confirmed cases have to be developed. It is important to identify mechanisms for laboratory confirmation.
• Is there a national public health laboratory?
• Is the laboratory capacity at peripheral/intermediate/central level?
• What are the procedures for packaging and shipment of specimens?
• Are rapid diagnostic tests available?

3 Surveillance indicators Indicators for action should be defined. For each health event under surveillance, the defined indicators allow the detection of potential outbreaks: increase in the number of cases, increase in mortality, detection of one case of a specific disease (e.g., hemorrhagic fever), increase of case fatality (e.g., increase in fatality in cases of diarrhea).

Incidence rate is the preferred indicator. It allows comparison between populations and time periods. In CE, in the absence of denominators to compute incidence rates, other indicators may be used. All of them have limitations and, consequently, decisions should be based on the combination of all of them.

Indicators used in complex emergencies are:
• Number of cases reported by week and by place (camp, district)
• Number of reporting units by week; especially at the beginning of the implementation of the new surveillance system, the number of reporting units changes from one week to the other; a change in the number of cases reported could reflect the change in the number of reporting units
• Incidence rates
• Proportional morbidity (number of cases reported of health event X/total number of consultations)

Figures 20.1a–20.1d show various surveillance indicators used in Albania during the Kosovar refugee crisis, where denominators were not available. In Figure 20.1a, we see a sharp increase of reported cases of diarrhea that might indicate an outbreak. However, the other indicators (stable proportional morbidity, increase in total number of consultations, and increase in number of units participating in the system) suggest that the increase in the number of cases of diarrhea may be explained by an increase in the population covered by the surveillance system.

To keep the system simple, cases are not reported individually but aggregated. Reporting should be done by age group and sex only if this breakdown of the data is useful for outbreak detection (e.g., increase of watery diarrhea in adults triggering a suspicion of cholera). Usually, data are reported in two age groups (<5 yr and ≥ 5 yr). If an outbreak investigation is launched, additional data are then collected (precise onset, location, age, etc).

4 Data source for each indicator For each indicator, the data source should be defined taking into account the health services delivery.

Data sources for reporting health events might include:
• National, district health centers
• Hospitals
• Medical NGOs
• Community leaders
• Laboratories

For other indicators that complement the event-based surveillance, data sources include:
• Agency in charge of population register
• Data for mortality: survey, home visitors, graveyard surveillance
• Water and sanitation agencies

In order to measure the magnitude of outbreaks, to observe trends of CD, and to compare CD occurrence in different populations over different periods of time, a denominator is needed. Special efforts and resources should be devoted to permanently update the denominator. Updating can be done by a census performed and regularly completed by community health workers (1 health worker per 1000 persons) or through repeated surveys using specific mapping and counting methods to estimate population size [9].

In CEs where international organizations intervene there is usually an information center where information coming from all organizations is centralized. The information centers have data on population figures, lists of NGOs, and geographical information systems. It is important to identify common variables included in the information center databases and in the surveillance system (e.g., identification of health centers) so that the information can be linked.

5 Surveillance form A simple one-page surveillance paper form could be used to collect and transmit surveillance data. The surveillance form includes time and place information and has to be translated into the local language. On the back of the form, case definitions and a number of telephone/fax or a way to contact the person or agency in charge of surveillance may be included. Examples of surveillance forms can be found in the WHO Communicable Disease Control in Emergencies field manual [2] or in early-warning surveillance

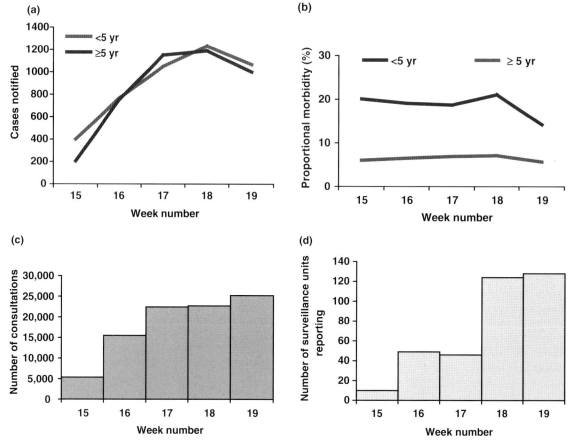

Fig 20.1 Indicators used in the Kosovar refugees early-warning system, Albania, 1999. (a) Number of cases of diarrhea among Kosovar refugees by week and age group, Albania, Weeks 15–19, 1999. (b) Proportional morbidity of diarrhea among Kosovar refugees by week and age group, Albania, Weeks 15–19, 1999. (c) Number of consultations among Kosovar refugees by week, Albania, Weeks 15–19, 1999. (d) Number of surveillance units participating in the Kosovar refugees surveillance system by week, Albania, Weeks 15–19, 1999.

guidelines available at WHO Web page (see appendixes).

As in any surveillance system, the revision and validation of forms is an essential step to improve data quality.

6 Data flow Data are transmitted from peripheral level to central level and feedback should come back to the peripheral level. The flow of data has to be realistic and defined taking into account the logistical constraints. All potential methods for data transmission should be considered: car, radio, lorry, fax, telephone, e-mail.

If possible, data should be collated and reported at least once a week. Alerts on rumors or confirmed serious events should be transmitted daily by any means (telephone, SMS, radio, e-mails). If mobile or landline telephones are available, a telephone staffed 24/7 must be available for urgent communications.

7 Analysis The analysis should be timely and simple. An electronic tool can be developed or adapted for data entry, automatic data analysis and, if possible, data transmission and automatic report. Free domain software can be used in these situations such as EpiData [11], Epi-Info [12], or R: [13]. For instance, in Banda Aceh (Indonesia), the data management, analysis, and reports of the surveillance/early-warning and response system developed after the December 2004 tsunami were performed with an application combining EpiInfo 6, EpiData 3.2, and Epi2000 with a link to mapping tools (HealthMapper 4.1 and ArcView 3.2a) [14].

The system should be stable, robust, and easy to maintain. A data manager is key to design and implement the system and to train others. Computerization of the surveillance system should be fully functional from the beginning of any crisis.

Analysis at the peripheral level is also recommended. Simple graphs (number of cases per day or week of selected CD) can be updated on a regular basis by community health workers or health staff at health posts and dispensaries.

8 Feedback Feedback is essential. Automatic reports could be generated if an electronic reporting tool is in place, including graphs, maps, and summary tables. Feedback should arrive to all partners and people participating in the surveillance system regularly. Alert bulletins can be distributed when needed and an epidemiological bulletin published every week. Periodic meetings where all partners are involved (e.g., weekly health sector meeting) are a good opportunity to present the results, define actions, and to motivate agencies to report (e.g., list of agencies reporting and not reporting can be presented as regularly done in Banda Aceh for the feedback of the surveillance results after the tsunami [14]).

9 Actions The level at which action should take place and responsibilities at each level should be defined and agreed upon. Rapid response teams have to be organized and kits for outbreak investigation and control prepositioned (e.g., rapid diagnostic tests, Cary-Blair, oral rehydration salts).

Piloting and implementation of surveillance systems

Once the protocol is agreed upon it should be presented at all surveillance levels. Field visits are necessary to explain the objectives and the procedures and to get comments from people working in the first line of the surveillance system. A pilot trial of the system is necessary to validate the procedures and to check the feasibility of the planned activities. It can be done in a selected area to determine whether case definitions are well understood, if the data flow is adapted to the situation, and if the data collection form needs to be adapted. Short training for data collectors and people working in the surveillance systems must be organized and repeated. Standard procedures and documentation should be made available at all levels (e.g., surveillance forms, case definitions, data flow, contacts of surveillance focal points, data management manual). The first weeks of the implementation are essential to motivate all partners at community, intermediate, and central level. Field visits should be scheduled to sensitize, train, and strengthen the surveillance network.

Monitoring, evaluation, and system modification

By definition, a CE situation is unstable, with population movements and arrival of new organizations in the field, and the surveillance system should include monitoring indicators to adapt the system, if needed. Some of the program indicators to be monitored are the proportion of units reporting (participation rate), timeliness, and completeness of forms. Population figures should be updated each time there are new estimates. This should represent a dedicated and sustained activity. Because of the rapid turnover of international staff, it is important to ensure that new staff are trained and understand their surveillance tasks.

After the acute phase the system can be adapted to a more stable situation. The surveillance objectives may be revised and other health events affecting the population included (e.g., tuberculosis, sexually transmitted infections). As the situation stabilizes, additional training of local epidemiologists could be organized. If the crisis is prolonged, it is recommended that an evaluation of the surveillance system be undertaken to assess its usefulness [15].

Some examples

Albania: surveillance system for refugees in an open situation

In 1999, following the North Atlantic Treaty Organization (NATO) bombing in Kosovo, Kosovar refugees fled to Albania (Plate 20.1). Albania was faced with an economic and social crisis and its public health surveillance system could not adapt to the crisis. In the first weeks, medical organizations working with refugees started collecting data in a non-standardized way. Data were not transmitted to National Institute of Public Health (IPH) in Tirana. Therefore, it was not possible to estimate the health status of the population or to define public health program priorities. Consequently, the IPH, with the support of the WHO and in collaboration with the Institut de Veille Sanitaire (French Public Health Institute), developed an emergency surveillance system for communicable diseases to detect and control potential outbreaks among the refugee population [16].

One of the challenges in Albania was that it was an open situation: refugees were not concentrated in an area but scattered all over the country and more than half of them were hosted by Albanian families and integrated into the local population. Therefore, the sources of surveillance information included medical agencies working in camps and Albanian health facilities (Plate 20.2). All health units had to report on a weekly basis the number of cases and deaths due to the nine health events included in the system to the district epidemiologists. The surveillance forms were transmitted from the districts to the IPH in Tirana by fax, through NGOs' cars, or any other available means. During field visits in the first days of data collection, the epidemiologists identified cases of measles in Kukes city. A measles vaccination campaign took place among Kosovar and Albanian children in the two affected districts.

During the crisis, Albanians public health staff and international organizations worked together to implement surveillance activities. This was essential to strengthen the Albania surveillance system. The crisis was short and refugees came back to Kosovo 2 months later. The surveillance system for the crisis was adapted to the Albanian context in order to complement the national surveillance system and strengthen the detection of outbreaks. As a consequence of the collaboration during the crisis, a partnership program was developed between the Institut de Veille Sanitaire (France) and the IPH, which, among other activities, included the training of Albanian epidemiologists in Europe.

This experience illustrates how crisis represent an opportunity to strengthen national capacities.

Basrah, Iraq: surveillance system for war-affected local population

The 2003 war in Iraq resulted in a disruption of health services, interruption of health programs, and looting of public health facilities. In April 2003, WHO, in collaboration with the Basrah Public Health Directorate, developed a communicable diseases surveillance system in Basrah Governorate [17]. The system was based on the National surveillance system that existed before the crisis: healthcare facilities had to report to the Public Health District and from the Public Health District data had to be transmitted to the Governorate. Because of the destruction of the Public Health Laboratory, laboratory diagnosis was limited in Basrah and the surveillance system was syndrome-based. Suspected cases of cholera were detected and samples were sent to Kuwait for confirmation.

A rumor verification system was set up to complement the weekly reporting of cases. For the first time in such an emergency, most of the international organizations present in the field had access to the Internet through satellite connections. Therefore, the international organizations were asked to report immediately all information on potential outbreaks, or rumors of outbreaks to the WHO office in Basrah. The information was disseminated through a distribution list sent to all partners, including UN agencies, NGOs, coalition forces, and donor agencies.

Before starting the data collection at Governorate level and despite the critical security situation, a 2-day surveillance workshop was organized in Basrah to which all district epidemiologists and international organizations were invited. The aim was to agree on the surveillance protocol, case definitions, and data flow. This workshop was essential to involve all partners in the surveillance system.

The main barrier in Iraq to implementation of an effective surveillance system was the lack of security. Epidemiologists could not move around the Governorate to follow up rumors, implement control measures, or carry out supervision visits. Ensuring security should be a priority in such contexts.

With all medical records and surveillance registries destroyed during the war and no access to most of the areas outside Basrah city, the role of local staff with a long working experience in the Governorate was essential to reactivate the surveillance system after the war.

Darfur 2003: surveillance system for an internal displaced population

After years of tribal conflicts in the Greater Darfur region (Sudan) between armed militia and local population, the situation deteriorated in February 2003. The Darfur population fled towns and villages, seeking refuge across the border in Chad and in settlements for internally displaced persons (IDP) within the three states of the Darfur region. The result was a displacement of an estimated 1.3 million people, with 2.2 million people being "war affected."

The sanitary and health conditions of the affected population were bad with poor accessibility to clean water, sanitation, and precarious food situation. In this context, it was essential to establish a system able to detect outbreaks of epidemic-prone diseases. In collaboration with the Federal Ministry of Health, an early-warning surveillance system was developed to cover the IDP in the accessible camps [18].

The affected population were not refugees, but displaced persons in their own country, and the surveillance system had to be a reinforcement of the routine Sudanese surveillance system and not a parallel system. The national communicable diseases surveillance system was reorganized in 2003, the events to be reported defined, and national guidelines with case definitions published. The National Public Health Laboratory in Khartoum was designed as the National Reference Laboratory for the whole country. In 2004, an early-warning system was developed for Darfur. Among the 22 health events included in the routine surveillance system, 12 were selected for the Darfur early-warning system according to their potential epidemic risk in camps: diarrhea, bloody diarrhea, measles, meningitis, malaria, acute flaccid paralysis, acute jaundice, acute respiratory syndrome, neonatal tetanus, unexplained fever, malnutrition, and injuries.

In the context of a Federal country, with difficulties in accessibility, the responsibility of surveillance and response was at the state level. From the three Darfur states, epidemiologists sent data to the Federal level using satellite e-mail connection.

The National Public Health Laboratory developed standard operating procedures for sending samples from Darfur to Khartoum. Media for specimen collection and transportation were positioned at the state level. With the support of WHO, a plan of action was developed to improve diagnostic capacities at camp level. Through the surveillance system, an outbreak of hepatitis E affecting internal displaced people was detected in July 2004 [7].

One limitation of the Darfur surveillance system was that many settlements were not accessible for humanitarian agencies due to security problems and therefore, no data on this part of the population could be obtained.

Lessons learnt, barriers, and success

It is now recognized that surveillance of infectious diseases is a key intervention to be implemented during the first phases of the emergency. It requires a network of motivated people from different organizations and disciplines, working together.

The surveillance should be based on a short list of priority diseases and additionally include mechanisms to report immediately unexpected events.

Surveillance systems for CD are just a component of elements contributing to control epidemics. Other essential information is necessary in order to interpret surveillance data and to define priority actions:
• Population data
• Mortality data
• Vaccination coverage
• Water and sanitation indicators
• Surveillance of malnutrition
• Drug supply, stockpiles

Mortality (expressed as number of deaths per 10,000 population per day) is the most important indicator in complex emergencies and defines the severity of the situation. Mortality figures are difficult to collect and cannot be estimated through surveillance data coming from health centers. A system should be in place to measure mortality (active surveillance, repeated surveys) and integrate it with the CD surveillance system.

Barriers

The main barriers in surveillance of CD in complex emergencies are:
• Lack of standardization in data collection, standard protocols
• Poor coordination among main organizations
• Lack of integration of information collected through the surveillance system and other public health indicators
• High turnover of international staff
• Lack of security for the affected population, local population, humanitarian workers
• Political conflicts between international agencies and local governments

Key issues in success

There are a number of key issues to be considered in complex emergencies for surveillance:
• Coordination among agencies, clear leadership of one institution
• Ensure security and accessibility to the affected population
• Integration of national counterparts since the beginning of the process
• Integration of surveillance indicators with other public health indicators
• Implementation of surveys to complement CD surveillance system data (rapid health assessments, nutritional surveys, mortality surveys, etc.)
• Training of human resources through supervision, field visits, short courses, guidelines
• Frequent feedback
• Good data management
• Integration of new technologies: Internet, mobile telephones, mapping tools

References

1 Chechhi F, Roberts L. HPN Network Paper 52. *Interpreting and Using Mortality Data in Humanitarian Emergencies: A Primer for Non-epidemiologists*. London: Overseas Development Institute; 2005.

2 Connolly MA (ed.). Communicable disease control in emergencies: a field manual. WHO/CDS/2005.27. Geneva: World Health Organization; 2005:295.

3 Burkle FM. Lessons learnt and future expectations of complex emergencies. *BMJ* 1999;**319**(7207): 422–6.

4 Toole MJ. Mass population displacement: a global public health challenge. *Infect Dis Clin North Am* 1995;**9**(2): 353–66.

5 Connolly MA, Gayer M, Ryan MJ, Salama P, Spiegel P, Heymann DL. Communicable diseases in complex emergencies: impact and challenges. *Lancet* 2004;**364**(9449): 1974–83.

6 Connolly MA, Heymann DL. Deadly comrades: war and infectious diseases. *Lancet* 2002;**360**(suppl):s23–4.

7 Guthmann JP, Klovstad H, Boccia D, *et al.* A large outbreak of hepatitis E among a displaced population in Darfur, Sudan, 2004: the role of water treatment methods. *Clin Infect Dis* 2006;**42**(12):1685–91.

8 Médecins Sans Frontières. *Refugee Health: An Approach to Emergency Situations*. London: Macmillan Education Ltd; 1997.

9 Brown V, Jacquier G, Coulombier D, Balandine S, Belanger F, Legros D. Rapid assessment of population size by area sampling in disaster situations. *Disasters* June 2001;**25**(2):164–71.

10 Chandramohan D, Maude GH, Rodrigues LC, Hayes RJ. Verbal autopsies for adult deaths: their development and validation in a multicentre study. *Trop Med Int Health* 1998;**3**(6):436–46.

11 Lauritsen JM (ed.). *EpiData Data Entry, Data Management and Basic Statistical Analysis System*. Odense, Denmark: EpiData Association; 2000–2006. Available from: http://www.epidata.dk. Accessed April 20, 2007.

12 Epi Info^{TM}, Version 3.3.2. Atlanta, GA: Centers for Diseases Control and Prevention. Available from: http://www.cdc.gov/epiinfo. Accessed April 20, 2007.

13 The R project for statistical computing. Available from: http://www.r-project.org. Accessed April 20, 2007.

14 Ministry of Health, Indonesia, World Health Organization assisted by Global Outbreak Alert and Response Network (GOARN) partners, UNICEF. Epidemic-prone disease surveillance and response after the tsunami in Aceh, Indonesia. *Euro Surveill* 2005;**10**(5):E050505.2. Available from: http://www.eurosurveillance.org/ew/2005/050505.asp#2. Accessed April 20, 2007.

15 Centers for Diseases Control and Prevention. Updates guidelines for evaluating public health surveillance systems. *MMWR* July 27, 2001;**50**:13.

16 Valenciano M, Pinto A, Coulombier D, Hashorva E, Murthi M. Surveillance of communicable diseases among the Kosovar refugees in Albania, April–June 1999. *Euro Surveill* 1999;**4**(9):92–5.

17 Valenciano M, Coulombier D, Lopes CB, *et al.* Challenges for communicable disease surveillance and control in southern Iraq, April–June 2003. *JAMA* 2003;**290**(5): 654–8.

18 Pinto A, Saeed M, El SH, Rashford A, Colombo A, Valenciano M *et al.* Setting up an early warning system for epidemic-prone diseases in Darfur: a participative approach. *Disasters* 2005;**29**(4):310–22.

Additional Web resources

World Health Organization, Health Action in Crisis Department: www.who.int/HAC. Accessed April 20, 2007.

United Nations High Commissioner for Refugees: www.unhcr.org. Accessed April 20, 2007.

United Nations Children's Fund: www. unicef. org. Accessed April 20, 2007.

United Nations Office for the Coordination of Humanitarian Affairs: http://ochaonline.un.org. Accessed April 20, 2007.

The International Emergency and Refugee Health Branch, Centers for Disease Control and Prevention, Atlanta: www.cdc.gov/nceh/ierh. Accessed April 20, 2007.

Standardized Monitoring and Assessment of Relief and Transitions: www.smartindicators.org. Accessed April 20, 2007.

Center for Research on the Epidemiology of Disasters: www.cred.be. Accessed April 20, 2007.

The SPHERE project: http://www.sphereproject.org. Accessed April 20, 2007.

MALARIA – SUSPECTED

- *Uncomplicated malaria*

Patient with fever or history of fever within the past 48 hours (with or without other symptoms such as nausea, vomiting and diarrhea, headache, back pain, chills, myalgia) in whom other obvious causes of fever have been excluded.

- *Severe malaria*

Patient with symptoms as for uncomplicated malaria, as well as drowsiness with extreme weakness and associated signs and symptoms related to organ failure such as disorientation, loss of consciousness, convulsions, severe anemia, jaundice, hemoglobinuria, spontaneous bleeding, pulmonary edema, and shock.

To confirm case:
Demonstration of malaria parasites in blood film by examining thick or thin smears, or by rapid diagnostic test kit for *Plasmodium falciparum.*

MEASLES Fever **and** maculopapular rash (i.e. nonvesicular) **and** cough, coryza (i.e. runny nose) or conjunctivitis (i.e. red eyes);

or

Any person in whom a clinical health worker suspects measles infection.

To confirm case:
At least a fourfold increase in antibody titer **or i**solation of measles virus **or** presence of measles-specific IgM antibodies.

MENINGITIS – SUSPECTED Sudden onset of fever (>38.0°C axillary) **and** one of the following:

- ☐ neck stiffness,
- ☐ altered consciousness,
- • other meningeal sign **or** petechial/purpural rash.

In children <1 year meningitis is suspected when fever is accompanied by a bulging fontanelle.
To confirm case:
Positive cerebrospinal fluid antigen detection **or** positive cerebrospinal fluid culture **or** positive blood culture.

Source: Case definitions are adapted from the *Communicable Disease Control in Emergencies: A Field Manual,* M.A. Connolly (ed.) Used with permission of the World Health Organization, Geneva, 2006.

Use of Electronic and Web-Based Means in Infectious Disease Surveillance

21 Use of the World Wide Web to enhance infectious disease surveillance

Nkuchia M. M'ikanatha, Dale D. Rohn, David P. Welliver, Toby McAdams & Kathleen G. Julian

Introduction

Although health departments have been reporting disease for decades, the Internet or the World Wide Web (Web) offers unprecedented opportunities to disseminate information, collect actual reports, and share results. The first challenge in disease reporting is to ensure that healthcare providers, infection control professionals, laboratorians, and others know how to report diseases including which diseases to report, when to report, which forms to use, and where to send them. Posting this information on health department Web pages provides easy and consistent access to the information. But posting the forms for disease reporting is only the beginning—the next challenge is to provide for Web-based submission of case reports. This can streamline data entry processes, allow for more rapid data collection, and simplify the submission process for users. Finally, timely data summaries can be made available on the Web, greatly increasing accessibility. Seeing the compiled and analyzed data, a wider range of persons can recognize the importance of disease reporting. All of these processes depend on a fairly new medium—the Web. Hiring Web specialists and developing close partnerships between these specialists and content experts such as epidemiologists can help health departments use the Web to its fullest potential.

This chapter provides an overview of the use of the Web to enhance infectious disease surveillance in the United States (US). The overview is not exhaustive, but instead highlights many examples of excellent use of the Web, lessons learned, and practical considerations. The lessons learned are offered to assist public health departments in the US and in other parts of the world to leverage use of this important communication medium.

The Internet transformation in healthcare information

The ongoing advances in Internet technology are altering information systems and societies profoundly. In many countries including the US, availability of government services on the Web has become a societal expectation. A 2004 United Nation's world public sector report observed, "Electronic distribution of government documentation and increasing public access to government information are being developed very quickly in many countries. Many governments have set up Web sites and connected databases and information systems to the Internet, thus enabling the public to search, locate, view and download government reports, studies, computer software, data files and databases" [1].

In the US, the Web is used as means for offering services by all levels of government. Federal agencies in the US, including the Centers for Disease Control and Prevention (CDC, http://www.cdc.gov), the National Institutes of Health (http://www.nih.gov), and the Agency for Healthcare Research and Quality (http://www.ahrq.gov/) use the Web to increase accessibility of trusted information targeted to patients and clinicians. Professional organizations such as the American Medical

Association offer Web-based member services, including access to online journals and practice guidelines [2].

Disease reporting information on the Web

Barriers to disease reporting include not knowing what, when, and how to report. Furthermore, reporting requirements and methodologies vary by state in the US. Healthcare providers may not know which diseases are reportable in their jurisdiction and health department phone numbers or case report forms may not be readily accessible [3]. However, the Web can be an excellent medium to provide practical disease reporting information that can be tailored to each jurisdiction.

Figure 21.1 illustrates results of a 2003 study on the use of the Web to promote physician reporting. The study found that health departments' Web sites had partial information regarding what, when, how, and where to report diseases. For ex-

ample, 84% (48) of the 57 US jurisdictions provided disease reporting information, although only 42% of these included online case-reporting forms [4]. Further review of state Web sites in 2006 suggests considerable progress has been made in providing practical reporting information. For example, the South Carolina Department of Health and Environmental Control's Web site provides a list of reportable diseases divided into three sections to identify diseases that should be reported immediately, within 24 hours, or within 7 days, along with instructions on when and how to report. Local jurisdiction phone numbers, fax numbers, and mailing addresses for reporting cases are provided on the reportable diseases list. Clinical and demographic information that is necessary for case reports is also indicated [5]. Case reporting forms can be easily downloaded from the Texas Department of Health's Web site [6] and faxed to the numbers provided on the form. The South Dakota Department of Health provides a list of reportable diseases in both HTML and printable PDF formats (Figure 21.2) [7]. On the Michigan Department

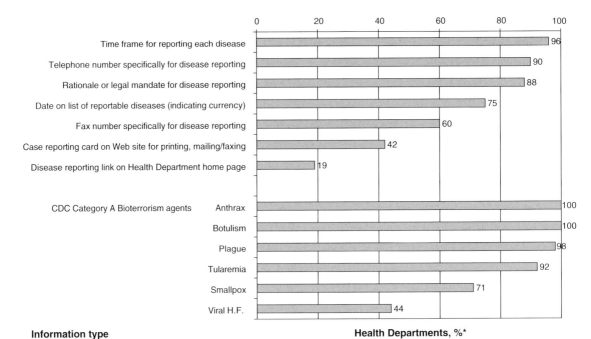

Information type

Health Departments, %*

Fig 21.1 Presence of disease reporting information on Health Department Web sites—United States, 2003. *Percentage of health jurisdiction Web sites for which the listed information type was found on the site, based on 48 sites having disease-reporting information. (Used with permission of the American Medical Association from Ref. [4].)

WHEN TO REPORT

Category I diseases are reportable immediately by telephone on recognition or strong suspicion of disease.

Category II diseases are reportable immediately by telephone, mail, or fax within 3 days of recognition or strong suspicion of disease.

WHAT TO REPORT: Disease reports must include as much of the following as is known:

- Disease or condition diagnosed or suspected
- Case's name, age, date of birth, sex, race, address, and occupation
- Date of disease onset
- Pertinent laboratory results and date of specimen collection
- Attending physician's name, address, and phone number
- Name and phone number of person making the report

HOW TO REPORT

 Secure website: www.state.sd.us/doh/diseasereport

 Telephone: 1-800-592-1804 confidential answering-recording device, or **1-800-592-1861** or **605-773-3737** for a disease surveillance person during normal business hours; <u>after hours</u> to report Category I diseases, call **605-280-4810**

 Fax: 605-773-5509

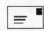 **Mail** or **courier,** address to: Infectious Disease Surveillance, Office of Disease Prevention, Department of Health, 615 East 4th Street, Pierre, SD 57501; marked *"Confidential Disease Report"*

Fig 21.2 Example of Web-based reporting instructions available on South Dakota Web site [7].

of Community Health's Web site, the reportable disease list indicates in bold green font the diseases for which an isolate or serum sample must be submitted to the state's public health laboratory [8].

In addition to provision of logistical reporting information, a brief description of the rationale for disease reporting can give healthcare providers a better understanding of its benefits, and therefore encourage reporting. The Arizona Division of Public Health Services' Web site describes the rationale for communicable disease reporting and includes links to specific state regulations [9].

State health departments' sites are also used to address privacy concerns related to implementation of the Health Insurance Portability and Accountability Act of 1996 (HIPAA), which became effective in 2003. Although HIPAA explicitly permits disease reporting to public health authorities

that is required by state laws or regulations, many jurisdictions encounter healthcare providers who are reluctant to report cases, citing the HIPAA rule as the reason. In conjunction with information on how to report diseases, the Michigan Department of Community Health's Web site addresses potential HIPAA-related concerns with reference to HIPAA and Michigan regulations [8].

Public health departments can also use the Web to support surveillance by posting clinical guidelines for diagnosis and management of diseases of public health importance. Clues to recognition of diseases (e.g., for anthrax, mediastinal widening on chest X-rays), and recommendations on diagnostic testing (e.g., for West Nile virus, cerebrospinal fluid for IgM ELISA with accompanying serum for IgM and IgG ELISA) can be readily provided on the Web. For example, the New York City Department of Health and Mental Hygiene's Bureau of

Reporting by healthcare providers to public health officials

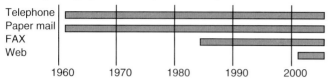

Reporting within public health agencies

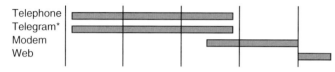

Fig 21.3 Historical development of disease reporting technologies.
*After 1989, telegram was used by one jurisdiction (territory) only.

Communicable Diseases Web site provides topical guidelines that discuss clinical diagnosis and management of specific diseases. For fall 2006, the Web site included guidance on when to suspect and how to report potential cases of avian H5N1 influenza, and specimens useful for diagnostic testing [10].

Secure Web-based submission of case reports

In the US, healthcare providers and laboratorians report cases of notifiable conditions to local or state health departments, who in turn voluntarily forward them to the CDC. The Web can provide an attractive means for reporting. Disease reporting in the 1960s, 1970s, and early 1980s depended on the telephone, paper mail, and telegrams (Figure 21.3). In contrast to electronic data collection, these methods allowed for collection of only the most basic information.

Widespread use of computers to facilitate disease reporting and other surveillance activities started in 1989 when all states began using the National Electronic Telecommunications Systems for Surveillance (NETSS). While case reports were still submitted by healthcare providers and laboratorians to the local jurisdictions by traditional means, with NETSS, case reports in a standard format (with many more details potentially added from investigations) were transmitted to the national level (CDC) via modem each week. By 2002, state reporting to CDC evolved to the point where all states were able to transmit NETSS-formatted data to the

CDC over a secure Internet connection, the CDC's "Secure Data Network" (SDN).

As the US progresses to full adoption of new standards for data composition and messaging defined by the principles of the National Electronic Disease Surveillance System (NEDSS) initiative (www.cdc.gov), case reports in many states can be automatically pulled from NEDSS-compatible state and local systems for daily secure transmission to the CDC over the Web. As more states and territories bring NEDSS-compatible systems online, automated secure Web-based reporting from states to the CDC will spread. At the same time, these new systems can often provide health departments with the capability to receive electronic laboratory and morbidity reports, improve data management, and incorporate reports for analysis and visualization of their data.

Modalities for healthcare provider and hospital reporting have evolved in a more additive fashion compared to the evolution of health department systems. The time-tested methods of paper forms, telephone (verbal), and fax reports have been used by healthcare providers for decades and will probably continue for years, although these modes are declining as electronic reporting becomes more widely available. The Web was first able to improve the reporting system by enabling states to post lists of reportable diseases and conditions, instructions for reporting, and reporting forms, as described previously. Provided that these Web sites can be easily located by users, the Web has the capacity to overcome some of the barriers to reporting.

By 2002, a small number of states began implementation of Web-based surveillance systems that supported health department users, but few if any permitted healthcare providers to access these systems. Automated reporting from laboratories has taken precedence over other types of provider reporting. However, in 2006, several states with NEDSS-compatible systems have established a means for direct provider entry. Often direct entry begins with hospital-based reporting by infection control professionals. Whether physicians in private practice will embrace Web entry of case reports is yet to be determined.

As part of the NEDSS initiative mentioned above, the CDC created and supported a prototype electronic surveillance system, named the NEDSS "Base

System," that some states have chosen to use for surveillance. However, most states are developing their own electronic systems that are compatible with the data standards of the NEDSS concept and are also Web-based. By September 2006, 13 states had implemented the NEDSS Base System and in 33 other states NEDSS-compatible systems were either fully deployed or in development (Figure 21.4). In states where either Base or NEDSS-compatible systems are deployed, progress has been made in several areas including timeliness, access to data by communicable disease investigators, data management, and use of data in outbreak investigation. For example, in New Jersey where a NEDSS-compatible, Web-based communicable disease surveillance system has been implemented,

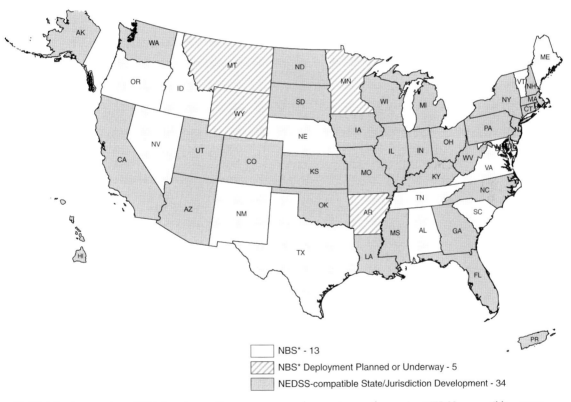

NBS* - 13

NBS* Deployment Planned or Underway - 5

NEDSS-compatible State/Jurisdiction Development - 34

Fig 21.4 Implementation of Web-based surveillance systems compatible with National Standards—United States, 2006. We used data presented by a Centers for Disease Control and Prevention official (CDC) at the 2006 Public Health Information Network Conference to indicate states using either National Electronic Disease Surveillance System (NEDSS)

base system or those using NEDSS-compatible systems developed by states. The data presented by CDC included both systems completed and those under development. The number of states with capability for direct reporting by physicians is unknown but suspected to be limited.
*NBS = NEDSS Base System, CDC-developed.

time to entry of new cases was reduced from an average of 28 days to an average of 3–5 days after illness onset [11]. In Oklahoma, where a NEDSS-compatible system has been implemented, a total of 164 infection-control practitioners and 210 laboratorians representing all Oklahoma hospitals are using the system to report cases [11]. Some states, such as Pennsylvania, have implemented a fully integrated, Web-based surveillance system that enables providers and laboratories to report electronically and that disseminates Health Alerts electronically [12].

While use of the Web for disease reporting offers the benefits described above, it is important to note potential challenges. In the design of Web-based reporting systems, designers must consider end users' different operating systems (Windows, Macintosh, etc.) and different access speeds to the Internet (dial-up modems versus high-speed broadband). Because of the importance of maintaining the security of electronic transactions of confidential health information, extensive resources must be directed to deployment of appropriate encryption and other security measures. Even for qualified users, the resulting protection can introduce cumbersome barriers, including the problems associated with password maintenance. At another level of complexity, digital certificates used to certify security of specific data entry computers require installation steps and renewal procedures that may require the support of information technology specialists. Web-based reporting systems may impose learning burdens on users. One practical approach to provider training is the use of systems such as Michigan's self-guided slide presentation [13].

In the experience of the NEDSS initiative in the US, significant large-scale challenges have been encountered as individual states hire information technology firms to design and implement electronic reporting systems. Several important potential problems can be averted by early involvement of stakeholders and end users in the design and testing phases. For example, without sufficient epidemiologist input, Web-based, disease-specific case report forms may lack sufficient details to capture pertinent clinical and epidemiologic information. If systems prove to be too cumbersome, instead of promoting surveillance, Web-based reporting may in itself become a barrier to disease reporting. End-

user input and pilot testing is therefore critical to the medium's success.

The costs for development of electronic reporting systems can be staggering. During 2002–2006, CDC distributed over $50 million to eligible states for the NEDSS initiative. However, these funds only partly covered the costs of systems to individual states. Problems can be encountered if the scope of the project is not clear upfront—for example, if not designed and budgeted in the early phases, it may be much more expensive to add chronic diseases data management modules to the core communicable diseases electronic surveillance program.

Use of the Web to disseminate surveillance information

In addition to ongoing data collection, analysis and dissemination of findings are also fundamental to surveillance methodologies expounded by Alexander Langmuir in the 1950s [14] (see also Chapters 1 and 39, Part 1). Surveillance programs must not become entrenched in data collection only, but they must also expend equivalent effort on analysis and dissemination of useful surveillance findings to persons who can undertake effective prevention and control activities [15]. In addition, lack of or inefficient feedback of data to reporters has been cited as one of several reasons why healthcare providers do not report cases [3]. A goal of surveillance should be provision of valuable surveillance data in a timely, pertinent manner not only to public health personnel, but also to healthcare providers.

To document the extent the Web was being used to disseminate surveillance information, we searched a random sample of 21 state health departments' Web sites between 2005 and 2006. Nearly all (95%) of the Web sites reported at least simple counts of some reportable diseases and the majority of the Web sites had specific data on recent enteric diseases (e.g., *Salmonella*, 74%), vaccine preventable diseases (e.g., pertussis, 71%), tuberculosis (88%), and vector-borne (e.g., West Nile virus, 94%). However, less than half (43%) of these Web sites reported antibiotic susceptibility data for any of the last 3 years and information regarding a current or recent outbreak (within the last 6 mo) was even more limited (33%).

Health departments that are currently disseminating surveillance information on the Web can serve as models for other jurisdictions. The New York City Health Department Web site offers alerts to physicians about current outbreaks, listed in reverse chronological order, for the preceding 2 years [16]. Examples of year 2006 New York City alerts include *Escherichia coli* O157:H7 infections associated with bagged, fresh spinach in multiple states, rabies-positive cats and raccoons on Staten Island, and a suspected meningococcal meningitis outbreak in Brooklyn. The Oregon Department of Human Services' Public Health Division has archives of monthly reports of notifiable diseases for each year back to 1997 with annual summaries analyzing data by county [17]. As of October 2006, monthly reports were available from as recently as August 2006. The Minnesota Department of Health Web site provides an annual report of antimicrobial susceptibilities of selected pathogens submitted to the Minnesota Public Health Laboratory in the preceding years back to 1998 [18]. The report includes number and percent of specific isolates tested and percent susceptible to specific antibiotics. The report also contains some description of the data—for example, the 2005 report indicated that only 34% of *Campylobacter* isolates from patients returning from foreign travel were susceptible to quinolones.

States are also developing innovative, interactive means of displaying surveillance data. The Tennessee Department of Health hosts an online database of surveillance data that can be queried to create easy-to-read reports customized by disease, county, and time period [19]. Additionally, mapping of surveillance data can be a particularly effective means of communication. CDC's national arbovirus surveillance program, in collaboration with mapping technologies of the United States Geological Survey, publishes very up-to-date county-specific maps of major arboviral diseases, including West Nile virus [20]. National or state maps can be easily customized by the Web site user to select for county-specific human, veterinary, bird, or mosquito arbovirus surveillance data.

The development of enhanced features for electronic surveillance databases should incorporate both increased Web-based reporting capacities and improved data dissemination features. Providing feedback to reporters requires that sites be designed with the providers' needs in mind. When linked with Web-based reporting, such feedback could include immediate verification of what has been reported, list of cases the provider reported previously, links to treatment guidelines and other recommendations, local antimicrobial susceptibility patterns, and information about the frequency and distribution of recent reports of the condition in the reporter's area. At the health department level, electronic surveillance databases must be easy to query by epidemiologists and other public health investigators. In addition to customized (ad hoc) reports, electronic surveillance systems should be able to automatically generate clearly formatted reports, graphs, and maps that can be used by disease investigators and healthcare workers.

Design considerations for use of the Web to support infectious disease surveillance

As discussed earlier in this chapter, the use of the Web can enhance infectious disease surveillance by promoting disease reporting and increasing communication of surveillance data. To achieve these desired objectives requires more than simply posting surveillance information on the Web. It is crucial to understand the unique requirements of this medium, including specific usability principles, which can guide development of sites that better address healthcare providers' needs. The site www.usability.gov provides a step-by-step Web usability guide for planning, testing, and refining Web sites. The following practical tips (Box 21.1) are offered to health departments who are developing and enhancing their Web sites on disease reporting and surveillance information.

Ease of navigation is an important feature of Web design. In addition to the general public, users on sites with health reporting and surveillance data will include busy clinicians with little time to search the Web site. While some infectious diseases surveillance Web pages will be of interest to the general public (e.g., geographic distribution of diseases such as Lyme disease and associated advice related to tick-borne disease prevention), effective Web sites should offer separate navigation pathways for healthcare professionals seeking more

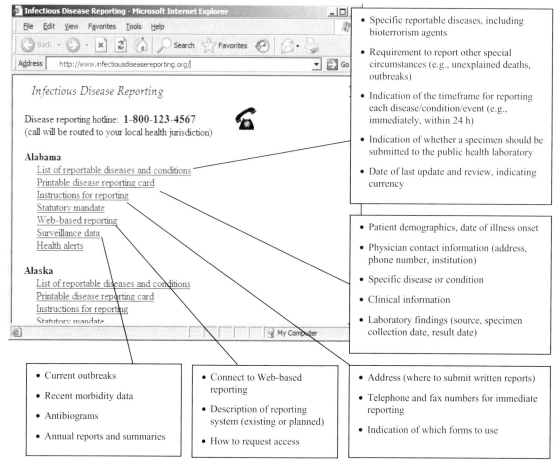

Fig 21.5 Example of a proposed national disease reporting site with links to state and local sites.

national map, users can click on a particular state to access links to a standard set of pandemic influenza preparedness materials from that state, including their pandemic influenza plan and historical information about the 1918 pandemic in that state. In general, information is posted and maintained by the states on their own state sites, rather than at the pandemicflu.gov site, thereby preserving local autonomy.

In a similar way, it would be helpful to offer clinicians a single toll-free telephone number to report cases that automatically routes to the appropriate local jurisdiction. An active model system, the American Association of Poison Control Centers' centralized toll-free number (1-800-222-1222) is currently used to route voluntary reports of poi-

soning exposures to the caller's nearest poison center [27].

Challenges to the creation of a centralized national disease surveillance Web site or toll-free number typically center on resources, including staff time and money. There have also been concerns that a national site would control state-level information. Linking to state and local sites rather than reposting materials on that site should alleviate most of those concerns.

Summary

The evolution of the Web as means for communication offers a practical, relatively inexpensive way to promote infectious disease surveillance through both data collection and distribution. The Web can readily provide clinicians with information on what, when, how, and where to report. Especially for emerging diseases and bioterrorism threats, the Web can support surveillance through publication of health alerts and public health guidelines with advice on disease recognition and diagnostic testing. With increasing efforts directed toward timely, efficient dissemination of surveillance data on the Web, clinicians and others can access information on current outbreaks, incidence and prevalence of reportable diseases, and antibiotic susceptibility patterns of recent isolates. The Web is also a practical technology that can be used to share surveillance information with neighboring public health jurisdictions, policy makers, and members of the public. Moreover, while requiring highly integrated and advanced information technology-public health collaborations, Web-based reporting systems may bypass the limitations of paper-based reporting modalities.

To enhance use of the Web in infectious disease surveillance, there is a need to more intensively address usability and accessibility. Such efforts should include users' perspective in all phases of the Web content development process. Usability tests should be considered for all levels of Web users, including epidemiologists, data analysts, healthcare providers, infection control professionals, laboratorians, data entry staff, and the general public. Content experts should be actively involved with Web development staff. It is essential to ensure that use of the Web is a helpful tool and not a new burden, particularly for frontline healthcare providers [28].

Increasing efforts devoted to building good, useful, accessible, multipurpose infectious disease surveillance Web sites will invite increased usage by healthcare workers. Once a Web site proves its usefulness, healthcare workers are more likely to return again to seek information, or to report cases of public health importance. Development of this virtual relationship creates a closer tie between the public health community and clinicians, thus increasing opportunities for healthcare worker education, contributions of healthcare workers to public health goals, and other collaborative efforts.

Acknowledgments

We thank C. Scott Danos (CDC) for helpful discussions and invaluable insights regarding the US National Electronic Disease Surveillance System initiative. We also acknowledge fruitful discussion and assistance provided by June E Bancroft and Kathy Livingston (Oregon Department of Human Services) and Elly Pretzel (Minnesota Department of Health). In addition, we thank Steven Rosenberry (Pennsylvania Department of Health) for assistance with mapping.

References

1 United Nations. *World Public Sector Report: Globalization and the State 2001*. New York: United Nations; 2004. Available from: http://unpan1.un.org/intradoc/groups/public/documents/UN/UNPAN012761.pdf. Accessed May 17, 2006.

2 American Medical Association. AMA Internet ID. Available from http://www.ama-assn.org/ama/pub/category/3133.html. Accessed May 17, 2006.

3 Konowitz PM, Petrossian GA, Rose DN. The underreporting of disease and physicians' knowledge of reporting requirements. *Public Health Rep* 1984;**99**:31.

4 M'ikanatha NM, Welliver DP, Rohn DD, Julian KG, Lautenbach E. Use of the Web by state and territorial health departments to promote reporting of infectious disease. *JAMA* March 3, 2004;**291**(9):1069–70.

5 South Carolina Department of Health and Environmental Control. List of reportable conditions in South Carolina. Available from http://www.scdhec.net/health/disease/docs/reportable_conditions.pdf. Accessed November 10, 2006.

6 Texas Department of State Health Services. Reporting Forms. Available from: http://www.dshs.state.tx.us/idcu/investigation/forms/. Accessed November 10, 2006.

7 South Dakota Department of Health. Reportable Diseases in South Dakota. Available from: http://www.state.sd.us/doh/Disease/report.htm. Accessed November 10, 2006.

8 Michigan Department of Community Health. Communicable Disease Reporting in Michigan. Available from: http://www.michigan.gov/mdch/0,1607,7-132-2945_5104-12538-,00.html#CD%20Reporting. Accessed on November 10, 2006.

9 Arizona Department of Health Services. Communicable Disease Reporting. Available from: http://www.azdhs.gov/phs/oids/dis_rpt.htm. Accessed October 17, 2006.

22 The Netherlands' Infectious Diseases Surveillance Information System (ISIS)

Arnold Bosman & Hans van Vliet

Introduction

Surveillance information must be reported in a timely fashion to those who can take appropriate actions. Though traditionally surveillance reports are published in journals and periodical papers, in recent years more often the Internet is used for distribution. The Infectious Diseases Surveillance and Information System (ISIS) was developed by the National Institute for Public Health and Environment (RIVM) of the Netherlands to provide an information technology (IT) infrastructure for the continuous collection and analysis of data and for the distribution of surveillance information. ISIS collects data from sentinel laboratories and mandatory notifications of infectious diseases. Through daily automated analysis and Web-based reporting, ISIS aims to provide the most recent information on infectious diseases in the Netherlands. Through the Web site www.rivm.nl/isis information is distributed to those professionals who "need to know" to allow them to undertake action.

Whereas most laboratories introduced data management systems to process diagnostic test results in the 1970s, these systems were often without a common standard for data coding or exchange protocols. As the computer systems in laboratories expanded and in some cases were integrated with hospital information systems, it became feasible to access them as data sources for surveillance.

In contrast to most laboratory surveillance systems that report only positive test results, the ISIS system receives daily files with all new test results from associated sentinel laboratories, both positive and negative. In this chapter we describe an outline of how data collection, analysis, and reporting takes place within ISIS for data on mandatory notifications and laboratory test results.

National context of ISIS

With approximately 16 million inhabitants, the Netherlands is a modestly sized country in the European Union. The Dutch healthcare system is a mixture of public and private care; everyone is covered by a basic medical insurance. Each citizen is supposed to be registered with one of the over 6700 general practitioners, who are responsible for family medicine and act as gatekeepers to the more specialized layers of the healthcare system. The healthcare system guarantees that everyone has access to medical care. With 93 hospital organizations covering 141 main locations and 38 ambulatory clinics the supply of medical care is quite differentiated. The 458 municipalities are responsible by law to deliver public healthcare. Municipalities are organized into 36 Municipal Health Services (MHS; Figure 22.1).

The Infectious Disease Law (1999) describes 35 diseases that are notifiable [1]. The list of notifiable diseases is divided into three categories: Group A covers diseases that need to be notified within 24 hours after suspicion of the diagnosis. The diseases in this group are poliomyelitis anterior acuta (as this has a high potential for outbreaks in this country with large pockets of low

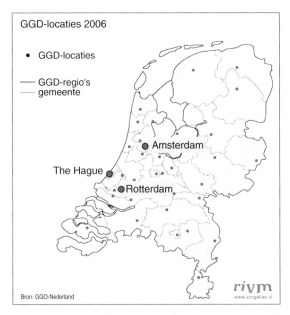

Fig 22.1 Locations of 458 municipalities and 36 Municipal Health Services (GGDs).

get sufficient surveillance information on notifiable diseases, RIVM has requested MHS to report additional data on a voluntary basis. MHS are the regional authorities responsible for receiving preliminary notifications in order to initiate immediate control measures. MHS send abstracts of these reports as soon as possible to the CMO at the Inspectorate of Healthcare and a voluntary report to RIVM.

Data collection: mandatory notification through Internet "OSIRIS"

MHS are asked to send a minimum data set on each notification received to the CMO and in addition, since the introduction of the Infectious Disease Law in 1999, to send more detailed data to RIVM. For tuberculosis only, MHS has agreed to send a detailed surveillance questionnaire for each patient with tuberculosis infection to the KNCV Tuberculosis Foundation, based in the Hague. RIVM analyzes and interprets all surveillance data on these notifiable diseases and disseminates surveillance information through the ISIS Web site to those who need to know.

In order to reduce the administrative burden, RIVM developed and introduced an Internet-based reporting system "OSIRIS" (Online System for Infectious disease Reporting within ISIS) in 2002 [2]. The IT group of the ISIS project at RIVM designed the system. The programming and development was outsourced to commercial IT companies. GGD Netherlands, the national society for MHS, coordinated the introduction of OSIRIS. Since 2002, all 36 MHS use OSIRIS to report notifiable diseases to the CMO, RIVM, and KNCV Tuberculosis foundation.

MHS staff only need to enter the data once on disease-specific electronic registration forms and the system distributes the data to the various organizations (CMO, RIVM, KNCV Tuberculosis Foundation). Physicians and laboratory staff continue to use paper, fax, and e-mail to send their notifications to MHS (Figure 22.2).

Authorized users at MHS, CMO, RIVM, and KNCV Foundation have password-protected access to the system. Once MHS receives a notification, they immediately enter the preliminary data online.

vaccine coverage), SARS, and smallpox. Group B covers shigellosis, botulism, typhoid fever, cholera, Creutzfeld–Jacob's disease (classical and variant), diphtheria, recurring fever, hepatitis A, hepatitis B, hepatitis C, rabies, pertussis, measles, meningococcal disease, paratyphoid fever A, B, and C, plague, tuberculosis, viral hemorrhagic fever, typhus, and foodborne illness. All physicians are required by law to notify the MHS of patients diagnosed with one of the diseases in Group A or B. Group C covers diseases that are only reportable by the laboratory that makes the diagnosis to MHS: brucellosis, enterohemorrhagic *Escherichia coli*, yellow fever, leptospirosis, malaria, anthrax, psittacosis, Q-fever, rubella, and trichinosis.

The Chief Medical Officer (CMO) at the Inspectorate for Healthcare is responsible for the monitoring of the execution of the Infectious Disease Law. All notifications need to be reported by MHS to the CMO as soon as possible. As surveillance is not an objective of the law, the minimum data set for notifications, as described in the law, is quite limited. The National Institute for Public Health and the Environment (RIVM) is responsible for national infectious disease surveillance. In order to

Table 22.2 Example of inclusion criteria for laboratory test results in the ISIS database to count patients with the case definition "gonorrhea."

Field	Allowed values for the ISIS case definition "gonorrhoea"
Subject	*Neisseria gonorrhoeae*
Material	Any
Origin	Any
Obtained by	Any
Method	"Bacterial culture" or "hybridization test" or "PCR"
Result	"Positive" or "isolated"
Patient	Any age, any gender
Aggregation window	30 days

this individual. The key cannot be converted back to the original data. As all laboratories connected to ISIS use the same algorithm to generate this key, it is possible to recognize test results that belong to the same patient while maintaining anonymity, even when tests are done in different laboratories. This is especially relevant since some test results need to be interpreted together with other tests in order to draw conclusions for diagnosis.

In order to be able to count "cases" using the ISIS laboratory results, RIVM has developed case definitions. These case definitions may lack high specificity at the patient level, yet for surveillance purposes they are expected to provide a good tool for monitoring trends. An example of such case definition is given in Table 22.2 for gonorrhea. Any patient with a positive result for culture, hybridization test, or PCR for *Neisseria gonorrhoeae* will be labeled "gonorrhea case" at the first positive test result.

The "aggregation window" is used to avoid counting patients with several positive tests within one disease episode more than once. For gonorrhea we determined (through consensus) with microbiologists that each positive test that followed within 30 days of a previous positive test for the same patient, should be considered to belong to the same episode of infection. As an example of the application of case definitions to the patients' test results, consider a hypothetical person from a high-risk group, who is tested positive for gonorrhea by PCR in "week 1" (see Figure 22.3). If the regular antibiotic treatment does not work, then the symptoms will remain, and the patient will present again for testing in "week 2." This time, bacterial culture plus tests for antimicrobial resistance are performed on the material of the swab: the culture is positive for *N. gonorrhoeae*. After prescription of the appropriate antibiotics, this patient is likely to be invited back 1 week later ("week 3") to confirm that the treatment has now been successful. Both PCR and culture are now negative. In "week 6" the same patient returns for new tests, as the symptoms have returned; it appears that not all sexual partners have been treated and the bacterial culture is again positive for *N. gonorrhoeae*.

How does the algorithm of ISIS apply the case definition to the test results of this hypothetical patient? The first positive test (PCR in week 1) complies with the case definition, which makes this patient count as a "case of gonorrhea." The second test (positive culture in week 2) also complies with the case definition, but falls within the aggregation window of 30 days after the last time that this patient was categorized as a "case." Therefore, this patient will not again be counted for the same diagnosis. The third and fourth tests are negative, so do

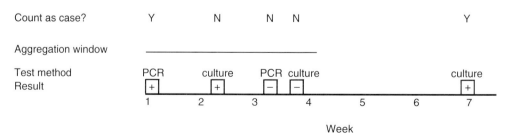

Fig 22.3 An example of five consecutive diagnostic test results for gonorrhea from a single patient within a period of 7 weeks and the interpretation of the ISIS case definition.

not comply with the case definition. The fifth test in week 6 does, and falls outside the aggregation window: the patient will now be labeled as "case of gonorrhea" for the second time in this example. With the case definitions in place, ISIS will count "episodes of infection" and is able to detect if patients experience multiple episodes of the same infection. The main reason, however, for developing the algorithm to apply case definitions, is to make sure that a patient is counted only once during an episode of infection, even though there may be several (different) positive test results in the database.

Some case definitions require that two or more test results of the same patient are interpreted together, such as with acute hepatitis B virus infections: if one patient has a test showing hepatitis B surface antigen in combination with IgM antibodies against hepatitis core antigen then the patient is labeled as "likely acute hepatitis B virus infection." These "surveillance case definitions" will be by no means as accurate at the individual level as true microbiological diagnosis; however, we assume that for surveillance purposes they will suffice.

We have also developed case definitions for certain syndromes. Since the ISIS laboratory data contain all negative test results, we have tried to define case definitions such as "suspected infection of the central nervous system," by looking at patients with microbiological tests on cerebrospinal fluid or "severe pulmonary infection" by selecting all patients who had a blood culture plus a test on pulmonary material within the same week. Though it has been possible to identify patients complying with those case definitions, more study is needed to determine the value for surveillance and early warning purposes.

Standardized reports

The data collected on notifications and laboratory test results, as described in the previous paragraphs, are stored in databases (an Ingres database for laboratory data and MS SQL Server for notifications) at the national level at RIVM. Both manual and automated analysis of surveillance data takes place within ISIS. The environment for analysis of data is a SAS Data Warehouse. For each of the notifiable diseases and each of the case definitions, standard-

ized reports are created daily, showing distribution per diagnosis of cases in time (week, month, and year) and place (MHS region), as displayed in Figure 22.4. In addition, age–sex distributions are produced for each disease [4].

For all notifiable diseases, a so-called "barometer" is produced daily, to indicate which diseases have a higher number than expected in the most recent 4-week period, and which have a lower number than expected (see Figure 22.5). The algorithm used is similar to the figure-one analysis that is used for weekly notification data in the *Morbidity and Mortality Weekly Report (MMWR)*, using Z scores.

Daily automated time series analysis

An early warning algorithm was developed for all surveillance data, in order to automatically detect any unexpected national increase in cases of any of the collected diagnoses [5]. The algorithm is a simple linear regression model, adjusted for seasonality, secular trends, and past outbreaks in a manner similar to that described by Farrington *et al.* and requires little parameter resetting or model checking [6]. Briefly, to calculate an expected total value for the current epidemiological week, a regression line is plotted through the totals in the nine epidemiological weeks centered on the same epidemiological week in the previous 5 years. For example, to calculate an expected value for week 20, a regression line is plotted through the values at weeks 16–24 of the previous 5 years as described by Widdowson *et al.* (2003). A threshold is calculated as 2.56 standard deviations above the expected value. Once an observed value is above this threshold, an alarm signal is generated on a Web page. The Web page with alarm signals is accessible only by a group of public health epidemiologists to facilitate their work to identify aberrations in the surveillance data in order to detect possible outbreaks or unexpected changes in trends.

Closing the surveillance circle: online interpretation of signals

Though a lot is gained by publishing automated surveillance reports online, in terms of timeliness they were relevant to public health. The analysts were also responsible for identifying and flagging news reports about any conditions that were notifiable under the International Health Regulations (i.e., cholera, plague, and yellow fever) or considered to have potentially serious public health consequences. Human analysis was carried out during "regular" daytime working hours. During public health emergencies (e.g., severe acute respiratory syndrome, SARS), however, the analysts' responsibilities were extended to 24/7 coverage, as they provided and disseminated status reports electronically on the situation around the clock.

News media sources and languages used to monitor relevant public health issues were expanded to be able to cover additional regions around the world. News media sources were originally limited to those in English and French. Later Arabic, Chinese (simplified and traditional), Russian, and Spanish sources were included. Additional analysts were recruited to process the non-English articles; their work consisted of reviewing and selecting relevant news reports, translating the headlines into English, and then disseminating to users electronically.

GPHIN Multilingual System (2004–Present)

Based on the experience gained from the prototype, the development of a multilingual platform was implemented in 2003 and launched in November 2004. This new multilingual system had to accommodate an increased volume of news reports and be able to adapt to the advanced information technologies and addition of languages.

Similar to the prototype version of GPHIN, the current GPHIN multilingual Internet-based system is composed of two critical and interdependent processes—an automated process and a human analysis process. The automated processes were implemented not to replace the GPHIN analysts but rather to assist them with tasks that computerized systems could accomplish much faster. For example, due to the increased volume of news reports daily, the categorization of news reports into taxonomy groups was automated. Key features of the multilingual platform include a relevancy scoring algorithm; machine translation engine; machine translation comprehensibility rating

algorithm; multilingual taxonomy; query function; and an archive.

Automated component

As shown in Figure 23.2, the automated process consists of a number of steps beginning with the monitoring for potential public health threats on a 24/7 basis. Through news aggregators, over 20,000 news media sources are monitored in eight languages (Arabic, Chinese—simplified and traditional, English, Farsi, French, Russian, and Spanish). Search syntaxes developed by GPHIN analysts are used to identify and gather relevant news reports; reports are then forwarded to the multilingual platform. News reports are further filtered and categorized according to the GPHIN system taxonomy. Categories in the taxonomy include human diseases, animal diseases, plant diseases, other biologics, chemical incidents, radioactive exposures, unsafe products, and natural disasters. In some cases news reports not captured by the automated process are manually entered into the GPHIN system.

Non-English news reports are automatically translated into English only. News reports in English are translated into all other non-English languages. The translated news reports provide the user with the essence of the article but are not the quality provided through professional translation. GPHIN's machine translation engines are powered by Nstein Technologies, Inc. (www.nstein.com/realtime.asp) and are designed to translate content at a fraction of the cost of professional translation. An algorithm rates the comprehensibility of a translated news report. Reports with low comprehensibility scores are reviewed and revised by analysts as needed.

A relevancy algorithm is then applied to prioritize the analysis of the news reports. Each news report is assigned a relevancy score based on keywords and terms present in the news report and in the GPHIN system taxonomy. News reports with a score of 30 or less are considered irrelevant and not available for viewing by users but are kept in the database. News reports with scores between 30 and 85 are reviewed by the analysts for relevancy before they are made available for viewing. During nonworking hours, the news reports that fall within this range are automatically made available

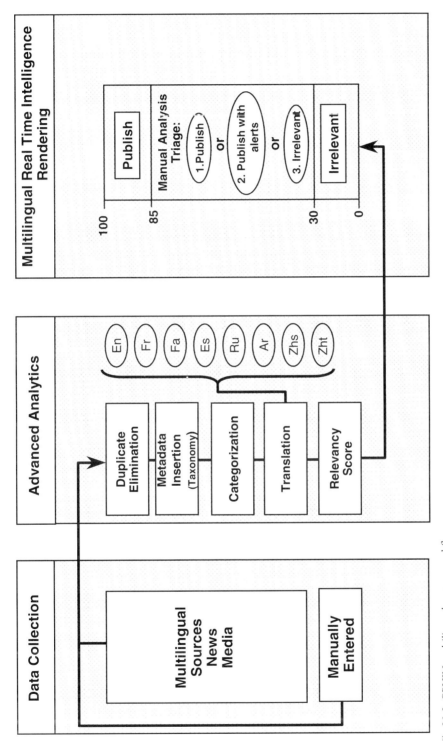

Fig 23.2 GPHIN multilingual system workflow.

monitoring of informal or unofficial sources of information such as news media. Based on the premise that no one institution will ever have the necessary resources to adequately respond to an outbreak of international concern, WHO established a network of partner institutions, the Global Outbreak Alert and Response Network (GOARN), that could be called upon to coordinate multidisciplinary international responses. As a partner of GOARN, the GPHIN system provides an efficient and reliable mechanism of access to the news media to assist in the early detection of relevant public health events.

On a daily basis, designated surveillance officers at WHO screen incoming e-mail communications and electronic information sources for reports of events of potential international concern. Sources of information are both formal and informal and include GPHIN, the WHO network, ministries of health and other government agencies or institutions, WHO Collaborating Centres, UN agencies, nongovernmental organizations, electronic discussion groups, news media, and personal communications.

When the source of information is informal, WHO seeks verification. Attempts to corroborate GPHIN reports are often performed or coordinated by WHO. An event is considered verified when the country's ministry of health (MOH), or the WHO country office on behalf of the MOH, provides information that confirms the occurrence of an outbreak, regardless of whether the etiology has been laboratory confirmed. An event is "discarded" when the MOH or the WHO country office on behalf of the MOH provides information that confirms the occurrence of a health event but adds that the occurrence was not serious, unusual, or unexpected. An event is "unverifiable" when WHO is unable to gather any further information despite repeated requests to the MOH. The vast majority of the verification process is conducted through electronic communication (e.g., e-mail) with telephone and fax communications used as secondary means.

CDC

In the United States, GPHIN is used extensively by the Centers for Disease Control and Prevention (CDC) through their Epidemic Exchange Program

(EpiX). EpiX provides a secure Web-based communication platform used by CDC officials, state and local health departments, poison control centers, and other public health professionals to access and share health surveillance information. Analysts at the CDC monitor and summarize GPHIN information about relevant public health events on a daily basis and post it on EpiX along with other sources of information. Over the past few years, GPHIN has become an important contributor to CDC's EpiX program. More recently EpiX has developed a module specialized in the collection and dissemination of relevant news media reports.

Successes and challenges

In the development of the GPHIN multilingual system, a set of criteria was established to ensure effectiveness and efficiency. The criteria were developed based on experience with the prototype and on the US CDC's guidelines for evaluating early-warning systems [10]. The following sections explore the criteria used to characterize the success of the GPHIN system.

Usefulness

The output of the GPHIN system has proven to be valuable both during and in the absence of a public health emergency. Since the WHO has the mandate to verify with countries any event that is of potential international concern, data were obtained from the WHO to assess what GPHIN's contribution has been in proportion to the other sources of information used by the WHO.

According to WHO data, from January 1, 1998, to December 31, 2005 (excluding events from February 10, 2003, to July 31, 2003, relating to the SARS outbreak), WHO identified 1752 events of potential international concern for which further information was sought. During this 5-year period, there were 136 additional events classified as "information only" that were excluded from the analysis. The initial reporting source is available for 1692 events, with data missing for 60 events in 1998 and 1999. News media was the initial reporting source for 787 (46%) of the events. GPHIN brought the media story to the attention of WHO in the vast majority of instances (649 or 82% of

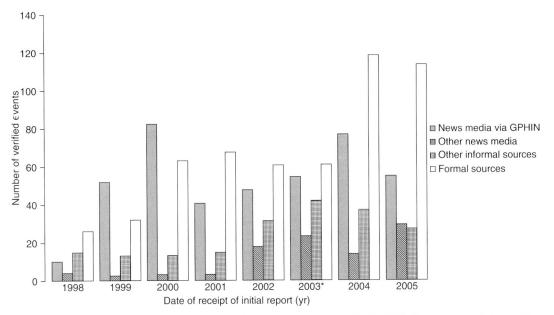

Fig 23.4 Number of verified events by year of receipt of initial report and source of initial report (*n* = 1256). *Excludes events related to SARS outbreak from February 10, 2003, to July 31, 2003. (Data source: World Health Organization.)

787 events) and its contribution is likely under-represented due to misclassification. Of the 1692 events, 1256 were verified (Figure 23.4). News media was the initial reporting source for 518 (41%) of the verified events and GPHIN played an important role by bringing the media story to the attention of WHO in 81% of these (422 of 518 verified events). The proportion of verified events for which news media was the initial reporting source has varied from year to year and it is difficult to interpret these variations given the changes of practice and personnel over this time period and the limitations of the two databases from which the data for this analysis were derived.

One of GPHIN's earliest significant achievements was in December 1998. Information gathered by the GPHIN system alerted the public health community to a new strain of influenza in northern China [11]. The GPHIN system was the first to provide preliminary information about the influenza outbreak in northern China. Other important contributions were during the SARS and avian influenza outbreaks beginning in 2003. In these situations, the media reports provided by GPHIN signaled significant changes in the evolution of the outbreak before WHO received official notification. The valuable contribution made by GPHIN was not only in the reporting on the magnitude of the outbreak, but also about related issues such as the type of control and prevention measures being considered and implemented by countries worldwide. The GPHIN analysts worked closely with the Department of Foreign Affairs and International Trade Canada to provide them with information to help determine what steps were needed to assist Canadians abroad. The GPHIN analysts provided similar support for the avian influenza outbreak in 2003. GPHIN continues to provide information about avian influenza outbreaks currently occurring around the world to officials in the Canadian Food Inspection Agency, the Food and Agriculture Organization of the United Nations, and the Office of International Epizootics.

While the information from news media is useful, there are ongoing challenges to ensure that the information is reliable and accurate. It is often difficult for GPHIN analysts to ascertain which

311

news reports provide accurate information. Over the years, analysts have become aware of news sources that may have motivations over and above providing news, including those that are political. The analysts consider this when sifting through numerous news reports. In addition, where possible, analysts select news reports in which the source for the information is an official from a healthcare organization, government, or international body such as WHO. There is value in receiving several different news sources report on an event. This enables the analysts and users to get a better picture of a situation. For example, one news report might focus on the clinical aspects of the cases involved in the outbreak, whereas another might focus on the type of control measures implemented and associated challenges.

One of the challenges with news reports is the false positives that occur occasionally. An important task of the GPHIN analysts is to understand the style of writing and the use of language in different regions of the world. For example, in some parts of the world, the majority of the initial reports of outbreaks are often described as "mysterious outbreaks" or "unusual disease." These outbreaks later turn out to be situations that are endemic and seasonal in that specific region. Another difficulty is deciphering the cause of an event when information has been incorrectly translated by the journalist from one language to another. A good example is an outbreak of chicken pox reported in Yemen, which was incorrectly translated from Arabic to English as smallpox. In Arabic, the word for chicken pox is very similar to the word for smallpox and can easily be misinterpreted. In this situation, the GPHIN analysts took less than 15 minutes to assess the accuracy of the news report. Subsequent news reports in Chinese and French clarified that the journalist had made an error and that the outbreak in Yemen was chicken pox. The initial report was therefore not sent as an alert to users but kept in the database with the other news reports for viewing. In a case such as this, GPHIN informs users that there was a journalist's error in the report.

Timeliness

As an early-warning system for potential public health threats, timeliness is paramount. A number of steps have been taken to meet this objective for GPHIN. One is to take advantage of today's advancements in communication and information technology to shorten the time between the publication and retrieval of the news reports. The GPHIN system gathers news reports every 15 minutes. Automated processing of the news reports means that they are ready for viewing in less than a minute. In some cases, news aggregators have agreements with news agencies that permit the retrieval of news reports a few hours or as early as a day or two prior to official publication.

New technologies are enabling faster dissemination of news. Technologies such as speech to text and text to speech are becoming more mature. For example, a statement made by an official during a press conference can automatically be transformed into text and disseminated worldwide. Also, any breaking news or alerts generated by the GPHIN system can be disseminated to users via cell phone, Blackberry^{TM}, and other digital tools.

Another approach is the use of different languages. Over the years it has been proven that monitoring news reports in different languages is necessary for the timely reporting of public health events. For example, early reports gathered by the GPHIN system in November 2002 about an atypical respiratory illness in mainland China were in Chinese [12]. The first report in English retrieved by the GPHIN system referring to the atypical outbreak in mainland China was not until January 2003. Similarly, the initial reporting of possible outbreaks of avian influenza in Azerbaijan and Iran were in Farsi.

A significant gap in GPHIN's early-warning capability lies in the timely identification of significant alerts by human analysts. Since generation of the alerts requires manual review by the analysts, there is a delay in alert distribution during nonworking hours in Canada. Thus, analyst coverage is not able to address the time zone differences of users worldwide. It is only during public health emergencies identified by PHAC officials or the WHO that the analysts work on a 24/7 basis to ensure that updated information is provided to users quickly. Solutions to address this gap are currently being considered and discussed.

Sensitivity and specificity

The GPHIN system must identify relevant information and separate it from the "noise" in the system. Several measures are in place to meet this objective. First, the search criteria developed by the analysts to monitor and retrieve relevant news reports involves a delicate balance between being too specific and being too general. The criteria are adjusted regularly to ensure that all public health issues of concern are captured. The next step is in the application of the relevancy scoring algorithm. It is an ongoing challenge to assign appropriate values that will be sensitive enough to distinguish a relevant from an irrelevant news report, taking into consideration the style of writing of the journalist. On an average, approximately 10% of 2000 articles processed are flagged as irrelevant. Noise reduction in the system can also be improved by eliminating duplicate news reports. The GPHIN system has been effective in reducing the number of news reports with nearly identical text. Over a period from January 1, 2005, to June 30, 2006, 1,334,784 news reports were retrieved by the GPHIN system and of these 338,660 (25%) were flagged as duplicates (Figure 23.5).

It is difficult for the automated processes described above to filter out news reports that are irrelevant because the journalist's choice of words or style of writing. For example, during sports games, the term "yellow fever" is often used to describe the temperament of the sports fans (Box 23.1, Article 1). When other terms such as "outbreak" and "struck" are included in news reports that are not health related (Box 23.1, Article 2), modifications to the exclusion search criteria are difficult to devise. GPHIN analysts are the final component that helps to ensure the relevance of news reports in the system.

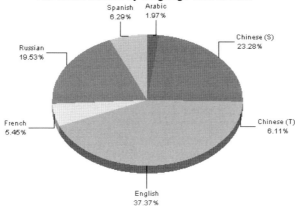

Net news stories by language distribution

	News stories	Duplicates	Net news stories
Arabic	19,634	0	19,634
Chinese (S)	313,658	81,795	231,863
Chinese (T)	74,402	13,562	60,840
English	541,149	168,918	372,231
French	72,987	18,669	54,318
Russian	230,668	36,076	194,592
Spanish	82,286	19,640	62,646
Total	**1,334,784**	**338,660**	**996,124**

Fig 23.5 Proportion of duplicate news reports—January 1, 2005, to June 30, 2006.

Box 23.1 Writing style of journalist.

Article 1: *Yellow fever*
November 18, 2003
Tampa Tribune
An *epidemic* of penalties has thwarted many drives, resulting in a three-game losing streak and essentially leaving the Bucs' season on *life support*

Article 2: *Yellow fever grips Oasis*
February 24, 2006
Kalgoorlie Miner
An *outbreak* of *yellow fever struck* the Oasis last Friday when John Paul College held its annual swimming carnival

---

Flexibility

The multilingual GPHIN system is scaleable and adaptable on many fronts. The search criteria can be easily adjusted with results evident within 30 minutes. For example, should a new disease be identified, the analysts will develop new search criteria to be used by the news aggregators in the eight languages. The new search criteria would, for example, include the symptoms and the geographic distribution of the disease. Within 30 minutes from the time of the update, relevant news reports about the new disease can be retrieved. In the meantime, while the changes are being automated, the analysts are able to manually gather information about the new disease directly from the databases of the news aggregators and immediately distribute these articles to the users. The multilingual platform is also scaleable. The platform was designed in modules making it relatively easy to add other modules and to incorporate new technologies or languages.

Stability

The stability of the GPHIN system requires not only that the platform is operational with limited downtime but also that there is adequate support staff to operate, maintain, and continue to enhance the system. The GPHIN system has been stable and robust. Maintenance activities that require downtime of the system for more than a few minutes are performed during a time of day when news reports disseminated by news media and use of the GPHIN system in all time zones are minimal. Support from the team of analysts and information technology specialists dedicated to GPHIN is essential to the stability of the system. The team of IT specialists who support the GPHIN system has been instrumental in managing technical difficulties that have arisen. The team continuously assesses the functionality of the GPHIN system to see where improvements can be made that are of benefit to the users and analysts.

Costs

The operational, upgrade, and development costs of the GPHIN system approach $3.5 million annually, a significant amount within the constraints of the budget of the Canadian government. A substantial proportion of the operational expenses are for the cost of licenses from news aggregators for use of the news reports, followed by the cost of licenses for the machine translation software for eight languages. Following the launch of the new GPHIN system, a subscription program was instituted that required users of the system to make financial contributions toward the continued enhancements of the GPHIN system. This has funded the successful implementation of required upgrades and enhancements, and ensured that the system is user-friendly and remains on the leading edge of global surveillance technology. However, shrinking budgets of public health institutions indicate a need to explore alternative sources of funding for GPHIN.

An organization may request access to GPHIN by contacting the program at:
Global Public Health Intelligence Network (GPHIN)
Centre for Emergency Preparedness and Response
Public Health Agency of Canada
100 Colonnade Road, Postal Locator 6201A
Ottawa, Ontario K1A 0K9
Canada
Tel: (613) 957-2715
Fax: (613) 952-8286
E-mail: GPHIN-RMISP@phac-aspc.gc.ca

Information about the organization including why and how it intends to use GPHIN information in the context of public health will be requested in order to determine the appropriate subscription package for the organization. It is important that potential users understand that in order to use GPHIN efficiently, there has to be capacity within the organization to ensure the ongoing and timely monitoring and follow-up of GPHIN incoming information.

Once there is agreement on how the GPHIN system will be used, a subscription agreement is then drawn up that outlines the type of service to be provided to the organization, policies on using the GPHIN content, and payment.

Future of the GPHIN program

The continuing trend of globalization coupled with gaps or failures within public health infrastructures means that global public health security is increasingly under threat. There is an ongoing need for mechanisms to help alert the public health community worldwide of potential threats.

GPHIN has demonstrated the capability to support the early-warning functions of surveillance systems and to complement formal surveillance systems in monitoring the evolution of disease outbreaks. At the heart of the International Health Regulations (2005) is the need to establish and ensure effective global surveillance for the early detection of public health emergencies of international concern (PHEIC) [13]. In order to meet this requirement, WHO Member States must build their surveillance and response capacity to detect, assess, and report events that may constitute PHEIC and to liaise with WHO. GPHIN will be able to contribute to the implementation of the International Health Regulations (2005) by strengthening the early-warning function of national surveillance systems. GPHIN may be especially useful in Member States with limited resources for surveillance infrastructure or with a reluctance to report events that may constitute PHEIC. As long as GPHIN maintains its competitive value, it will continue to play an important role in global public health surveillance in providing WHO and other public health institutions with relevant and timely information from news media sources.

The GPHIN program can be enhanced to provide more support to the Canadian and international public health community. It can continue to establish collaborative arrangements and networks with experts in the areas of public health that the GPHIN system covers. This would help guide the improvement in monitoring, gathering, and analysis of public health threats worldwide. For example, the GPHIN system could enhance its role in monitoring for epizootics and zoonotics that are linked to a risk to human health. The GPHIN system is one of the sources of information used by the Food and Agriculture Organization of the United Nations and the Office of International Epizootics for monitoring livestock and emerging transboundary diseases.

Continued advances in communications and information technology will serve to make more news readily available. It is a challenge to the public health community to use information from the news media effectively and efficiently. While the value of the news media is recognized, the idea of using news media as an informal source of information in global public health surveillance has not been fully embraced by many in the public health community. Without this source of information, however, there will be a critical gap in the ability to detect potential public health threats worldwide—especially in areas where public health infrastructures are weak or nonexistent. While motivations for the news media and the public health community may differ (i.e., increased readership and profit for media versus effective health communications), it is possible for representatives from these two distinct fields to cultivate a positive relationship. Establishing a way to work together would increase the opportunities to use news media as a medium for monitoring and detecting potential public health threats [14].

The public health community must understand the importance of a bidirectional passage of information. It is only recently that the public health community recognized the benefits of working with the news media to help dispel false rumours about public health events or threats and to provide the general public with accurate information quickly [15,16]. Some news media agencies have also recognized the importance of their role in presenting accurate information to the public—the public health community should capitalize on building relationships with these more responsible news agencies.

Information is the primary tool of public health surveillance. As data from different sources such as syndromic surveillance systems, geographic information systems, and epidemiologic studies become readily available, new ways to manage and process the information must be adopted. The challenge is how to use all the different sources and types of information (formal versus informal, structured versus unstructured) in a useful, efficient, and timely way to detect, verify, analyze, assess, and investigate public health events that may have serious consequences.

Summary

This chapter includes discussion of the ability of the innovative multilingual GPHIN system to use news media and make valuable contributions to global public health surveillance. GPHIN has helped change the way global health surveillance is organized and practiced [17]. It has helped to revitalize international monitoring of disease outbreaks; it also weakens the ability of governments to control or conceal reports of disease outbreaks. Last, it has provided WHO with new forms of leverage in its efforts to encourage Member States to confirm and act on outbreaks occurring within their borders [17].

The GPHIN system will continue to exist as long as there is an increased threat to global health security due to globalization and weak or nonexistent public health infrastructures. It is now a functional element within the Web of interrelated subsystems and networks which make up the global public health surveillance structure. With the continued advances in communications and information technologies, the GPHIN system will continue to evolve as its ability to monitor and gather preliminary information about important public health events is enhanced effectively.

Acknowledgments

The authors are indebted to Drs. Uhthoff, Guerrero, Ni, and Xu; Ms. Ghiasbeglou; Ms. Ghanem; Ms. Rodionova; Mr. Blench; and Mr. Dubois for their zealous dedication and contribution to global public health surveillance. They also acknowledge Drs. Nowak's and Lake's contributions to the development of the GPHIN prototype. The authors thank Drs. Buehler, M'ikanatha, and Lynnfield for their support and careful manuscript review.

References

1 Langmuir AD. The surveillance of communicable diseases of national importance. *N Engl J Med* 1963;**268**(4):182–92.

2 World Health Organization. Report of the technical discussions at the twenty-first World Health Assembly on national and global surveillance of communicable diseases. A21/Technical Discussions/5; May 18, 1968.

3 Lederberg J, Shope RE, Oaks SE (eds.) *Emerging Infections: Microbial Threats to Health in the United States.* Washington, DC: National Academy Press; 1992.

4 World Health Organization. Communicable disease prevention and control: new, emerging and re-emerging infectious diseases. Report by the Director-General 48th World Health Assembly. A48/15; February 22, 1995.

5 Health Canada, 1998. Connection for better health: strategic issues. Interim Report. Available from: http://www.hc-sc.gc.ca/hcs-sss/pubs/ehealth-esante/1998-connect-connexe-achi-ccis/index_e.html#letter. Accessed June 27, 2006.

6 Health Surveillance Working Group. The Strategic Plan April 1 2000 to March 31 2003: the network for health surveillance in Canada. Available from: http://www.phac-aspc.gc.ca/csc-ccs/pdf/NHSC-strategic-plan_e.pdf. Accessed June 27, 2006.

7 Heymann DL, Rodier GR. WHO Operational Support Team to the Global Outbreak Alert and Response Network. Hot spots in a wired world: WHO surveillance of emerging and re-emerging infectious diseases. *Lancet Infect Dis* December 2001;**1**:345–53.

8 Grein TW, Kamara KO, Rodier G, *et al*. Rumors of disease in the global village: outbreak verification. *Emerg Infect Dis* March–April 2000;**6**(2):97–102.

9 Public Health Agency of Canada. Health Canada's preparedness for and response to respiratory infections season and the possible re-emergence of SARS; Fall/Winter 2003–2004. Available from: http://www.phac-aspc.gc.ca/sars-sras/ris-sir/index.html#22. Accessed July 9, 2006.

10 Centers for Disease Control and Prevention. Framework for evaluating public health surveillance systems for early detection of outbreaks: recommendations from the CDC Working Group. *MMWR Morb Mortal*

Wkly Rep 2004;**53**(RR5):1–11. Available from: http://www.cdc.gov/mmwr/preview/mmwrhtml/rr5305a1.htm. Accessed July 6, 2006.

11 Balkisson D. Canada begins global inspection for infection; March 12, 1999. Available from: http://www.carleton.ca/Capital_News/12031999/f4.htm. Accessed July 6, 2006.

12 Heymann DL, Rodier G. Global surveillance, national surveillance, and SARS. *Emerg Infect Dis* February 2004;**10**(2):173–5.

13 Baker M, Fidler D. Global Public Health Surveillance under New International Health Regulations. *Emerg Infect Dis* July 2006;**12**(7):1058–65.

14 Southwell, BG. Communication of information about surveillance and outbreaks. In: M'ikanatha, NM. Lynfield R, Van Beneden CA, De Valk H (eds.), *Infectious Disease Surveillance*. London: Blackwell; 2007:417–426.

15 Garrett L. Understanding media's response to epidemics. *Public Health Rep* 2001;**116**(suppl 2):87–91.

16 Samaan G, Patel M, Olowokure B, *et al.* Rumor surveillance and avian influenza H5N1. *Emerg Infect Dis* March 2005;**11**(3):2192–5.

17 Mykhalovskiy E, Weir L. The global public health intelligence network and early warning outbreak detection: a Canadian contribution to global health (Commentary). *Can J Public Health* 2006;**97**(1):42–4.

24 National notifiable disease surveillance in Egypt

Frank Mahoney, Rana A. Hajjeh, Gerald F. Jones, Maha Talaat & Abdel-Nasser Mohammed Abdel Ghaffar

Introduction

The development of surveillance systems that provide quality data to local and national health authorities on a timely basis is a high priority in public health. This chapter describes the reorganization and enhancement of communicable disease surveillance in Egypt including the transition from paper-based to computerized reporting. The early adoption of computers in the health sector has primarily been in the areas of personnel management, accounting, and monitoring the administration of clinical services, with limited emphasis on management of public health data [1,2]. In the early 1980s, the utilization of computers to support public health activities in Egypt became evident, particularly to assist in the analysis and management of statistics such as vital records and immunization coverage data. By the mid to late 1980s, computers became more widely used to support research efforts in epidemiology and demography with rapid growth in utilization after establishment of the Field Epidemiology Training Program (FETP) in 1993 [3]. The FETP program has been actively involved in the development of the National Egyptian Diseases Surveillance System (NEDSS) in Egypt.

NEDSS evolved out of activities supported by the Egyptian Ministry of Health and Population (MOHP), the World Health Organization (WHO), and United States (US) government agencies in the late 1990s. During that time, there was considerable interest in the area of communicable disease surveillance after publication by the Institute of Medicine on the Global Threat of Emerging Infectious Diseases [4]. Recognizing the mutual objectives of the MOHP, WHO, and USG technical partners, a working group was formed to coordinate assistance in the area of disease surveillance. Chaired by the WHO country representative to Egypt, the group organized and supported an in-depth review of the communicable disease surveillance system in Egypt and subsequently developed a long-term plan and budget to strengthen surveillance. This plan evolved over time and was extremely useful in managing diverse resources available to the MOHP, including support from the World Bank, the US Agency for International Development (USAID), and the US Department of Defense Global Emerging Infections Surveillance System (GEIS). USAID played a key role in providing financial support; the main technical partner was the US Naval Medical Research Unit No. 3 with considerable input from the US Centers for Disease Control and Prevention (CDC).

Background: communicable disease surveillance in Egypt

With a population of more than 72 million persons, Egypt is one of the most populous countries in the Middle East. The MOHP is organized into 255 administrative districts located in 27 governorates. Surveillance for communicable diseases is a high priority because infectious diseases continue to be a leading cause of death and disability. Traditionally, communicable disease surveillance has been restricted to the collection of data from public sector facilities and focused on monitoring hospital admissions to a network of 108 infectious disease hospitals throughout the republic. These "fever hospitals" are designated as the primary referral centers for treatment of patients with priority infectious diseases. Other reporting sources include public sector health units and MOHP general hospitals. Reporting from the general hospitals is ad hoc at best and there is considerable underreporting from public sector clinics. University and private sector hospitals do not report communicable diseases to the MOHP and there is no legislation requiring private providers to report. Surveys on health-seeking behaviors suggest that the majority of patients with febrile illness seek care from private sector providers and population-based surveillance studies indicate that 50–60% of patients with diseases such as typhoid fever and brucellosis are managed in the primary care private sector [5,6]. Thus, there is considerable underreporting in the MOHP surveillance system.

In the fall of 1999, WHO organized a mission to conduct an in-depth review of the communicable disease surveillance system in Egypt. Findings from this review included the following constraints:
• Several different "official" lists of reportable diseases with >50 reportable conditions including many with limited public health importance
• No standardized case definitions of reportable diseases
• A paper-based reporting system of aggregate data to the national level
• Limited analysis and feedback of data at all levels
• Poor quality of data without laboratory confirmation of disease
• Multiple reporting systems that often included discrepant results

The consultation outlined a plan to strengthen the surveillance system with the following key recommendations:

A. Development of an organizational structure for surveillance at the district, governorate, and national levels

B. Implementation of a process to review and revise the list of reportable diseases

C. Development of surveillance guidelines with standardized case definitions and case investigations

D. Training to strengthen epidemiology and laboratory capacity at all levels

E. Improved reporting from private sector providers

F. Computerization of data at all levels to facilitate data analysis and feedback

Strategic approach for strengthening surveillance

Following the in-depth review, WHO organized a surveillance working group with program heads from the disease control programs in the MOHP (e.g., immunizations, tuberculosis, vector-borne diseases, HIV, foodborne diseases) and key technical partners. This group implemented a strategy to strengthen surveillance over the next several months.

Prioritization of diseases for reporting

The surveillance working group reviewed and revised the list of notifiable diseases based on a structured process to evaluate the public health importance of each disease (www.who.int/csr/resources/publications/surveillance/). While the report from the WHO mission recommended restricting the list of reportable disease to no more than 16 priority conditions, the surveillance working group recommended a list of 28 priority diseases including 14 Group A diseases that were to be immediately reported to the District Health Office, 7 Group B diseases to be reported weekly, and 6 Group C diseases that were to be reported on a monthly basis (Table 24.1).

The group also reviewed reporting forms for each disease and reached a consensus on core data elements that would be reported for all diseases and supplemental information that would be collected for selected diseases. A plan was outlined for the development of software to support management of information in this new approach for communicable disease surveillance.

Organizational structure for surveillance

To facilitate human resource development, the Minister of Health issued a decree calling for the

with plans to install such systems throughout the country.

USAID supported the purchase of computers, servers, and other critical equipment and provided resources for training and logistic support. To ensure sustainability of program support, USAID support was linked to efforts by the MOHP to establish a line item in the MOHP budget for operational activities of the ESU. In addition, the MOHP supported recruitment of new staff, renovations of district health offices, and installation of phone lines and equipment.

Guidelines development

Surveillance guidelines were developed and adapted to different practice settings and distributed to diverse reporting sources. Case definitions were based on WHO criteria including recommended laboratory criteria for reporting suspect, probable, and confirmed disease (www.who.int/csr/resources/publications/surveillance/). During the development of software, these definitions were used to develop automatic data validation routines on data entry and to provide feedback on errors on case investigation forms and reports.

Software development

Development team
To facilitate the computerization of data, a software development team was organized with primary responsibility for development assigned to the US CDC in collaboration with technical experts from the MOHP and NAMRU-3.

System requirements
Because of limited experience with computer use at all levels, the design team envisioned a system that would be workable and acceptable to persons with minimal experience and would include an Arabic interface and menu-driven data entry screens. The MOHP wanted a surveillance system that was sensitive to detect disease changes in a community as well as timely enough to ensure the information could be acted upon quickly. Considerable time was devoted to outlining system requirements that would be responsive to these general needs as well the needs

of different disease control programs. As anticipated, the needs evolved over time and the system requirements were reflected in multiple versions of the software being developed. End-user input was obtained during site visits to provincial and district health offices as well as through a systematic review of system components at the national level. System requirements were developed and agreed upon in writing as each version was developed (see Appendix).

Database architecture and design
Based on core features, design requirements, existing information technology (IT) infrastructure, and data management capacity, the team elected to work in a provider–client model using a compiled application in Sequence Query Language (SQL) (Figure 24.2). The front-end of the system utilized Microsoft Access for development of the user interface with MS SQL Server (and Microsoft Desktop Engine (MSDE)) as the back-end for data management. The database was developed with a modular design modeled after National Electronic Telecommunications System for Surveillance (NETSS) in the US where modules can be added/linked without affecting the overall database structure. Each module was developed to be maintained independently. Thus, data-specific modules or updated modules can be added or deleted to the system.

MS SQL was selected as a database engine based on several features. It allowed for seamless integration with operating systems that were used in Egypt including MS Office Suite. The application could be scalable from a simple workstation to a large application with anticipated evolution of the system over time. MS SQL was being supported by Microsoft in Egypt with training and certification courses which had been attended by MOHP personnel. It was anticipated that development costs would be low since MSDE was freely distributed with MS SQL server and only a limited number of licenses for MS SQL would be needed. Other appealing features of MS SQL included the ability to export to several different programs using MS Excel messaging and performance features including processing speed and the capacity to handle large numbers of records. It was anticipated the software could be migrated to a

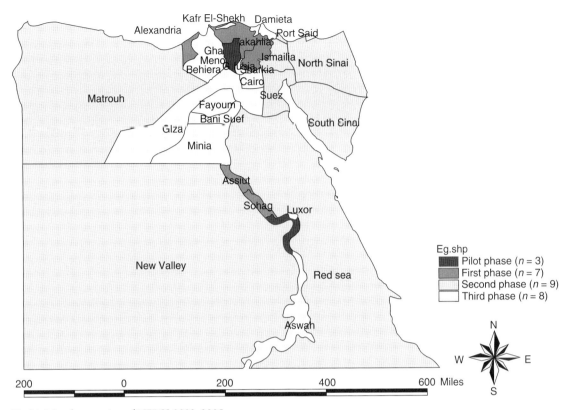

Fig 24.2 Implementation of NEDSS 2002–2005.

Web-based environment over time, pending interest and needs of the MOHP.

The relational database was designed with a core data entry screen and disease-specific data entry screens. A five-field key was established as a unique identifier to link the core screen to supplement disease-specific case information. The software was designed with business rules and pick-lists to facilitate data entry by novel users and to minimize errors. Pick lists were used in a hierarchical fashion from governorate down to the village level to establish residence. In addition, code was written to filter appropriate responses for selected diseases. Population tables were included to calculate and map district-level incidence additional features included aberration detection routines and outbreak alerts.

Data security features included the assignment of a password login for all users and assigned admin-istrators roles at all levels. Menu-driven feedback reports are available at all levels. At any point in the system, users can click on an icon and switch from an Arabic or English environment. Feedback reports are available at all levels in both languages. In fever hospitals with >50 beds ($n = 57$), code was written to accommodate data entry at the facility level using the hospital admissions and discharge log books as a source of reports.

Strengthening laboratory-based surveillance

In parallel with efforts to strengthen epidemiology capacity, the MOHP upgraded laboratories to support reporting of laboratory-confirmed disease. Most of these efforts were directed to providing equipment and training in the provincial level public health laboratories and laboratories in the infectious disease hospitals with >50 beds. Guidelines were developed with standardized procedures for processing of clinical samples using MOHP-approved diagnostic algorithms and reagents. Multiple workshops were conducted to standardize practices and improve services with emphasis on laboratory management. The Central Public Health Laboratory developed logistic capacity to ensure adequate supplies of basic diagnostic reagents and supplies (e.g., blood culture media, serology reagents, consumable supplies) and implemented a quality assurance program with supervision and monitoring visits. Using input from MOHP laboratory personnel, "SLIME" (Software for Laboratory Information Management in Egypt) software was developed with features that supported reporting of notifiable diseases.

Piloting and implementation of NEDSS

The beta version of the software was released in 2001 in three governorates. Based on feedback from the pilot utilization, the software was debugged and Version 1 was released in 2003. Several lessons were learned in the release of the beta version including problems with lack of dedicated staff, inadequate space for setup of computers and data entry, and limited access to phone lines. Software bugs included problems with report generators and file transfer protocols.

Training of master trainers was used to install the software in a phased manner over a 3-year period (Figures 24.2 and 24.3). In each phase, computers were delivered and infrastructure established to support reporting in nine provinces. After training

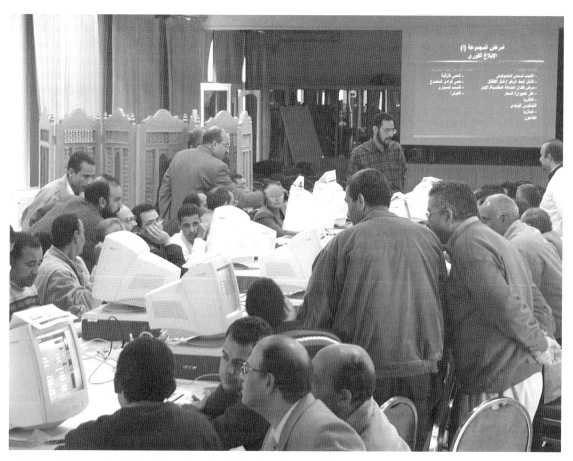

Fig 24.3 Training session for district and provincial level surveillance officers in Egypt.

and installation, follow-up visits were conducted after 1–2 months to provide on-site training and troubleshoot problems.

Training was conducted using a multidisciplinary team of clinicians, epidemiologists, and IT personnel from the ESU and NAMRU-3. Information management specialists were trained to install and maintain the software at the national and provincial levels. An epidemiology course on surveillance was organized for provincial and district surveillance officers with specific orientation to new surveillance guidelines and reporting system. A follow-up course focused on NEDSS data entry and data management at all levels. An example of the data screen is shown in Figure 24.4. Courses were initially conducted with provincial level staff who then assisted with training of district-level staff in their own province. Since many of the district health

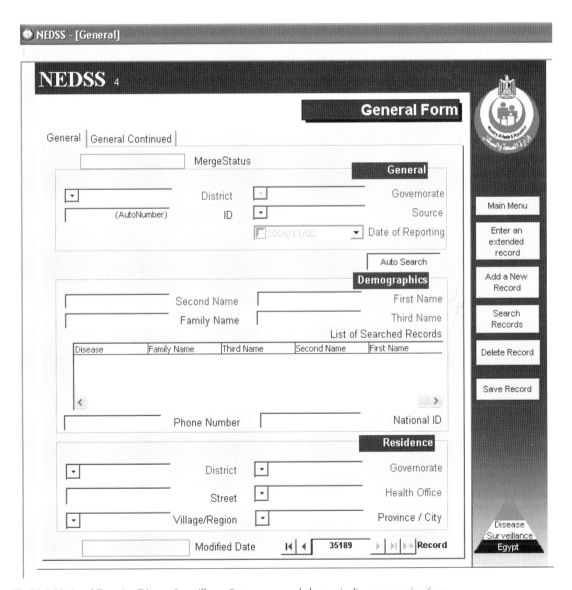

Fig 24.4 National Egyptian Disease Surveillance System—general electronic disease reporting form.

Table 24.2 Timeline and monitoring of key process indicators for implementation of electronic reporting in Egypt, 2002–2006.

Process indicators	Timeline				
	2002 (Beta)	2003 (Phase 1)	2004 (Phase 2)	2005 (Phase 3)	2006
Percent of governorates ($n = 27$) with NEDSS functioning	7.5%	33%	66%	100%	100%
Percent of governorates with dial-up connectivity	NA	30%	100%	100%	100%
Percent of governorates with servers	NA	NA	41%	100%	100%
Districts ($n = 243^*$) with NEDSS functioning	7%	34%	73%	100%	100%
Percent of districts with dial-up connectivity	0	0	31%	100%	100%
Timeliness of reports from governorates	NA	NA	19%	74%	85%
Completeness of reports from governorates	NA	NA	18%	59%	100%
Number of persons trained at the governorate and district level	82	282	606	834	867

*Two new districts were established in 2006.

personnel were novel users, NEDSS training included orientation to and use of computers and emphasized data entry, routine analysis and interpretation of data, backup of data, and file transfer procedures.

Monitoring and evaluation, system modification

The transition to NEDSS was monitored with joint supervisory visits by technical teams from the MOHP and NAMRU-3. These visits included monitoring progress in data collection, entry, transfer, and feedback to reporting sources and included considerable on-the-job training. The MOHP has followed a number of process indicators to monitor implementation of NEDSS (Table 24.2).

In 2006, a routine system of monitoring and supervision was implemented to ensure sustainability of NEDSS implementation relying on the Governorate Surveillance Coordinators to visit various reporting sources every 2 months. Standard data collection tools were developed for use by governorate-level staff that were trained on calculating performance indicators to identify strengths and weaknesses in system implementation.

Discussion and lessons learned

There were a number of lessons learned in the implementation of NEDSS that may be of use to other countries considering development of electronic reporting systems.

Developing consensus and timelines to change from a paper-based to a more efficient and accurate electronic reporting system

The change from paper-based reporting to NEDSS in Egypt has been challenging. NEDSS is the first information management system to be widely distributed within the health sector where there is an entrenched and labor-intensive bureaucracy maintaining paper-based systems. The introduction of computers to manage information has been viewed with suspicion, particularly, if district and provincial managers cannot "see" what has been recorded in a computer. The current culture of communication in the MOHP places a great deal of emphasis on placing seals or stamps on "official" information, and it has been difficult to gain this recognition for data that are electronically transmitted. To assure colleagues about the accuracy of the information, the ESU has spent considerable efforts to validate accuracy of information including quantitative comparisons of NEDSS with source data. On a macroscale, a change in the political environment and wide-scale adoption of computerized health information systems is just now penetrating the health sector.

Identifying resources to support implementation at all levels

Investment in public health surveillance systems is challenging in countries with limited resources and where there is a rapidly growing population with increased demand for new technology and advanced clinical services. This competition for resources is a key constraint in the development of information systems that do not generate income. There has been long-standing support from WHO and other international partners for surveillance activities; however, it is often restricted to specific disease programs and funding lines. US support for communicable disease surveillance became available after publication of a Presidential Directive (NSTC-7) that declared that international capacity for infectious disease surveillance was inadequate to protect the health of the US population. NSTC-7 specifically directed US government agencies to work together to strengthen surveillance capacity internationally. It is estimated that the total cost from external partners to support this project was $2.5 million. USAID and the World Bank provided much of the support.

This project also required considerable investment in human resources. Generally, the MOHP was able to assign existing staff as surveillance coordinators at the provincial and district levels. However, it was difficult to identify staff at the healthcare facility level, prompting the MOHP to support the establishment of new data management positions. This was a high priority for the MOHP given the considerable interest at the global level on rapid communication of surveillance information [7–9].

Anticipating problems with transparency in reporting and developing methods to edit records at different levels

Transparency in reporting has been a difficult issue to manage. In the past, surveillance information was not easily accessed and editing of information occurred at different levels. NEDSS has been designed such that the "truth" resides at the district level and that records cannot be changed once they have been sent forward to the provincial and national health offices. For diseases where reporting may have significant economic or political implica-

tions, district health officers usually do not report before receiving the approval from the central authorities; as in many countries, information on the occurrence of selected diseases is often restricted to those with a "need to know."

In addition to adjusting to this new transparency in disease reporting, the inability to edit records at a higher level has been problematic, particularly for disease control programs when supplemental information on case reports may be available at a higher level. For example, serologic testing for measles is conducted at the national laboratory and results are sent to the federal focal point for measles. It has been challenging to route this information back to the district level and update the case record. Indeed, it has been challenging to route laboratory information within the same institution into NEDSS, prompting the software development team to write programs to merge information from SLIME with NEDSS at the healthcare facility level.

Developing flexibility in the flow of information

Other challenges with the current architecture of NEDSS include the inability to transfer case records between districts. This transfer may occasionally be necessary when, for example, patients seek care in healthcare facilities located in neighboring districts. The current design of NEDSS does not allow flow of information between districts electronically; thus, paper notification is required to establish a case record in the district of residence.

Avoiding "data collection paralysis" through work force development and support

Health information systems include two key interrelated components including the process of compiling and presenting information in a "usable" format and the process of using this information for data-based decision making [10,11]. Generally, NEDSS has been very successful in improving and streamlining the process of data collection; however, it has been much more difficult to demonstrate the usefulness of the system in efforts to improve public health programs. This "data collection mode paralysis" was also a key constraint identified during the original assessment of the surveillance system and is a common problem, especially in newly

327

established surveillance systems in countries with limited resources.

Effective surveillance at the district level requires a workforce with a broad range of clinical, epidemiologic, and analytical skills [12]. The establishment of district and provincial surveillance officers as the primary "users" of surveillance information is a new concept in Egypt. In the past, surveillance for communicable diseases was a highly centralized process with most of the information being sent to the MOHP-CDC for in-depth analysis and response. The decentralization of this responsibility has been challenging since district health offices often have broad range of program responsibilities and limited resources and incentives to respond to communicable disease surveillance information. During deployment, most of the NEDSS training focused on the process of routine surveillance and outbreak response with limited emphasis on case investigation and case management. Other than HIV and tuberculosis, most of the disease control programs offer limited guidance on case management and response at the community level.

Persons responsible for managing disease control programs should be engaged and take ownership of surveillance activities

The limited utilization of NEDSS for public health action also stems from the organizational structure of the ESU. The ESU was modeled after the Epidemiology and Program Office in the CDC [13] in the US with the intention to create a surveillance activity to serve diverse MOHP programs, including those for injuries and chronic diseases. Unlike the Epidemiology and Program Office, however, the ESU was created outside the MOHP-Communicable Disease Control department and under the supervision of the First Undersecretary of Health; thus, there is a separation of persons responsible for collecting of data from those who are responsible for responding to the data. This fragmentation is further exacerbated by the separation of key program staff such as the Expanded Program on Immunization being located in the Department of Maternal and Child Health and outside of the MOHP-CDC. This separation of surveillance staff from disease control program staff has been dysfunctional, particularly since both groups are part of a larger bureaucracy and have limited interactions and/or opportunities to work together.

Ensuring access and effective utilization of NEDSS data

Currently, there are four to five epidemiologists working on NEDSS at the national level. The roles and responsibilities of these staff are not well defined and their capacity to provide meaningful oversight and analysis of information is limited. In particular, while basic reports are routinely generated, there is very limited interpretation of data to monitor the impact of public health programs. The ESU staff provides access to NEDSS for all disease control programs but has not had the time to assist program managers in data analysis and interpretation and it has been challenging to get focal points for different disease control programs to use NEDSS to facilitate better public health response to surveillance information. For example, there is very limited analysis of data from the extended records despite considerable efforts in including this information in NEDSS.

The MOHP is more "right-sized" in the field of information technology and is able to troubleshoot and maintain NEDSS as a reporting system with good IT staff available at the national and provincial levels. Thus, most of the field support for NEDSS is information technology-related with limited emphasis on responding to surveillance information. The development of an effective epidemiologically oriented workforce is probably the most challenging long-term development issue identified in this project.

Future directions

To strengthen human resource capacity, the MOHP is planning to improve access and in-depth analysis of NEDSS data to disease control program managers at all levels. These program managers are being tasked to assist in the revision of guidelines and the provision of training to implement and monitor the response side of the surveillance activities. Merging of the ESU and MOHP-CDC would greatly facilitate better utilization of NEDSS (see Box 24.1).

Box 24.1 Key priorities for better utilization of NEDSS.

• Improving access of data to disease control programs.
• Work force development
• Flexibility in the flow of information
• Automated reporting of private sector laboratories

Developing capacity to edit data at the central level is a high priority. This would require including a data reconciliation feature so that information that is changed in a case record can be transmitted back to the district level. This would require a feature to allow the district health officers to take note of the edited records and approve the changes. The development of a two-way flow of information in NEDSS would also provide district health officers with visibility of case reports on residents who may seek care in neighboring districts or remote referral centers. It is anticipated that NEDSS will be migrated to a Web-based surveillance system to accommodate these features.

The development of SLIME software and support for MOHP laboratories has greatly improved laboratory confirmation of nationally notifiable diseases. However, there are a considerable number of private laboratories and hospitals that do not report. Engagement of these private sector laboratories in automated reporting is a high priority for the MOHP and expected to improve the timeliness and completeness of infectious disease reports [14].

The current architecture of NEDSS is restricting further development to meet other needs of the MOHP, particularly in the areas of chronic disease surveillance, provision and utilization of services, and monitoring healthcare outcomes. There are inherent limitations in the structure of case-based reporting systems. Development of a registry-based health information system using a unique identifier to establish a record for each case-patient would allow for reporting of multiple events in the same person. Integration of surveillance into a comprehensive health information system would allow for better definition of disease burden for acute and chronic diseases and provide the opportunity to link access to services to healthcare outcomes. It is appealing to consider the design of such systems for countries like Egypt that are transitioning from paper to computer-based health information systems. However, there needs to be much broader engagement and commitment from national authorities on the value of investing in comprehensive health information systems to realize these benefits.

References

1 Wilson R. Using computers in health information systems. In: Lippeveld T, Sauerborn R, Bodart C (eds.), *Design and Implementation of Health Information Systems*. Geneva: World Health Organization; 2000:198–212.

2 Lippeveld T, Sauerborn R, Sapirie S. Health information systems—making them work. *World Health Forum* 1997;**18**(2):176–84.

3 Hatch D, Imam IZ. Collaboration: the key to investigations of emerging and re-emerging diseases. *East Mediterr Health J* 1996;**2**(1):30–6.

4 Lederberg J, Shope RE, Oaks SC. *Emerging Infections: Microbial Threats to Health in the United States*. Washington, DC: Institute of Medicine; 1992.

5 Crump JA, Youssef FG, Luby SP, *et al*. Estimating the incidence of typhoid fever and other febrile illnesses in developing countries. *Emerg Infect Dis* 2003;**9**(5):539–44.

6 Srikantiah P, Girgis FY, Luby SP, *et al*. Population-based surveillance of typhoid fever in Egypt. *Am J Trop Med Hyg* 2006;**74**(1):114–9.

7 Fidler DP. Germs, governance, and global public health in the wake of SARS. *J Clin Invest* 2004;**113**(6):799–804.

8 Jebara KB. Surveillance, detection and response: managing emerging diseases at national and international levels. *Rev Sci Tech* 2004;**23**(2):709–15.

9 Thiermann A. Emerging diseases and implications for global trade. *Rev Sci Tech* 2004;**23**(2):701–7.

10 Lippeveld T, Sauerborn R. A framework for designing health information systems. In: Lippeveld T, Sauerborn R, Bodart C (eds.), *Design and Implementation of Health Information Systems*. Geneva: World Health Organization; 2000:15–32.

11 Hopkins RS. Design and operation of state and local infectious disease surveillance systems. *J Public Health Manag Pract* 2005;**11**(3):184–90.

12 Weinberg J. Surveillance and control of infectious diseases at local, national and international levels. *Clin Microbiol Infect* 2005;**11**(suppl 1):12–4.

13 Centers for Disease Control and Prevention. Guidelines for evaluating surveillance systems. *MMWR Morb Mortal Wkly Rep* 1988;37(suppl 5):1–18.

14 M'Ikantha NM, Southwell B, Lautenbach E. Automated laboratory reporting of infectious diseases in a climate of bioterrorism. *Emerg Infect Dis* 2003;9(9):1053–7.

Appendix: System requirements for NEDSS

Beta Version 1

Design: Key design features included the following:

1 Use of industry standard protocols for connectivity, communication, messaging, and data migration

2 User access rights for maximum security

3 Built-in bilingual functionality (To maintain one code base and alleviate the problem of developing two separate versions (English and Arabic), an independent language module was developed. The translation module provides dynamic language translation for any screen of the system, including reports)

4 Rapid communication of information collected

5 Quality assurance checks

6 The ability to incorporate data from different sources

7 The ability to combine information over time

8 Capacity for long-term data storage and retrieval

9 Multilevel modules for analysis and visualization of data

10 System backup and restore utilities

11 Self-initiated quality control and system checks

Deployment: Version 1 was installed on desktop computers in 27 governorate health offices, and 246 district health units over a 2-year period.

Messaging: The Messaging module facilitates extraction and consolidation of data from disparate locations to a single location upon one click of a button. Another added feature of the module is the ability of central level to extract data for any its subordinates in case of any data loss. There are also certain rules built—that ensure proper data transmission and data merge for a specific governorate. Data transmission and data merge are the two main submodules of Messaging.

Data Transmission: Data transmission provides the user the ability to extract data and send to a hierarchal location. Data can be extracted by specifying selection criteria (e.g., by range of dates, by disease, by disease category, or by location). All transmitted files are encrypted, compressed, and password protected. For contingency purposes, messaging provides data file transmission via diskette. Data files sent are moved to an archive for any future reference.

Data Merge: Data merge provides user ability to merge data from the data files received from subordinate locations. Merge process is then initiated which will unlock, decompress, and decrypt the data file. Data are then compared against existing data and merged accordingly into the local database. Reports list the subordinate sites that did and did not report. Data files once merged are moved to an archive subdirectory for future reference.

Reports Module: Two components for reporting for "General" and "Detailed" reports were developed. General reporting produces summary tables within a specified time (week, month, or year) for all diseases for all or specified governorates and all or specified districts. The reports were designed for a minimum interaction to produce reports for novice users. The detailed reporting produces summary tables and graphs of notified cases of diseases by sex, place, time, disease status, and disease outcome over a specified period in time. Reports can be generated down to the level of the reporting source.

Version 2

User Roles and Rights/System Authentication: The user management module was developed to limit access to certain modules/components of the system to unauthorized users. The roles management module was developed to function in conjunction with the user module that provides system authentication and login rights for each user.

System/Code Maintenance: A module was developed to give the MOHP complete autonomy of codes for the system including a database management tool to modify and maintain data table contents. New disease codes and geographic jurisdictions can be created or modified and the user can add or modify new or existing diseases, specimens, laboratory tests, test results. Codes for governorates, districts, and reporting sources can also be modified and the user can set up different business rules to specify what action needs to be taken or occur as a result of information that is entered.

Deduplication Module: This utility allows the user to automatically generate a list of all potential duplicate records. The user can decide whether to merge two records by selecting one out of the two potential duplicate records or leave the record as they exist.

Ad Hoc Query Module: The ad hoc query tool was created to allow access to the entire disease database. Menu-driven prompts allow the user to create a selection criterion or query. This query generates a subset of the disease database that is loaded into Microsoft Excel. This tool enables the users of the application to graphically specify the conditions (e.g., outcome, case status) of the query, the variables to be included in that query, and the disposition of the results. The results may be displayed as "Pivot Tables" or "Pivot Charts." Pivot tables and Pivot Charts are interactive. Once produced, the results can be "pivoted" (Change the X and Y axes). The resulting chart or table can be formatted as various types, bar, pie, and many types of 3-D effects.

Epi Info Link Module: The link to Epi Info Analysis allows direct access to the MS SQL Server database for the generation of output such as record lists, graphs, or tables. Push-of-a-button technology allows users to connect to the MS SQL Server database and read general disease table in the appropriate language selected. All features of Epi Info are available.

Backup and Restore Module: The electronic surveillance system provides a backup and restore module that provide an important safeguard for protecting critical data stored in the database. The system has been designed to perform complete system backups every 3 hours. The backup utility also allows users to backup the database on demand.

Export Module: The export module gives users the ability to export from the MS SQL Server database to produce files such as Access, Comma Delimited, Fixed Length, and Excel for use in other database and statistical packages.

System Update Methodology: System Updates module allows updates made at the Central jurisdiction to be propagated to the lower jurisdictions. Updates can be transferred by dial-up networking or by floppy disk. This methodology reduces the amount of effort necessary to deploy changes in a timely fashion.

Version 3

Analysis, Visualization, and Reporting (AVR): Version 3 includes updated modules on the analysis, visualization, and reporting (AVR) of data to allow the user to customize reports to formats suitable for different levels of decision makers and stakeholders. The modules allow the user to calculate rates of disease over time, cause-specific mortality rates, case-fatality ratios.

NEDSS On-Line Help: NEDSS On-Line Help is a tool available to users in either Arabic or English and uses Microsoft Help Viewer.

Enhanced Search Module: The search module provides a user-friendly tool to search in either Arabic or English for all fields on the "General Form" data entry screen.

Version 4

Version 4 includes changes in data elements to be reported based on requests from specific disease control programs. One additional disease has been included (suspect Avian Flu) and automated data analysis routines to detect aberations in disease incidence and outbreaks has been included. Version 4 also includes an automated production of a disease surveillance bulletin.

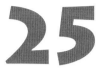

25 Electronic reporting in infectious disease surveillance

PART 1: Basic principles of electronic public health surveillance

Gérard Krause & Hermann Claus

Introduction and definitions

Electronic collection, processing, and dissemination of information have the potential to greatly improve the power and efficiency of public health surveillance systems, particularly data quality and timeliness. Flexibility, data security, and ethical issues can cause greater challenges in electronic systems compared to traditional systems. Electronic surveillance refers to systems where digitized information is transmitted. In this chapter we will not discuss the transmission of information via digital telephones, and transmission of word processor files or scanned graphs via e-mail attachments. Electronic processing may include a single transmission process from a local to a state health department, but can also cover the complete process from a laboratory information system to a surveillance report published on the Internet.

Electronic surveillance distinguishes itself from conventional surveillance by the method of data transmission. The steps of this process are diagnosis, notification, reporting, and publication. Diagnosis of a specific disease or infection occurs through the laboratory or clinical techniques or both. Notification is the process of bringing the diagnosis to the attention of the public health system. In general, this occurs at the level of the local public health department, although it will vary from country to country and state to state. Typically, it is at the local level that immediate prevention and control measures are instituted and further investigations are done. The process following notification is called reporting in this chapter and refers to forwarding the information received by the primary recipient of the notification (e.g., the local public health department) to the health authority of the next administrative level (e.g., the district health department, state health department, or federal health agency). Data quality control, epidemiological analysis, and interpretation take place prior to publication. Publication occurs when the data are made generally available; an example would be yearly epidemiological reports. In principle, all three elements—notification, reporting, and publication—can be performed electronically.

Syndromic surveillance is often confused with electronic surveillance as syndromic surveillance is often implemented through electronic data processing [1]. However, syndromic surveillance can be done on a paper-based system and simply differs from conventional surveillance system in that it processes the raw, uninterpreted occurrence of symptoms and excludes any clinical or laboratory-based diagnostic process [2].

Increasing information need

Demands for surveillance systems are increasing for a variety of reasons. The dynamic of an infectious disease outbreak greatly depends on the mobility of persons and vectors (e.g., foods). Modern means of travel and transport, together with increasing globalization in literally every aspect of life, have increased the potential for infectious diseases to spread rapidly across borders as exemplified by the SARS epidemic (3; see also Chapter 39, Part 2). Also, there is widespread concern that the risk for intentional release of pathogens has increased and this has mobilized attention and funds to develop electronic surveillance systems. These demands are added to a cultural demand for instantaneous access to information, including epidemiological information on infectious disease [4]. Public health action has always been influenced by public expectations and electronic mass media accelerate this process. Often the public media transport information on infectious disease events to the national and international level earlier than an established surveillance system. PROMED and the World Health Organization's GOARN system are examples of harnessing public media reports for surveillance purposes [5,6].

Instead of replacing conventional surveillance systems, rapid mass media actually add an additional task to surveillance—the task of rapidly ruling out proclaimed but nonexisting public health risks. Additional challenges also result from the freedom of information legislation that is installed in over 40 countries. These regulations oblige public agencies to release information to the press or to the individual citizen upon request [7]. Although this transparency is to be supported as long as principles of confidentiality of individuals are adhered to, the major challenge is a technical one. A public health agency can no longer limit its resources to the analysis and reporting of issues prioritized by its own criteria, but personnel resources must be invested to serve information requests that might not be seen as a public health priority by the agency in charge. This increases the need to automatically analyze data or to proactively make detailed data available.

There are international regulations that require electronic collection of surveillance data. Decision 2119/99/EC and Directive 2003/99/EC of the European Union (EU) oblige EU Member States to report surveillance data on infectious diseases to a designated EU agency [8,9]. Although the regulations do not specify that this information must be transferred electronically, it would be almost impossible and certainly very inefficient to collect data

from 25 Member States with an overall population of 457 million on paper-based spreadsheets. Electronic surveillance has become a necessity. The question is which parts of the surveillance process should be automated and to what extent should information be digitized.

Digitization of information and media disruption

The initiation of data collection—when a pathogen is detected in a sample or when a diagnosis is made—is when qualitative information first needs to be translated into digitized information. Implementation of an electronic surveillance system is a good opportunity to systematically revise and standardize the information to be collected. The temptation to increase the capacity of computerized systems to collect all available information without limitation and without categorization should be resisted. One of the challenges in implementing an electronic system is to define how much detail is needed and how it should be categorized. Whenever the number of healthcare providers and other data sources is large and their organizational structure complex and individualized, it is difficult to integrate them into one uniform electronic system [2]. In such situations conventional notification by healthcare providers via phone, fax, or letter to the local health department may be the preferred approach [10]. Media disruption occurs, for example, when information entered into one database (e.g., physicians entering data for accounting purposes), is sent to the health department in such a format that it must then be transfered manually into another electronic database. This should be avoided whenever possible as it is resource and time consuming, and can be a source of error. On the other hand, if media disruption occurs at the appropriate level, it can be integrated into a quality control procedure that is necessary anyway.

A "Round-Robin" test for case definitions for notifiable diseases conducted in all local health departments in Germany indicated that case definitions are essential for assuring a high positive predictive value of a surveillance system but are difficult to execute on preprogrammed algorithms. Local health department staff must individually interpret incoming data [11]. In general, the information needs to be translated into the electronic system manually. In this test case, the clinical diagnosis made by the physician was entered into the system. This process is sensitive to errors, expensive, and difficult to control because it occurs in the periphery of the system and many persons are involved (e.g., physicians and nurses). For this reason it appears logical that electronic surveillance systems connect to health related databases that have already been installed for reasons other than for surveillance, such as hospital-based information systems used for billing or internal quality control. It must be kept in mind that information collected for billing or other purposes may introduce certain biases or random errors that may not be tolerable for epidemiologic analysis [10]. A surveillance system that connects to existing laboratory information systems has the benefit that data can be directly processed and forwarded electronically [12,13]. However, this carries the risk that clinical information that is not part of the laboratory information system will be ignored. In addition data from small laboratories (e.g., those specialized in the diagnosis of specific pathogens) without compatible electronic information systems may be excluded.

In Germany, the Regional Physicians Associations at the level of federal states (Bundesländer) maintain a complex system to monitor and manage financial compensation for medical services provided by general practitioners containing data on diagnoses and treatments [14]. The Robert Koch Institute is extracting and processing these data in order to complement the existing surveillance system for infectious diseases for epidemiological analysis [14]. Although the Regional Physicians Associations' databases use the International Classification of Disease codes, it is difficult to compute the incidence rate of a specific infectious disease. Gastroenteric illnesses, for example, are almost never distinguished by pathogens, yet the causative agent is essential information for an infectious disease surveillance system. For this reason the database is useful only for surveillance of certain vaccine-preventable diseases.

Timeliness

Timeliness in surveillance can be greatly improved by the application of electronic transmission of information. Although transmission via phone or fax offers an advantage over mail, the main advantage of electronic surveillance systems is that mathematical algorithms and semiautomatic decision instruments can more easily process digitized information. The fewer the media between and within the notification, the transmission, and the reporting process the shorter the delay. One of the delays that cannot be influenced is that from onset of symptoms to diagnosis of the disease [2]. This delay varies greatly depending on pathogens [15]. The delay in notification is perhaps the most critical as it defines the timeliness by which the public health service can initiate public health interventions [16]. Some laboratory information systems are able to automatically send out a notification as soon as a notifiable pathogen has been detected [13].

Electronic patient management systems will increasingly be used to remind physicians that an event is notifiable. This is likely to shorten notification delay and can also increase compliance.

The benefit of Web-based reporting is that one media disruption is avoided. However, the notifier will generally have to open a Web-based application and manually enter data into the Web interface that are already available in another electronic or paper-based documentation system. Therefore, a stand-alone Web-based notification system may not improve timeliness and may negatively affect the completeness of notification, flexibility and representativeness of reporters, because it requires Web access and Web competency.

As soon as epidemiologically relevant data are entered in the electronic system, the delay for transmission and reporting will depend mainly on the time required for data quality control and epidemiological analysis. Quality control can be automated using quality control algorithms and automated statistical analyses, but depending on the local situation it may warrant manual analysis before the information is forwarded to a central national or international surveillance centre where automated procedures are in place. Epidemiological analysis requires involvement of qualified epidemiologists.

During the FIFA Football World Cup 2006 in Germany, the SurvStat database was updated daily with all notifiable diseases [17–19]. All case reports that had passed the automated quality control algorithms were directly transmitted to the national surveillance agency and were made available to the public with a maximum delay of 1 day. After the World Cup the reporting frequency was reduced to a weekly update, as this facilitated synchronization with manual quality control procedures. Based on the positive experience of the enhanced surveillance during the World Cup, North Rhine-Westphalia (the largest of the 16 states in Germany) decided to report notifiable diseases daily on a routine basis.

Data confidentiality and ethical issues

Electronic public health surveillance systems must be compliant with existing laws and regulations on data security and confidentiality. Adequate systems must be in place to prevent unauthorized persons from accessing the database, and any information that is not absolutely necessary for infectious disease control must not be collected in the first place. Existing laws convey that linkage of databases that may lead to the collection of such "unnecessary" data must be avoided. A general obligation of civil servants to confidentiality is necessary but not sufficient. Data flow and databases must be designed such that inappropriate linkage of databases is technically impossible unless disproportional efforts are applied. In many countries national public health agencies are not allowed to receive names, complete birth dates, or addresses of notified cases. The local health departments are the institutions in charge of contacting the affected person(s) and executing direct infectious disease control measures. In other countries, such as Sweden, unique personal identification numbers issued to all Swedish residents are used at state and national level as a unique identifier for cases in the surveillance system [20]. These different legal requirements will obviously lead to different technical solutions. In Germany, a unique identifier is generated by hash code that cannot be reidentified, thus assuring that cases are not counted twice yet also preventing any identification of the individual [14].

Electronic transmission of data can add a layer of security not present in standard transmission. Accidental dialing of a wrong fax number may cause confidential information to be sent to unauthorized recipients. Disease notifications mailed by postal service may be intercepted and misused. Safety requirements for electronic surveillance systems will need to increase as technical possibilities for misuse increase as well. Beyond legal restrictions it should be clear that the best protection against any misuse is to limit the information collected to what is absolutely necessary for the surveillance function at the specific level. Sometimes efforts to guard against misuse may have unforeseen consequences. When new infectious disease control laws were enacted in Germany in 2001, it was believed by the legislators that notifications of hepatitis C needed particular data protection measures due to difficulty in distinguishing chronic from acute diseases. The law contained a specific paragraph specifying that names and other personal identifiers had to be deleted after 3 years from records kept at the local health department level. Unfortunately, this measure generated the problem that local health departments may not be able to identify repeated testing on individuals, leading to double reporting.

Technical approaches

The challenges of establishing an electronic surveillance system are not so much caused by the implementation of the appropriate information technology but more by the necessity to establish adequate procedures and structures by which data management is organized. The following questions should be answered to clarify the design of the database:
• Exactly what data are to be retrieved?
• How are the fields and respective values defined?
• How are older entries saved?
• How will corrections be documented?
• To what extent are data inconsistencies controlled?
• How are respective algorithms defined? Who defines them?
• How is change-management realized? Are changes in definitions documented? Do they apply to older data retrospectively? Is there a defined translation algorithm in place?

• Are the different types of administrators and users defined for the different functions (data entry, quality control, data management, scientific interpretation, publication, use)?

Once these questions are answered, the choice of adequate information technology is relatively straightforward. It is recommendable that one of the widely available database systems (e.g., Oracle, Informix, SQL Server, mySQL, PostgreSQL) be chosen to allow interoperability. XML standards (XSD, XSLT) should be applied for data definitions in order to maintain independence from different platforms. A powerful development platform should be used (e.g., Windows versus Linux, commercial versus open source, client application versus Web application). Of course, additional tools need to be carefully chosen in order to be compatible with the system (e.g., mapping tools, statistical software). It is also important to make sure that tools will be available in the future and will be adequately developed further by the software producers.

Today's information technology allows the implementation of any kind of data security measures regardless of where the data are physically stored and how the data are transported electronically. Deciding between Intranet, Internet, or e-mail-based data transport is no longer a matter of data security but of available infrastructure and other resources. The major determinant for information technology of electronic surveillance systems is acceptability by stakeholders and users in applying electronic signatures and coding mechanisms. Another important issue is the ownership of the data, which often determines where the data are physically stored. In federal countries such as the United States and Germany, national surveillance systems rely on a network of databases in each of the different states. Data needed at the national

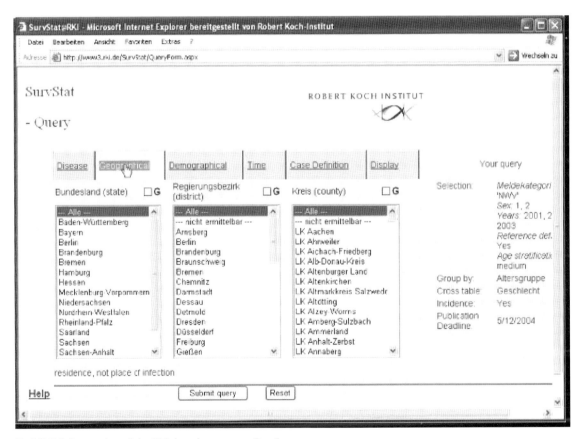

Fig 25(1).1 Screen shot of the Web-based query page SurvStat.

level are then extracted from these databases into a central national database. This way the states retain ownership and responsibility for the data within their states. A centralized database (e.g., Sweden) is likely to be more economical compared to a distributed database (e.g., Germany) [19,20].

For publication of surveillance data, printed formats may continue to play an important role. A survey of a large representative sample of general practitioners in Germany showed that these doctors preferred to receive epidemiological data in a printed form rather than having to search for it on the Internet [21]. A survey recently conducted among recipients of the yearly epidemiological report sent out by the Robert Koch Institute in Germany found that the majority of respondents wanted the data in a printed format, in addition to

being available on the Internet. However, the Internet has become a major format for publishing of epidemiological data [22].

Although summarized reports and tables on public health surveillance are commonly available on the Internet, truly interactive databases available through the Internet are not yet widely available. In focused group discussions officers from local health departments throughout Germany, wanted epidemiological details of their local areas [23]. The assessment revealed that the only solution to cover the diverse needs was to provide an interactive database that allows a variety of individual queries and that is available through the Internet. The result is SurvStat [24], accessible at http://www3.rki.de/SurvStat (Figures 25(1).1 and 25(1).2).

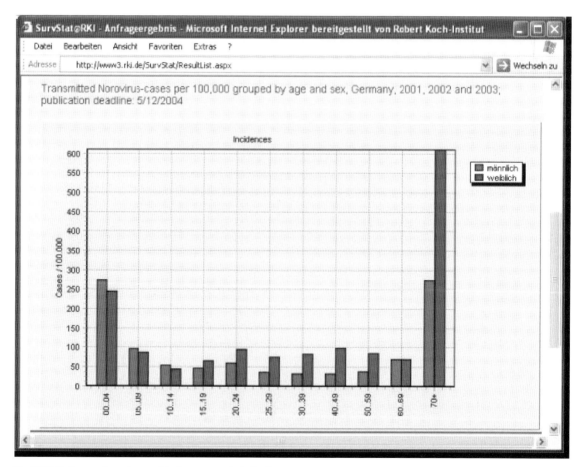

Fig 25(1).2 Screen shot of a graphical query result in SuvStat.

Such approaches carry many advantages and some risks. If databases with raw data are made available to the public, such a tool can cover many inquiries. This will save resources as public health administrations will not have to respond to inquiries. Making data available to the scientific community will allow experts to make use of the data, to conduct investigations, and to discover potential flaws in the data quality. On the other hand, making differentiated databases available also carries the risk that interest groups or individuals will misinterpret the data either because technical knowledge needed to analyze the data is not available or because data are being intentionally misused for political purposes [22].

Conclusions

Application of information technology for the surveillance of infectious diseases is a natural consequence of increased information demands and improved availability of the respective technology. However, issues of data ownership and data confidentiality may be the limiting factor in applying the available technical possibilities. The most important challenge in implementing an electronic surveillance system is to clearly define the functions, the content, and the procedures within the surveillance system. Application of the most modern information technology may well mask, but not necessarily solve problems resulting from inconsistent handling of data or lack of clear definitions.

References

1 Green MS, Kaufman Z. Surveillance for early detection and monitoring of infectious disease outbreaks associated with bioterrorism. *Isr Med Assoc J* 2002;**4**(7):503–6.

2 Daniel JB, Heisey-Grove D, Gadam P, *et al.* Connecting health departments and providers: syndromic surveillance's last mile. *MMWR Morb Mortal Wkly Rep* 2005;**54**(suppl):147–50.

3 Goddard NL, Delpech VC, Watson JM, Regan M, Nicoll A. Lessons learned from SARS: the experience of the Health Protection Agency, England. *Public Health* 2006; **120**(1):27–32.

4 Choi BC. Public health practitioners can learn from the weather forecasters. *J Epidemiol Community Health* 2004;**58**(6):450.

5 Madoff LC, Woodall JP. The internet and the global monitoring of emerging diseases: lessons from the first 10 years of ProMED-mail. *Arch Med Res* 2005;**36**(6):724–30.

6 Formenty P, Roth C, Gonzalez-Martin F, *et al.* [Emergent pathogens, international surveillance and international health regulations (2005)]. *Med Mal Infect* 2006;**36**(1):9–15.

7 Wikipedia Contributors. Freedom of information legislation. *Wikipedia, The Free Encyclopedia*; 2006. Available from: http://en.wikipedia.org/w/index.php?title=Freedom_of_information_legislation&ol did=72543846. Accessed August 31, 2006.

8 Decision No 2119/98/EC of the European Parliament and of the Council of 24 September 1998 of setting up a network for the epidemiological surveillance and control of communicable diseases in the Community. Available from: http://europa.eu.int/eur-lex/pri/en/oj/dat/1998/l_268/l_26819981003en00010006.pdf#search=%22Commission%20Decision%202119%22. Accessed August 31, 2006.

9 Directive 2003/99/EC of the European Parliament and of the Council of 17 November 2003 on the monitoring of zoonoses and zoonotic agents, amending Council Decision 90/424/EEC and repealing Council Directive 92/117/EEC. Available from: http://europa.eu.int/eur-lex/pri/en/oj/dat/2003/l_325/l_32520031212en00310040.pdf. Accessed August 31, 2006.

10 M'ikantha NM, Southwell B, Lautenbach E. Automated laboratory reporting of infectious diseases in a climate of bioterrorism. *Emerg Infect Dis* 2003;**9**(9):1053–7.

11 Krause G, Brodhun B, Altmann D, Claus H, Benzler J. Reliability of case definitions for public health surveillance assessed by Round-Robin test methodology. *BMC Public Health* 2006;**6**(1):129.

12 Widdowson MA, Bosman A, van SE, *et al.* Automated, laboratory-based system using the Internet for disease outbreak detection, the Netherlands. *Emerg Infect Dis* 2003;**9**(9):1046–52.

13 Zucs AP, Benzler J, Krause G. Mandatory disease reporting by German laboratories: a survey of attitudes, practices and needs. *Euro Surveill* 2005;**10**(1):26–7. Available from: http://www.eurosurveillance.org/em/v10n01/1001-223.asp. Accessed August 31, 2006.

14 Schrauder A, Kappelmayer L, Reiter S, Krause G, Benzler J. Surveillance of vaccine preventable diseases—a new approach in Germany [abstract] 2005. In: *10th EPIET Scientific Seminar*, Mahon, Menorca, Spain, October 13–15, 2005.

specific standards relevant to ELR [6], such as use of the Logical Observation Identifier Names and Codes (LOINC®) and Systematized Nomenclature of Medicine (SNOMED®) as a uniform way to code test result data (LOINC and SNOMED will be discussed later in this chapter. See Chapter 24 for more information about the NEDSS initiative.) CDC has provided funding to many states for the development of ELR systems. In 2005, 24 US jurisdictions had operational ELR systems [7].

Considerations in designing an ELR system

There are a number of steps to take and decisions to make when a public health agency decides to implement ELR (Box 25(2).1). First, a major consideration is the national standards for electronic medical information exchange (e.g., American National Standards Institute Health Level 7 (HL7), a major messaging format that will be discussed later in this chapter). Since many laboratories report to more than one jurisdiction and since laboratories cannot efficiently maintain more than one standard for file formats, codes, and messaging, it is important to be informed about and utilize the current national standards and practices.

Second, it is critical to ensure that there is adequate legal authority for laboratory reporting. Are laboratory reports that are indicative of conditions of public health importance legally reportable by clinical laboratories? Can the health department require reporting in a particular format or within a specific time frame? These factors must be established early in the process. In the US, each state establishes the reporting requirements for physicians, hospitals, and laboratories. Most states require laboratory reporting of test results that indicate a diagnosis of a reportable disease. For select diseases that require immediate public health intervention, (e.g., botulism or measles), laboratories are often required to telephone the test results to local or state public health officials in addition to subsequently submitting the routine detailed test report.

Third, adequate and sustainable funding must be available. The CDC provides some funding through the NEDSS initiative. States and larger local jurisdictions will also need to contribute funding since NEDSS funding has not increased in recent years.

A fourth key factor is that development of ELR systems requires a collaborative approach–state and local health departments and public and private clinical laboratories must be involved to ensure success. Also, a complete and functional ELR system cannot stand alone, but must link to other public health systems to facilitate response and ultimately lead to data to inform public health and clinical decision making. Collaborative development of methods to interlink systems must be considered during ELR planning. This aspect is discussed further below. Finally, it should be recognized that ELR

Box 25(2).1 General considerations for developing an electronic laboratory reporting system.

- What electronic reporting standards will be used?
- What is the legal authority for collecting laboratory reports?
- Which test results will be reported? For example:
  - Infectious disease
    - Culture
    - Serology
  - Chronic disease
    - Pathology for cancer

- Hemoglobin A1c for diabetes
  - Environment-related disease
    - Lead, heavy metals, water testing
  - Animal test results
    - Rabies
    - Mosquitoes (West Nile virus, etc.)
- What frequency of reporting is needed?
- What is the content of the reports?
- How will the quality of the reporting be monitored over time?

system development is a process and a "final" system will probably never be achieved; the system will undergo constant development as laboratory tests change and as information technology and standards change. In New York, the process described below began in the mid-1990s and is still evolving and developing.

Test report considerations

In designing an ELR system, the first test report-related decisions that must be made are which test results will be reported, the frequency of reports, and the content of the reports. A system that handles only human infectious disease test results may be relatively simple, whereas a system that handles other reports—for example, diagnostic pathology reports for state cancer registries containing open text fields, childhood lead poisoning test reports where parental information is critical, environmental sample test results, or animal test results—may need to be more sophisticated in design. The frequency of reporting should also be considered early in the planning phase. Many infectious disease results are needed by public health staff within 24 hours so that interventions, such as preventive treatment of close contacts, can be promptly instituted. However, some chronic infectious disease test results, such as HIV serology or CD4 lymphocyte counts, may not be needed immediately. In these situations, transmitting test results in batches every few days or weeks can save laboratories time and simplify public health processing of reports. Finally, the content of the reports should be based on what information laboratories can realistically be expected to have. Most laboratory reports for public health surveillance purposes generally need, at minimum, to include patient and physician information, specimen type, test type and result, and dates of specimen collection and test completion.

Technical considerations

There are three important technical areas to consider in developing an ELR system: the format of reports, coding of test type and results, and messaging (which refers to how reports are securely transmitted from laboratory to health department). These issues are best handled by experts in information technology, but it is very important for public health staff who use the electronic surveillance systems to have a basic knowledge of how they affect ELR performance.

Format refers to how each report is structured in electronic form. To have a workable surveillance system, all parties must agree on the record format so that they can communicate. There are different formats, each with its strengths and weaknesses. One of the simplest is direct data entry via the Internet: laboratory staff enters data into a fixed data entry screen. This method is very time-consuming if there are a large number of reports to be entered. Another common format is a fixed-length American Standard Code for Information Interchange (ASCII) file. Such a file, with one text line for each laboratory result, can be constructed at the laboratory from previously entered data using common software packages and transmitted via a secure means to the health department. It is also relatively simple and commonly used, but is not very flexible since it cannot be adapted to varying message contents. A third, more flexible and robust format which is especially useful for systems with multiple test types, is the HL7 format, which has emerged as the standard for exchange of clinical information [8]. HL7 is a defined set of rules for sending simple text characters in groups that represent data fields. HL7 has a variable length message and thus has the potential to meet many different messaging needs. HL7 is also more difficult to implement since there are multiple message types and a "reader" is required to parse the message into meaningful units of information. As with any electronic standard, HL7 format is evolving; there are several versions currently being used and improved versions are being developed. A significant challenge in ELR system development is to decide which version of HL7 to use and when to upgrade to newer versions. Although many laboratories do not currently utilize HL7 format, it is increasingly becoming the standard for ELR and is used by most large laboratories and vendors of medical information systems. Implementing HL7 for ELR, and deciding which version to use, require expert consultation.

The lack of standardized coding to report test results creates another challenge for electronic reporting. Many laboratories use either text (e.g., "*Staphylococcus aureus* detected") or their own individual proprietary coding system to designate results. This situation makes it difficult to process large numbers of test results electronically, without writing a computer program to translate each laboratory's results into standard codes. Some public health departments in the US are writing for each laboratory "crosswalk tables" which "translate" laboratory tests into codes. Other public health departments require that laboratories take on this task and translate their results into a standard format before transmitting their results. There are two commonly used coding standards that are increasingly becoming national standards for laboratory reporting. The first is the LOINC system, which includes codes for different types of medical observations, including laboratory tests [9]. The second is the SNOMED coding system, which is used to identify specific test results (e.g., specific bacteriologic organisms). The two systems are best used together to give a complete description of the laboratory test done and the test results. Figure 25(2).1 shows how these codes can be used to specify test results. Until all laboratories are capable of sending results using these codes, public health agencies will also have to be flexible in accepting results in other code systems or in text.

The third major technical consideration is the secure transfer of confidential test results with patient identifying information from laboratories to public health departments. Routine e-mail and Internet transfer are generally not secure. However, there are industry standards for the safe transfer of confidential information that should be incorporated into ELR system design. One example of specifications for the secure electronic exchange of information is the Electronic Business eXtensible Markup Language (ebXML) [10]. The CDC has developed specifications for automated system-to-system exchange of information, based on ebXML. An added challenge is the frequent need to distribute selected test results in a secure form to certain program areas or jurisdictions. Authentication of system users (e.g.,

Spreadsheet 1

A Disease Name	B LOINC Codes	LOINC Names/Name	C Report Criteria
Brucellosis	6328-9	BRUCELLA SP AB	>1:160
Brucellosis	6326-3	BRUCELLA ABORTUS ABJGM	Positive
Brucellosis	9496-1	BRUCELLA CANIS ABJGM	Positive
Brucellosis	551-2	BRUCELLA CULTURE	Brucellosis organism list

Spreadsheet 2

List Name	Findings/Organisms	SNOMED Code
Brucellosis organism list	*Brucella abortus*	L-13202
Brucellosis organism list	*Brucella canis*	L-13206
Brucellosis organism list	*Brucella melitensis*	L-13202

Fig 25(2).1 Example of LOINC and SNOMED coding for clinical laboratory results. Portions of two related spreadsheets that were jointly developed by the CDC, the CSTE, and the Association of State and Territorial Public Health Laboratory Directors. They illustrate how LOINC codes alone specify a positive brucellosis antibody test result (first three entries in Spreadsheet 1) or a positive *Brucella* culture (fourth entry) and how the addition of a SNOMED code specifies the specific species of *Brucella* cultured. (Source: *Annals of Internal Medicine*, Vol. 127, No. 8, Part 2, 1997. Used with permission of the American College of Physicians.)

through the use of passwords or digital certificates) and verification of receipt of files are important aspects of designing secure messaging capability.

There are several other technical issues that need to be considered. Maintaining a help desk will be necessary to provide ready assistance by telephone to answer technical and reporting questions from both laboratories and public health users of the system. Disaster recovery planning is critical to any system; it is necessary that data be recovered in the event of a system failure. Related to this is a plan for archiving files for long-term storage. Edit checking for incomplete data fields or incompatible data entries may be built into the system, if desired. It may also be desirable to include automatic alerting capabilities so that whenever certain test results of urgent public health importance are received, the appropriate person is immediately notified automatically. For example, the New York State ELR system is programmed to generate automatic telephone alerts when a laboratory report of a disease requiring urgent attention such as meningococcal meningitis is received (see below).

Process for implementing ELR

The process (Box 25(2).2) for implementing ELR is just as important as the design decisions. ELR involves getting different types of reports from multiple laboratories that use different information management systems to many different end users rapidly and securely. Designing and implementing any large electronic information system involving multiple participants requires careful planning and manage-

ment. The project manager is the person who coordinates all aspects of development and implementation. Project management has evolved into a specialty with its own methods and techniques. The project manager oversees the definition of the project's specific objectives to avoid conceptual confusion, ensures the fiscal commitment necessary for success, develops the timetable for completing each deliverable during the process, and watches for and coordinates response to difficulties as they arise.

Planning an ELR system must involve all stakeholder groups from the beginning. The meetings, chaired by the project manager, are often referred to as joint application development sessions (JAD sessions). These sessions include discussions of the objectives of the project, with very detailed decisions about the business rules for the system. These meetings must be attended by technical informatics experts and staff knowledgeable about laboratory testing and public health surveillance procedures. The public health and laboratory program needs should drive the design decisions with the technical informatics staff providing expert consultation on how to meet program needs. For example, surveillance staff can explain how laboratory results need to be processed to generate a suspect case report needing public health investigation. This may entail an electronic solution so that the laboratory report automatically generates an electronic case report, which avoids unnecessary data reentry. Likewise, public health laboratory staff may wish to electronically access information collected by surveillance staff and link it to information on specimens that have been submitted for testing at the laboratory. Including representatives of all user

---

Box 25(2).2 A process for implementing an electronic laboratory reporting system.

- Planning phase
  - Designate responsible unit(s) and appoint project manager
  - Conduct user group JAD sessions
  - Provide executive leadership
  - Ensure financial support
- Development and implementation phase
  - Institute a change control process to enable modifications during development
  - Conduct a pilot phase to debug the system

and ensure the system is meeting program goals
  - Conduct training
  - Certify laboratories to submit electronic data
- Operations phase
  - Operate a Help Desk to assist laboratories with questions
  - Conduct a quality assurance program to ensure complete, timely, and accurate reporting

345

groups ensures that the final system meets as many needs as possible. Users included in design decisions can also understand the compromises that invariably have to be made. The support of executive leaders, including top management, and a solid financial commitment to support the system's development and ongoing future maintenance needs are essential.

Other important process considerations include change control, piloting the system, training, certification of laboratories for using the system, and monitoring the system for quality assurance. Change control refers to an explicit written process for changing the original design of the system during development and implementation. As development proceeds, changes will invariably be needed; key participants need to know about the changes and have the opportunity to comment on them before they are approved. Before the system is fully implemented, there should be a pilot test of the system to identify any problems so that they can be corrected before full implementation.

Training of all users before they are expected to use the system is critical for success. Without good user training and a commitment on the part of users, the system will not function well or even be used. Also, before each laboratory is allowed to stop sending paper reports to public health authorities, there needs to be a certification process that ensures that each laboratory is sending valid, complete, and timely reports electronically. This certification process should be explicitly defined before implementation of the system. Lastly, once the system is running, there needs to be a monitoring system that periodically evaluates each laboratory's electronic submissions to ensure the quality of submitted reports. Some of the questions to consider include: Are all the reports being received or are some being missed? Is the information in each report complete? Are the reports coming in promptly? Initial and ongoing quality assurance is critical in ELR, just as it is with any reporting system.

Case study: New York's electronic clinical laboratory reporting system

The New York State's ECLRS provides a case study for the development of a state-based system. With the full support of the state health commissioner and with a commitment of several million dollars of state funding, the project was launched over a 3-year development period. The health department contracted the development to an outside vendor and followed the project management process described above.

ECLRS is built on the state's existing Web-based Health Information Network (HIN) that allows all county, regional, and state health departments, hospitals, laboratories, and other health providers to exchange information securely. This system uses a thin client, Web browser/server model, with HTTPS connections (the Secure Socket Layer encrypted protocol). The HIN is described in detail elsewhere [11]. Most laboratories do not have the capability of submitting results in HL7 format and New York wanted a system that could be implemented rapidly by many laboratories. ECLRS does not require the use of HL7, but is able to process HL7 messages. ECLRS also accepts messages in a standardized ASCII format that can be generated by many software packages. To encourage use of ECLRS by small laboratories which may not utilize HL7 nor ASCII format or may not wish to develop necessary interfaces, the system also has a direct Web-page entry screen (Figure 25(2).2). Web entry has proven to be extremely popular for the many laboratories that have very few test results to report to public health authorities.

The need for report routing affected several design decisions. ECLRS automatically forwards selected test results to the appropriate public health program area at the state level and to the appropriate local county health department, of which there are 58 in New York State (Figure 25(2).3). Some laboratories use LOINC and SNOMED codes, which make it easy to identify what the report is and to which public health program it should go. However, most laboratories do not use these codes. For these laboratories, New York designed ECLRS so that laboratories could submit separate files (e.g., files each for sexually transmitted diseases, tuberculosis, lead, other communicable disease results) that allow for appropriate routing of reports based on the type of file that is submitted.

Under New York regulation, each communicable disease report also needs to go to the county

Fig 25(2).2 Part of the Internet data entry screen from the New York State Electronic Clinical Laboratory Reporting System.

health department where the patient resides. However, large national laboratories do not have demographic information linked to the test result at the time of reporting. To partially solve this problem, ECLRS forwards the report to the local jurisdiction based on a hierarchical decision tree according to available information: first to the county of patient residence if the information is available, next to the jurisdiction of the physician, and lastly to staff at the state health department who telephone the submitting laboratory to ask for the jurisdiction so that the report may be appropriately forwarded. This process is not ideal and can involve considerable staff time in assigning reports.

ECLRS also has automatic alerting capabilities. When a laboratory report for a disease requiring urgent public health attention is received, the system generates automatic telephone calls to staff at the county health department of the patient's residence. Experience with this alerting capability has shown that most of the time local public health staff are already aware of the test result due to a telephone report from the laboratory. Thus, ELR automatic alerting provides a back-up notification system for urgent test results.

New York has implemented the following certification process before laboratories may discontinue sending their reports on paper. Laboratories begin

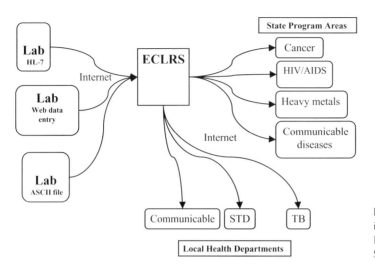

Fig 25(2).3 Diagram showing the flow of information in the New York State Electronic Clinical Laboratory Reporting System.

by sending reports both by paper and through ECLRS. Usually, two or three local health departments agree to monitor the completeness and accuracy of the electronic reports by comparing them to the paper reports. Once the electronic reports have been shown to match (or even exceed) the quality of the paper reports, the laboratory is certified and is allowed to discontinue reporting by paper.

To monitor the quality of reporting after a laboratory is certified, each laboratory's reports are continuously evaluated by the New York State ECLRS staff for any changes in the frequency and number of reports (that might suggest missing submissions), for completeness of data elements, and for timeliness. As an additional check on the completeness of laboratory reporting, the following process has also been instituted. The New York State Health Department regulates and approves all laboratories that perform diagnostic testing on New York residents. As part of that program, New York investigators make site visits to every laboratory every 2 years. During those visits, they review laboratory logs and abstract a sample of test results that should have been reported via ECLRS. These test results are then compared against archived ECLRS files to ensure that they were reported. Laboratories with missing reports are contacted and reporting problems are corrected.

New York has evaluated the effect of ECLRS on reporting for one large national laboratory and found that the median time from specimen collection date to its report to the local public health jurisdiction decreased from 14 to 5 days [10]. The percent of reports with missing data elements was 4% for patient date of birth (compared with 6% with paper reports) and was 51% for patient address (compared with 17% with paper reports). Electronic reporting can greatly reduce delays in reporting, but obtaining complete information electronically continues to be a challenge for some laboratories [12]. By comparison, an evaluation of electronic disease reporting from three clinical laboratories in Hawaii showed that electronic reporting resulted in a 2.3-fold increase in the number of reports, that electronic reports arrived an average of 3.8 days earlier than conventional reports, and that they were more complete [3].

Summary: lessons learned

Electronic laboratory reporting has the potential to significantly improve public health surveillance by speeding reports, decreasing staff time and cost in reporting, and increasing accuracy of the information. However, the experience of implementing ELR in New York is reminiscent of a quotation from Benjamin Disraeli: "What we anticipate seldom occurs; what we least expected generally happens [13]." Implementing ELR has proven more challenging than most public health officials had anticipated. Eventually, we can expect that all laboratories and healthcare providers will use common standards, which will promote efficient and easy exchange of medical information. Until then, implementing ELR will continue to have its challenges, but it can be done and is well worth the effort.

In the interest of providing guidance to those who are embarking on a new ELR system, here are some lessons that have been learned by those who have implemented ELR in New York:

• Involve all actual and potential system users *early* in the planning process and keep them informed as development proceeds. This effort will pay off in the long run by increasing user satisfaction and by avoiding mistakes that may require system redesigns.

• Allow more time for development than you expect. You will probably need it.

• Be flexible as you implement ELR. Currently, there is great variation among laboratories in file format and coding. The more flexibility in the ELR system, the more laboratories will be able to use it rapidly.

• Always have a trial period before discontinuing paper reports for each laboratory. It may not be possible for electronic reports to totally replace paper reports for some laboratories.

• If your ELR system generates 24/7 alerts for urgent reports, be prepared for the continuing need for human-to-human communication. Most computer-generated alerts turn out not to be public health emergencies that need immediate action.

In conclusion, ELR provides significant advantages to the public health surveillance enterprise. Laboratory reports are critical to initiating public health investigations and interventions in many cases. Assuring complete and timely laboratory reporting is a critical step to realizing this promise. However, there are significant issues for state and local health departments in planning and implementing these complex systems. Collaboration is necessary, not only among state and local health departments and clinical laboratories, but also among epidemiologists, public health field staff, and health information technology specialists. NEDSS provides critical standards to allow ELR systems to be developed in many state and local jurisdictions,

while still permitting collation of data into a national system. Many states and other countries are embarking on this process. Their success will be critical to successful public health efforts to prevent and control disease in the future.

References

1 Silk BJ, Berkelman RL. A review of strategies for enhancing the completeness of notifiable disease reporting. *J Public Health Manag Pract* 2005;**11**(3):191–200.

2 Half of US doctors don't have digital records. *Reuters* June 2006. Available from: http://msnbc.msn.com/id/13192489. Accessed June 28, 2006.

3 Effler P, Ching-Lee M, Bogard A, Ieong M, Nekomoto T, Jernigan D. Statewide system of electronic notifiable disease reporting from clinical laboratories. *JAMA* November 17, 1999;**282**(19):1845–50.

4 Panackal AA, M'ikanatha NM, Tsui F, *et al.* Automatic electronic laboratory-based reporting of notifiable infectious diseases at a large health system. *Emerg Infect Dis* July 2002;**8**(7):685–91.

5 M'ikanatha NM, Southwell B, Lautenbach E. Automated laboratory reporting of infectious diseases in a climate of bioterrorism. *Emerg Infect Dis* September 2003;**9**(9):1053–7.

6 Centers for Disease Control and Prevention. Progress in improving state and local disease surveillance—United States, 2000–2005. *MMWR Morb Mortal Wkly Rep* 2005;**54**:822–5.

7 Magnuson JA. Summary: 2005 ELR national snapshot survey [monograph online] Available from: http://www.coast2coastinformatics.com/2005ELRSurvey.html. Accessed June 28, 2006.

8 Health Level Seven, Inc. *Health Level Seven*. Ann Arbor, MI: Health Level Seven, Inc; 2003. Available from: http://hl7.org/. See also: http://www.ansi.org/default.aspx/. Accessed October 6, 2006.

9 McDonald CJ, Huff SM, Suico JG, *et al.* LOINC, a universal standard for identifying laboratory observations: a 5-year update. *Clin Chem* 2003;**49**(4):624–33.

10 The OASIS ebXML Joint Committee for OASIS. The Framework for eBusiness [monograph online]. Available from: http://www.ebxml.org/. Accessed October 12, 2006.

11 Gotham IJ, Smith PF, Birkhead GS, Davisson MC. Policy issues in developing information systems for public health surveillance of communicable diseases. In: O'Carroll PW, Yasnoff WA, Ward ME, Ripp LH, Martin EL (eds.), *Public Health Informatics and Information Systems*. New York: Springer-Verlag; 2003:537–73.

12 Smith PF, Chang H, Noonan-Toly C, Shannon R, Fisher C. Evaluation of data quality from an electronic laboratory reporting system, New York State. In: *International Conference on Emerging Infectious Diseases, Program and Abstracts Book*, Atlanta, GA; 2004:66–7.

13 *The Oxford Dictionary of Quotations*, 3rd edn. Oxford: Oxford University Press; 1979:186.

Additional Web resources

SNOMED® International, a division of the College of American Pathologists: www.snomed.org

CDC's National Electronic Disease Surveillance System Lab Reporting: www.cdc.gov/ nedss/elr/index.html

CDC's PHIN: Vocabulary Standards and Specifications: www.cdc.gov/phin/vocabulary/index.html

Public Health/Health Administration (PH/HA) Electronic Laboratory-based Reporting: http://phha.mlanet.org/ activities/elr.html

Health Level 7: http://www.hl7.org/

Logical Observation Identifiers Names and Codes (LOINC®)—Regenstrief Institute, Inc: http://www .regenstrief.org/loinc/

NYS Electronic Clinical Laboratory Reporting System–ECLRS: http://www.health.state.ny.us/professionals/ reportable_diseases/eclrs/index.htm

ebXML—eXtensible Markup Language: http://www.ebxml .org/

26 Implementing syndromic surveillance systems in the climate of bioterrorism

Julie A. Pavlin & Farzad Mostashari

Introduction

The need to rapidly detect an outbreak caused by bioterrorism, as well as natural outbreaks of new and old disease pathogens, has prompted a search for faster and more reliable methods for disease surveillance. The feasibility of intentional use of lethal pathogens to spread disease and disrupt social systems was demonstrated in the anthrax letter attacks of 2001. Even prior to 2001, many hospital and outpatient systems had converted to electronic registration and billing systems; often preliminary and confirmatory diagnoses and even patient chief complaints are entered into accessible databases. With this information available, researchers had already begun to develop data mining tools to extract data in formats usable for surveillance and to analyze large, continuous data sets for aberrations that could be indicative of a disease outbreak.

"Syndromic surveillance" typically refers to the automated analysis of routinely collected health-related data that are available even before specific diagnoses are made. Examples include early, nonspecific diagnoses, such as "cough" entered as chief complaint in an Emergency Department electronic medical record, or "pneumonia, not otherwise specified" entered in a billing database. Syndromic systems typically use electronically collected and disseminated data, but can include paper-based methods such as manual daily reviews of death certificates for potentially infectious causes. Although pioneering research articles in the field of syndromic surveillance date to the 1980s [1], the rapid expansion of the field in recent years can be attributed to

(1) increasingly available and timely electronic data, (2) advances in informatics and statistics for data extraction, normalization, and detection of aberrations in temporal or spatial data, and (3) growing concerns about the threat of epidemics, influenza pandemics, and bioterrorism. Several of the existing syndromic surveillance systems were developed in the late 1990s with funding from bioterrorism grants [2]. The debate continues, however, on whether syndromic surveillance systems can detect acts of bioterrorism [3–10]. There have been retrospective demonstrations [11], and statistical algorithms can detect shifts in disease counts early in an epidemic curve, but few systems have been able to demonstrate prospective early recognition in a manner that has led to effective intervention. In Chapter 33 our colleagues provide an in-depth review of evaluation methods for outbreak detection using these systems. Valid arguments exist that syndromic surveillance systems may not detect outbreaks faster than traditional methods, and even with advance warning, they may not assist with disease mitigation [6]. However, syndromic surveillance systems may be able to provide information that can assist with multiple public health functions.

With every new technology, there are phases of maturity and adoption by users, developers, and the public, sometimes described as the "Hype Cycle" [12]. First, there is a trigger or breakthrough that generates significant interest, and then a peak of inflated expectations, followed by a trough of disillusionment as the technology fails to meet expectations. For those who continue pursing the technology, there is a slope of advancement, as the practical

351

applications are understood, and a plateau of productivity as the benefits are accepted. We believe that we are now on the slope of advancement in the field of syndromic surveillance, although many questions remain unanswered.

In recent years, the community of syndromic surveillance researchers and practitioners from the fields of informatics, statistics, epidemiology, and public health have implemented and optimized components of syndromic surveillance systems, which we will summarize here. We believe that this accumulated experience can serve as a basis for building and operating syndromic surveillance systems that are cost-effective and productive contributors to public health surveillance activities nationwide.

Syndromic surveillance informatics: data sources

Data types

Traditional surveillance for infectious disease outbreaks usually consists of positive laboratory tests or at least cases that meet a clinical case definition. In contrast, syndromic surveillance is based on data received before a definitive diagnosis. As such, any syndromic system should complement traditional surveillance programs. Furthermore, if state and local syndromic surveillance systems result in strengthened technical abilities and data relationships with local clinical partners, the development of electronic laboratory reporting of reportable diseases could be greatly facilitated.

Data that arise from an interaction with the medical system, but that do not include confirmed diagnoses, can include early, nonspecific diagnoses, such as "upper respiratory infection," or procedures from initial encounters, such as "throat culture." They can be recorded as text in an electronic record, or through codes such as the International Classification of Diseases (ICD) or Current Procedural Terminology (CPT). These data can also include chief complaints from patients presenting for care, or initial impressions from emergency medical personnel on ambulance runs. Preclinical information obtained about the health of a population before a medical visit includes over-the-counter pharmacy sales for items such as cough syrup or antidiarrheal medication and calls to nurse advice lines or doctor's offices for information. These types of data occur early in the illness process but are usually nonspecific.

Other types of data that can be included in a syndromic system are from behavioral changes. If there is widespread illness in a population, it is possible that measurable changes can be detected in sewage generation [13] or school [14] or work absenteeism [15]. These data are very nonspecific and have been found to be less than reliable for disease detection, but become more reliable when combined with data from other sources. The recent acceleration in the adoption of electronic records increases both the opportunity and challenges for syndromic surveillance's secondary use of complex data.

Data normalization and syndrome categorization

One of the major challenges addressed by syndromic surveillance-related informatics has been methods for normalizing, standardizing, and categorizing of clinical and administrative data in order to repurpose it for public health. In order to be analyzed for statistical anomalies, the indicator health events represented by syndromic data must be grouped. A syndrome grouping schema based on ICD-9 codes, with an emphasis on bioterrorism detection, is available (www.bt.cdc.gov).

Many electronic databases are difficult to use because of a lack of standardized vocabulary. Even when standards exist, they are often corrupted by local implementations and dummy codes. Free-text data (most commonly from emergency department chief complaints) must be normalized to account for common misspellings, abbreviations, and regional vernacular differences. Software tools are available, including New York City's simple SAS-based phrase and keyword searching program and its derivatives [16], the ESSENSE program's weighted keyword search [17], and the Real-time Outbreak Detection System (RODS) laboratory's CoCo Bayesian text classifier [18].

Data acquisition

With the increasing use of clinical information systems and the movement toward interoperability and data standards, the problem of available data has changed from not enough to too much. There are a number of factors to consider when targeting data for acquisition:

1 *Timeliness.* Timeliness of data varies. For example, the data on over-the-counter pharmacy sales in the National Retail Data Monitor (NRDM) is generally available within 24 hours [19]. In contrast, it can take up to 5 days for receipt of 70% of a day's encounters to populate the BioSense surveillance system (a syndromic surveillance system developed by the Centers for Disease Control and Prevention (CDC), using national data sources) [20]. Surveillance goals and public health workflows will dictate the timeliness required. If the goal is gaining a few hours advantage on detection of bioterrorism attacks, "real-time" data transmission is needed. If the goal is general outbreak detection and monitoring of health trends involving daily analyses, then batched file transfers (typically run as part of early morning reporting and archiving batch processes) are sufficient. If the goal is following influenza trends, data with up to a week's delay are suitable.

2 *Data completeness and reliability.* Different data sources are associated with varying levels of data quality. Unstructured data must be evaluated for how often "dummy codes" or uninterpretable values are used and the prevalence of missing data. Any systematic bias in missing data must be determined (e.g., more severely ill patients, Sundays). Once data transmission is established, it is also worth evaluating the ongoing reliability of the data stream.

3 *Data quality.* Manual chart review of a sample of cases, with sensitivity and specificity estimated against a clinical gold standard, can assist in this evaluation. In order to access how accurately the trends in data correspond to epidemiologic phenomena, a time series of data should be compared to known seasonal trends for the particular illnesses, such as influenza and gastrointestinal illness, at the community level.

4 *Flexibility.* One of the main advantages of syndromic surveillance systems over traditional diagnostic surveillance is the potential to rapidly and flexibly examine trends in emerging health issues of topical concern. The richness and information content from a data source can vary in this respect. For example, a pick-list driven chief complaint field can be an improvement over free-text chief complaints for normalization and interpretability, but will not enable as broad a range of ad hoc analyses. Examples might include searches for uncommon combinations ("blood" and "cough") or for keywords such as "heroin," "fireworks," or specific event names such as "Olympics."

5 *Investigability.* When aberrations are detected, how feasible is investigation and response? Although syndromic data does not typically include obvious identifiers, is there a link to enable individuals to be identified in the event of a concerning cluster? Ideally, in-depth clinical information can be accessed quickly, if needed.

6 *Usefulness.* Usefulness is the extent to which the above factors meet surveillance goals and expectations.

A variety of data sources have been evaluated for their utility in syndromic surveillance systems. Reviews for many data sources have been published [2,10,11]. Table 26.1 highlights research on the validity and usefulness of specific data types. Results vary with the population under surveillance and source of the data, but in general, the closer the data source is to a medical encounter (chief complaints, provider initial diagnoses, laboratory test orders), the more reliable the information. When considering a new syndromic surveillance system, costs of and opportunities provided by available data sources should be evaluated against desired goals. For example, a large integrated healthcare delivery system with a single electronic medical record system that dominates the healthcare market in the geographic area is a promising data source to pursue. At the current time, for most localities emergency department chief complaint data have provided the appropriate mix of availability, timeliness, flexibility, and the ability to investigate.

Syndromic surveillance statistics: temporal and spatial cluster detection

Automated analysis of prospective time series health data for detection of temporal and spatial clustering has received much attention since the advent of syndromic surveillance. Many statistical methods have been developed and published. Available and commonly used statistical algorithms include the CDC's Early Aberration Reporting System (EARS) suite based on the CuSum process

Table 26.1 Examples of data types used in syndromic surveillance, their strengths, and weaknesses.

Data type	Analysis results
Absenteeism	School absenteeism in elementary students detected some influenza peaks
	Elementary school absences more reliable for detection of seasonal respiratory outbreaks
School nurse reports	Can provide early indication of influenza [21]
Over-the-counter (OTC) medication sales	OTC sales can provide indication of communitywide illness, such as influenza and gastrointestinal disease, but may not be as sensitive as emergency department surveillance [22]
	Correlation present between cold medications and influenza activity, but did not predict in advance [23]
	OTC sales can forecast influenza-like illness (ILI) incidence by 1–3 wk [24]
Nurse advice lines	Predictive of physician encounters for respiratory and lower and upper gastrointestinal disease [25]
	Increase in calls for ILI preceded increase in visits by 1–3 wk in England and Wales, but unlikely to detect a historic cryptosporidiosis outbreak [26,27]
Calls to poison control centers	Calls for unintentional food poisoning were not duplicative of cases reported to the health department—may represent a useful addition to surveillance data [28]
Companion animal surveillance	Nationwide surveillance for syndromes possible through veterinary clinic and diagnostic laboratory chains [29]
Ambulance dispatch	Sensitive to community-wide respiratory outbreaks [30]
	More sensitive for severe illness and in the elderly [31]
	Provided strongest signal-to-noise ratio for respiratory disease caused by wildfires [21]
Emergency department chief complaints	Reported gastrointestinal (GI) outbreaks did not correlate with syndromic signals, and syndromic signals occur frequently, are difficult to investigate, and can only be a supplement to traditional systems [32], but in the same system, detected widespread increase in diarrhea after power outage and assisted with systematic investigation [33] and detected norovirus outbreak [34]
	Chief complaints are accurate when compared to discharge diagnoses, can detect outbreaks, sensitivity/specificity ranges 30–75%/93–99% for different syndromes, precedes hospital admission by 10.3 days for respiratory and 29 days for GI outbreaks [35]
	Respiratory symptoms correlate with virologic test results in a pediatric population [36]
Diagnostic codes (e.g., ICD) from outpatient visits	Detected ILI at the same time as sentinel providers and an increase in positive laboratory tests [37]
	Sensitivity low in retrospective analysis of GI outbreaks when 8% of population under surveillance [38]
	Sensitive in primary care setting in Singapore [39]
Laboratory test orders	Stool cultures and fecal white blood cell (WBC) correlate with gastrointestinal diagnoses; throat cultures correlate with influenza outbreaks [40]
Prescriptions	Medicaid data readily available, picked up increase in macrolide prescriptions after a case of pertusis reported [41]
Hospital admissions	Surveillance for fever and rash picked up cases compatible with initial presentation of smallpox; excess admissions for pneumonia correlate with physician visits, and positive laboratory tests [42]

control algorithms (www.bt.cdc.gov), autoregressive moving average time series methods [43], rule-based anomaly detection [44], and scan statistics (www.satscan.org) [45]. Although the optimal analytic method is dependent on the type of data and analytic goals, we can make certain generalizations:

1 *The importance of the "expected."* Fundamentally, all statistical methods for outbreak detection compare observed rates or counts of syndromic events to what would be expected in the absence of a disease outbreak. The methods differ in how they arrive at this expected, for example, in the baseline period used, in weight given recent events versus past events, and in accounting for seasonal or cyclical trends.

2 *Role of baseline data.* Many of the health surveillance algorithms used in the past required 3–5 years of baseline data. In fact, due to changing consumer or health delivery patterns, coding schema, and information systems, "baseline" data from 3 to 5 years prior may no longer be comparable to current data as methodologies change significantly over time. Fortunately, algorithms used today require much shorter periods of time for definition of baseline data [46].

3 *Controlling for volume.* Syndromic counts can be affected by consumer and health-seeking behavior to a much greater extent than traditional surveillance data. Days of week effects are the most dramatic example of this. Most analytic approaches incorporate the overall volume of events in calculating a particular syndrome's expected rate of occurrence. The simplest and perhaps most common way to accomplish this is to use the ratio of the syndrome of interest to all events (or "other" syndromes).

4 *Difficulty of evaluating performance of analytic methodology.* Although different analytic methods often find different temporal and spatial clusters in the same data, it is very difficult to evaluate the superiority of one method over another, in part due to problems in capturing all three relevant attributes—sensitivity, specificity, and timeliness—simultaneously. The absence of "gold standard" outbreaks also contributes to the difficulty of objectively evaluating algorithm performance. Many algorithms have been evaluated using outbreak simulations with real or simulated background data [47–49], although the generalizability of such stud-

ies can be questioned. The algorithm judged superior tends to be that which best matches the type of simulated outbreak used.

Syndromic surveillance in practice: public health utility

Early recognition

The most commonly promoted use of syndromic surveillance in a bioterrorism situation is for early detection of an attack. Timely knowledge of an increase in disease incidence would certainly assist in mobilizing resources and potentially decrease associated morbidity and mortality.

There are many examples of retrospective studies showing that syndromic surveillance can provide early warning of large community-wide disease outbreaks when compared to traditional disease reporting. Data from emergency department logs, ambulatory visits, ambulance dispatches, and pharmaceutical sales, when properly cleaned and analyzed, have shown marked aberrations coincident with seasonal outbreaks of influenza and viral gastroenteritis (Table 26.1). Helping to drive the enthusiasm for syndromic surveillance development, many policymakers, commercial vendors, and public health practitioners have expressed optimism that syndromic surveillance systems could detect the prodromic phase of a bioterrorist attack with widespread (aerosolized or large food or waterborne) agents prior to notification by traditional reporters. Furthermore, it is assumed that this alerting could motivate earlier etiologic diagnoses, and the institution of preventive measures such as vaccination and prophylaxis, as well as prioritization of these measures to affected communities in time to reduce morbidity and mortality.

However, as outlined by Buehler *et al.*, the characteristics of an outbreak that make it most likely to be detected by syndromic surveillance are (1) narrow distribution of the incubation period, (2) longer prodrome, (3) absence of a clinical sign that would speed diagnosis, and (4) diagnosis is dependent on the use of specialized tests that are unlikely to be ordered [6]. Certainly, not all bioterrorism-caused outbreaks will have these characteristics. In addition, early detection may or may not assist with determining whether the outbreak is the result of an intentional biological attack. Any disease outbreak must be investigated by appropriate public health officials, and law enforcement will only be involved if evidence arises that point to illegal activity. Early detection alone does not ensure recognition of a biological attack, but data in a syndromic system may help find clues that suggest an intentional event.

Resource allocation

The infrastructure and relationships developed for syndromic surveillance can be leveraged during emergencies to assess not only disease rates and impact, but also the flow of resources. If data sources are available that cover the majority of an affected region's population, it may be possible to find who (by geographic location, age, gender, etc.) needs attention first. During the 2001 anthrax letter attacks, New York City's nascent pharmacy surveillance system provided useful information regarding prescriptions filled and available stock on hand for ciprofloxacin and doxycycline. Data in syndromic surveillance systems could assist emergency and public health responders allocate limited resources.

Tracking outbreaks and evaluation of countermeasures

Once an outbreak is recognized, available countermeasures must be put in place to decrease morbidity and mortality and prevent further spread. Data in a syndromic surveillance system can evaluate the effect of these countermeasures. Starting in 2004, the CDC tracked influenza activity across the nation using both syndromic and traditional influenza surveillance data. The goal of this initiative was to examine the potential effects of the vaccine shortage and to provide information that could be used during an influenza pandemic to target resources. In the event of a bioterrorist attack, as in a pandemic attack, countermeasures that may include prophylaxis, vaccines, quarantine, and treatment will need to be assessed rapidly using data flows that are already in place.

Case finding

The ready availability of syndromic data can provide powerful support to epidemiologic investigations and outbreak management. For example, in New York City's attempts to expand case finding for cutaneous anthrax, the public health department investigated individual emergency room visits with a mention of "spider bite" or "anthrax." Cases of rash febrile illness among children in a particular area were also examined. By using indicators of more severe disease, such as inpatient diagnoses, small numbers of significant cases could be detected. If a disease is diagnosed of particular public health importance, whether from concern for bioterrorism or of a potentially lethal and virulent disease such as avian influenza, syndromic data from recent emergency room and outpatient visits can quickly locate potential cases.

Reassurance during threats

Monitoring population health in real time with a system that can detect large increases in prodromic illness provides reassurance during periods of high concern. Many systems activated or increased vigilance during the worldwide SARS outbreak, including the military and health departments in Wisconsin and New York City [50,51]. Local health departments have also instituted systems for increased monitoring during high-profile events like the Republican National Convention and the Salt Lake City Olympics. Other periods of high concern may include situations where bioterrorist agents have been deployed on a small scale, such as the anthrax letter attacks, or after the potential ricin exposure in North London [52]. With the use of environmental sensors for bioterrorism detection in large metropolitan areas, potential alerts can be shared with public health officials who can then carefully monitor syndromic data in the same geographic area.

Challenges

Privacy

Most syndromic surveillance systems do not reveal patient identity, but owners of data, who are responsible for maintaining confidentiality, are justifiably concerned and may not be willing to provide information. Furthermore, patients who feel that their medical privacy might be compromised may take privacy-protective behaviors and, for example, avoid medical appointments [53]. The Health Insurance Portability and Accountability Act (HIPAA) allows unfettered public health reporting to agencies authorized to receive them [54], but it is incumbent on these public health authorities to request the minimum data necessary for this purpose. The HIPAA "safe harbor" standards for anonymity require the removal of several fields (e.g., date of service) essential for prospective disease surveillance. Consequently, researchers and other developers of surveillance systems will typically require "business associates" or "limited data set" agreement to access potentially identifiable information.

Population representativeness

For any type of surveillance system, one of the most important aspects is how representative the data are of the population under surveillance. If only a small group of patients from a medical group practice is included in the surveillance, the system is not a reliable monitor of a major metropolitan area. Most syndromic surveillance systems do not have the exposure needed to detect all outbreaks. Even in New York City's emergency department surveillance system, where 90% of visits are covered, 0 of 49 gastrointestinal outbreaks reported were detected by the system. This was due to a combination of factors: for example, many patients did not go to emergency rooms or went to facilities not covered by the system [32]. In the simulation for a bioterrorist attack at the Mall of the Americas in Minneapolis, the syndromic surveillance system only covered 9% of patients; therefore, it would take a large number of patients infected before the tested system would alarm [8].

To maximize effectiveness, syndromic surveillance systems should capture a majority of medical encounters in a given geographic area. If they do not include representation from all ethnic neighborhoods and socioeconomic groups, even large outbreaks can be missed. Systems with limited patient population information can still be of use, but only in the event an outbreak starts or spreads to this group.

Breakdown of communications in a disaster

One hallmark of syndromic surveillance is that the data are usually collected for other purposes than disease surveillance—for billing, sales records, insurance claims, resource management, etc. Therefore, the data may not capture information that could be useful in investigating disease outbreaks (e.g., recent travel or other exposures); however, it is not generally susceptible to bias. Despite the automatic, electronic nature of syndromic surveillance, there exists the possibility that communications and data transmission could fail during a disaster, such as a large bioterrorism attack. This could be due to simultaneous cyber attacks or to the fact that there is always a person involved in the data capture chain, and during a time of crisis, data entry may not occur.

Costs

Many negative reviews of syndromic surveillance have emphasized the cost [2,4]. Few studies have detailed the costs involved in establishing and running a syndromic system, but some have evaluated the cost and time spent investigating false alarms [20,32]. By using precollected data and available analytic methods, costs in setting up syndromic systems can be reduced. In addition, federal systems are now in place that can be provided free of charge to health departments and are expanding geographic coverage.

Legal agreements between data providers (hospitals), data processors, researchers, and health departments can add significantly to the cost of a system. When Pennsylvania set up a syndromic surveillance system using a university-based platform, legal agreements were needed with each of 138 hospitals, their data processors, the university analyzing the data, and health departments to delineate responsibilities of each party, and create a limited data use agreement, even though HIPAA allowances were in place (G. Schuyler, personal communication, September 2006). The design phase was very labor-intensive, with two Web casts required for hospitals to understand the process and two full-time staff dedicated to simply answering phone queries from concerned hospital representatives. Once set up, the system worked well. It has since been converted to a stand-alone for-profit company for data analysis. This move required new legal agreements. Whether syndromic systems are worth the investment will only be determined as systems actually perform in outbreak detection and personnel and system costs are evaluated over the long term.

Conclusion

Several of the existing syndromic surveillance systems were developed with funding from bioterrorism grants. It is, however, necessary to move the syndromic surveillance field away from a focus solely on bioterrorism detection. No system will detect every case of bioterrorism and a system must be able to detect naturally occurring diseases in order to detect a bioterrorist attack. In addition, use for endemic and epidemic natural-occurring disease detection will increase applicability and therefore overall usefulness. Expansion of syndromic surveillance systems for diseases other than infectious, such as injuries, heart disease, and mental illness, will also increase utility and decrease overall cost.

We feel that development is needed in multiple areas. These include the linking of rapid diagnostic tests and associated data to syndromic alerts, the use and evaluation of multivariate methods of data analysis and comparison, the sharing across jurisdictions of population health knowledge and situational awareness to improve response, and the involvement of healthcare providers in the surveillance system network to allow incorporation of surveillance and outbreak data in clinical decision making. For those considering developing a new system, exploring tools already available can greatly speed progress and decrease costs. In addition, using already collected, free data will greatly decrease expenditures, especially recurrent costs after system development. We believe that syndromic surveillance systems can be operated cost-effectively and can be productive contributors to public health surveillance activities.

References

1 Hannoun C, Dab W, Cohen JM. A new influenza surveillance system in France: the-Ile-de-France "GROG." 1. Principles and methodology. *Eur J Epidemiol* 1989; 5(3):285–93.

2 Bravata DM, McDonald KM, Smith WM, *et al.* Systematic review: surveillance systems for early detection of bioterrorism-related diseases. *Ann Intern Med* 2004; **140**:910–22.

3 Sosin DM. Syndromic surveillance: the case for skillful investment. *Biosecur Bioterrorism Biodefense Strategy Pract Sci* 2003;**1**:247–53.

4 Reingold A. If syndromic surveillance is the answer, what is the question? *Biosecurity Bioterrorism Biodefense Strategy Pract Sci* 2003;**1**(2):77–81.

5 O'Toole T. Emerging illness and bioterrorism: implications for public health. *J Urban Health* 2001;**78**(2):396–402.

6 Buehler JW, Berkelman RL, Hartley DM, Peters CJ. Syndromic surveillance and bioterrorism-related epidemics. *Emerg Infect Dis* 2003;**9**(10):1197–204.

7 Dembek ZF, Cochrane DG, Pavlin JA. Syndromic surveillance [letter]. *Emerg Infect Dis* 2004;**10**(7):1333–4.

8 Nordin JD, Goodman MJ, Kulldorff M, *et al.* Simulated anthrax attacks and syndromic surveillance. *Emerg Infect Dis* 2005;**11**(9):1394–8.

9 Kaufmann AF, Pesik NT, Meltzer MI. Syndromic surveillance in bioterrorist attacks. *Emerg Infect Dis* 2005; **11**(9):1487–8.

10 Berger M, Shiau R, Weintraub JM. Review of syndromic surveillance: implications for waterborne disease detection. *J Epidemiol Community Health* 2006;**60**:543–50.

11 Pavlin JA. Medical surveillance for biological terrorism agents. *Hum Ecol Risk Assess* 2005;**11**(3):525–37.

12 The Gartner Group. Understanding hype cycles. Available from: http://www4.gartner.com/pages/story.php.id .8795.s.8.jsp#1. Accessed October 4, 2006.

13 Li C-S, Aggarwal C, Campbell M, *et al.* Site-based biosurveillance [abstract]. *MMWR Morb Mortal Wkly Rep* 2004;**53**(suppl):249.

14 Besculides M, Heffernan R, Mostashari F, Weiss D. Evaluation of school absenteeism data for early outbreak detection—New York City, 2001–2002 [abstract]. *MMWR Morb Mortal Wkly Rep* 2004;**53**(suppl):230.

15 Wagner M, Pavlin J, Brillman JC, Stetson D, Magruder S, Campbell M. *Synthesis of Research on the Value of Unconventional Data for Early Detection of Disease Outbreaks*. Washington, DC: Defense Advanced Research Projects Agency, BioALIRT Program; 2004.

16 Heffernan R, Mostashari F, Das D, Karpati A, Kuldorff M, Weiss D. Syndromic surveillance in public health practice, New York City. *Emerg Infect Dis* 2004;**10**(5):858–64.

17 Sniegoski CA. Automated syndromic classification of chief complaint records. *JHAPL Tech Dig* 2004; **25**(1): 68–75.

18 Tsui F-C, Espino JU, Dato VM, Gesteland PH, Hutman J, Wagner MW. Technical description of RODS: a real-time public health surveillance system. *J Am Med Inform Assoc* 2003;**10**:399–408.

19 Wagner MM, Tsui F-C, Espino J, *et al.* National Retail Data Monitor for public health surveillance. *MMWR Morb Mortal Wkly Rep* 2004;**53**(suppl):40–2.

20 Sokolow LZ, Grady N, Rolka H, *et al.* Deciphering data anomalies in BioSense. *MMWR Morb Mortal Wkly Rep* 2005;**54**(suppl):133–40.

21 Magruder SF, Marsden-Haug N, Hakre S, *et al.* Comparisons of timeliness and signal strengths for multiple syndromic surveillance data types—San Diego county, July 2003–July 2004 [abstract]. *MMWR Morb Mortal Wkly Rep* 2005;**54**(suppl):193.

22 Das D, Metzger K, Heffernan R, Balter S, Weiss D, Mostashari F. Monitoring over-the-counter medication sales for early detection of disease outbreaks—New York City. *MMWR Morb Mortal Wkly Rep* 2005; **54**(suppl):41–6.

23 Ohkusa Y, Shigematsu M, Taniguchi K, Okabe N. Experimental surveillance using data on sales of over-the-counter medications—Japan, November 2003–April 2004. *MMWR Morb Mortal Wkly Rep* 2005;**54**(suppl): 47–52.

24 Vergu E, Grais RF, Sarter H, *et al.* Medication sales and syndromic surveillance, France. *Emerg Infect Dis* 2006;**12**(3):416–21.

25 Magruder S, Henry J, Snyder M. Linked analysis for definitions of nurse advice line syndrome groups, and comparison to encounters. *MMWR Morb Mortal Wkly Rep* 2005;**54**(suppl):93–7.

26 Doroshenko A, Cooper D, Smith G, *et al.* Evaluation of syndromic surveillance based on national health service direct derived data—England and Wales. *MMWR Morb Mortal Wkly Rep* 2005;**54**(suppl):117–22.

27 Cooper DL, Verlander NQ, Smith GE, *et al.* Can syndromic surveillance data detect local outbreaks of communicable disease? A model using a historical cryptosporidiosis outbreak. *Epidemiol Infect* 2006;**134**(1): 13–20.

28 Derby MP, McNally J, Ranger-Moore J, *et al.* Poison control center-based syndromic surveillance for foodborne illness. *MMWR Morb Mortal Wkly Rep* 2005; **54**(suppl):35–40.

29 Glickman LT, Moore GE, Glickman NW, Caldanaro RJ, Aucoin D, Lewis HB. Purdue University-Banfield National Companion Animal Surveillance Program for emerging and zoonotic diseases. *Vector Borne Zoonotic Dis* 2006;**6**(1):14–23.

30 Mostashari F, Fine A, Das D, Adams J, Layton M. Use of ambulance dispatch data as an early warning system for communitywide influenza like illness, New York City. *J Urban Health* 2003;**80**(suppl 1):i43–9.

31 Greenko J, Mostashari F, Fine A, Layton M. Clinical evaluation of the Emergency Medical Services (EMS) ambulance dispatch-based syndromic surveillance system, New York City. *J Urban Health* 2003;**80**(suppl 1):i50–6.

32 Balter S, Weiss D, Hanson H, Reddy V, Das D, Heffernan R. Three years of emergency department gastrointestinal syndromic surveillance in New York City: what have we found? *MMWR Morb Mortal Wkly Rep* 2005;**54**(suppl):175–80.

33 Marx MA, Rodriguez CV, Greenko J, *et al.* Diarrheal illness detected through syndromic surveillance after a massive power outage: New York City, August 2003. *Am J Public Health* 2006;**96**(3):547–53.

34 Centers for Disease Control and Prevention. Norovirus activity-United States 2002. *MMWR Morb Mortal Wkly Rep* 2003;**52**:41–5.

35 Chapman WW, Dowling J, Ivanov O, Olszewski B, Wagner M. Three stages of evaluation for syndromic surveillance from chief-complaint classification—Pennsylvania and Utah [abstract]. *MMWR Morb Mortal Wkly Rep* 2005;**54**(suppl):185.

36 Bourgeois FT, Olson KL, Brownstein JS, McAdam AJ, Mandl KD. Validation of syndromic surveillance for respiratory infections. *Ann Emerg Med* 2006;**47**(3):265–71.

37 Ritzwoller DP, Kleinman K, Palen T, *et al.* Comparison of syndromic surveillance and a sentinel provider system in detecting an influenza outbreak—Denver, Colorado, 2003. *MMWR Morb Mortal Wkly Rep* 2005; **54**(suppl):151–6.

38 Yih WK, Abrams A, Danila R, *et al.* Ambulatory—care diagnoses as potential indicators of outbreaks of gastrointestinal illness—Minnesota. *MMWR Morb Mortal Wkly Rep* 2005;**54**(suppl):157–62.

39 Ang BCH, Chen MIC, Goh TLH, Ng YY. An assessment of electronically captured data in the Patient Care Enhancement System (PACES) for syndromic surveillance. *Ann Acad Med Singapore* 2005;**34**:539–44.

40 Peterson D, Perencevich E, Harris A, Novak C, Davis S. Using existing electronic hospital data for syndromic surveillance [abstract]. *J Urban Health* 2003;**80**(suppl 1): i122–3.

41 Chen J-H, Schmit K, Chang H, Herlihy E, Miller J, Smith P. Use of Medicaid prescription data for syndromic surveillance—New York. *MMWR Morb Mortal Wkly Rep* 2005;**54**(suppl):31–4.

42 Hadler JL, Siniscalchi A, Dembek Z. Hospital admissions syndromic surveillance—Connecticut, October 2001–June 2004. *MMWR Morb Mortal Wkly Rep* 2005;**54**(suppl):169–74.

43 Reis BY, Mandl KD. Time series modeling for syndromic surveillance. *BMC Med Inform Decis Making* 2003;**3**:2.

44 Wong WK, Moore A, Cooper G, Wagner M. WSARE: what's strange about recent events? *J Urban Health* 2003;**80**(suppl 1):i66–75.

45 Kulldorff M. Prospective time-periodic geographical disease surveillance using a scan statistic. *J R Stat Soc* 2001; **A164**:61–72.

46 Burkom H, Murphy SP, Shmueli G. Automated time series forecasting for biosurveillance. Robert H. Smith School Research Paper No. RHS 06-035 August 2006. Available from SSRN: http://ssrn.com/abstract=923635. Accessed January 8, 2007.

47 Mandl KD, Reis B, Cassa C. Measuring outbreak-detection performance by using controlled feature set simulations. *MMWR Morb Mortal Wkly Rep* 2004; **53**(suppl):130–6.

48 Buckeridge DL, Burkom H, Moore A, Pavlin J, Cutchis P, Hogan W. Evaluation of syndromic surveillance systems—design of an epidemic simulation model. *MMWR Morb Mortal Wkly Rep* 2004;**53**(suppl):137–43.

49 Kulldorff M, Zhang Z, Hartman J, Heffernan R, Huang L, Mostashari F. Benchmark data and power calculations for evaluating disease outbreak detection methods. *MMWR Morb Mortal Wkly Rep* 2004;**53**(suppl):43–6.

50 Steiner-Sichel L, Greenko J, Heffernan R, Layton M, Weiss D. Field investigations of emergency department syndromic surveillance signals—New York City. *MMWR Morb Mortal Wkly Rep* 2004;**53**(suppl):184–9.

51 Foldy SL, Barthell E, Silva J, *et al.* SARS surveillance project—internet-enabled multiregion surveillance for rapidly emerging disease. *MMWR Morb Mortal Wkly Rep* 2004;**53**(suppl):215–20.

52 Cooper DL, Smith G, Baker M, *et al.* National symptom surveillance using calls to a telephone health advice service—United Kingdom, December 2001–February 2003. *MMWR Morb Mortal Wkly Rep* 2004; **53**(suppl):179–83.

53 Bishop LS, Holmes BJ, Kelley CM. National consumer health privacy survey 2005. California HealthCare Foundation, November 2005. Available from: http://www.chcf.org/documents/ihealth/ConsumerPrivacy2005ExecSum.pdf. Accessed November 12, 2006.

54 Broome CV, Horton HH, Tress D, Lucido S, Koo D. Statutory basis for public health reporting beyond specific diseases. *J Urban Health* 2003;**80**(suppl 1): i14–22.

Additional Web resources

International Society for Disease Surveillance (ISDS) homepage: www.syndromic.org.

Centers for Disease Control and Prevention (CDC): www.cdc.gov/EPO/dphsi/syndromic.htm; http://www.bt.cdc.gov/surveillance/ears/; http://www.cdc.gov/biosense/.

Department of Defense (DoD): www.geis.fhp.osd.mil/GEIS/SurveillanceActivities/ESSENCE/ESSENCE.asp.

North Carolina (State): http://www.ncedd.org/.

National Bioterrorism Demonstration Project (Health Plan Data): http://www.btsurveillance.org/.

Real-time Outbreak Detection System (RODS) Laboratory (Academic): http://www.rods.health.pitt.edu/.

United Kingdom: www.hpa.org.uk/infections/topics_az/primary_care_surveillance/NHSD.htm.

Methods for Surveillance Data Analysis, Communication, and Evaluation

27 Software applications for analysis of surveillance data

John H. Holmes, Dale D. Rohn & Joseph M. Hilbe

Surveillance is, by definition, information-intensive, in that its essential function is to gather information about the health of the public. To address data-related demands, increasingly sophisticated and user-friendly information technology tools are becoming more widely available. This chapter introduces the reader to readily accessible information management and analysis software, some of which do not require fees. Table 27.1 lists some of the more popular open-source (free) software tools that can be used in analysis of surveillance and other epidemiologic data. These resources are primarily distributed through the Web—full programs can be downloaded. For some applications, versions exist which are translated into a range of languages.

Proprietary software packages that are suitable for epidemiologic data analysis are available. Three packages are often used due to their extensive analytic tools, wide acceptance in the public health community, and availability of ongoing user support. These packages are SAS (http://www.sas.com/), SPSS (http://www.spss.com/), and Stata (http://www.stata.com/). All three provide a robust array of analytic tools that operate in an interactive graphical user interface environment, including Windows, Macintosh, or Unix (including Linux). They support a wide variety of data visualization and graphing tools, batch processing (which allows users to write programs for efficient analyses), and a variety of data formats. A comparison of common statistical and epidemiologic analysis software packages and programs is provided in Table 27.2.

Finally, while still being tested to establish its role in surveillance, data mining is a unique type of data analysis for which software is available. Instead of being hypothesis-driven (as conceived and directed by humans), data mining utilizes computer programs to seek patterns in large data sets. An open source tool is the Weka data mining suite (http://www.cs.waikato.ac.nz/ml/weka/), a package that includes data preparation and reduction, analysis, and visualization. It is written in Java and runs on all platforms. Commercial tools include SPSS Clementine (http://www.spss.com/clementine/) and SAS Enterprise Miner (http://www.sas.com/technologies/analytics/datamining/miner/). Data mining requires substantial expertise in understanding the algorithms, their uses and limitations, as well as an intimate familiarity with the data being mined.

As illustrated in this chapter, a variety of software applications are useful for infectious disease surveillance. In the future, new tools currently in various stages of development may become more widely available. For example, as is discussed in Chapters 22 and 23, automated methods are being developed that search electronic data to identify "spikes," or deviations, from baseline disease activity that may suggest an outbreak. While interpretation by humans will remain necessary, computerized tools promise to facilitate the analysis of the tremendous quantities of public health data that are collected.

Table 27.1 Commonly used open-source (free) software tools for analysis of infectious diseases surveillance data.

Epi Info™	Widely used epidemiologic data management and analysis software; includes tools for designing data collection forms, performing data entry with error and logic checking, analysis, graphing, and reporting. Supports sophisticated tools for mapping and geocoding that use the Environmental Systems Research Institute, Inc. mapping standards. Users can download free maps as "shapefiles" and link these directly to Epi Info data files to create visual representations of infectious disease outbreak patterns. Runs under Microsoft Windows. http://www.cdc.gov/epiinfo/
EpiDATA Entry and EpiData Analysis (EpiData)	Epidemiologic data collection, entry, analysis, and reporting suite similar to Epi Info but also includes strong data encryption, double-entry with 100% verification, and import and export of data from additional formats with variable and value labels. Runs under Windows. http://www.epidata.dk/
Analysis Software for Word Based Records (AnSWR)	Comprehensive software tool for performing qualitative and quantitative analysis of text-based data. Suitable for collaborative or group-based analyses where analysts in different locations are working on the same document. Runs in a networked client-server environment under Windows. Excellent alternative to proprietary qualitative analysis software. http://www.cdc.gov/hiv/software/answr.htm
CDC EZ-TEXT	Qualitative analysis program. Support for developing questionnaires and codebooks are included, allowing seamless data entry and analysis in the same software environment. Runs only on single computers and does not require a server. http://www.cdc.gov/hiv/software/ez-text.htm
CLUSTER	Software includes 12 statistical methods that analyze the significance of a cluster using techniques that evaluate clustering in time and space. Runs under Windows. http://www.atsdr.cdc.gov/HS/cluster.html
Open Source Epidemiologic Statistics for Public Health (OpenEpi)	Suite of analytic tools for epidemiologic analysis that can be run from a browser interface online or locally. Written in Java, highly transportable between platforms. Useful for analyzing person-level and count-level data. http://www.openepi.com/Menu/OpenEpiMenu.htm
WinEpiScope	Developed by CLIVE, a consortium of veterinary schools in the United Kingdom. Supports a wide variety of epidemiologic analysis tools useful for infectious disease surveillance, including tools useful for a wide variety of study designs. Runs under Windows. http://www.clive.ed.ac.uk/cliveCatalogueItem.asp?id=B6BC9009-C10F-4393-A22D-48F436516AC4
Computer Programs for Epidemiologic Analyses (PEPI)	Suite of statistical tools for epidemiologic analysis. Supported under Windows. http://sagebrushpress.com/pepibook.html
The Medical Algorithms Project (MAP)	Extensive software resource for all types of medical computations. Numerous calculators specific to infectious disease analysis are available. Typically run under Microsoft Excel as downloadable spreadsheets with formulas and prompts for data entry. http://www.medal.org/visitor/www/inactive/ch23.aspx

Table 27.2 Comparison of common statistical and epidemiologic analysis software packages and programs.

	Software	Database[a]	Data entry[b]	Import export[c]	Data management[d]	Reporting[e]	Graphics	Statistical analysis[f]	Epidemiologic analysis[g]	Computing environment[h]	Network capable[i]	Cost/licensing[j]
Commercial	SAS	No	Graphical	Yes	Yes	Yes	Extensive	Extensive	Extensive	Unix MS Windows OS X	Yes	Expensive/annual
	SPSS	No	Graphical	Yes	Yes	Yes	Extensive	Extensive	Yes	Unix MS Windows OS X	Yes	Expensive/annual
	Stata	No	Spreadsheet	Yes	Yes	Yes	Extensive	Extensive	Extensive	Unix MS Windows OS X	Yes	Moderate/perpetual
	EpiInfo	Yes	Graphical	Yes	Yes	Yes	Yes	Yes	Extensive (see Figures 27.1–27.3)	MS Windows	No	Free/none
Free	EpiData	Yes	Yes	Yes	Yes	Yes	Yes	Yes	Yes	MS Windows	No	Free/none
	AnSWR	No	Yes	No	No	Yes	No	No	No	MS Windows	Yes	Free/none
	EZ-Text	No	Yes	No	No	Yes	No	No	No	MS Windows	No	Free/none
	CLUSTER	No	No	No	No	No	No	Limited	Limited	MS Windows	No	Free/none
	OpenEpi	No	No	No	No	Yes	No	Yes	Yes	MS Windows	No	Free/none
	Win EpiScope	No	No	No	No	Yes	No	Yes	Extensive	MS Windows	No	Free/none
	PEPI	No	No	No	No	No	No	Yes	Extensive	MS Windows	No	Free/none

[a] Indicates whether or not software supports creation of relation databases.

[b] Creation and editing of forms for data entry with or without data checking (range or logic checks). Graphical interfaces support Windows-style objects such as buttons, combo boxes, and pull-down menus.

[c] Supports importing from or exporting to data sets and files of various formats.

[d] Allows user to manipulate data (creating new variables, queries, data views, and data sets for analysis or use by other software).

[e] Supports creation of user-defined report formats for printing to screen, files, or printout.

[f] Tools for analysis including univariate, bivariate, and multivariate procedures.

[g] Tools for epidemiologic analysis, including risk and odds estimates, incidence and prevalence measures, and rates and proportions.

[h] Type of computer systems that support the software.

[i] Software runs on a client-server or peer-to-peer network.

[j] Cost per user and requirements for licensing, if needed.

FREQ Q6Villag STRATAVAR = Q8III

Next Procedure
Village, III?=Yes
Village, III?=No

Village, III?=Yes

Forward

Village	Frequency	Percent	Cum Percent
Newera	4	12.1%	12.1%
Rwenbinyoni	7	21.2%	33.3%
Rwenshama	22	66.7%	100.0%
Total	33	100.0%	100.0%

95% Conf Limits

Fig 27.1 An example of a frequency distribution from an EPI Info Analysis Output Window. From an EPI Info training manual available on the Centers for Disease Control and Prevention's Website at: http://www.cdc.gov/cogh/descd/.

Here is what your 2x2 table will look like. You can see that it is a table comparing one variable with two values as possible answers with another variable with two variables as a possible answer; hence, a two-by-two (2x2) table.

Q27HMATO : Q8ILL

Q8ILL

Q27Hmato	Yes	No	TOTAL
Yes	28	26	54
Row %	51.9	48.1	100.0
Col %	84.8	78.8	81.8
No	5	7	12
Row %	41.7	58.3	100.0
Col %	15.2	21.2	18.2
TOTAL	33	33	66
Row %	50.0	50.0	100.0
Col %	100.0	100.0	100.0

Fig 27.2 An example of a risk factor analysis table produced using EPI Info. The 2 × 2 table tells us that of the 54 people who ate matooke, 28 became ill while 26 did not. Of the 12 people who did not eat hot matooke, 5 became ill while 7 did not. From an EPI Info training manual available on the Centers for Disease Control and Prevention's Website at: http://www.cdc.gov/cogh/descd/.

Single Table Analysis

	Point Estimate	95% Confidence Interval Lower	Upper	
PARAMETERS: Odds-based				
Odds Ratio (cross product)	1.5077	0.4252	5.3458	(T)
Odds Ratio (MLE)	1.4984	0.4122	5.7607	(M)
		0.3575	6.7885	(F)
PARAMETERS: Risk-based				
Risk Ratio (RR)	1.2444	0.6075	2.5492	(T)
Risk Difference (RD)	10.1852	-20.7294	41.0997	(T)

(T=Taylor series; C=Cornfield; M=Mid-P; F=Fisher Exact)

STATISTICAL TESTS	Chi-square	1-tailed p	2-tailed p
Chi square - uncorrected	0.4074		0.5232889021
Chi square - Mantel-Haenszel	0.4012		0.5264529161
Chi square - corrected (Yates)	0.1019		0.7496188489
Mid-p exact		0.2724281422	
Fisher exact		0.3754075862	

Fig 27.3 In this example, the odds ratio is 1.5077; 95% confidence interval—Taylor series is 0.4252–5.3458; two-tailed p-value—Chi square uncorrected is 0.5232 round. From an EPI Info training manual available on the Centers for Disease Control and Prevention's Website at: http://www.cdc.gov/cogh/descd/.

28 Analysis and interpretation of reportable infectious disease data

Mindy J. Perilla & Elizabeth R. Zell

Introduction

A goal of disease surveillance is to provide public health agencies and their partners with objective measures of the health events that are occurring in a population and the rates at which these events occur over time. When case definitions and data collection are standardized, these measures can be compared across seasons, years, and locations. Data about infectious diseases in a community are collected by public health agencies through disease reports and submitted for analysis through surveillance systems. As discussed in earlier chapters, surveillance systems take various forms. Population-based surveillance, for example, requires that information be garnered in such a manner that it represents all members of a community, whereas sentinel surveillance involves the collection and interpretation of data from a smaller, defined subset of the population. Passive surveillance relies on the people and institutions in a community who identify the presence of diseases, such as clinicians and laboratorians, to inform public health agencies that a disease event has occurred, while active surveillance systems rely on public health agencies to contact and communicate with clinicians and laboratorians regularly to ascertain if there have been any occurrences of specific disease events. Regardless of the methods used to conduct surveillance for reportable infectious diseases, it is the analysis of collected data and subsequent interpretation of these analyses that permit public health authorities to infer the health status of a population. This chapter presents basic tools to bring surveillance data from its elemental form, where it represents individuals, through a process of aggregation, analysis, and interpretation so it can be used in a population-based context appropriate to public health.

Goals of analysis and interpretation of surveillance data

The goals of analysis and interpretation of surveillance data may differ by public health authority. In the United States (US), local and county health departments conduct routine surveillance to identify disease trends, recognize problems in the community or in the surveillance system, and ascertain the need to respond to a disease of public health concern. State health departments conduct similar tasks and also review data aggregated from local health departments to be aware of health conditions occurring across jurisdictions within a state. State and local health departments may analyze regional data to identify risk factors for disease and to shape and evaluate public health interventions or local policies. Data are further aggregated at the national level, enabling analysts to look for patterns across regions. Analyses of these larger populations over longer time periods help frame research questions for further investigation and can guide development of public health policies.

By monitoring the *status quo* of a population's health through effective surveillance, public health agencies can define a baseline level of disease events. When reports are aggregated and analyzed, the results can then be compared and interpreted relative to the established baseline. Disease rates can be monitored for unexpected fluctuations, emerging problems (e.g., antimicrobial resistance) can be identified, and the impact of prevention strategies (e.g., vaccination programs) can be measured. Regular attention to surveillance data can help inform public health practitioners of issues and assist in guiding the allocation of public health resources [1–3].

Data elements

Although public health surveillance focuses on health of a population, individual persons experience the disease event. Individual case reports are investigated to better classify case status, and similar disease events are aggregated for analysis and interpretation. The individual components that make up disease reports can be considered "data elements." An example of a data element collected in routine surveillance is "reporter category" with potential values being "physician," "laboratory," etc.

Public health agencies typically use standard disease case report forms and specify information required from disease reporters in order to standardize collection, storage, and analysis of data. Standardized report forms and databases used to record disease reports typically have fields for common variables or data elements such as patient demographics (name, address, date of birth), laboratory test result and clinical symptoms (used to classify the individual as having a suspected or confirmed infection), the date of symptom onset or laboratory testing, and information identifying the reporter and reporting agency. (An example of a case report form is included in Chapter 14.) Report forms and databases often collect other information useful for disease investigation such as vaccination history, recent antibiotic use, source of drinking water, any association with a child-care facility, and so on.

Data elements can be continuous, categorical, or open-ended. Continuous variables have a range of values of measurement (e.g., age, distance); categorical variables place data into a limited number of groups or categories (e.g., sex, race, questions to which the response can be "yes," "no," or "unknown"); and open-ended variables do not have a discrete set of possible answers but are open text fields that allow the person entering data to write in a response (e.g., a description of what the case patient did in the 24 hours prior to onset of illness). Open-ended variables are the least frequently used type of variable because these data are more difficult to include in routine analyses.

In a disease investigation, some data elements may be used at the local level and then removed or "stripped" from a data set when it is shared with higher-level jurisdictions (e.g., transmitted from the state level to the federal level). The elements of data most commonly removed from shared data sets are identifier variables, such as the name and address of a case patient. This information is pertinent to the detailed investigation of a case, and is transmitted to the national level only if national authorities are participating in the direct case investigation. More general information about the case, such as county of residence, upholds privacy rules for data sharing, is useful for monitoring the spread of disease or identifying geographic differences in disease incidence, and is usually included among data transmitted to the national level.

When data sets are shared across agencies, it is important for data elements that were used to define or categorize a case to remain in the data set. Similarly, jurisdictions often provide coinvestigators with the inclusion and exclusion criteria they have used in order to ascertain that there is consistency in the sensitivity and specificity of how cases are defined.

Numerators and case definitions

Public health measures often refer to numerators and denominators, where the numerator is the aggregate number of cases or events observed, and the denominator is the count of the comparison population or the total population in an area over the time in which the cases or events were observed. Depending upon the disease, numerators may represent only confirmed cases or both confirmed and probable cases. Not all reports received by surveillance systems represent actual cases of disease. Reports that do not meet criteria to be counted as cases are excluded from the numerator.

Consistency in case definitions is important because it results in a measure that is independent of individual investigators and permits data from different places to be aggregated for further analysis.

For example, if a case of influenza is defined by laboratory data in one area, by fever in another, and nasal congestion and cough in a third, combining data from the "cases" identified at the three different locations would be misleading and could lead to faulty, misinformed public health decision making. However, use of a standard case definition allows investigators to combine all cases and to draw conclusions about the larger pool of affected individuals. If a disease is nationally notifiable, there will often be guidance from the national level regarding a case definition, the sorts of questions to be asked, and the data to be collected for analysis. In addition to standardized case definitions, there may also be tools to help conduct similar investigations across sites.

Denominators: identifying the reference population

Surveillance systems receive information about cases, but comparison groups are important to the calculation of summary measures of analysis and their interpretation. The cases and comparison groups represent different components of the same population. Cases comprise the numerator and the population from which they were drawn (i.e., the catchment area covered by the surveillance system) comprises the comparative denominator.

Denominator data can come from a variety of sources. Some common useful data sources for denominators are census data and vital statistics data. For example, if a surveillance system is designed to capture reports of conditions in a city, the appropriate denominator would be the city population as measured by the most recent census. If a system were designed to measure cases of neonatal tetanus or neonatal group B streptococcal infections in a state (or province) in a year, the appropriate denominator would be the number of live births in that state (province) for the year. However, if a system were designed to measure only infections among patients in a hospital's surgical ward in a given month, the denominator would be the total number of patients who had been on that ward in that month. Sometimes the denominator is not available for the same time frame as that of the numerator or case count, at which time the most recent official population estimates can be used.

Census data provide overall counts and one can stratify census population data by categories such as gender, age, and race/ethnicity. Furthermore, other socioeconomic measures may be collected by the census and may be useful for ecologic analyses, such as associations of a disease with regions of a city that have greater household crowding. The government of a country typically conducts census counts on a periodic basis and in some places interim demographic and health survey data are collected with the assistance of external agencies. Census population counts do not reflect counts of live births or deaths, but these measures are available through vital statistics offices. It is important to use a denominator measure appropriate for the population from which cases were derived in order to make valid comparisons that can contribute to evidence-based decisions. Together, the case-count numerators and the pertinent denominators can be used to create summary measures of analysis.

Routine surveillance monitoring

Surveillance systems typically collect data on an ongoing basis and it is important to review the data regularly. Routine monitoring of surveillance data allows identification of trends or patterns among notifiable diseases. In order to identify patterns, it is helpful to have comparative measures. Comparisons can be made to existing baseline data and, within a given time frame, comparisons may be made within a population using variables such as season, race, gender, or age group.

When baseline data are available, it is helpful to compare similar time frames. If looking at quarterly data, for example, one can compare adjacent quarters within a year and the same quarter over several years. This will assess whether issues are related to season or to surveillance artifacts at the end of a reporting time frame when cases are "due" to be closed. When baseline surveillance data are not available, analysts may compare characteristics of cases to the overall population. For example, in 1980 in the US, staphylococcal toxic shock syndrome was epidemiologically linked to the use of highly absorbent tampons after it was noticed that cases occurred among menstruating women but not among other groups of women or men [4].

369

Advances in technology have led to increased access of epidemiologically pertinent supplemental laboratory data by public health analysts. Laboratory tools that are useful for disease surveillance include bacterial culture, antigen testing, antimicrobial susceptibility testing, serologic testing, serotyping, and molecular methods like polymerase chain reaction (PCR) and pulse-field gel electrophoresis (PFGE). In 2006, examination of PFGE patterns led to the detection of an *Escherichia coli* O157:H7 outbreak in the US; the resultant epidemiologic investigation of cases implicated consumption of raw spinach and spinach was removed from market shelves nationwide [5]. Molecular methods of surveillance are discussed in greater detail in Chapter 30.

In routine surveillance monitoring, cases need to be evaluated in their epidemiological context. For example, hepatitis B virus (HBV) is spread through contact with infected body fluids. An increased incidence of acute HBV infection among older members of the population would be unexpected and could indicate the cross-contamination of medication vials or instruments in a medical care setting [6]. Public health analysts should be aware of the different tools available to a surveillance system and consider the findings of routine analyses relative to the expected distribution of cases of disease in a population.

Units of time

Prior to the interpretation of data, it is important to identify appropriate units of time. Data can be presented as weekly, monthly, quarterly, or annual measures. However data are aggregated, it is wise to use standardized units. Calendar months are standard across locations (that use the same calendar) but, because different months contain different numbers of days (e.g., February typically has three fewer days than March), measures are subject to variations even if the number of reports per day is consistent over time. In response to such variations in calendar measures, the US Centers for Disease Control and Prevention (CDC) defines standardized week-units that run from Sunday to Saturday, independent of the Gregorian calendar. This standard time unit, the morbidity week, is used by health departments at the local, state, and national levels and

its use permits aggregations of data without concerns of differential temporality. It can be helpful to combine standard morbidity weeks into quarters of 13 weeks each, and to define week groupings that represent seasons of the year for analytic purposes. It should also be noted that because calendar years do not have exactly 52 weeks (365 days/7 days per week = 52.18), and because of the occurrence of leap years (when February has 29 days instead of 28) on a 4-year cycle, the standard morbidity-week calendar periodically contains 53 weeks in the morbidity year.

Assessing data quality

Public health data analysts must become familiar with data for their population of interest. An initial step is to look at completeness of data and the overall distribution of values in the set. Generally speaking: know your system and know your diseases.

An initial assessment of data quality can be obtained by looking through data records by hand or with the assistance of analytic computer software to ensure that the data are "clean"; that is, that the data accurately represent what was intended to be recorded. One way to check data is to look for "outlier" values. Outliers are individual values found at the extremes of the overall distribution of values among a data set. Examples include illnesses usually screened for in women that are reported in men, illnesses reported for persons outside the age group usually affected, and reports of illnesses uncommon in a region. Another common data error is duplicate reports stored as separate records. However, be attentive when de-duplicating records: it is not uncommon for siblings to have the same reportable illness at the same time, and records for twins can appear to be a duplicate report for the same individual. It is also important to identify and assess missing data values and decide how to manage them, whether by further investigation or exclusion. Approaches to working with data containing unknown values are discussed further in the (*supplemental analyses*) section of this chapter.

Data quality issues can also arise from changes in case ascertainment, disease awareness, or reporting practices by the community. A shift in the number (either an increase or a decrease) of reported cases may reflect the true situation, or can be a surveillance artifact. When a case definition changes, for example, there can be a change in the number of cases; the change in cases reported may not warrant an immediate public health response, but the change in case definition should be documented so that surveillance data can be properly interpreted in the future. Occasionally, there is increased community awareness of disease (e.g., during a campaign focusing on measles elimination) that leads to a change in care-seeking and reporting behaviors. A change in activity by reporters themselves, such as when a commercial laboratory starts or stops reporting laboratory results, or when new personnel at reporting institutions are unfamiliar with disease reporting requirements, may result in a significant change in the numbers of reported cases. Therefore, it can be helpful to monitor activity of reporters and contact them if there is a change in what your surveillance system is receiving.

Addressing data quality can take time, but a little bit of up-front attention to your data is less time-intensive than following up on false findings with a full-scale public health response. Anomalies in data trends can identify outbreaks, glitches in the reporting system, and areas that need further evaluation. Tables and graphs of data may also help to identify aberrances and shape analyses.

Data presentation in graphical form

Charts, tables, and graphs can be helpful tools for public health analysts. They may be used in the course of an ongoing analysis to help shape the direction of an investigation, in the interpretation of data, and as a useful means to relay information.

Different audiences may need to see data presented in different ways in order to better understand its implications. Statisticians might prefer tables of calculated values so they can draw their own in-depth conclusions whereas policymakers may prefer analyses presented with charts and graphs. For all presentations, titles should be used and each axis should be clearly labeled with values and units of measurement.

Use of standard colors or patterns across groupings can enable your audience to assess the story your data tells in an easy glance. Because graphical presentation aims for clear, straightforward in-

terpretation, three-dimensional (3-D) or other visually busy representations available in some computer graphing tools should be avoided. When using color in graphical presentations, it is important to remember that people viewing the presentation may not be able to see color due to lack of an adequate quality color print-out or due to color-blindness. It is therefore a good idea to create color-pattern schemes that are easily differentiated in the scales of black, grey, and white. Maps can be useful for public health analyses, but are beyond the scope of this chapter and are addressed in Chapter 31 in detail.

There are different ways to present frequencies, distributions, and other measures visually [7]. Commonly used charts and graphs include line graphs, vertical bar charts, histograms, horizontal bar charts, and pie charts. Chart types can be combined to represent more detailed findings (Figure 28.1). For example, line graphs superimposed on bar charts can show case counts and rates simultaneously in a straightforward manner; stacked bar charts can show subcomponents of a measure (e.g., male and female) by putting two colors in one bar to represent the different categories. Bar charts can also be used to create variants of things like population pyramids, showing distribution of an event by age and gender. Lines can also be used to indicate ranges, such as confidence intervals or calculated threshold boundaries, on a graph. In general, some helpful parameters for how to present data include using line graphs for data measuring change over time, bar charts for data with counts or categorical outcome characteristics, and pie charts to represent data tallying to 100%. When summing values to 100%, the relative contribution of each component may not be easily differentiated; if so, graphical methods other than pie charts should be considered.

One graphical presentation particular to public health is that of the epidemic curve, or "epi-curve" (Figure 28.2), commonly used in outbreak investigations. Although the purpose of an epi-curve is to show the incidence of cases over time, and time is represented on the x-axis, a histogram is used rather than a line graph. Individual cases are represented as box-units stacked at the time of incidence (e.g., symptom onset) so that the count for the time can be read on the y-axis. The units of time used in an

371

Table 28.1 *Streptococcus pneumoniae*, Active Bacterial Core surveillance (ABCs): US, 2005.

Calendar quarter	Cases	Percent	Cases/100,000 population
January–March	1408	36.03%	5.06
April–June	988	25.28%	3.55
July–September	420	10.75%	1.51
October–December	1092	27.94%	3.93
Total	*3908*	*100.00%*	*14.05*

ABCs surveillance area population: 27,816,784.

fourth calendar quarters and lowest in the third quarter of each year due to the seasonality of *S. pneumoniae*, a respiratory infection with low disease incidence in the warmer months.

Percents and proportions

Percent (or proportion × 100%) is the number of cases in a defined time frame (e.g., first quarter of the year) divided by the total number of cases in a defined time frame (e.g., an entire year). As shown in Table 28.1, the third quarter of each year has the lowest percent of annual cases in addition to the lowest disease counts; this shows how more than one measure can be used to illustrate a finding from your surveillance system. However, as overall disease incidence changes, a constant or increased percent of a particular subset of cases may be indicative of something new. For example, antibiotic resistant *S. pneumoniae* was initially identified as an emerging problem because the percentage of resistant cases increased over time. However, with widespread use of the pediatric pneumococcal conjugate vaccine, a marked reduction in invasive pneumococcal disease, including antibiotic resistant disease, has been observed. Monitoring changes in the percentage of resistant cases can assist in identifying new resistance problems in *S. pneumoniae* serotypes not included in the current pediatric vaccine.

Disease rates

Rates of disease are very useful measures and can be calculated when the population can be defined for a

surveillance area and denominators or population counts are available. Two types of rates are often used: incidence rates and prevalence rates [1,9]. Incidence is defined as new cases of disease per population unit (over time) and is commonly used for infectious diseases with the exception of those that result in chronic infections.

Incidence rate
$$= \frac{\text{Number of NEW cases in defined time frame}}{\text{Population at risk}} \times 10^n$$

Prevalence rates include all persons who have ever had a disease, and are more commonly applied in analyses of chronic diseases, but are useful measures for some diseases of infectious etiology and chronic outcome, such as hepatitis B, hepatitis C, and HIV. (The analysis of HIV surveillance data is discussed in detail in Chapter 29.)

Prevalence rate
$$= \frac{\text{Total number of cases in defined time frame}}{\text{Population at risk}} \times 10^n$$

Incidence and prevalence rates are commonly calculated as cases per 100,000 (i.e., 10^5) population. The rates presented in this chapter apply to new cases of infectious disease and all rates used henceforth will be incidence rates.

For diseases of neonates, incidence rates are typically calculated as cases per 1000 (i.e., 10^3) live births; this is in part because a single birth cohort is smaller than other populations, and using this sort of scale yields more meaningful and readily interpreted measures. Examples of diseases for which a live births denominator would be used include early-onset group B streptococcal infections, defined as occurring in the first 7 days of life (0–6 days of age), late-onset group B streptococcal infections (occurring in the 7th to 89th days of life), neonatal tetanus, and congenital syphilis [10].

Surveillance systems are often passive systems, relying on clinicians or laboratories to identify and report cases to a public health authority, and do not capture all cases for the population of interest. However, if the reporting is consistent over time it provides useful information. If the catchment area for surveillance is well-defined and a population denominator is available, "crude" rates can be calculated. These observed crude rates are useful measures but are often not sufficient indicators of the total actual burden of disease. In this situation, analysts may wish to "adjust" or "standardize" observed rates to the distribution of the population of interest in order to better estimate actual disease burden [11].

Time periods used in analyses

Monitoring disease over time is a useful and often critical component of surveillance systems, and it is important to consider the time period included in analytic measures. There are differences in what one might be able to learn from evaluating disease by day, week, month, quarter, or year. These are important issues one needs to contemplate when deciding how to shape surveillance systems to help best monitor disease over time.

Once the unit of time has been decided, a graph of case counts or incidence rates by the unit of time assists in understanding the information available. Often there is great day-to-day or week-to-week variation in the time-based measures. This can be related to disease epidemiology (e.g., some diseases have seasonal variation), related to reporting logistics (e.g., reporting of incident weekend cases at the beginning of the next week), or other factors. If this is true for a given data set, one may wish to consider moving averages. A moving average can be defined retrospectively as the mean of the previous n data points. Consider, for example, a 10-day moving average in mid-June. June 15th would be represented by the mean average data from days 10 through 19, June 16th would average data from days 11 through 20, and so on. Application of a moving average may allow for the better visualization of disease over time by smoothing out the "noise" or variation in case counts or disease rates [12]. Furthermore, moving measures can guide development of possible threshold measures. Public health officials at the local, state, and national levels may find threshold calculations useful for the detection of increases in disease incidence that exceed expected variations. Such increases can signify an outbreak of disease, or at least an area warranting closer attention. Some syndromic surveillance systems use moving averages in the determination of potential outbreaks [13]. Moving averages are also used in time

series analyses. Time series analyses are addressed in many texts (e.g., [12]) and computer software applications are available to assist analysts with this approach, but these are beyond the scope of this chapter.

Supplemental analyses of surveillance data

Tracking disease trends and monitoring changes that occur for a population as a whole is very informative. However, there are times when subgroup analyses are useful and should be done as part of routine monitoring. It can be helpful to know if a disease is affecting one component of your population more than others, as sometimes diseases do not occur equally across the population distribution. Subgroup analysis of surveillance data can promote better understanding of disease epidemiology.

When one thinks of subgroup analyses, it is useful to frame things in the framework of *What*, *Who*, *When*, and *Why*.
- "What" could be the disease of interest, or some aspect of the disease presentation.
- "Who" might be a particular age group, race, or gender.
- "When" would be a specified period of time.
- "Why" can address the reasons for the "what," "who," and "when"; e.g., whether an outbreak of a vaccine-preventable disease is the result of failure to vaccinate or vaccine failure.

Often, subgroup analyses can be conducted in the context of routine surveillance. It is important to know the summary measure of how many cases are occurring in a location, but it can also be important to know who is being affected by the disease. Many diseases have different incidence rates by age group, race, and gender. For example, prior to vaccine introduction, *S. pneumoniae* had higher incidence of disease in young children and the elderly, and this could not have been detected without the use of analyses that looked for differences by age [14]. Another example of a difference detected by subgroup analysis is that rates of the sexually transmitted infection with *Chlamydia trachomatis* tend to be higher in females than males, and also higher in adolescents and young adults than in older and younger age groups (see Figure 28.1b).

Differences detected by subgroup analyses can help shape more focused outreach, prevention, and control efforts, and lead to better-informed policy.

When a surveillance system routinely captures not just case counts but also basic characteristics of individuals (e.g., age, race, and gender), it is possible to conduct analyses of subgroups relative to the population of infected individuals. However, in order to monitor changes in rates of disease within subgroups, it is important to have denominator data reflective of those same subgroups. That is, if appropriate denominators are not available, analyses are possible but only at the level of proportions among the population with disease. For example, without denominators one can determine that among cases of disease X, 62% of cases belong to a certain racial group. With appropriate denominators, the analyst can look further to see if the distribution of disease (e.g., incidence) is equal across the population distribution: i.e., does that racial group comprise approximately two-thirds of the population, or does the population consist of only 15% of that racial group. Comparison to the pertinent population permits calculation of rates and can help identify disparities that may be addressed with a public health response.

Surveillance systems serve an important role in documenting the impact of public health activities on disease incidence. Supplemental analyses may be conducted, therefore, to measure changes accompanying new or improved interventions for disease reduction, such as the introduction of new vaccines, screening tools, or prophylaxis guidelines. One method involves comparison of rates between two time periods as a percent change. To illustrate, percent change for a baseline and intervention period rate of disease would be calculated as:

Percent change
$$= \frac{R_{\text{post-intervention}} - R_{\text{pre-intervention}}}{R_{\text{pre-intervention}}} \times 100\%$$

where $R_{\text{pre-intervention}}$ is the old (baseline) rate of disease and $R_{\text{post-intervention}}$ is the rate of disease temporally associated with the intervention. Other approaches for evaluating changes in disease rates include rate differences, differences in proportions, and relative risks for comparing rates in different subgroups [11,15,16].

Public health analysts are also often interested in detecting disease trends. The most commonly used approach is a statistical test for linear trend that requires two components of the chi-square (χ^2) test [10]. More advanced analytic methods are available [12,17] but detailed descriptions of these methods go beyond the scope of this chapter.

An aspect of data quality that affects analyses but can be difficult to manage is missing data. Missing data can further impact the analysis and interpretation of disease trends by subgroup because of the decreasing sample sizes found in subanalyses. If one excludes those cases with missing data, the resultant rates of disease can be misleading, with some groups under-represented. Accounting or adjusting for missing (unknown) data can be done through what are called imputation methods. However unknowns are dealt with, the methods should be well-defined and described for the audience to properly interpret. Imputation can be as simple as distributing the unknowns in the population according to the known proportions for the rest of the population with reported values. Other methods are more complex and beyond the scope of this chapter [18,19].

Although surveillance can contribute to shaping the understanding of disease epidemiology, the methods and context of data collection differ from those used in epidemiologic studies. The analysis of epidemiologic data is addressed in many texts (e.g., [2,9–11,16,20). However, the application of statistical methods to the analysis of surveillance data is controversial, with questions arising about the proper use of tests for statistical significance and p-values. Surveillance data can be drawn from an entire population or, as discussed above, it can represent a subset of the population. Some analysts believe that a year's worth of surveillance data, for example, represents a random sample from the population with disease over all years of disease occurrence and so it is acceptable to calculate p-values and apply other statistical tests. In contrast, others believe that surveillance data is an important source of information but that it represents a non-random population, so it is inappropriate to apply measures of statistical significance to its assessment. Instead of statistical tests of significance, confidence intervals may provide a better framework for evaluating and interpreting data from a surveillance system over time. Further elaboration on this topic is beyond the scope of this chapter. No matter the methods used, public health analysts need to be able to move the data from the stage of analysis to that of interpretation, so they and others can learn from it.

Interpretation

Appropriate interpretation of surveillance data requires an in-depth knowledge of all aspects of the reporting system from which the data are obtained and of the specific infectious disease under surveillance. When reviewing data collected from an established surveillance system it is also helpful to review routinely generated disease reports—annual numbers of cases or incidence rates, age and sex distributions, seasonal patterns—to know what might be expected and therefore what is out of the ordinary.

An understanding of the reporting community and population under surveillance is essential. In both passive and active surveillance systems a reportable infectious disease is recognized only when the ill person seeks medical care and, in the case of laboratory-based surveillance, when a healthcare provider orders the appropriate diagnostic test. The completeness of disease detection therefore reflects local healthcare-seeking behaviors and clinical testing practices. For example, most diarrheal illnesses are markedly under-reported as patients often do not seek care for transient infections and providers often treat empirically, if at all (see Chapter 5).

Knowing the demographics of the specific population under surveillance allows the public health analyst to determine how broadly the findings from the surveillance data can be generalized to other populations. Population-based surveillance data with its theoretic 100% case detection should be the easiest to interpret; the incidence and descriptive epidemiology of the reportable disease under surveillance should reflect the true disease distribution and risk factors among persons in the entire geographic area surveyed. If the differences and similarities between the surveillance population (e.g., a state) and a larger geographic area (e.g., a country) are known, the disease incidence rates and total disease burden of the larger population may be estimated. For example, national incidence rates and disease burden can be estimated from a state or multiple states that are under active, population-based surveillance when the observed age- and race-specific incidence rates are assumed to be representative for the disease under surveillance. In contrast, generalizability or extrapolation of findings obtained from analysis of sentinel surveillance is often limited; the population surveyed may be restricted to one age group (e.g., children), an urban population, or to hospitalized patients which represent more severe manifestations of the disease under surveillance.

When interpreting surveillance data, other limitations should also be kept in mind. These include the possible bias inherent in data collection methods, seasonal variations, sub-population surveyed, and disease trends specific to particular geographic regions [1,20]. Many diseases are seasonal; influenza and other viral respiratory infections occur more commonly in the winter while many diarrheal illnesses are more frequent during warmer, summer months. Annual rates should not be extrapolated from data obtained from a single season. Rate calculations of regionally endemic diseases (e.g., coccidiomycoses and other regional fungal infections) should be limited to the appropriate geographic areas.

Changes in disease rates may be indicative of a true change or may represent artifact, as discussed in (*Assessment of data quality*) above. An acute increase in the rate of a disease may indicate an outbreak. Alternatively, media coverage or changes in the reporting system including new personnel or new laboratory tests may lead to increased reporting. A true long-term increase in cases may represent a shift in disease epidemiology, such as disease caused by emergence of new serotypes of a previously vaccine-controlled bacterium. Increases could also represent a shift in risk factors, as seen with cases of *Pneumocystis* pneumonia and Kaposi's sarcoma in young men in the early 1980s, which helped lead to the identification of HIV/AIDS. A decrease in cases may represent successful uptake of a prevention method, such as a vaccine.

Surveillance data are valuable tools to monitor the impact of prevention methods. If rates begin to rise despite use of a previously successful prevention method, resources can be targeted to determine the reason for the epidemiological shift and to develop new interventions. The data can then be used to monitor the impact of the new interventions. Surveillance data should be interpreted with care. Analysts can assist in the appropriate interpretation of data and in the dissemination of analyzed data in printed and oral presentations and publications. Data should be used to inform policy-makers so that decisions can be evidence-driven.

Conclusions

Surveillance is an important tool used to improve public health. It entails the collection of data through reporting systems, investigation and classification of cases, and the aggregation of similar disease events for analysis and interpretation, with the application of standardized case definitions permitting data from different sources to be combined for valid comparisons. Analysts working with reportable infectious disease data have many options for how to analyze and to describe surveillance data, so it is important to consider the story to be conveyed to the audience and then use the appropriate tools to do so. The use of basic measures such as incidence rates and proportions, as well as more advanced rate comparisons over time can help in the development and evaluation of disease impact, prevention, and control strategies. On occasion, interpretation and discussion of findings from routine analyses may suggest the need for a more in-depth look at a potentially emergent public health concern. Analysis of data from surveillance systems and interpretation of results in a manner appropriate to the context in which data were collected can provide public health personnel with data for decision-making in a resource-efficient manner and can help inform and shape both immediate responses and long-term policies.

References

1 Teutsch SM, Churchill RE (eds.). *Principles and Practice of Public Health Surveillance*, 2nd edn. New York: Oxford University Press; 2000.

2 Thacker SB, Wetterhall SF. Data sources for public health. In: Stroup DF, Teutsch SM (eds.), *Statistics in Public Health: Quantitative Approaches to Public Health Problems*. New York: Oxford University Press; 1998.

3 Buehler JW. Surveillance. In: Rothman KJ, Greenland S (eds.), *Modern Epidemiology*. Philadelphia: Lippincott-Raven Publishers; 1998.

4 Shands KN, Schmid GP, Dan BB, *et al.* Toxic-shock syndrome in menstruating women: association with tampon use and *Staphylococcus aureus* and clinical features in 52 cases. *N Engl J Med* 1980;**303**:1436–42.

5 Centers for Disease Control and Prevention. Ongoing Multistate Outbreak of *Escherichia coli* serotype O157:H7 infections associated with consumption of fresh spinach—United States, September 2006. *MMWR Morb Mortal Wkly Rep* 2006;**55**(38):1045–6.

6 Centers for Disease Control and Prevention Transmission of hepatitis B and C viruses in outpatient settings—New York, Oklahoma, and Nebraska, 2000–2002. *MMWR Morb Mortal Wkly Rep* 2003; **52**(38):901–6.

7 Tufte ER. *The Visual Display of Quantitative Information*, 2nd edn. Cheshire, CT: Graphics Press; 2001.

8 Rosenstein NE, Perkins BA. Update on *Haemophilus influenzae* serotype b and meningococcal vaccines. *Pediatr Clin N Am* 2000;**47**(2):337–52.

9 Armitage P, Berry G. *Statistical Methods in Medical Research*, 3rd edn. Cambridge: Blackwell Science; 1994.

10 Bracken MB (ed.). *Perinatal Epidemiology*. New York: Oxford University Press; 1984.

11 Fleiss JL, Levin B, Paik MC. *Statistical Methods for Rates and Proportions*, 3rd edn. New York: John Wiley & Sons; 2003.

12 Box G, Jenkins GM, Reinsel G. *Time Series Analysis: Forecasting and Control*, 3rd edn. New Jersey: Prentice Hall; 1994.

13 Burr T, Graves T, Klamann R, Michalak S, Picard R, Hengartner N. Accounting for seasonal patterns in syndromic surveillance data for outbreak detection. *BMC Med Inform Decis Mak* 2006;**6**:40–9.

14 Robinson KA, Baughman W, Rothrock G, *et al.* Epidemiology of invasive *Streptococcus pneumoniae* infections in the United States, 1995–1998: opportunities for prevention in the conjugate vaccine era. *JAMA* 2001; **285**(13):1729–35.

15 Martin SM, Plikaytis BD, Bean NH. Statistical considerations for analysis of nosocomial infection data. In: Bennett JV, Brachman PS (eds.), *Hospital Infections*, 3rd edn. Boston: Little, Brown & Co; 1992.

16 Rothman KJ, Greenland S (eds.) *Modern Epidemiology*, 2nd edn. Philadelphia: Lippincott-Raven Publishers; 1998.

17 Kim HJ, Fay MP, Feuer EJ, Midthune DN. Permutation tests for joinpoint regression with applications to cancer rates. *Stat Med* 2000;**19**:335–51. [Erratum: *Stat Med* 2001;**20**:655.]

18 Little RJA, Rubin DB. *Statistical Analysis with Missing Data*, 2nd edn. New York: John Wiley & Sons; 2002.

19 Schafer JL. *Analysis of Incomplete Multivariate Data*. New York: Chapman and Hall; 1997.

20 Jekel JF, Elmore JF, Katz DL. *Epidemiology, Biostatistics, and Preventive Medicine*, 2nd edn. Philadelphia, PA: WB Saunders; 2001.

the surveillance data it holds by limiting reporting of any identifying information into the national system and maintaining various legal protections.

Adjustments to the data

Two statistical adjustments are made to the data in the case-based HIV/AIDS reporting system in the US to help the analyst account for two limitations of the surveillance system: the temporal delay between case diagnosis and case report and the increasing difficulty for the system to ascertain accurate transmission-risk behavior information.

Reporting delay adjustment

Although the median delay between diagnosis and report to the health department is 4 months, this delay varies by demographic group [13]. To account for the delay, HIV/AIDS case data are adjusted using a maximum likelihood statistical procedure, taking into account differences in reporting delays among exposure, geographic, racial/ethnic, age, sex, and vital status categories [14]. This method uses past patterns of reporting delays to predict the number of cases diagnosed by characteristic that are expected to be reported over the following 5 years.

Risk redistribution

At the start of the AIDS epidemic, when efforts were underway to describe the epidemiology of an unknown pathogen, most medical records contained information on transmission-related behaviors. Over time this information has been increasingly scarce and by 2004, 35% of HIV cases reported to CDC did not contain risk factor information [15]. In the face of a growing number of cases initially reported without behavioral risk, CDC developed statistical methods to mitigate bias introduced into the data from missing transmission category [13]. Using historical patterns of classification of cases reported without risk factor information, the proportion of cases eventually classified into a known transmission category is calculated. These fractions are then used to distribute current cases without reported risk factor information into transmission categories, stratifying by sex, race, and region. While risk factor is not imputed for individual cases, the distribution of cases into transmission categories is adjusted and confidence intervals

can be computed to describe the uncertainty in the estimate [16]. This method requires two major assumptions. First, it assumes that the distribution of true transmission category among cases reported without risk factor information is homogeneous over time. Second, the method assumes that cases reported without risk factor information that are eventually classified into a transmission category are representative of all such cases.

Basic approach to analysis of surveillance data

There are three basic steps in approaching the analysis of case-based and other types of surveillance data.

1 *Develop an analysis plan*. First, an analysis plan should be developed that outlines the key questions of interest and identifies variables necessary to answer these questions. The steps in the plan should include:

a List the questions that surveillance data can help answer. This should be done in consultation with the final data users to ensure their data needs are met. Surveillance data are especially useful for describing the epidemiology—person, place, and time—of the disease in question. For example, if an agency that is planning to implement a new HIV prevention program would like to know which risk group is experiencing the greatest number of new HIV diagnoses in the most recent years, analysis decisions will need to be made about whether to stratify the data by sex, race, and perhaps geographic region.

b Define the variables needed to answer the questions. For instance, a program may wish to compare the number of diagnoses in a particular year by sex, age, race, or ethnicity.

c Create table shells without data and sample graphs to ensure that the appropriate questions are being asked and that all the data will be used.

d Identify personnel with appropriate epidemiologic and statistical skills, as well as any special computer software needs. For complex analyses, it is important to involve statisticians from the start in order to ensure that appropriate methods are used based on the characteristics of the data.

e Allocate sufficient funds and time for analysis. Data cleaning and management, including cross-checking, recoding, and creating composite indicators from two or more variables, often take more time than the actual analysis.

2 *Explore the data.* The second step is to explore the data. Thorough data exploration is the most important step in understanding and presenting a coherent picture of disease incidence and prevalence. Once the data have been collected and cleaned, an epidemiologist or statistician should examine and explore the data to understand the data coding and detect any errors. This should be followed by producing frequency distributions of key variables and by recoding the data to create any new summary indicators that may be useful in the analysis. Basic analyses typically encompass the person, place, and time dimensions of epidemiologic inquiry.

This initial data exploration is often called univariate analysis. Univariate analysis is the most basic—and often the most important—type of analysis. It refers to the distribution of a single variable, which can be expressed either as a proportion if the variable is categorical (e.g., the proportion of persons with HIV infection who are men who have sex with men [MSM]) or as a central tendency, such as mean, median, or mode, if the variable is continuous (e.g., age at diagnosis, or CD4 cell count at diagnosis). Measures of dispersion such as standard deviation and standard error are also used at this stage of data exploration. It is during this initial phase of the analysis that cases or values of variables are identified that stand out from the rest, termed outliers. It is important to assess whether these outlying values are valid or instead are the result of coding errors.

If the sole purpose of the analysis is to examine changes in characteristics of cases over time, statistical techniques including chi-square tests for trend or time-series analysis can be used to determine whether the observed changes over time in proportions or means occurred by chance alone or more likely reflect a true biological or sociological trend.

If, however, the purpose of the analysis is to examine the relationship between an outcome and certain case characteristics, the next task in data exploration is to examine the relationships between key variables. This step in data exploration is called bivariate analysis. Bivariate analysis refers to an analysis of the association between two variables. An initial assessment of the relationship between a case characteristic (predictor or independent vari-

able) and an outcome (dependent variable) is often done using a $2 \times n$ table. For example, an analysis looking at whether sex is related to late HIV diagnosis would include constructing a 2×2 table of sex (male, female) and timing of HIV diagnosis (less than 12 mo before AIDS diagnosis; greater than or equal to 12 mo before AIDS diagnosis). In addition, bivariate analyses are done on key predictor variables of interest to identify possible confounders in the analysis. It is important to identify if two predictor variables are related to each other, as this will inform further analyses and the interpretation of the findings.

The appropriate statistical test to determine whether bivariate associations are due to chance alone depends on the type of variable (categorical or continuous), the number of categories if the variable is categorical, and whether the distribution is normal if the variable is continuous. Standard tests include chi-square tests for analysis of the association between two categorical variables, Student's *t* test for analysis of the association between a dichotomous and a continuous variable, and correlation coefficients for analysis of the association between two continuous variables.

3 *Perform analysis.* The next step is to perform the epidemiologic and statistical analyses. The intent of the analysis may be to examine the difference in an outcome of interest between demographic or transmission risk groups. For example, consider the question of whether cases with certain risk characteristics are more prone to certain opportunistic illnesses. Observing that Kaposi's sarcoma occurred predominantly among MSM compared with injection drug users (IDU) and decreased over time coincident with changing sexual behavior were important observations that led to our understanding of human herpes virus 8 as an opportunistic infection [17–19].

It is important to account for potential confounders when examining a relationship between an outcome and case characteristics in order to avoid spurious conclusions. There are several ways to account for confounders, including stratification, direct and indirect standardization, and multivariate analysis [20]. Multivariate analysis refers to the simultaneous analysis of the association between multiple predictor variables and an outcome variable.

descriptive titles and labels that can stand-alone. Resources exist which provide general guidance on data display [49].

Tables

Single-variable tables list a single variable (e.g., age group), and the number and percentage of cases within each category. Multivariable tables, or contingency tables, are used more frequently and examine the association between two or more variables. By convention, outcome variables are placed in columns and predictor variables in rows. If the table is examining the association between different predictor variables, the variable of greater interest often goes into columns. For example, in a combined biological and behavioral survey that examined the relationship between the predictor variable "used condom at last intercourse with nonsteady partner" and the outcome variable HIV, there would be three columns—HIV-infected, HIV-uninfected, and total. If examining HIV case reporting trends in women by age group, years would most likely be in columns and age group in rows.

Graphs and charts

Perhaps the most frequently used graph in surveillance epidemiology is the scale line graph, which depicts frequency distributions over time. In scale-line graphs, the y-axis (vertical axis) represents frequency and the x-axis (horizontal axis) represents time. An example of this type of graph is shown in Figure 29.1, which shows numbers of AIDS cases and deaths on the left y-axis and the number of persons living with AIDS (prevalence) on the right y-axis. In general, the y-axis should be should be shorter than x-axis and should start with 0. One can then determine the range of values needed and select an appropriate interval size. Finally, if the y-axis is too great with both very high and very low values, a logarithmic scale can be used.

The cumulative frequency curve, representing either continuous or categorical data, shows the effect of the addition of each subsequent variable on the x-axis on the total number of events on the y-axis; the right-hand-most variable should sum to 100%. Survival curves are used to demonstrate the percentage of subjects remaining unaffected by unit of time. In surveillance, survival curves have been

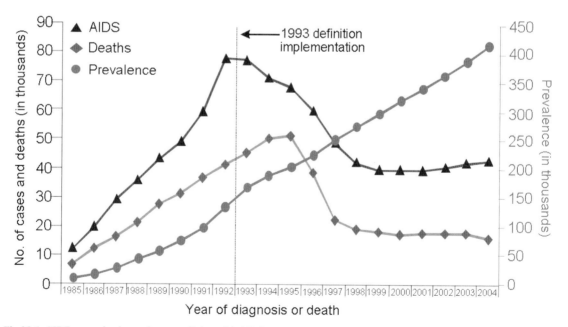

Fig 29.1 AIDS cases, deaths, and persons living with AIDS, 1985—2004, United States.
Note: data have been adjusted for reporting delays.

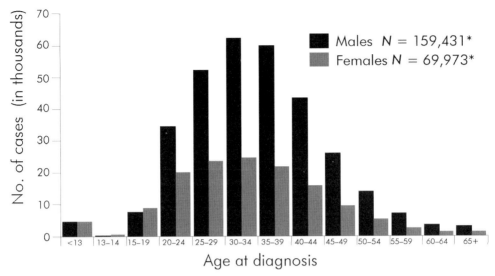

Fig 29.2 Reported cases of HIV infection (not AIDS) by age group and sex, cumulative through 2004—42 areas. *Note*: Data from 42 areas with confidential name-based HIV infection reporting as of December 2004. *Excludes 7 persons of unknown sex.

used extensively to graph the time from one sentinel event to another, such as HIV diagnosis to AIDS diagnosis or AIDS diagnosis to death. As described earlier, typically Kaplan-Meier statistics are used and survival graphs can show more than one line, such as survival before 1996 and survival from 1996 on.

Whisker and box plots are also used to graphically represent continuous data, especially if the data are nonparametrically distributed. The "whisker" is a line that shows the range of values on a vertical line, and the "box" shows the values that comprise between 25 and 75% of all the observations. A horizontal line in the box shows the median value. These have been used from laboratory values, such as CD4 counts or plasma viral loads.

Histograms display a frequency distribution by means of rectangles whose widths represent class intervals and whose heights represent corresponding frequencies. An example of this is HIV cases by age group at diagnosis, where age groups are not necessarily all the same number of years, such as <13 years, 13–14 years, 15–19 years (see Figure 29.2).

Pie charts are circular graphic representations that compare subclasses or categories to the whole class or category using different colored or patterned segments. An example is the distribution of HIV/AIDS cases by transmission risk category, where each slice of the pie chart represents a different transmission risk behavior (see Figure 29.3).

Effective presentation of analytic results is critical in order to communicate the important story that surveillance data can tell. It is incumbent upon the public health scientist to provide clear and accurate results to persons who use these data for decisions.

Conclusion

Surveillance data are fundamental to public health practice and can provide answers to important public health questions. Case-based HIV surveillance systems have certain characteristics that must be considered during analysis, interpretation, and presentation of data. Analyses of case-based systems range from basic descriptive epidemiology—person, place, and time—to complex inferential statistical modeling. Results from these analyses can provide answers to a full range of questions related to HIV risk behaviors, acquisition, diagnosis, progression, mortality, and survival. It is through

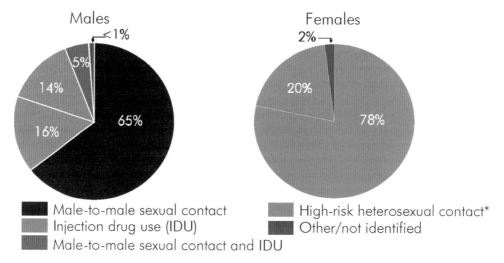

Males

Females

Males legend:
- ■ Male-to-male sexual contact
- ■ Injection drug use (IDU)
- ■ Male-to-male sexual contact and IDU

Females legend:
- ■ High-risk heterosexual contact*
- ■ Other/not identified

Fig 29.3 Proportion of HIV/AIDS cases among adults and adolescents, by sex and transmission category 2004—35 areas.
Note: Data include persons with a diagnosis of HIV infection regardless of their AIDS status at diagnosis. Data from 35 areas with confidential name-based HIV infection reporting since at least 2000. Data have been adjusted for reporting delays and cases without risk factor information were proportionally redistributed.
*Heterosexual contact with a person known to have or at high risk for HIV infection.

the collection and analysis of high quality data that critical public health problems are identified, evaluated, and ultimately prevented.

References

1 Janes GR, Hutbagner L, Cates W, Jr, Stroup D, Williamson GD. Descriptive epidemiology: analyzing and interpreting surveillance data. In: Teutsch SM, Churchill RE (eds.), *Principles and Practice of Public Health Surveillance*, 2nd edn. Oxford: Oxford University Press; 2000.

2 Nurminen M. Linkage failures in ecological analysis. *World Health Stat Q* 1995;**48**:78–84.

3 Mortimer JY, Salathiel JA. 'Soundex' codes of surnames provide confidentiality and accuracy in a national HIV database. *Commun Dis Rep CDR Rev* 1995;**5**:R183–6.

4 Centers for Disease Control and Prevention. Current trends: revision of the case definition of acquired immunodeficiency syndrome for national reporting—United States. *MMWR Morb Mortal Wkly Rep* 1985;**34**:373–5.

5 Institute of Medicine. *Measuring What Matters: Allocation, Planning, and Quality Assessment for the Ryan White CARE Act*. Washington, DC: National Academies Press; 2003.

6 Centers for Disease Control and Prevention. Current trends: update on acquired immune deficiency syndrome (AIDS)—United States. *MMWR Morb Mortal Wkly Rep* 1982;**31**:507–8, 513–4.

7 Centers for Disease Control and Prevention. Current trends: classification system for human T-lymphotropic virus type III/lymphadenopathy-associated virus infections. *MMWR Morb Mortal Wkly Rep* 1986;**35**:334–9.

8 Centers for Disease Control and Prevention. Revision of the CDC surveillance case definition for acquired immunodeficiency syndrome. *MMWR Morb Mortal Wkly Rep* 1987;**36**(RR-17):1–15S.

9 Centers for Disease Control and Prevention. 1993 Revised classification system for HIV infection and expanded surveillance case definition for AIDS among adolescents and adults. *MMWR Morb Mortal Wkly Rep* 1992;**41**(RR-17):1–19.

10 Centers for Disease Control and Prevention. Guidelines for national human immunodeficiency virus case surveillance, including monitoring for human immunodeficiency virus infection and acquired immunodeficiency syndrome. *MMWR Morb Mortal Wkly Rep* 1999;**48**(RR-13):1–28.

11 Gostin LO, Lazzarini Z, Neslund VS, Osterholm MT. The public health information infrastructure. A national review of the law on health information privacy. *JAMA* 1996;**275**:1921–7.

12 Centers for Disease Control and Prevention. *Technical Guidance for HIV/AIDS Surveillance Programs, Volume III: Security and Confidentiality Guidelines*. Atlanta, GA: US Department of Health and Human Services, Centers for Disease Control and Prevention; 2006. Available from: http://www.cdc.gov/hiv/topics/surveillance/resources/guidelines/guidance/index.htm. Accessed April 25, 2007.

13 Klevens RM, Fleming PL, Li J, *et al*. The completeness, validity, and timeliness of AIDS surveillance data. *Ann Epidemiol* 2001;**11**:443–9.

14 Green T. Using surveillance data to monitor trends in the AIDS epidemic. *Stat Med* 1998;**17**:143–54.

15 McDavid K, McKenna MT. HIV/AIDS risk factor ascertainment: a critical challenge. *AIDS Patient Care STDS* 2006;**20**:285–92.

16 Song R, Hall HI, Frey R. Uncertainties associated with incidence estimates of HIV/AIDS diagnoses adjusted for reporting delay and risk redistribution. *Stat Med* 2005;**24**:453–64.

17 Rutherford GW, Schwarcz SK, Lemp GF, *et al*. The epidemiology of AIDS-related Kaposi's sarcoma in San Francisco. *J Infect Dis* 1989;**159**:569–72.

18 Moore PS, Gao SJ, Dominguez G, *et al*. Primary characterization of a herpesvirus agent associated with Kaposi's sarcomae. *J Virol* 1996;**70**:549–58.

19 Strathdee SA, Veuglelers PJ, Moore PS. The epidemiology of HIV-associated Kaposi's sarcoma: the unraveling mystery. *AIDS* 1996;**10**(suppl 1):S51–7.

20 Szklo M, Nieto JF. *Epidemiology: Beyond the Basics*. Gaithersburg, MD: Aspen Publishers; 2000.

21 Amato DA. A generalized Kaplan–Meier estimator for heterogeneous populations. *Commun Stat A Theory Methods* 1988;**17**:263–86.

22 Finkelstein DM, Muzikansky A, Schoenfeld DA. Comparing survival of a sample to that of a standard population. *J Natl Cancer Inst* 2003;**95**:1434–9.

23 Lemp GF, Payne SF, Neal D, Temelso T, Rutherford GW. Survival trends for patients with AIDS. *JAMA* 1990;**263**:402–6.

24 Lee LM, Karon JM, Selik R, Neal JJ, Fleming PL. Survival after AIDS diagnosis in adolescents and adults during the treatment era, United States, 1984–1997. *JAMA* 2001;**285**:1308–15.

25 Lee LM, McKenna MT. Monitoring the incidence of HIV infection in the United States. *Public Health Rep* 2007;**122**(suppl 1):72–9.

26 Rangel MC, Gavin L, Reed C, Fowler MG, Lee LM. Epidemiology of HIV and AIDS among adolescent and young adults in the United States. *J Adol Health* 2006;**39**:156–63.

27 Giovannetti L, Crocetti E, Chellini E, Martini A, Balocchini E, Constantini AS. [Andamenti temporali di incidenza e mortalità per AIDS in Toscana (1987–2000)]. *Epidemiol Prev* 2004;**28**:100–6.

28 Cressie NAC. *Statittics for Spatial Data*. New York: John Wiley and Sons; 1993.

29 Langford IH, Leyland AH, Rasbash J, Goldstein H. Multilevel modeling of the geographical distributions of diseases. *Appl Stat* 1999;**28**(Pt 2):253–68.

30 Lee LM, Lobato MN, Buskin SE, Morse A, Costa S. Low adherence to guidelines for preventing TB among persons with newly diagnosed HIV infection, United States. *Int J Tuberc Lung Dis* 2006;**10**:209–14.

31 Lee LM, Lehman JS, Bindman AB, Fleming PL. Validation of race/ethnicity and transmission mode in the US HIV/AIDS reporting system. *Am J Public Health* 2003;**93**:914–7.

32 Hall HI, Li J, Campsmith M, Sweeny P, Lee LM. Date of first positive HIV test: reliability of information collected for HIV/AIDS surveillance in the United States. *Public Health Rep* 2005;**120**:89–95.

33 Cohen J. A coefficient of agreement for nominal scales. *Ed Psychol Meas* 1960;**20**:37–46.

34 Youden WJ. Index for rating diagnostic tests. *Cancer* 1950;**3**:32–5.

35 Jara MM, Gallagher KM, Schieman S. Estimation of completeness of AIDS case reporting in Massachusetts. *Epidemiol* 2000;**11**:209–13.

36 Hall HI, Song R, Gerstle JE, III, Lee LM; HIV/AIDS Reporting System Evaluation Group. Assessing the completeness of reporting of human immunodeficiency virus diagnoses in 2002–2003: capture–recapture methods. *Am J Epidemiol* 2006;**164**:391–7.

37 Hook EB, Regal RR. Capture–recapture methods in epidemiology: methods and limitations. *Epidemiol Rev* 1995;**17**:243–64.

38 Centers for Disease Control and Prevention. Human immunodeficiency virus infection in the United States: a review of current knowledge. *MMWR Morb Mortal Wkly Rep* 1987;**36**(suppl S-6):1–48.

39 Brookmeyer R. Reconstruction and future trends of the AIDS epidemic in the United States. *Science* 1991;**253**:37–42.

40 Mokotoff E, Glynn MK. Surveillance for HIV/AIDS in the United States. In: M'ikanatha NM, Lynfield R, Van Beneden C, de Valk H (eds.), *Infectious Disease Surveillance*, 1st edn. Oxford: Blackwell Publishing; 2007:201–211.

41 Centers for Disease Control and Prevention. Human immunodeficiency virus (HIV) risk, prevention, and testing behaviors—United States, National HIV Behavioral Surveillance System: men who have sex with men, November 2003–April 2005. *MMWR Morb Mortal Wkly Rep* 2006;**55**(SS-6):1–16.

42 Janssen RS, Satten GA, Stramer SL, *et al.* New testing strategy to detect early HIV-1 infection for use in incidence estimates and for clinical purposes. *JAMA* 1998;**280**:42–8.

43 Song R, Karon JM, White E, Goldbaum G. Estimating the distribution of a renewal process from times at which events from an independent process are detected. *Biometrics* 2006;**62**:838–46.

44 Sullivan PS, Karon JM, Malitz FE, *et al.* A two-stage sampling method for clinical surveillance of individuals in care for HIV infection in the United States. *Public Health Rep* 2005;**120**:230–9.

45 Lee LM, Fleming PL. Estimated number of children left motherless by AIDS in the United States, 1978–1998. *J Acquir Immune Defic Syndr* 2003;**34**:231–6.

46 Kochanek KD, Murphy SL, Anderson RN, Scott C. *Deaths: Final Data for 2002. National Vital Statistics Reports: Vol 53 No 5.* Hyattsville, MD: National Center for Health Statistics; 2004.

47 Pastor PN, Maukuc DM, Reuben C, Xia H. *Chartbook on Trends in the Health of Americans. Health, United States, 2002.* Hyattsville, MD: National Center for Health Statistics; 2002.

48 Anderson RN, Smith BL. *Deaths: Leading Causes for 2002. National Vital Statistics Reports: Vol. 53 No 17.* Hyattsville, MD: National Center for Health Statistics; 2005.

49 Peavy JV, Dyal WW, Eddins DL. *Descriptive Statistics: Tables, Graphs, and Charts.* Atlanta, GA: Centers for Disease Control and Prevention; 1986.

30 Use of molecular epidemiology in infectious disease surveillance

John Besser

Introduction

Molecular epidemiology is the application of nucleic acid-based detection and analytic methods to the study of diseases in populations. Molecular epidemiological methods are used in the surveillance of infectious diseases to identify etiology, physical sources, and routes of disease transmission. In addition, these methods can be used to define the molecular basis for characteristics relevant to disease control and prevention, including virulence, antibiotic resistance, and antigenicity [1]. Molecular methods have gradually moved from the research laboratory into clinical and public health laboratories, and are affecting surveillance systems at multiple levels.

Scientists have over 100 years of experience with microbial culture and classical identification schemes, but less than 10 years of experience with most molecular detection and identification assays. Molecular tools have revealed essentially limitless variation in the microbial world, prompting challenges in data interpretation. These challenges can be considerable in outbreak investigations, but are even greater in surveillance where significant trends are intertwined with endemic disease.

Classifications

Molecular epidemiology enables classification of microorganisms as part of epidemiological inference. The following terms are part of the basic language of the field (adapted from Refs. [2] and [3]). Although these definitions seem straightforward, in practice it is challenging to fit microorganisms into the neat categories that these terms suggest.

- *Species:* A formal taxonomic unit defined by a set of characteristics common to each member of that unit, subordinate to genus, and superior to subspecies classifications (e.g., subtype, serotype, and strain) Some definitions include ability to interbreed.
- *Subspecies:* A general term for classification below the level of species.
- *Subtype:* A group of microorganisms that share a genetic variation that distinguishes them from other members of their species, serotype, or other subspecies classification. A set of molecular markers and often a specific method are used as part of the subtype definition.
- *Serotype:* Classification based on shared antigenic characteristics.
- *Strain:* The term is most commonly used to define groups of microbial cells or isolates within the same taxonomic classification that share a phenotypic or genotypic trait that suggests a common origin. The term may also refer to a stock maintained in culture and successively passaged.
- *Clone:* The recent prodigy of a single microbial cell. The term "clonal" is often used to describe groups of organisms that are functionally indistinguishable, or that have low degrees of genetic diversity.

The goal of classification in molecular epidemiology is to describe genetic differences between pathogens in order to explain patterns of disease. Tools of microbial taxonomy, the formal science of classification based on present-day characteristics,

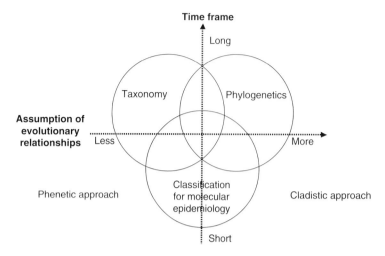

Fig 30.1 The relationship between the microbial classification for taxonomy, phylogenetics, and molecular epidemiology.

and phylogenetics—the science of evolutionary relationships—are used to achieve this goal. While taxonomic and phylogenetic classifications and those based on molecular epidemiological data are interrelated, the terms are not interchangeable. Genetic differences between organisms may or may not reflect taxonomic differences or infer phylogenetic relationships. This distinction is important when describing similarities between surveillance strains. In general (but not always), taxonomy and phylogenetics involve differences between organisms that arise over long time frames, whereas molecular epidemiology generally involves relationships that evolve over relatively short time frames (Figure 30.1). Molecular methods are now used in all three disciplines.

Microbial agents are placed in taxonomic schemes as a convenient form of scientific communication. Identification by species (e.g., *Yersinia pestis*, *Campylobacter jejuni*) or subspecies (e.g., *Salmonella* Typhi, *Escherichia coli* O157:H7, vancomycin-resistant *Staphylococcus aureus*) not only helps in the clinical management of the respective diseases, but also defines the denominator for pathogen-specific surveillance programs. The concept of "species," relatively easy to define in multicellular, sexually reproducing life forms with long generation times, is far less clear in the microbial world. In animals, systematic genetic mixing occurs during sexual reproduction, but relatively little change and no propagated genetic change occurs

during the millions of cell cycles between generations. In contrast, propagated genetic change in microbes is more-or-less continuous, with small, incremental genetic changes occurring during each cell cycle (Figure 30.2). Genetic material is exchanged between microorganisms, often at multiple taxonomic levels through a variety of mechanisms. Molecular biology has made it clear that microbial life is infinitely complex in the natural environment and that no scheme can fully describe natural relationships.

Surveillance programs, reporting rules, and regulations are based on precise taxonomic definitions, but these definitions fit biological reality only in a general sense. For example, the United States Food and Drug Administration (US FDA) has legally defined a zero tolerance for *Listeria monocytogenes* in cooked or ready-to-eat foods [4], but permits the presence of *Listeria innocua*, a genetically similar microorganism. Isolates have been identified which share characteristics of both, creating a diagnostic and regulatory conundrum [5]. Microbiology laboratories usually provide species identification based on a "best-fit" with phenotypic and/or genotypic markers, but species definitions are imprecise.

There is even more confusion at the subspecies level. For long-established programs such as *Salmonella* surveillance, precise definitions of serotypes have been developed over time based on antigenic makeup [6]. The PulseNet program has defined subtypes based on specific pulsed-field gel

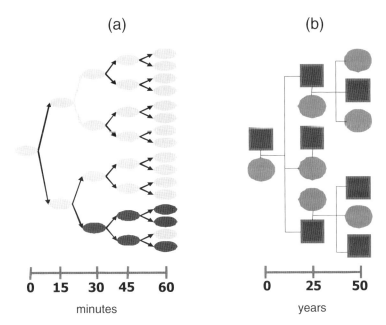

Fig 30.2 Comparison of bacterial (a) and human (b) pedigrees.

electrophoresis (PFGE) patterns using standardized methods [7]. Subtypes of HIV are determined by sequence alignment with reference strains [8,9]. However, for most microorganisms standard markers are lacking. Due to continuous variation, the concepts of "strain" and even "clone" become fuzzy at a molecular level. While the concept of species, serotype, and strain continue to be important for communication and form the foundation of many surveillance programs, it is important to recognize that classification schemes for microorganisms are convenient constructs rather than laws of nature.

Microbial ecology and subspecies classification

The goal of classification in molecular epidemiology is to use relationships between microorganisms as indirect markers for patterns of transmission events or trends that affect human or animal health. This epidemiological inference adds an additional layer of uncertainty as it involves the intersecting worlds of microbial ecology and human activity. With rare exceptions, the ecology of the disease under surveillance is broader than the cases under investigation, and many links in the chain of transmission may be unknown or unknowable. However, we can use subsets of information for detection and investigation of disease events. For instance, *Salmonella* may be transmitted from its primary reservoir to a variety of products, cross-contaminate ready-to-eat food products, amplify in improperly prepared food, persist for long periods of time in the food preparation environment, and transmit person-to-person or through animals. At any time, multiple routes of transmission may occur. Convergence of multiple transmission events is even a possibility, and multiple types of agents may be involved in single outbreaks.

In spite of the inherent complexity of *Salmonella* ecology and most other diseases, we can still detect and investigate an individual event, such as a restaurant outbreak, by tracking a specific marker organism. Molecular assays used as part of subtype surveillance programs can be used to make sense out of a complex system by refining the case definition. They take advantage of genetic changes that occur in microorganisms to a greater or lesser extent in a continuous and predictable manner. Transmission events can be identified within the milieu of microbial surveillance data by choosing

395

genetic marker(s) of strain relatedness that reflects the transmission event of interest. Narrow case definitions, such as one that includes a PFGE subtype, can be used to group together cases more likely to be related to each other. If the marker is properly chosen, using agent-specific case definitions during hypothesis generation and testing can increase the sensitivity of outbreak detection and strengthen measures of association. Once an outbreak has been detected, the case definition can be widened to understand as much of the larger system as possible. Thus, surveillance and outbreak investigations may at different times require different tools and approaches. In the 1998 international outbreak of *Shigella sonnei* and enterotoxigenic *E. coli* associated with parsley, multiple strains of bacteria were involved due to contact of product with fecally contaminated water [10]. In the initial phase of investigation, however, the multijurisdictional nature of the outbreak was determined through identification of matches of one specific strain.

The ability to understand the complexities of disease events varies greatly by agent. For instance, smallpox transmission was straightforward to monitor and became an ideal target for eradication because most or all cases have recognizable symptoms and humans are the only known reservoir. Disease events such as botulism poisoning or pulmonary infection with weaponized anthrax are noticed even without pathogen-specific surveillance. In contrast, a large percentage of individuals carrying or infected with influenza, *Salmonella*, or *Streptococcus pyogenes* have no symptoms or do not seek medical care, and may have complex interactions with animal reservoirs, making it difficult or impossible to understand the source of the outbreak. For these types of diseases, refining the case definition by subspecies characterization may be the only way of identifying significant trends that are themselves part of the overall microbial ecology.

Molecular markers

It is technically possible, although currently not practical, to measure differences or similarities between microorganisms using whole genome or proteome sequencing. Currently, molecular markers are used to sample the genome or proteome for characteristics of interest. Examples of markers include restriction fragments produced as part of PFGE or restriction length polymorphism analysis (RFLP), variable number tandem repeats (VNTR) used for multilocus VNTR analysis (MLVA), polymorphic sequences used for multilocus sequence typing (MLST), single nucleotide polymorphisms (SNPs), and influenza neuraminidase sequences used to measure antiviral agent susceptibility. As with any sampling method, markers should represent the population, in this instance the full genetic or protein complement of the microorganism, in a way that best answers the question. How well a molecular marker serves that goal depends on (a) the nature of the microbial characteristic represented by the marker, (b) the diversity of alleles and rate of change of the marker in its natural environment, (c) the persistence of individual alleles over time, and (d) how well the marker and others in the typing system define the population of interest. For example, the molecular marker for *emm* sequencing, a method used for surveillance of *Strep. pyogenes* infections, is in a region of DNA that codes for the streptococcal M protein. Although this is only one of the estimated 1865 protein-coding genes of *Strep. pyogenes* [11], sequence differences coding for this protein are thought to be a primary determinant of virulence [12], and therefore this gene is a useful marker for disease tracking [13]. Strains that are distinguished by *emm* sequencing can be used as markers for the spatial and temporal movement of *Strep. pyogenes*. Additionally, knowing the M type can allow the connection of current infections with a historical database of strain types based on M protein. The *emm* sequencing method is sensitive enough to detect classical M types, and not so sensitive that differences obscure the relationships under study. A finer level of genetic comparison or an additional marker might be preferable if the primary surveillance goal was to examine very short term evolutionary changes, such as teasing apart closely related transmission events, or tracking changes in drug resistance mechanisms.

Subtyping systems such as MLST, MLVA, and PFGE rely on markers from multiple loci to define the genotypes of interest. The population structure of each microbial taxon determines the degree of linkage that can be expected between loci [14]. For "clonal" population structures for organisms such as *Salmonella* spp. and *E. coli*, which have relatively low rates of horizontal gene transfer, the relationship between loci within a particular lineage remains relatively stable. "Panmictic" population structures such as that of *Neisseria gonorrhoeae* are characterized by high rates of horizontal gene transfer and relatively random distribution of alleles between loci. Thus, markers from the same set of loci in two genera may give very different levels of discrimination and subtype stability.

Genetic markers can be chosen to fit the time frame under study. For long-term trends, genetic loci such as those coding for housekeeping genes can be chosen, since most mutations in these genes are lethal and evolution is slow. Genes coding for surface antigens exposed to the immune system are good for short-term evolutionary trends. Potential markers can be scored for diversity, evenness, and richness in the population of interest using measures such as Simpson's and Shannon's indices [15,16]. The art of molecular biology for surveillance involves finding the right set of markers that balance discrimination and stability in a manner that best addresses the question being asked.

Subspecies classification for surveillance

Molecular methods are increasingly being used as part of routine surveillance to classify microorganism to the subspecies level in order to identify outbreaks or other trends against a background of sporadic disease or to answer specific research questions. They have become important for surveillance of common conditions, such as diarrheal disease or influenza, and for answering questions not readily determined from clinical presentation, such as drug resistance or antigenic relationship to vaccine.

Salmonella serotype surveillance is one of our oldest surveillance programs, and has been an integral part of our national food safety program for over 60 years. It is one of the best examples of how identification to the subspecies level can be used to identify and clarify epidemiological associations. Antigenic relationships have been sufficiently stable over time to be used in scientific discourse and courtroom testimony. Surveillance for *Salmonella* Typhi began in the US in 1912 and a nationwide

program for routine identification of other common *Salmonella* serotypes was established in 1963 [17]. Although other pathogens such as norovirus and *C. jejuni* cause far more cases of gastrointestinal disease than *Salmonella* [18], *Salmonella* serotype surveillance became one of the most productive pathogen-specific surveillance programs. Problems such as microbial contamination of sprout seeds and subsequent growth during germination [19], contamination of ice cream during bulk transport after terminal pasteurization [20], and plumbing anomalies in a Chicago-area dairy [21] have been discovered and remediated because of *Salmonella* serotype surveillance. Serotype surveillance takes advantage of the fact that salmonellae are not randomly distributed (i.e., cases that share a particular serotype are more likely to share a common source). Including serotype information as part of the case definition increases the sensitivity of cluster detection, as increases in the incidence of individual serotypes may be differentiated from background sporadic cases and other outbreaks. Once a cluster has been detected, use of a serotype-specific case definition during hypothesis generation and testing increases the statistical association between illness and the contaminating exposure, making it more likely that a common link can be identified. Another example of subspecies surveillance is for *E. coli* serotype O157:H7. Surveillance for this subspecies began in many US states after a large, multistate outbreak in 1993 [22].

Since the discovery of DNA there has been a gradual move toward the use of molecular methods for classification of microorganisms, both above and below the species level. In some instances, molecular tests have been developed to replace standard antigen-based methods in order to maintain continuity with acquired wisdom and historical databases. Examples include molecular *Salmonella* serotyping [23], *Neisseria meningitidis* serogrouping [24,25], and *emm* sequencing, a surrogate for *Strep. pyogenes* M-typing [26].

There has been considerable effort to subtype organisms for which there were no available or commonly used serological methods. In the 1990s, the US Centers for Disease Control and Prevention (CDC) and US health departments began exploring the use of molecular subtyping such as PFGE, as a routine surveillance tool to detect and investigate outbreaks of infectious diseases [27,28]. In 1996, CDC initiated PulseNet, a US molecular subtyping network, to provide testing standards, coordinated communication, and a national database of subtype patterns for rapid state-to-state comparison of findings. In the early 2000s PulseNet expanded worldwide with subtyping centers in Canada, Europe, Latin America, and Asia Pacific including China [29]. Since its inception, PulseNet has been directly responsible or played a key role in the detection of many national and international outbreaks of foodborne disease, and has contributed to declines in the incidence of listeriosis and *E. coli* O157 infections [29,30]. Through integration with regulatory monitoring programs, human cases have been more easily linked to animal and food sources.

Molecular methods have been used for HIV strain/susceptibility [9], norovirus surveillance [31], and in hospital programs to monitor strain variation of methicillin-resistant *Staph. aureus* (MRSA) and vancomycin-resistant enterococcus [32,33]. Other uses have included monitoring of inducible clindamycin resistance in *Staph. aureus* and *Strep. pyogenes* [34,35] and resistance to neuraminidase inhibitors in influenza A virus [36]. The "Harmony" project in Europe has databases for molecular subtype data with a focus on organisms important to hospital infection control, including hepatitis B virus, *Legionella pneumophila*, *Mycobacterium tuberculosis*, MRSA, *Pseudomonas aeruginosa*, measles virus, and norovirus [37].

Match interpretation

An important application of molecular epidemiology is the use of the natural genetic variability of microorganisms to tease out recent epidemiological events or trends. Interpretation of molecular subtype matches or mismatches in surveillance data sets can impact whether or not investigations are initiated, can drive public health and regulatory action or inaction, and may have legal consequences.

In general, pairs or groups of microbial subtypes are considered "indistinguishable," "similar," or "different" [14]. At the simplest level, cases with indistinguishable subtypes are more likely to be associated than cases with similar or different subtypes. "Similar" subtypes are those that are only slightly different from each other and are close enough to be potentially accounted for by normal genetic variability, such as the variability that may occur within the time frame of an outbreak. Such cases are less likely to share a common epidemiological association than those with indistinguishable subtypes, but more likely to be associated than cases with "different" subtypes. While indistinguishable microbial subtypes suggest an increased probability of epidemiological association, quantitatively determining the strength and confidence of an association based on a subtyping test is more problematic than it is with human "DNA fingerprinting," against which microbial subtyping is frequently compared.

MLVA, which is used for human "DNA fingerprinting" is similar to tests used in microbial subtyping [38]. For humans, the population frequencies of the paired alleles found at various genetic loci are determined, and are used to design assays that can differentiate between humans with a high and definable level of confidence. This type of analysis is used to evaluate biological material collected at a crime scene. The probability that a match between the biological material or "evidence" and a particular individual is based upon a chance per millions or billions of occurrences that the match is coincidental with somebody else who is not an identical twin. The high degree of confidence is made possible by human biology, ecology, and the relative simplicity of the question being asked. The offspring of humans have relatively large genetic differences from each other and from their parents when compared with bacteria and their progeny. This is due to systematic genetic mixing during sexual reproduction, which occurs at rare intervals when measured against our own lives. Throughout our lives, cells are continually produced asexually, but the rate of mutation is very small due to robust DNA repair mechanisms, and mutations that occur are not further propagated. In spite of the high degree of confidence that DNA evidence offers for human typing, it cannot stand alone. Temporal, geographic, biological, and social factors must be factored into the final decision of guilt or innocence. For instance, the suspect needs to have been alive at the time of the crime, not have an identical twin, and must have been in a location where committing the crime would have been possible.

Methods used to track infectious disease for prevention and control purposes are often similar or identical to those used for human typing. However, the associations of interest in disease surveillance are more complex, involving the relationship among microorganisms with their own genetics and ecology, and patterns of human or animal behavior and susceptibility to disease. The factors that define the associations include everything that influences the epidemiology of the disease, including the larger ecosystem within which the microorganisms reside. Under the general heading of "microbes" is a diverse group of life forms, including viruses, bacteria, parasites, and fungi. These life forms span the genetic spectrum, and each offers its own interpretive challenges. Microorganisms have various strategies for genetic mixing which are similar to our own to a greater or lesser extent.

How much value can we assign to a microbial molecular match or mismatch? As described above, confidence levels for human "DNA fingerprinting" assays are extremely high, where the goal is simply to measure identity between two human specimens that can be uniquely differentiated from each other through the use of stable markers. In contrast, the goal of surveillance is usually to examine trends or to detect transmission events indirectly through the use of the inherent variability of microbial markers that exist within a large and complex disease system. Interrelated factors which influence the significance of a subtype match or mismatch include factors such as (a) genetic diversity of the agent investigated with the markers used, (b) the prevalence of the strain(s) in question, and (c) the genetic stability of the markers used to compare strains. For instance, a match between two isolates of a rare strain in a diverse population of strains is more significant than a match between two isolates of a common strain in a population with little diversity. A mismatch between strains defined by a relatively unstable marker is less significant than a mismatch between strains defined by a highly stable marker. While subtype matches can be compelling, they cannot "stand alone" as proof or disproof of association. They must be interpreted in the context of epidemiological factors. The interrelationships between the strength of the microbiological and epidemiological evidence will be discussed in the following sections.

Specific probabilities are not assigned to the laboratory test itself, as is done in human DNA fingerprinting, because of the inherent complexity of the system. Quantitative measures that may be available include (a) the overall measures of association, such as the odds ratio and p value in a case-control or case-to-case comparison study and (b) the prevalence of the agent in the population under study. The odds ratio and p value represent the sum of the epidemiological factors that make up the association, including the molecular test used to refine the case definition. For example, if the association between illness due to a specific pathogen strain and a particular exposure in a well-designed outbreak case-control study has an elevated odds ratio and p value of 0.005, the chance that the odds ratio was due to random variation is 1/200. As will be discussed later, refining the case definition by using greater molecular test discrimination may under some circumstances improve measures of association. However, significance measures in infectious disease outbreaks are not likely to approach what is found in human DNA fingerprinting for a number of reasons, including (a) uncertainty due to unknown, and often unknowable microbial interactions, and (b) microbial genetic variability. This variability both limits achievable significance levels and is the very quality exploited by molecular subtyping tested to tease recent disease events from background noise.

The prevalence of the agent in the population under study, although not a factor when calculating the significance of an association between disease and exposure affects those measures indirectly. The more common the agent, the more likely that sporadic, unrelated cases will cluster together with outbreak cases (type 1 probability error). In real life situations, the prevalence of the agent is not normally known, and measures of association may not be available when actions need to be taken. Unlike criminal law, where much is riding on a quantitative assessment of a match, public health actions may need to be taken using only common sense and sound epidemiology.

Finally, if we can strengthen the measures of association by refining the case definition with molecular subtyping, can we disprove an apparent association by using alternate tests or additional markers? If alternate methods add new biological

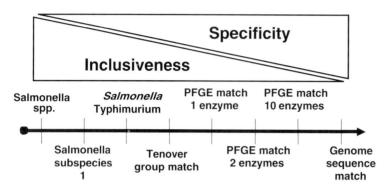

Agent/Case definition

Fig 30.3 *Salmonella* Typhimurium case definition based on pathogen classification level. On the left is an inclusive but nonspecific agent definition "*Salmonella* spp." On the right is a completely specific and noninclusive agent definition based on a full genome sequence of every isolate.

information that cause reinterpretation of the basic epidemiological model, they can be used to disprove the association. For instance, molecular subtyping, transposon typing, and analysis of molecular virulence determinants in human and animal isolates of vancomycin-resistant enterococci (VRE) in Europe and the US revealed different sets of microbial subpopulations which challenged the prevailing epidemiological model that explained the rise of nosocomial VRE in the US [39]. In the absence of this type of information, can simple enhancement of strain discrimination further prove or disprove a significant association?

Strain discrimination and epidemiological case definition

Molecular testing is used in surveillance to isolate a signal, such as a trend or cluster of disease, from background noise. Our ability to differentiate infectious disease events from sporadic disease is affected by the discriminatory power of the subtyping method in addition to the other factors described. But how much strain discrimination is really necessary?

The genetic makeup of all living things change during every cell division, and using molecular methods it is theoretically possible to differentiate every cell from every other cell. In the era of molecular biology, it is increasingly becoming necessary to make choices about microbial classification as

part of surveillance activities. How microorganisms are classified is particularly important for pathogen-specific surveillance where the agent is used as part of the case definition. For any disease under surveillance there is a spectrum of potential agent classifications that may be used. Using *Salmonella* surveillance as an example, at one end of the spectrum is an all-inclusive but nonspecific agent definition, such as a *Salmonella* spp. not otherwise differentiated (Figure 30.3). This agent definition maximizes the likelihood of a type I probability error, the suggestion that there is an epidemiological relationship when in fact there is not (false positive association). It also increases the likelihood of a type II probability error, the suggestion that there is not an epidemiological relationship when in fact there is (false-negative association), since the inclusion of misclassified cases decreases the signal-to-noise ratio, masking trends such as outbreaks. On the other end of the spectrum of potential definitions is a completely specific and noninclusive definition based on 100% whole genome sequence identity. Using this agent definition, every isolate from every patient would be different from every other isolate, eliminating clustering and maximizing strain diversity and type II probability error. A method to measure relatedness between strains would be necessary to make any sense out of the data. Somewhere in between these two extremes is a level of strain classification that minimizes both types of probability error, and is most effective at addressing a particular surveillance or investigation goal.

Utility of additional strain discrimination

Epidemiologists and regulatory officials are often faced with difficult decisions that depend, on part, on interpretation of microbiological surveillance data. For example, should a product be recalled based on investigation findings using a single enzyme PFGE case definition or should a second PFGE enzyme result be obtained first?

A number of factors are important to consider when determining the level of strain discrimination needed for surveillance program design, public health intervention, or regulatory action.

1 *The nature of the surveillance goal or the question being asked:* If the surveillance goal is detection of outbreaks and identification of a common source, finer-level classification increases the specificity of the case definition, which may, to a point, increase the sensitivity of cluster detection and the statistical association between illness and exposure. The detection of *E. coli* O157:H7 outbreaks through PFGE surveillance are good examples [28]. Additional strain discrimination may not be indicated for other surveillance goals, such as monitoring trends over time or over large geographic areas, investigation of isolated outbreaks associated with a common event, or determining the scope of an infectious disease problem.

2 *The number of cases:* Increasing the discrimination of a properly designed subtyping method refines the case definition by including only those cases most likely to be related to a common source. In the process, truly associated cases may be eliminated from the study. For instance, PFGE subtype variability has been documented among truly associated cases in well-characterized point source outbreaks [40]. When the number of cases is very small, the impact of individual misclassified cases is large, whether they are falsely included in the case definition, or falsely excluded from the case definition.

3 *Phase of outbreak investigation:* Reingold described 10 steps in outbreak investigations [41]. The steps in which agent classification plays a role includes (not necessarily in this order): (a) establish case definition(s); (b) establish the background rate of disease; (c) find cases, decide if there is an outbreak, define scope of the outbreak; (d) generate hypotheses; (e) test hypotheses; (f) collect and test environmental samples. For outbreaks detected by pathogen-specific surveillance, where agent information is the primary mechanism for linking cases, additional strain discrimination increases the specificity of the case definition for hypothesis generation and testing, and increases the confidence of a link with environmental samples. The value of increased subtype discrimination for determining the scope of an outbreak is more complex. Its value depends on a number of factors described below, such as the prevalence of the agent, the prevalence of the exposure, and the imperative for identifying all cases. Thus, for a multijurisdictional outbreak with a common subtype, a relatively common exposure, and a low imperative for identifying all possible cases, increased system-wide subtype discrimination may improve the overall understanding of the event. For an outbreak with a rare, serious disease such as botulism or anthrax or an unusual exposure, the use of a wider rather than narrower agent definition may be indicated.

4 *The prevalence of a presumptive exposure:* In a cluster investigation, the prevalence of a suspect exposure in the population under investigation drives the overall measures of association at least as much as the specificity of agent definition, and impacts the need or lack of need for additional strain discrimination. In outbreaks due to high prevalence exposures, such as hamburger consumption in the US, it is difficult to demonstrate a meaningful difference between cases and controls unless (a) the number of cases (and controls) is high, or (b) the case definition is very specific, i.e., there are few misclassified cases. Increased subtype discrimination is one way to reduce the number of falsely classified cases that, if the subtyping test is properly designed, will reduce the number of nonexposed cases more than exposed cases (for a true exposure). If the exposure is rare, or if the exposure information is very specific, the value of additional strain discrimination is reduced.

5 *Specificity of the exposure information:* The specificity of exposure information gathered as part of surveillance and outbreak investigations helps define the exposure prevalence, and therefore affects measures of association in the same manner as exposure prevalence. For example, in the nationwide outbreak associated with cake batter ice cream prepared by a retail chain [42], the exposure

information collected could have been less specific ("ate ice cream"), more specific ("ate ice cream Chain A"), or highly specific ("ate cake batter ice cream from Chain A"). Increasing the specificity of exposure information has a similar impact as increasing agent discrimination on measures of association. Thus, a highly specific exposure profile may mitigate the need for additional strain discrimination.

6 *Significant or likely findings:* Once a significant common source or trend has been identified using one agent definition, additional strain discrimination is unlikely to further validate the association, unless an alternate hypothesis is being considered. The epidemiological context defines the significance of an association rather than any particular level of strain discrimination [43]. Therefore, strain discrimination should not be a prerequisite for public health intervention or regulatory action. In the nationwide outbreak associated with cake batter ice cream, investigators encountered a rare subtype, a rare, specific exposure among cases but not controls, and a plausible mechanism of dissemination, making further strain discrimination unnecessary. The PulseNet system has a policy that two restriction endonucleases should be used in each determination for selected surveillance pathogens, but the intention of this policy is to make higher strain resolution data readily available when needed, not as criteria for action [44].

7 *The prevalence of the agent (as defined by the laboratory test) in the population:* If an agent is common, the chance that unrelated sporadic cases of disease are inadvertently included in a cluster investigation is high, which lowers measures of association between cases connected to a common source. Conversely, if an agent is rare, the chance of inadvertent inclusion is low, making further subtyping less important. For example, in the 2006 outbreak of *E. coli* O157:H7 due to contaminated spinach, the case definition included a specific PFGE type, which was identified on average 21 times per year prior to the outbreak, or 0.7% of patterns submitted annually to the PulseNet database ([45], personal communication). If the normal prevalence of the strain had been 25% instead of 0.7%, type 1 probability error would have been proportionately more important. Similarly, the chance that cases of invasive disease due to *Strep. pyogenes* in a tem-poral cluster are related to a common transmission event is weaker, all other factors being equal, for a commonly identified invasive strain such as *emm* type 1, versus a less common strain such as *emm* type 18.

8 *The genetic stability and population structure of the agent:* The value of added discrimination, and indeed the value of subtyping at all, is affected by the population structure of the agent, which is influenced by its innate genetic stability.

Measures of relatedness

For some specific surveillance goals, it is useful to "lump" rather than "split" subtype data (i.e., consolidate individual subtypes into larger groups by measuring relatedness between individual strains) and cluster analysis. Potential reasons for measuring relatedness includes (a) tracking broad geographic or temporal trends, (b) widening the case definition for investigations where capturing all possibly associated cases is more important than eliminating possibly unrelated cases (minimizing type II probability error), (c) tracing infectious disease events backwards in time, and (d) surveillance of a disease where the causative agent is genetically unstable with respect to the marker/method used.

Examples of broad trends evaluated through the use of relatedness measures include the use of PFGE or sequence-based strain clustering algorithms to monitor the geographic distribution of *Francisella tularensis* strains in the US [46], influenza A virus type H5N1 in Asia [47], and patterns of horizontal transfer of resistance genes in *Salmonella* Typhimurium [48]. Increasing the sensitivity of the case definition and tracing disease events backward in time series are sometimes useful in forensic investigations, to determine the scope of an outbreak, to identify an environmental source, or when the number of cases is small but the implications of omission are great. A widely publicized use of this type of analysis is the investigation of possible HIV transmission from a Florida dentist to his patients [49]. Relatedness measures are often used for understanding transmission patterns of *Enterococcus faecium*, which has high background rates of recombination [50].

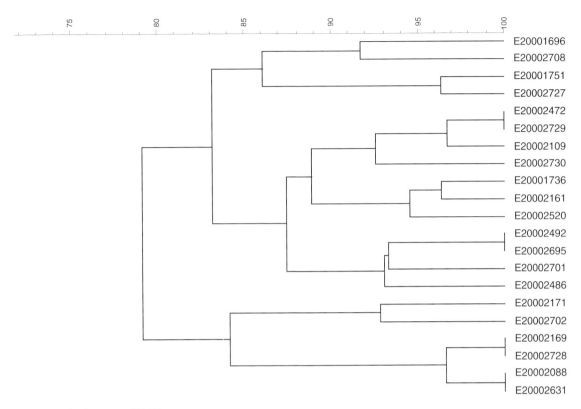

Fig 30.4 A dendrogram of PFGE patterns.

Determining relatedness and clustering

There are a large number of mathematical models used to estimate relatedness and clustering, each with their own assumptions, approximations, and limitations. Software commonly used for analysis of molecular surveillance data will readily draw graphical representations of strain relatedness and assign values that may or may not be useful for epidemiological inference.

Two broad approaches are used to describe and quantify the relatedness between microorganisms. *Phenetic* approaches assign numeric values to traits such as colonial or cellular morphology, biochemical characteristics, antimicrobial susceptibility, or electrophoresis patterns, and use these values as a basis for defining similarity or distance without consideration of evolutionary relationships. This is the theoretical framework for numerical taxonomy. PFGE dendrograms depict strain relationships

based on pattern differences which may or may not reflect evolutionary distance, and as such resemble phenetic representations (Figure 30.4). *Cladistic* approaches use an evolutionary model to predict the phylogenetic relationship between organisms (Figure 30.1). This requires that the data be oriented in an evolutionary "direction." These are often represented as genetic trees, such as cladograms and phylograms where the lines represent genetic relationship and distance. A good example of cladistic analysis is the investigation of vaccine-derived polio infections, where sequence divergence from the vaccine strain was used to estimate the time that the virus has circulated [51]. In this investigation, sequence-based microbiological data was combined with epidemiological information about cases. An evolutionary model assumed that strains evolved from the vaccine strain in the direction of more similar to less similar in a predictable manner. Molecular methods such as PFGE, MLVA, and

403

sequence-based methods can potentially be used in phenetic or cladistic analyses, but some molecular methods are more amenable to cladistic analyses than others.

If there is a research question involving relatedness or clustering of strains, often the approach is driven by the type of available data, such as the subtyping method, the extent and type of epidemiological information, and the absence or presence of an evolutionary model. For example, in a study of *Salmonella* Typhimurium resistance trends [52], several factors dictated a phenetic-like approach to comparing strains. Data were collected as part of routine surveillance and PFGE was the subtyping method used. PFGE electrophoresis patterns measure genetic relatedness indirectly, and it is not possible to say exactly how strains are different at the sequence level. The higher level of uncertainty makes it difficult to draw phylogenetic inference on broad surveillance data without additional epidemiological information. With a large, widely acquired surveillance data set of a relatively common, disease such as multidrug-resistant *Salmonella* Typhimurium, there was insufficient epidemiological information that could be used to orient data into an evolutionary model that predicts how molecular resistance determinants are gained and lost. In contrast, tracking new or rare diseases such as H5N1 influenza A virus with sequence-based methods are more amenable to cladistic analyses. The rarity of the disease makes it possible to draw meaningful connections between cases, specific genetic variation, and an evolutionary model. In one study, distinct clades were found to have evolved in two nonoverlapping regions of Asia, with strains affecting humans confined to a single, relatively homogeneous clade with a single antiviral susceptibility profile [47]. In the tree diagram representing these data, the branches actually represent phylogenetic distance.

Tenover and his colleagues used a cladistic approach to answer questions about interpretation of PFGE patterns in the outbreak setting during the development of PulseNet [53]. The specific goal was to assess the likelihood of genetic relatedness among epidemiologically related strains. The authors established a hierarchy of relatedness based on the least number of mutations that could account for observed pattern differences between an outbreak strain and other potentially related strains. Thus, exact pattern matches were termed "probably" related. Patterns with one- to three-band differences, the number that could result from single mutations, were determined "likely" related. Isolates with four- to six-band differences, which would require at least two mutations were termed "possibly" related. The number of possible mutations that could account for differences is much larger and difficult to define. However, focusing on the least possible of mutations serves the particular application, which involves assessing the risk of relationship to the outbreak strain. The authors recognized that this type of analysis might be less useful for general surveillance where there is generally insufficient information, such as relationships among cases to an outbreak, to overcome uncertainty in the subtyping method. Another issue with the use of these criteria for surveillance involves *transitivity*. Data from gel electrophoresis methods such as PFGE is continuous rather than discrete, and small errors in lane assignments create situations where pattern A = B and B = C, but A ≠ C. Finally, use of the Tenover scheme without a specific goal in a surveillance setting would reveal a complex web of relationships, making interpretation problematic for all but the smallest data sets.

Dendrograms are commonly generated to visually represent strain relatedness among large PFGE data sets, and used similarly for MLVA or other non-sequence-based surveillance data. While the Tenover assignments are based on the least number of mutations which could account for the observed banding difference between strains, this assumption cannot be made on general surveillance data, where a three-band difference between patterns could equally be due to one, two, three, or even more mutations. Phenetic analyses ignore this problem and assess the similarity or distance between the patterns, rather than attempting to infer genetic distance. In the absence of a very specific question or epidemiological information, this is probably as good an approximation as any. With some of the clustering algorithms described below, the order that the data are input affect how the tree is drawn. In spite of their limitations, dendrograms are useful for visualizing broad clustering trends, but researchers should be cautious about assigning significance to individual data points.

Terminology of relatedness measures and cluster analyses

A feature used to define a subtype is known as a *character*, and the possible values for that character are its *character states*. The organism is defined by a set of character states known as the operational taxonomic unit, or OTU. Thus, for *Salmonella* Typhimurium MLVA, the characters are the individual loci, the character state is the value at each locus (the allele, or number of repeat sequences), and an OTU is a particular pattern of values that defines a strain. Determining relatedness between OTUs involves defining the character states (not a trivial task with gel electrophoresis methods such as PFGE), applying a mathematical algorithm to compare strains, cluster analyses, graphical representation such as dendrograms or phylogenetic trees, and tree testing. Two of the most common indices used to assess similarity and distance are the Jaccard and Dice coefficients [3], which give weight to positive character states (such as the presence of a band on a gel). Sequence-based data are compared by alignment tools such as CLUSTAL [54].

The most common phenetic clustering methods are *hierarchical*, which use similarity coefficients to create nested groupings in which a single OTU can share characteristics with more than one grouping of OTUs. The most frequently applied clustering algorithms are the nearest neighbor method and the unweighted pair-group method using arithmetic averages (UPGMA). The most important cladistic methods used to infer epidemiological relationships include *parsimony* analysis, *maximum likelihood* analysis, and neighbor joining [14].

Summary

The decision to lump subtype data (e.g., consolidate strains into larger groupings) or split subtype data (e.g., add additional markers or methods to increase discrimination) when investigating clusters or outbreaks is based on a number of factors. There are a few practical generalizations that can be used as part of the decision process prior to taking public health action.

1 Increased agent discrimination beyond what is provided by the standard validated surveillance subtyping method is most likely to be useful or needed when (a) an investigation is in hypothesis generation or testing phase, (b) the subtype is common, or (c) the presumptive exposure is common or the exposure information is nonspecific. The number of cases under investigation may affect the usefulness of additional discrimination, as the effects of random variation are greater when the number of cases is very low.

2 In general, the types of investigations that benefit most from increased agent definition are (a) clusters detected through pathogen surveillance, where the agent is the principal factor linking cases (b) when a common source is suspected between two or more spatially or temporally separated outbreaks (however detected), especially when the agent is the primary linking element.

3 Once a statistically significant and epidemiologically plausible exposure has been identified in an investigation, increased discrimination is unlikely to be necessary before taking public health action, unless a specific alternate hypothesis is being considered.

4 Decreased discrimination or using measures of similarity may be useful (a) for determining the scope of an outbreak (especially if the exposure is rare), (b) for exploring broad trends, such as geographical segregation, strain evolution, or association between subtypes and a factor not directly tested (such as antibiotic resistance), (c) when the implicated agent is known to be genetically unstable with the available subtyping tests, and (d) when the consequences of not including cases is high, and/or when the number of cases is small (e.g., SARS, botulism, or pulmonary anthrax).

References

1 Levin BR, Lipsitch M, Bonhoeffer S. Population biology, evolution, and infectious disease: convergence and synthesis. *Science* February 5, 1999;**283**(5403):806–9.

2 Garmel GM. *Dorland's Illustrated Medical Dictionary*, 30th edn. Philadelphia, PA: WB Saunders; 2003.

3 Riley, LW. *Molecular Epidemiology of Infectious Diseases: Principles and Practices*. Washington, DC: American Society for Microbiology; 2004.

4 Federal Register, Volume 66 Number 44, March 6, 2001; page 13545–13546; Docket No. 99N–1168; DOCID: fr06MR 01–110.

5 Johnson J, Jinneman K, Stelma G, *et al.* Natural atypical *Listeria innocua* strains with *Listeria monocytogenes* pathogenicity island 1 genes. *Appl Environ Microbiol* July 2004;**70**(7):4256–66.

6 Popoff, MY, Le Minor L. *Antigenic Formulas of the Salmonella serovars*, 7th revision. Paris: World Health Organization Collaborating Centre for Reference and Research on *Salmonella*, Pasteur Institute; 1997.

7 Swaminathan B, Barrett TJ, Hunter SB, Tauxe RV; CDC PulseNet Task Force. PulseNet: the molecular subtyping network for foodborne bacterial disease surveillance, United States. *Emerg Infect Dis* May–June 2001;**7**(3): 382–9.

8 Myers RE, Gale CV, Harrison A, Takeuchi Y, Kellam P. A statistical model for HIV-1 sequence classification using the subtype analyser (STAR). *Boinformatics* September 1, 2005;**21**(17):3535–40.

9 Sides TL, Akinsete O, Henry K, Wotton JT, Carr PW, Bartkus J. HIV-1 subtype diversity in Minnesota. *J Infect Dis* July 1, 2005;**192**(1):37–45.

10 Naimi TS, Wicklund JH, Olsen SJ, *et al.* Concurrent outbreaks of *Shigella sonnei* and enterotoxigenic *Escherichia coli* infections associated with parsley: implications for surveillance and control of foodborne illness. *J Food Prot* April 2003;**66**(4):535–41.

11 TIGR Comprehensive Microbial Resource (CMR) Home Page. Available from: http://cmr.tigr.org/tigr-scripts/CMR/CmrHomePage.cgi. Accessed October 10, 2006.

12 Martin JM, Green M. Group A streptococcus. *Semin Pediatr Infect Dis* July 2006;**17**(3):140–8.

13 Li Z, Sakota V, Jackson D, Franklin AR, Beall B; Active Bacterial Core Surveillance/Emerging Infections Program Network. Array of M protein gene subtypes in 1064 recent invasive group A streptococcus isolates recovered from the active bacterial core surveillance. *J Infect Dis* November 15, 2003;**188**(10):1587–92.

14 Clinical and Laboratory Standards Institute. *Molecular Methods for Bacterial Strain Typing: Proposed Guideline*. CLSI document MM11-P. Wayne, PA: Clinical and Laboratory Standards Institute; 2006.

15 Hunter, PR, Gatson MA. Numerical index of the discriminatory ability of typing systems: an application of Simpson's index of diversity. *J Clin Microbiol* 1988;**26**:2465–66.

16 Shannon, CE, Weaver W. *The Mathematical Theory of Communication*. Urbana, IL: University of Illinois Press; 1949.

17 Swaminathan B, Barrett TJ, Fields P. Surveillance for human *Salmonella* infections in the United States. *J AOAC Int* March–April 2006;**89**(2):553–9.

18 Mead PS, Slutsker L, Dietz V, *et al.* Food-related illness and death in the United States. *Emerg Infect Dis* 1999;**5**(5):607–25.

19 Stewart DS, Reineke KF, Ulaszek JM, Tortorello ML Growth of *Salmonella* during sprouting of alfalfa seeds associated with salmonellosis outbreaks. *J Food Prot* May 2001;**64**(5):618–22.

20 Hennessy TW, Hedberg CW, Slutsker L, *et al.* for the Investigation Team. A national outbreak of *Salmonella enteritidis* infections from ice cream. *N Engl J Med* May 16, 1996;**334**(20):1281–6.

21 US Food and Drug Administration. Bad Bug Book. Available from: http://www.cfsan.fda.gov/~mow/intro.html. Accessed October 10, 2006.

22 Bell BP, Goldoft M, Griffin PM, *et al.* A multistate outbreak of *Escherichia coli* O157:H7-associated bloody diarrhea and hemolytic uremic syndrome from hamburgers: the Washington experience. *JAMA* November 2, 1994;**272**(17):1349–53.

23 Kim S, Frye JG, Hu J, Fedorka Cray PJ, Gautom R, Boyle DS. A multiplex PCR based method for the identification of common clinical serotypes of *Salmonella enterica* subspecies enterica. *J Clin Microbiol* October 2006;**44**(10): 3608–15.

24 Meningococcal Reference Unit; Gray SJ, Trotter CL, Ramsay ME, *et al.* Epidemiology of meningococcal disease in England and Wales 1993/94 to 2003/04: contribution and experiences of the Meningococcal Reference Unit. *J Med Microbiol* July 2006;**55**(Pt 7): 887–96.

25 Mothershed EA, Sacchi CT, Whitney AM, *et al.* Use of real-time PCR to resolve slide agglutination discrepancies in serogroup identification of *Neisseria meningitidis*. *J Clin Microbiol* January 2004;**42**(1): 320–8.

26 Beall B, Facklam R, Hoenes T, Schwartz B. Survey of *emm* gene sequences and T-antigen types from systemic *Streptococcus pyogenes* infection isolates collected in San Francisco, California; Atlanta, Georgia; and Connecticut in 1994 and 1995. *J Clin Microbiol* May 1997;**35**(5): 1231–5.

27 Barrett TJ, Lior H, Green JH, *et al.* Laboratory investigation of a multistate food-borne outbreak of *Escherichia coli* O157:H7 by using pulsed-field gel electrophoresis and phage typing. *J Clin Microbiol* December 1994;**32**(12):3013–7.

28 Bender JB, Hedberg CW, Besser JM, Boxrud DJ, MacDonald KL, Osterholm MT. Surveillance by molecular subtype for *Escherichia coli* O157:H7 infections in Minnesota by molecular subtyping. *N Engl J Med* August 7, 1997;**337**(6):388–94.

29 Swaminathan B, Gerner-Smidt P, Ng LK, *et al.* Building PulseNet International: an interconnected system of laboratory networks to facilitate timely public health recognition and response to foodborne disease outbreaks and emerging foodborne diseases. *Foodborne Pathog Dis* Spring 2006;**3**(1):36–50

30 Tauxe RV. Molecular subtyping and the transformation of public health. *Foodborne Pathog Dis* Spring 2006;3(1):4–8.

31 Blanton LH, Adams SM, Beard RS, *et al*. Molecular and epidemiologic trends of caliciviruses associated with outbreaks of acute gastroenteritis in the United States, 2000–2004. *J Infect Dis* February 1, 2006;193(3):413–21.

32 Austin DJ, Bonten MJ, Weinstein RA, Slaughter S, Anderson RM. Vancomycin-resistant enterococci in intensive care hospital settings: transmission dynamics, persistence, and the impact of infection control programs. *Proc Natl Acad Sci U S A*. June 8, 1999;96(12):6908–13.

33 Cameron RJ, Ferguson JK, O'Brien MW. Pulsed-field gel electrophoresis is a useful tool in the monitoring of methicillin-resistant *Staphylococcus aureus* epidemic outbreaks in the intensive care unit. *Anaesth Intensive Care* October 1999;27(5):447–51.

34 Chavez-Bueno S, Bozdogan B, Katz K, *et al*. Inducible clindamycin resistance and molecular epidemiologic trends of pediatric community-acquired methicillin-resistant *Staphylococcus aureus* in Dallas, Texas. *Antimicrob Agents Chemother* June 2005;49(6): 2283–8.

35 Desjardins M, Delgaty KL, Ramotar K, Seetaram C, Toye B. Prevalence and mechanisms of erythromycin resistance in group A and group B Streptococcus: implications for reporting susceptibility results. *J Clin Microbiol* December 2004;42(12):5620–3.

36 Monto AS, McKimm-Breschkin JL, Macken C, *et al*. Detection of influenza viruses resistant to neuraminidase inhibitors in global surveillance during the first 3 years of their use. *Antimicrob Agents Chemother* July 2006; 50(7):2395–402.

37 Health Protection Agency. Microbial Identification and Typing Databases. Available from: http://www.hpa.org.uk/cfi/bioinformatics/dbases.htm. Accessed September 29, 2006.

38 Johansson A, Farlow J, Larsson P, *et al*. Worldwide genetic relationships among *Francisella tularensis* isolates determined by multiple-locus variable-number tandem repeat analysis. *J Bacteriol* September 2004; 186(17):5808–18.

39 Bonten MJ, Willems R, Weinstein RA. Vancomycin-resistant enterococci: why are they here, and where do they come from? *Lancet Infect Dis* December 2001;1(5): 314–25.

40 Bielaszewska M, Prager R, Zhang W, *et al*. Chromosomal dynamism in progeny of outbreak-related sorbitol-fermenting enterohemorrhagic *Escherichia coli* O157:NM. *Appl Environ Microbiol* March 2006;72(3): 1900–9.

41 Reingold AL. Outbreak investigations—a perspective. *Emerg Infect Dis* January–March 1998;4(1):21–7.

42 FDA News. July 1, 2005. FDA Issues Nationwide Alert on Possible Health Risk Associated with Cold Stone Creamery "Cake Batter" Ice Cream. Available from: http://www.fda.gov/bbs/topics/news/2005/NEW01200.html. Accessed October 16, 2006.

43 Hedberg CW, Besser JM. Commentary: cluster evaluation, PulseNet, and public health practice. *Foodborne Pathog Dis* Spring 2006;3(1):32–5.

44 Besser JM. PulseNet Gestalt. 10th Annual PulseNet Update Meeting. Association of Public Health Laboratories. Available from: http://www.aphl.org/conferences/pulsenet_update_meeting_2006/. Accessed October 10, 2006.

45 Centers for Disease Control and Prevention (CDC). Ongoing multistate outbreak of *Escherichia coli* serotype O157:H7 infections associated with consumption of fresh spinach–United States, September 2006. *MMWR Morb Mortal Wkly Rep* September 29, 2006;55(38):1045–6.

46 Farlow J, Wagner DM, Dukerich M, *et al*. *Francisella tularensis* in the United States. *Emerg Infect Dis* December 2005;11(12):1835–41.

47 World Health Organization Global Influenza Program Surveillance Network. Evolution of H5N1 avian influenza viruses in Asia. *Emerg Infect Dis* October 2005; 11(10):1515–21.

48 Lawson AJ, Dassama MU, Ward LR, Threlfall EJ. Multiply resistant (MR) *Salmonella enterica* serotype Typhimurium DT 12 and DT 120: a case of MR DT 104 in disguise? *Emerg Infect Dis* April 2002;8(4):434–6.

49 Ou CY, Ciesielski CA, Myers G, *et al*. Molecular epidemiology of HIV transmission in a dental practice. *Science* May 22, 1992;256(5060):1165–71.

50 Ruiz-Garbajosa P, Bonten MJ, Robinson DA, *et al*. Multilocus sequence typing scheme for *Enterococcus faecalis* reveals hospital-adapted genetic complexes in a background of high rates of recombination. *J Clin Microbiol* June 2006;44(6):2220–8.

51 Kew OM, Sutter RW, de Gourville EM, Dowdle WR, Pallansch MA. Vaccine-derived polioviruses and the endgame strategy for global polio eradication. *Annu Rev Microbiol* 2005;59:587–635.

52 Wedel SD, Bender JB, Leano FT, Boxrud DJ, Hedberg C, Smith KE. Antimicrobial-drug susceptibility of human and animal *Salmonella* Typhimurium, Minnesota, 1997–2003. *Emerg Infect Dis* December 2005;11(12):1899–906.

53 Tenover FC, Arbeit RD, Goering RV, *et al*. Interpreting chromosomal DNA restriction patterns produced by pulsed-field gel electrophoresis: criteria for bacterial strain typing. *J Clin Microbiol* September 1995;33(9): 2233–9.

54 Chenna R, Sugawara H, Koike T, *et al*. Multiple sequence alignment with the Clustal series of programs. *Nucleic Acids Res* 2003;31:3497–3500.

31 Use of geographic information systems and remote sensing for infectious disease surveillance

Edmund Seto, Chester G. Moore & Richard E. Hoskins

Introduction

Geographic information systems (GIS) and aerial and satellite imagery ("remotely sensed" imagery) are contributing new tools to the surveillance for many types of infectious diseases. Before the GIS era, investigators used map pins and Mylar sheets overlaid onto printed maps to track outbreaks. In the past there was no possibility of rapid sharing of maps, no way to estimate various characteristics of one geography in terms of another, no possibility of integration of data across map layers via map algebra, and nowhere near the level of spatial analysis and spatial statistics that is now available with (often free) software.

With the arrival of GIS, and especially GIS for non-GIS specialists, at long last "where" becomes an equal partner with the other three parts of the epidemiologic investigational quartet: the others being "who," "what," and "when." GIS helps to answer the questions: Are there clusters of cases? Where are the clusters? Is the center of disease transmission moving in time and space? The application of GIS and spatial analysis to public health has numerous books, training, and Web sites. A small sample is shown in Table 31.1 Use of GIS and remote sensing technology will likely be a required core skill in public health training in the future.

In this chapter we provide a brief overview of the application of GIS and remote sensing, with emphasis on the latter. Then, we present an example of the application of GIS and remote sensing to schistosomiasis—this can serve as a model for other types of surveillance where environmental factors are an important consideration in understanding the disease process.

GIS: What can it do?

A GIS is a relational database software with location as the organizing entity. It has an elaborate front-end that allows operations on spatially referenced data, leading to "spatial analysis" as supported by its quantitative cousin, "spatial statistics." The working medium is a map. Although spatial analysis and spatial statistics can be very complex and may only be accessible to specially trained researchers, much of it is tutored common sense.

Maps, produced with GIS-based visualization and analytical tools, depicting hosts, vectors, human residences, the terrain where they live, and disease rates, can lead the investigator to a greater understanding of an infectious disease process in a population in space and time. Furthermore, the aerial and satellite images produced by remote sensing contain a wealth of additional information for infectious disease surveillance [1].

For the GIS beginner, point and thematic maps might seem to be the endpoint of GIS. However, there is much more beyond making a map of disease location and incidence: GIS is an integrator. It can display and operate on data that might be *only* related geographically. There are hundreds of GIS-supported operations that can be used on a map. Through the synergy of spatially referenced data, externally linked data, and spatial tools, new information can be generated which is unobtainable in

Table 31.1 Selected sources of information for GIS training and applications to health.

Title	Description	URL
ESRI Public Health	Health GIS portal, GIS articles on application to health	http://www.esri.com/industries/health/business/publichealth.html
Loma Linda University	Certificate program in public health GIS	http://www.llu.edu/llu/sph/geoinformatics/chg06.html
International Journal of Health Geographics	Online, free journal for applications of GIS and spatial analysis to health	http://www.ij-healthgeographics.com/
Health-Related University GIS Courses	List of programs offering GIS use in health training	http://www.esri.com/industries/health/news-community/university-courses.html
Health GIS conference	GIS and health conference with workshops and papers	http://www.esri.com/events/hug/index.html
Pan American Health Organization	GIS in public health and epidemiology	http://www.paho.org/English/SHA/shasig.htm
John Snow & Cholera	The often retold Snow story is a prime example of effective spatial analysis	http://www.ph.ucla.edu/epi/snow.html
healthmaps@u.washington.edu	Public health and GIS listscrve in the US	http://mailman1.u.washington.edu/mailman/listinfo/healthmaps
geo-health-bounces@flinders.edu.au	Public health and GIS listserve in Australia	https://listserver.flinders.edu.au/mailman/listinfo/geo-health
Public Health GIS News and Information	Centers for Disease Control and Prevention	http://www.cdc.gov/nchs/gis.htm

any other way. For example, by overlaying disease incidence data with climate data, we may understand environmental correlates to disease transmission [2,3]. By using buffer analyses (a buffer consists of equidistant lines enclosing point, line or polygon features (e.g., a 1-mile buffer constructed around known mosquito habitats to identify residential areas at greatest risk)), we can consider how proximity affects a disease process. The simplicity with which these analyses can be performed in GIS allows for exploratory spatial data analysis, whereby spatial patterns and relationships can be hypothesized, detected, and described. More sophisticated analyses include spatial statistical methods, such as cluster analyses aimed at detecting significant disease clusters in space and time, and spatial regression aimed at testing the associations between various spatial factors and disease incidence [1].

These analytical operations can be applied to surveillance for vector-, air-, and waterborne diseases. Perhaps the most important promise of GIS/remote sensing is that it can help predict the future course of an outbreak. Knowing where the cases are is fundamentally useful, but knowing where they are likely to occur next is what we really need. Are we headed toward an epidemic? What is the likelihood that West Nile virus (WNV) will appear in a community with particular landscape ecology? What are the areas of high risk for infection? What climate conditions support the disease process? And in the future, what is the role of climate change? The analysis of spatial patterns of infectious diseases can lead to a deeper understanding of disease pathways, and how to control them.

GIS layers for infectious disease mapping

To make useful maps for infectious disease surveillance, we need GIS layers which have data connected to them. For example:

Point data: disease cases and controls, birth and death certificates, hospitals, businesses, dead bird locations, well heads, clinics, biohazards, air and water quality testing sites

409

Line data: roads, rivers, railways, pipelines, emergency response routes

Polygon data: county or census tract boundaries and data, incorporated boundaries of towns, zip codes, planning areas, land parcels

Image data: Aerial photographs, satellite imagery in raster (also called grid or matrix) format. Raster data consists of a continuous layer of cells of uniform size and shape, each having a specific assigned value (e.g., brightness, elevation)

Vector-borne diseases

WNV is a mosquito-transmitted disease that has been addressed with GIS maps and operations (http://westnilemaps.usgs.gov/). GIS has been used to model mosquito populations in British Columbia [4] and to support a WNV surveillance program in Pennsylvania [5].

At the local level, the vector-borne (e.g., WNV) mapping process could be as follows:
• Data on mosquitoes are collected: Abundance of vector species at different locations, virus infection rates, flight range, temperature sensitivity, and insecticide resistance.
• In the case of WNV, dead bird surveillance data provides another GIS layer that can indicate areas where infection risk is potentially high for humans.
• The age distribution of vulnerable human populations is mapped from census data. For WNV, older persons may be more likely to have severe disease.
• Human cases of the disease (e.g., WNV) are geocoded and mapped.
• Mosquito larval habitats are identified, mapped, and evaluated for type of control (e.g., source reduction, insecticide treatment).
• The landscape composition is determined from aerial photos and satellite data with respect to vegetation and aquatic distribution relevant to mosquitoes.
• Buffers are created around potentially susceptible populations. Depending on the flight range of different vectors, suitable buffers are created from the vector breeding sites as well.
• If vulnerable populations are within flight range of potentially infected mosquitoes, then suitable preventive and control measures can be taken.

To be truly effective, data must be shared between agencies. This requires planning, coordination, and agreement on standards for reporting data across political boundaries. One such program is ArboNET, a Web-based arbovirus reporting system developed by the United States Centers for Disease Control and Prevention (US CDC), the state health departments, and the US Geological Survey (USGS). ArboNET provides data to monitor the geographic and temporal spread of WNV and other arboviruses in the US. It serves as an aid in identifying areas at increased risk for human infections and developing strategies to prevent arbovirus infections in humans or domestic animals [6,7].

WNV-related data (bird deaths, sentinel bird flock serology, mosquito infections, and human and domestic animal cases) are collected at the local level and reported to the state health department. The data are checked for accuracy at the state level, and then transmitted via one of several secure data transfer schemes to the CDC. County-level data are then transmitted to the USGS Web site, where it is integrated into the GIS database for posting as Web maps (Disease Maps 2006: http://diseasemaps.usgs.gov/) (Plate 31.1). Current maps are available at http://diseasemaps.usgs.gov/ and can be easily customized by Web users to select, for example, specific regions containing more-detailed county-level data.

Another good example of the application of GIS in vector-borne disease monitoring can be found in the maps of the California Vectorborne Disease Surveillance Gateway (CSG), operated jointly by California Mosquito and Vector Control Programs, the California Department of Health Services, and the Center for Vectorborne Diseases at the University of California–Davis (California Vectorborne Disease Surveillance System: http://vector.ucdavis.edu/arbo.html).

Airborne diseases

Airborne diseases are spread when particles bearing pathogens are expelled into the air due to coughing, sneezing, or talking. Examples are measles, varicella, tuberculosis, and some cases of severe acute respiratory syndrome (SARS) and influenza. The World Health Organization, for example, posts on

the Web frequently updated maps demonstrating the distribution of avian influenza H5N1 activity in space and through time. Further GIS layering of these types of diseases might include the following:
• Human and zoonotic cases of the disease are geocoded and mapped.
• Population data is mapped for most vulnerable populations and population density. If appropriate, immunization rates by age group are mapped.
• Cluster analyses are carried out to verify regions with higher than expected disease activity.
• Control measures are implemented in areas of disease clusters and preventive measures are implemented for at-risk populations.

Waterborne diseases

Cholera is an example of a classic waterborne disease, causing massive epidemics in Asia and South America within the recent past. GIS and remote sensing have been used effectively in understanding the dynamics of the cholera organism and in predicting cholera activity [8]. Schistomiasis will be discussed later in this chapter. GIS layers for these and other waterborne diseases might include the following:
• Natural water sources are marked on the map of the given region. These are further classified as running, stagnant, salt- or freshwater.
• Controlled water sources such as wells, water supplies, reservoirs, or sewage treatment plants are mapped.
• Buffers are created for these water bodies to establish areas prone to waterborne microorganisms, depending on the pipe network and flow condition.
• The distribution of populations vulnerable to these diseases is identified and mapped.
• Depending on these results, suitable control and preventive measures are taken.

Remote sensing and infectious diseases

Along with advances in GIS technology and the increased availability of spatial data, has been the increasing application of remote sensing to infectious disease surveillance. The term *remote sensing*, first used in the 1960s [9], evolved from older aerial photography and weather and spy satellite technology, and describes the acquisition and analysis of data obtained from a remote or distant target [10]. While some early studies from the late 1970s applied remote sensing to diseases such as malaria, the field grew considerably in 1985 with the creation of National Aeronautics and Space Administration's (NASA) Center for Health Applications of Aerospace Related Technologies (CHAART: http://geo.arc.nasa.gov/sge/health/chaart.html). The objective of the center was to expand the use of remote sensing to human health via education and training, and applied research. In fact, many of CHAART's collaborations with numerous universities and foreign institutes led to the growth of studies during 1990s, which included studies on cholera [8], malaria [11–18], Rift Valley fever [19–21], Lyme disease [22,23], and schistosomiasis [24–33]. Much of this early research focused on the use of remote sensing to identify environmental conditions associated with vector habitats that play a role in disease transmission.

Washino and Wood [34] and Hay *et al.* [35] have reviewed the evolution of literature on remote sensing in human health. In this chapter, we concentrate on the benefits and limitations of remote sensing surveillance approaches, introduce common methodologies for application of remote sensing data with examples from the infectious disease literature, and highlight future directions for remote sensing in health surveillance.

Potential benefits of remote sensing health surveillance

Remote sensing potentially can offer an efficient way to assess disease risk over large geographic areas including parts of the world where human and economic resources and infrastructure do not exist to support traditional disease reporting surveillance systems. Remote sensing is particularly well-suited to monitor diseases that are strongly tied to environmental determinants. Investigations concerning Rift Valley fever are good examples [36–38].

Rapid advances in remote sensing technology offer a bright future for disease surveillance [39]. Particularly exciting are new satellite-based sensors with improved imaging capabilities that potentially create new ways to study the spatial–temporal distribution of disease outbreaks, spread, and reemergence. While new sensors are exciting, space agencies apparently are not ignoring the old ones. In fact, many new satellites that carry sensors with new capabilities also carry sensors primarily aimed at extending the legacy of environmental measurements made by sensors on older satellites that may be reaching the end of their life span.

What is often not realized is that most, if not all remote sensing data, are archived and accessible via Internet search engines, such as the USGS's Earth Observing System Data Gateway (http://edcimswww.cr.usgs.gov/pub/imswelcome/). These archived data provide health researchers with historical environmental data, which can be used in retrospective analyses of environmental determinants of disease transmission. For example, NASA's Landsat program has a legacy of documenting changing land use and land cover since the early 1970s (http://landsat.gsfc.nasa.gov/).

How does remote sensing work?

Most of the satellite-based sensors used in disease studies are passive sensors that measure electromagnetic radiation naturally present in the environment. In contrast, active sensors both emit energy and measure the same energy that is reflected off of remote objects. The sun is typically the main energy source for passive remote sensing. The sun's radiation passes through and is scattered by the atmosphere. When the radiation reaches the surface of the earth, it is absorbed, transmitted through, and reflected off of land cover. The reflected fraction of the radiation passes back through the atmosphere and is measured by a satellite sensor.

The sun emits electromagnetic radiation that varies across a broad spectrum of wavelengths. Although the human eye can only see radiation within a narrow range of wavelengths (visible light ranges from short wavelength blue light, 0.4 μm, to long wavelength red light, 0.7 μm), many sensors are designed to measure not only visible light, but also other wavelengths. By measuring the amount of reflected energy at different wavelengths, it is possible via remote sensing to differentiate between various land cover types. For instance, by comparing reflected energy in both the visible (0.4–0.7 μm) and the near-infrared wavelengths (0.8–1.1 μm), it is possible to discriminate between various types of vegetation [10].

The reflected data recorded by the sensor are typically provided as a raster data set (e.g., an image file). Raster data sets consist of information stored in a rectangular grid of *pixels*. Each pixel corresponds to measurements made at a specific geographic area on the earth. The size of the pixel is related to a sensor's *spatial resolution*. Some coarse resolution sensors collect data for relatively large pixels (e.g., Advanced Very High Resolution Radiometer (AVHRR) 1.1-km pixels; http://noaasis.noaa.gov/NOAASIS/ml/avhrr.html), while other high-resolution sensors collect data for very small pixels (e.g., IKONOS 1-m panchromatic and 4-m color and near-infrared pixels; http://www.geoeye.com/). IKONOS is a commercial satellite launched in 1999. If the geographic area for a pixel contains multiple small landscape features, the reflectances are averaged together. Hence, coarse resolution images may often appear "blurry" due to the lack of resolving power and the averaging of reflectances over relatively large pixel areas. Although it may seem that high-resolution data would always be preferred for a surveillance application, in fact, there are trade-offs to be considered. Because IKONOS is a high-resolution sensor, each scene it produces is smaller, few images are available, and data are relatively expensive. In contrast, the AVHRR sensor is designed to provide daily global images. AVHRR images, while coarser in resolution, are available for free. Hence, high-resolution data are largely limited to small area studies, which attempt to understand very local transmission factors, such as identifying landscape and land use features that define important areas for transmission, whereas large-area national-level surveillance often utilizes coarser resolution images.

Another consideration in choosing remote sensing data is *spectral resolution*, or the number of wavelength bands at which reflected energy is measured for each pixel. Different land cover types vary in how they interact with and reflect the sun's energy. Some types of land cover reflect more radiation in certain wavelengths than others. A sensor that takes more samples along the wavelength spectrum is said to have a greater *spectral resolution*, which directly relates to its ability to differentiate between different land cover types. The Landsat Thematic Mapper (TM) sensor (http://landsat.gsfc .nasa.gov/) measures seven wavelength bands, providing good data for discerning subtle differences in vegetation and other land cover. In addition, its moderately high (30-m) spatial resolution, 16-day revisit time for successive images, decent coverage (170 × 183 km), and low cost have made it very popular for regional-level studies.

Although health researchers should consider the numerous trade-offs between sensor data in spatial and spectral resolution, image coverage and cost, and temporal frequency and availability, in practice often the two critical limiting factors for disease surveillance are the spatial scale and temporal frequency. National-level and/or daily imaging for surveillance applications are available only with coarser resolution sensor data. Coarse is a relative term, however, which is changing with time and new sensor technology. New MODIS data (http://rapidfire.sci.gsfc.nasa.gov/gallery/) at 250- and 500-m spatial resolutions are replacing AVHRR for global surveillance applications. Moreover, we are starting to see the benefits of using multiple sensor data together for many applications. For instance, the need to respond quickly to recent tsunami and hurricane disasters triggered the combined use of numerous sensor types to more comprehensively assess damage (Federal Emergency Management Agency (FEMA), Mapping and Analysis Center, Hurricane Katriana; NOAA Emergency Response Imagery, http:// ngs.woc.noaa.gov/eri_page/index.html). Future research in sensor nets and data fusion will most likely improve multisensor approaches to surveillance.

Analysis methods

Image analysis methods for disease surveillance range widely in complexity. Simple visual interpretation of remote sensing images can be very useful. The human eye can often identify an incredible amount of information from images, including new roads and urban development, and vegetation patterns and destruction. Overlaying and visually comparing images from different dates can allow

an analyst to rapidly assess the quantity and nature of land cover and land use change, which may be associated with reemerging disease, or to develop hypotheses as to why reemergence has occurred.

Image enhancement is another method that is commonly used in disease surveillance. An example of image enhancement is the processing of the original spectral reflectance data into vegetation indices that emphasize differences between vegetation types. Vegetation indices generally capitalize on differences in absorbance and reflectance between healthy and unhealthy or different types of vegetation in the visible and near-infrared spectrum [10]. A common vegetation index is the Normalized Difference Vegetation Index (NDVI), which is computed from near-infrared and red energy recorded by the sensor as (near IR − red)/(near IR + red). NDVI has been used in a number of studies, such as those identifying mosquito [11,12,15,17,18,40], fly [27,41,42], and tick habitats [22,23]. In the Wood *et al.* study [11], for example, NDVI was used for a mosquito study in California using airborne Multi-Spectral Scanner (MSS) data designed to simulate Landsat TM. Using discriminant analysis they found that higher NDVI was associated with high mosquito-producing rice fields, with an overall accuracy of 75%.

Remote sensing data may lead to environmental indices other than vegetation indices. These include meteorological variables such as land surface temperatures and rainfall [43], soil moisture maps [30], and elevation models derived from digital photogrammetry methods [44]. In the study by Xu *et al.* [44], elevations were computed from stereo-paired images from the Advanced Spaceborne Thermal Emission and Reflection Radiometer (ASTER) sensor. ASTER is an imaging instrument flying on Terra, a satellite launched in December 1999 as part of NASA's Earth Observing System (http://asterweb.jpl.nasa.gov/). Elevations were then used to inform the hydrological flow of larval stages of the *Schistosoma* parasite between villages, such that more informed regional disease control strategies could be designed.

Multispectral classification methods have also been applied to disease surveillance. The goal of image classification is to convert the recorded spectral radiances into meaningful information, such as thematic maps of different land cover classes. There are two general approaches to image classification: supervised versus unsupervised [10]. Both are statistical algorithms that are commonly available within image-processing software. In supervised classification, an analyst "trains" a classification by tracing a set of areas in the image that are representative of land cover types of interest (e.g., areas associated with vector breeding areas). The training areas define reference spectral signatures for each class. For example, a reference spectral signature for a rice field class might be defined by the mean and variance of recorded radiation for each wavelength band across all rice field training pixels. Classification of remaining pixels in the image occurs by an automated comparison of the pixel's spectral signature to that of the all reference signatures. A pixel will be labeled as belonging to a rice field if its spectral signature is most similar to that of the reference rice field signature.

Unsupervised classification is based on multivariate clustering algorithms to define a set of discrete land cover classes in the image. Often in unsupervised classification an analyst will specify some parameters that control the clustering process, such as the number of expected classes, and threshold values for within and between class variances that control how classes are generated. An automated iterative process is generally used to identify areas in the image that are spectrally different from one another, and mark these as different classes. It is the job of the analyst to label these areas as meaningful land cover classes.

Both classification methods are of use in disease surveillance. If sufficient field knowledge exists on the ecology of the vector to develop good training signatures, it may be possible to attempt a supervised classification to identify vector habitats [32,45]. However, unsupervised classifications may be more appropriate when the ecology of disease transmission is not clear. Studies of the latter type often use unsupervised classification to map large regions into distinct ecological zones. Disease incidence data are then overlaid on top of these zones to determine the extent to which transmission occurs in each of the zones. For instance, unsupervised Iterative Self-Organizing Data Analysis Technique clustering was used in a study to classify the country of Chad into ecological zones based on remote sensing-derived AVHRR data: surface temperature, rainfall, and elevation [46,47]. Schistosomiasis transmission was found to be most prevalent in the Sahelian zone and the Logone and Chari basins in the west of the country.

Case study: schistosomiasis early warning system for China

Today, roughly 40 million Chinese are at risk for infection by *Schistosoma japonicum*, a parasite that cycles through its various life stages in snails and their freshwater habitats [48]. Increased awareness of infectious diseases has motivated new large-scale disease control campaigns including the development of an early warning system for schistosomiasis reemergence in China. Remote sensing can potentially play an important role in such a warning system because schistosomiasis transmission is strongly conditioned by environmental factors. These factors define the presence of snail habitats as well as land use conditions that place villagers at risk of infection, such as the extent of irrigated agriculture, cattle grazing, and fishing areas. Chinese researchers at the Chinese Center for Disease Control and Prevention and US-based researchers have been actively developing such a remote sensing surveillance system.

Numerous studies demonstrate how snail habitats can be identified via remote sensing. In Egypt, Malone [30] used diurnal images to derive soil moisture maps that explain the presence of snails. In China, NDVI has been used to quantify snail habitats in marshland and lake environments [28,33], while in hilly and mountainous irrigated agriculture areas, the combined use of supervised and unsupervised classification also has been used [32].

A recent longitudinal study [49] of snail habitats in the Poyang Lake environment suggests that climate and seasonal flooding affect snail populations. Climate conditions early in the year affect how spring snail populations reemerge from over wintering conditions. During the summer monsoon season however, snail populations depend less upon climate and more upon the severity of flooding which disrupts and redistributes snail populations. Indeed, in China, many schistosomiasis outbreaks follow immediately after major flood events. The US-funded Tropical Medicine Research Center in

Shanghai has developed a method of tracking the effect of flooding on snail habitat areas through real-time mapping of cumulative water coverage. This can be more accurate than following water level gauges due to tidal effects and continual land use changes. Such a map was created from daily MODIS remote sensing data, at 250-m spatial resolution (Plate 31.2). For any given day of the year, such a map can identify areas that have received sufficient moisture levels to be high-risk snail habitats.

Presence of snails is but one factor in a warning system. Another factor relates to assessing parasite exposures for both human and animals. Within the Poyang Lake environment, exposure primarily occurs within marshlands of the lake where villagers take their cattle out to graze. If parasitized snails are also present, during grazing both humans and their cattle can become infected. Hence, an early warning system might consider, in addition to snail habitat areas identified via remote sensing, a GIS that includes human and animal populations as attributes, and their historical infection levels, as well as a spatial analysis that determines the spatial coincidence between snail habitats and cattle grazing areas. Other factors such as where and when various disease control activities were conducted, as well as changing land use, sanitation practices, and water resource development may also affect how such a system might assess overall village-level risk of infection for Poyang Lake.

At the heart of the early warning system is a need for some way to integrate the various pieces of information, such that each potential environmental change has a resultant effect on the probability of an outbreak. Multivariate regression models might be used to "fit" observed relationships. However, given rapid economic development, which is resulting in unprecedented agricultural changes and improvements in living conditions, there may be little data to fit such models. Instead, dynamic epidemiologic mathematical models that are based on a mechanistic understanding of how transmission occurs may be used to simulate disease transmission within village populations [50]. Such models can take as input spatially explicit time-varying data to assess risk [51–53].

To be effective, such a system requires a considerable amount of data connectivity and automation. For instance, interagency agreements must be in place such that climate data, remote sensing data, and human and animal census data can be readily accessed. There must be understanding, commitment, and protocols established for geocoding data that are not otherwise regularly entered into a digital format, such as human and cattle treatment data. Moreover, there must be clear guidelines for how such a system can be used to guide disease prevention measures.

Limitations and important steps for the future

There are several limitations in the application of GIS to disease surveillance. In many cases, disease case data are reported without any indication of spatial location. In addition, when location is indicated, it may have no relation to place of exposure. Surveillance for abundance and infection rates in disease vectors often is conducted without regard for appropriate sampling strategies. For example, local mosquito control programs place traps where they can be conveniently serviced, or where the technician "knows" the most mosquitoes will be collected. Vector abundance data collected over a long time period can be very useful in mapping risk. However, sampling sites that were in rural areas 10 years ago may be in the center of an urban area today, making interpretation of patterns extremely difficult. Finally, the ecological scale of the infectious disease system determines the scale at which data must be collected [54]. In the case of some arboviruses, such as St. Louis encephalitis and eastern equine encephalomyelitis, transmission may be confined to small areas of a square kilometer or less. There may not be sufficient sampling within such areas—and in surrounding uninfected areas—to measure any spatial patterns. Good planning and attention to proper sampling design can overcome many of these problems.

In remote sensing studies, scale is important. If the process is operating at a finer scale than the remote sensing imagery can resolve, there is little hope of getting meaningful relationships. With many vector-borne diseases, there appear to be multiple scales that are important [54]. Moreover, it may be misleading to think that remote sensing disease surveillance is as easy as running the latest satellite images through some magical classification system. Indeed, remote sensing, due to its ecologic nature, cannot account for all the myriad individual-level factors that affect transmission (see Chapter 9).

Moreover, even if one focuses only on vector populations (which arguably should be much better correlated than disease incidence with environmental conditions), the success of remote sensing surveillance largely depends upon our understanding of vector ecology. Consider one of the earliest remote sensing disease studies. Wagner *et al.* [55] used color-infrared photography to map forested and open wetlands, marshes, and residential areas for mosquito control in Saginaw and Bay Counties in Michigan—areas that had recently been struck with an epidemic of mosquito-borne St. Louis encephalitis. Their understanding of mosquito flight distances, and the distance between mosquito habitat areas and the residential areas that condition mosquito exposure was factored into their analysis to create control priorities for the two counties. As this simple example and the more complicated case study above suggest, it may be more appropriate to think of remote sensing as just one part of a larger information system that is based on a mechanistic understanding of how disease transmission occurs, and includes other pieces of information that informs surveillance and control.

Other more practical limitations exist with remote sensing. In the past, the cost and availability of data and appropriate hardware/software has largely relegated remote sensing disease surveillance to research, rather than routine practice. However, this is becoming less of a problem with time. Still, as the number of different types of sensor data increases, it places the burden upon health professionals to become sufficiently skilled to assess the many trade-offs involved with particular data sets. Moreover, despite little conceptual change in digital image processing methods over the past 10 years, the application of these methods requires substantial training in specialized software. One of the reasons why CHAART was such an important development for the field of disease surveillance was because it fostered interdisciplinary partnerships between remote sensing experts and disease experts to effectively develop surveillance solutions. If progress is to occur within the field, there must be a continued effort to educate a larger body of health professionals on the opportunities for remote sensing, increase the number of health professionals with specific GIS/remote sensing skills, and create more opportunities for collaborative partnerships that can lead to sustained application of remote sensing data to surveillance.

References

1 Bailey TC, Gatrell AC. *Interactive Spatial Data Analysis.* London: Longman Addison-Wesley Pub Co; 1995.

2 Parmenter RR, Yadav EP, Parmenter CA, Ettestad P, Gage KL. Incidence of plague associated with increased winter–spring precipitation in New Mexico. *Am J Trop Med Hyg* 1999;**61**:814–21.

3 Glass GE, Cheek JE, Patz JA, *et al..* Using remotely sensed data to identify areas at risk for hantavirus pulmonary syndrome. *Emerg Infect Dis* 2000;**6**:238–47.

4 Tachiiri K, Klinkenberg B, Mak S, Kazmi J. Predicting outbreaks: a spatial risk assessment of West Nile virus in British Columbia. *Int J Health Geogr* 2006;**5**(1):21.

5 Craglia M. *GIS in Public Health Practice.* Boca Raton: CRC press; 2004.

6 Marfin AA, Petersen LR, Eidson M, *et al..* Widespread West Nile virus activity, eastern United States, 2000. *Emerg Infect Dis* 2001;**7**(4):730–35.

7 Marfin AA, Gubler DJ. West Nile encephalitis: an emerging disease in the United States. *Clin Infect Dis* 2001; **33**(10):1713–9.

8 Colwell RR. Global climate and infectious disease: the cholera paradigm. *Science* 1996;**274**(5295):2025–31.

9 Campbell JB. *Introduction to Remote Sensing*, 2nd edn. New York: Guilford Press; 1996.

10 Jensen JR. *Introductory Digital Image Processing: A Remote Sensing Perspective*, 2nd edn. Upper Saddle River, NJ: Prentice-Hall; 1996.

11 Wood B, Washino R, Beck L, *et al.* Distinguishing high and low anopheline-producing rice fields using remote sensing and GIS technologies. *Prev Vet Med* 1991; **11**:277–88.

12 Wood BL, Beck LR, Washino RK, Hibbard KA, Salute JS. Estimating high mosquito-producing rice fields using spectral and spatial data. *Int J Remote Sens* 1992;**13**(15): 2813–26.

13 Pope KO, Rejmankova E, Savage HM, Arredondo-Jimenez JI, Rodriguez MH, Roberts DR. Remote sensing of tropical wetlands for malaria control in Chiapas, Mexico. *Ecol Appl* 1994;**4**(1):81–90.

14 Rejmankova E, Savage HM, Rejmanek M, Aredondo-Jimenez JI, Roberts DR. Multivariate analysis of relationships between habitats, environmental factors and occurrence of anopheline mosquito larvae *Anopheles albimanus* and *Anopheles pseudopunctipennis* in southern Chiapas, Mexico. *J Appl Ecol* 1991;**28**(3):827–41.

15 Rejmankova E, Savage HM, Rodriguez MH, Roberts DR, Rejmanek M. Aquatic vegetation as a basis for classification of *Anopheles albimanus* Weideman (Diptera: Culicidae) larval habitats. *Environ Entomol* 1992;**21**(3):598–603.

16 Beck LR, Rodriguez MH, Dister SW, *et al*. Remote sensing as a landscape epidemiologic tool to identify villages at high risk for malaria transmission. *Am J Trop Med Hyg* 1994;**51**(3):271–80.

17 Rejmankova E, Roberts DR, Pawley A, Manguin S, Polanco J. Predictions of adult *Anopheles albimanus* densities in villages based on distances to remotely sensed larval habitats. *Am J Trop Med Hyg* 1995;**53**(5):482–8.

18 Roberts DR, Paris JF, Manguin S, *et al*. Predictions of malaria vector distribution in Belize based on multispectral satellite data. *Am J Trop Med Hyg* 1996;**54**(3):304–8.

19 Linthicum K, Bailey C, Tucker C, *et al*. Towards real-time prediction of Rift Valley fever epidemics in Africa. *Prev Vet Med* 1991;**11**:325–34.

20 Linthicum KJ, Bailey CL, Davies FG, Tucker CJ. Detection of Rift Valley fever viral activity in Kenya by satellite remote sensing imagery. *Science (Washington DC)* 1987;**235**(4796):1656–9.

21 Linthicum KJ, Bailey CL, Tucker CJ, *et al*. Application of polar-orbiting, meteorological satellite data to detect flooding of Rift Valley Fever virus vector mosquito habitats in Kenya. *Med Vet Entomol* 1990;**4**(4):433–8.

22 Kitron U, Kazmierczak JJ. Spatial analysis of the distribution of Lyme disease in Wisconsin. *Am J Epidemiol* 1997;**145**(6):558–66.

23 Daniel M, Kolár J. Using satellite data to forecast the occurrence of the common tick *Ixodes ricinus* (L.). *J Hyg Epidemiol Microbiol Immunol* 1990;**34**(3):243–52.

24 Brooker S, Hay SI, Issae W, *et al*. Predicting the distribution of urinary schistosomiasis in Tanzania using satellite sensor data. *Trop Med Int Health* 2001;**6**(12):998–1007.

25 Brooker S. Schistosomes, snails and satellites. *Acta Trop* 2002;**82**(2):207–14.

26 Cross ER, Sheffield C, Perrine R, Pazzaglia G. Predicting areas endemic for schistosomiasis using weather variables and a Landsat data base. *Mil Med* 1984;**149**(10): 542–4.

27 Cross ER, Newcomb WW, Tucker CJ. Use of weather data and remote sensing to predict the geographic and seasonal distribution of Phlebotomus papatasi in southwest Asia [see comments]. *Am J Trop Med Hyg* 1996;**54**(5):530–36.

28 Guo JG, Vounatsou P, Cao CL, *et al*. A geographic information and remote sensing based model for prediction of *Oncomelania hupensis* habitats in the Poyang Lake area, China. *Acta Trop* 2005;**96**(2–3):213–22.

29 Davis GM, Wu WP, Liu HY, *et al*. Applying GIS and RS to the epidemiology of schistosomiasis in Poyang Lake, China. *Geogr Inf Sci* 2002;**8**(2):67–77.

30 Malone JB, Huh OK, Fehler DP, *et al*.. Temperature data from satellite imagery and the distribution of schistosomiasis in Egypt. *Am J Trop Med Hyg* 1994;**50**(6):714–22.

31 Malone JB, Abdel-Rahman MS, El Bahy MM, Huh OK, Shafik M, Bavia M. Geographic information systems and the distribution of *Schistosoma mansoni* in the Nile Delta. *Parasitol Today* 1997;**13**(3):112–9.

32 Seto E, Xu B, Liang S, *et al*.. The use of remote sensing for predictive modeling of schistosomiasis in China. *Photogramm Eng Remote Sens* 2002;**68**(2):167–74.

33 Zhou X, Dandan L, Huiming Y, *et al*. Use of Landsat TM satellite surveillance data to measure the impact of the 1998 flood on snail intermediate host dispersal in the lower Yangtze River Basin. *Acta Trop* 2002; **82**(2):199–205.

34 Washino RK, Wood BL. Application of remote sensing to arthropod vector surveillance and control. *Am J Trop Med Hyg* 1994;**50**(6, suppl):134–44.

35 Hay SI, Packer MJ, Rogers DJ. The impact of remote sensing on the study and control of invertebrate intermediate hosts and vectors for disease. *Int J Remote Sens* 1997;**18**(14):2899–930.

36 Anyamba A, Chretien JP, Formenty PB, *et al*.. Rift Valley Fever potential, Arabian Peninsula. *Emerg Infect Dis* 2006;**12**(3):518–20.

37 Anyamba A, Linthicum KJ, Tucker CJ. Climate-disease connections: Rift Valley Fever in Kenya. *Cad Saud Publica* 2001;**17**(suppl):133–40.

38 Linthicum KJ, Anyamba A, Tucker CJ, Kelley PW, Myers MF, Peters CJ. Climate and satellite indicators to forecast Rift Valley fever epidemics in Kenya. *Science* 1999;**285**(5426):397–400.

39 Hay, SI, Graham AJ, Rogers DJ (eds.). Global mapping of infectious diseases: methods, examples and emerging applications. *Adv Parasitol* 2006;**62**.

40 Wood BL, Beck LR, Washino RK, Palchick SM, Sebesta PD. Spectral and Spatial characterization of rice field mosquito habitat. *Int J Remote Sens* 1991;**12**(3):621–6.

41 Rogers DJ, Randolph SE. Mortality rates and population density of tsetse flies correlated with satellite imagery. *Nature (London)* 1991;**351**(6329):739–41.

42 Rogers D, Randolph S. Satellite imagery, tsetse flies and sleeping sickness in Africa. *Sist Terra* 1994;**3**:40–3.

43 Hay SI, Lennon JJ. Deriving meteorological variables across Africa for the study and control of vector-borne

infrastructure provided by the Mayor's Office of Emergency Management. Recognized and trusted health officials were available to speak with members of the press, and technical capacity existed for holding press conferences. Continued maintenance of communication capacity rather than an effort to establish such capacity in the face of an acute crisis, then, was crucial to success in this case.

The preexisting communication plan that worked well in 1999 in New York City includes a series of recommendations that are useful to recount here. These include the following, as has been summarized in World Health Organization guidance [29]:
• Attempt to communicate as quickly as possible after an incident.
• Understand that the tone of the first communication effort is critical.
• Say what you know, what you do not know, and what you are doing.
• Explain that information may change when you know more.
• Acknowledge the probability of public fear, even if the risk is small.

"Mad cow" disease and media coverage

The occurrence of variant Creutzfeldt–Jakob disease (CJD) in Europe and the US, where most epidemiological attention has focused, is extremely rare compared to other infectious diseases. Variant CJD is a prion disease that causes a rapidly progressive and fatal encephalopathy in humans. Media focus on the bovine disease (bovine spongiform encephalopathy (BSE), or "mad cow disease" in popular parlance) has been occasionally intense since the 1990s, especially whenever a new case of BSE is discovered in domestic cattle. Because of the suggested link between consumption of beef and development of variant CJD, a case of mad cow disease allows journalists to talk about a looming and dramatic health threat with a catchy name.

Changes in public opinion and behavior in the face of such media coverage, moreover, has suggested at least some vulnerability to dramatic images of the bovine threat, as Pennings and colleagues [30] discuss. In Germany, for example, beef consumption following the first documented case of BSE in 2000 declined. Beef consumption did not decline dramatically in the US and elsewhere at the time; however, following the 2003 discovery of BSE cases in Canada and the US, beef consumption apparently has also been affected.

At the same time, of course, beef consumption has not disappeared. In fact, the inverse side of the decline also provides an interesting example of the complicated nature of population risk perceptions. It is an open question whether such variation in response reflects reasoned risk assessment, desensitization as a result of repeated exposure to risk amplification, or varying emphasis by the media on the connection of the bovine disease to variant CJD. What is clear, however, is that human perception and response is not necessarily a stable mirror image of available information. Moreover, in concert with new epidemiological information, the sheer volume of media coverage can apparently amplify or attenuate existing belief intensity.

Lessons learned and recommendations

Working partnerships with journalists

It is clear that public health professionals are limited in their ability to reach wide swaths of audience members on their own and that audience members are not simple blank slates for influence. Moreover, the required step of working with media outlets itself brings some potential for missteps. Nonetheless, public health officials can attempt to plan in advance for communication activities, both with regard to routine surveillance and in response to specific outbreaks.

Observations about the nature of health news suggest a series of recommendations. Chances are that media organizations are not likely to change in structure or tendency any time soon, although some efforts are underway to improve the training of health journalists, e.g., the University of Minnesota's graduate courses on health journalism (see http://www.sjmc.umn.edu). What is perhaps more useful at this stage is for *public health officials* to take the lead to work constructively within the media constraints outlined in Table 32(1).1. When public health officials and journalists collaborate, stellar coverage is possible. In the early 1990s, for example, efforts of the US Centers for Disease Control and Prevention (CDC) to work with reporters

Table 32(1).1 Constraints facing journalists and recommendations for public health officials.

Constraint on journalists	Recommendation for health professionals
Limited source availability	Designate trained officials as media contacts
Need for newsworthiness	Scale back expectations for consistent, long-term coverage
	Promote information accuracy when coverage is prominent
Difficulty of communicating science	Conduct formative research for message development
Need for balance and conflict focus	Coordinate study results announcements when possible

Table 32(1).2 Important goals for health communication efforts.

Goal	Explanation
Accuracy	Content presented should not include any factual errors
Availability	Content should be easily available to all members of intended audiences, should be presented in a timely manner, and should be available for repeated engagement when appropriate
Balance	Benefits and risks of recommended actions should be discussed when appropriate
Consistency	Message presentations should be as consistent as possible over time
Respect for cultural diversity	Efforts should address people in ways that resonate with their perspective
Understandability	Language level and format should be appropriate for intended audience and reflect pretesting whenever possible
Use of appropriate evidence	Evidence base for effort should have undergone rigorous review

Note: Adapted from *Healthy People 2010.* See www.healthypeople.gov for details.

to highlight the emergence of antibiotic resistant organisms led to a Pulitzer Prize for the *Atlanta Journal and Constitution*'s piece on the topic [14]. Such cooperation does require active planning and foresight, but the result can be message communication of a sort unmatched by any other technique.

Establishing goals for message presentation

In addition to encouraging greater coordination with journalists, public health workers can also strive for specific goals in their communication planning and message presentation (see Table 32(1).2). Heeding cultural differences, for example, can help public health workers create messages that respect, and resonate with, audience members' perspectives on disease.

Building on such ideas, Freimuth *et al.* [14] review some important general ideas that are directly relevant for communication about infectious disease. Not surprisingly, they point out that effective health communication efforts employ message presentations that are simple, clear, and understandable (as you might assess with message pretesting studies with potential audience members). Importantly, though, they also emphasize that fear stirred by emotionally provocative language and imagery is unlikely to produce the intended response if not accompanied by information on what an individual can do to reduce their risk. This conclusion is consonant with a number of recent health commu-

nication studies [31,32] that have demonstrated a tendency among threatened audiences to denigrate or dismiss the message in question as a way of defending themselves. Health communication professionals working in the arena of infectious disease have particular reason to be cautious, given how frightening the prospect of disease transmission can be.

Talk about avian influenza, for example, should be accompanied by discussion of what individuals can do. Simply crafting a press release suggesting that "bird flu is set to arrive in the United States soon" is not likely to be as useful as a more detailed approach that includes recommendations for policymakers or for individuals. Of course, effective individual-level response is not always readily conceivable. At the same time, the numbing effect of repeated exposure to warning messages that include no steps for practical action can diminish the public health message.

Recent work by Seeger [33] to compile best practices in crisis and emergency risk communication offers the following:

• Craft messages with compassion, concern, and empathy.
• Acknowledge that, accurate or not, a public's perception is its reality.
• Tell people what they can do to reduce their harm.

Selecting channels

Which channels should public health professionals use in trying to reach audiences? A wide literature suggests that the most effective communication efforts are those that engage multiple channels of information [34]. From that perspective, choices about which channels to emphasize in communication planning should focus on which *combination* of channels to use rather than on which single channel to employ.

Moreover, we should recognize that channel selection should be a function of audience media use patterns—meaning we should carefully decide who comprises the audience for a particular public health message and then investigate their specific media diet—rather than being a function of steadfast and universal recommendations about which channels "work best." Imagine, for example, a situation in which public health officials need to reach migrant farm workers in California with specific behavior recommendations. Chances are that simply issuing a press release to newspapers in English would not be nearly as useful as a strategy that included outreach to Spanish-language radio stations and other similar outlets.

Of particular prominence in recent discussion about channel selection is the emergence of the Internet as an option for health communication

---

Box 32(1).1 Using the Internet for public health.

Increasingly, people are turning to the Internet for information about health and medicine. As of 2006, for example, more than 100 million Americans reported having accessed the Internet in search of health information [35]. At the same time, the quality of such information varies quite a bit [35]. How should public health professionals envision the Internet as a tool for their communication efforts?

Public health officials over time have found innovative ways to tap the immediacy and the resiliency of the Internet to provide dependable and accessible communication tools. Following 2005 landfall of Hurricane Katrina in the southeastern US, for example, an array of public health threats faced residents, volunteer recovery workers, and government officials, including the need for hand washing, mold avoidance, and tetanus-containing vaccines. In order to provide up-to-date recommendations in these areas, the staff at the US CDC developed a special section of their Web site (http://www.bt.cdc.gov/disasters/hurricanes/index.asp) to answer questions that local health officials, reporters, and members of the general public might have.

Internet sites offer such opportunities to post a wide variety of audio and visual materials for repeated and frequent access by a variety of audiences. This offers an improvement in information access relative to the ephemeral nature of a broadcast news conference. Moreover, public health workers who craft such information sites can have relatively extensive control over what is presented.

At the same time, we must consider issues of content selection and audience reach. Given the incredible volume and diversity of that information, the chance that necessary or desired audience members will visit your careful crafted Web site without special motivation or interest is slim. As a result, those who want to reach large audiences online are increasingly relying on releasing information to popular third-party Web sites, whether they are run by traditional media organizations with an online presence or by newly emergent online entities. In this way, the Internet environment can resemble the mass media news environment—with all of its opportunities and pitfalls—that we discuss throughout this chapter.

---

efforts. As noted earlier, the new medium offers a number of advantages and disadvantages. Certainly, many people are excited about the possibilities offered by the Internet, but at the same time our enthusiasm should be tempered by the realization that posting infectious disease information online is no guarantee it will reach the right people at the right time (see Box 32(1).1).

Summary

In this chapter, I have argued that the success of large-scale communication efforts regarding surveillance and outbreaks is a function of the performance of several groups, including health professionals, mass media professionals, and the lay people that populate relevant general audiences. We should not blame any one of those groups solely for the state of public understanding of infectious disease or for aggregate patterns of human behavior relevant to such disease. The experience of each group offers both opportunities and constraints for improving communication. Health professionals are likely only to be as effective in communication as their own information resources allow and so we must continue to build local and national information networks *before* acute episodes occur. Journalists and media professionals certainly do not always discuss infectious disease optimally, but they are also constrained by time and budget considerations and can benefit from proactive effort on the part of health agencies to help them cover emerging issues. Members of the general public are vulnerable to the perception-warping effects of dramatic examples and emotionally provocative messages. At the same time, they often seek accurate and straightforward information in times of crisis. By being cognizant of these communication issues, public health professionals can begin to tap the impressive but nuanced power of contemporary media to mitigate harm from infectious diseases.

References

1 Gellert GA, Higgins KV, Lowery RM, Maxwell RM. A national survey of public health officers' interactions with the media. *JAMA* 1994;**271**(16):1285–89.

2 Friedman SM, Dunwoody S, Rogers CL (eds.). *Scientists and Journalists: Reporting Science as News.* New York: The Free Press; 1986.

3 National Science Board. Science and Engineering Indicators 2004: Science and Technology, Public Attitudes and Understanding. NSB 04-01; May 2004. Available from: http://www.nsf.gov/statistics/seind04/c7/c7h.htm. Accessed April 21, 2007.

4 Wallack L. Mass media and health promotion: promise, problem, and challenge. In: Atkin C, Wallack L (eds.), *Mass Communication and Public Health: Complexities and Conflicts.* Newbury Park, CA: Sage; 1990: 41–51.

5 Greenberg RH, Freimuth VS, Bratic E. A content analytic study of daily newspaper coverage of cancer. In: Nimmo D (ed.), *Communication Yearbook 3.* New Brunswick, NJ: Transaction Books; 1979:645–54.

6 Klaidman, S. *Health in the Headlines: The Stories behind the Stories.* New York: Oxford University Press; 1991.

7 McGreevy D. Risks and benefits of the single versus the triple MMR vaccine: how can health professionals reassure parents? *J R Soc Promo Health* 2005;**125**(2): 84–6.

8 Mercado-Martinez FJ, Robles-Silva L, Moreno-Leal N, Franco-Almazan C. Inconsistent journalism: the coverage of chronic diseases in the Mexican press. *J Health Commun* 2001;**6**:235–47.

9 Pickle K, Quinn SC, Brown JD. HIV/AIDS coverage in black newspapers, 1991–1996: implications for health communication and health education. *J Health Commun* 2002;**7**:427–44.

10 Schwitzer G. Ten troublesome trends in TV health news. *BMJ* 2004;**329**:1352.

11 Wilkins L. Plagues, pestilence, and pathogens: the ethical implications of news reporting of a world health crisis. *Asian J Commun* 2005;**15**(3):247–54.

12 Turner RH. Media in crisis: blowing hot and cold. *B Seismol Soc Am* 1982;**72**(6):s19–28.

13 Danovaro-Holliday MC, Wood AL, LeBaron CW. Rotavirus vaccine and the news media, 1987–2001. *JAMA* 2002;**287**(11):1455–62.

14 Freimuth V, Linnan HW, Potter P. Communicating the threat of emerging infections to the public. *Emerg Infect Dis* 2000;**6**(4):337–47.

15 Glik D, Berkanovic E, Stone K, *et al.* Health education goes Hollywood: working with prime-time and daytime entertainment television for immunization promotion. *J Health Commun* 1998;**3**(3):263–82.

16 Southwell B. Risk communication: coping with imperfection. *Minn Med* 2003;**86**(12):14–6.

17 Southwell BG. Between messages and people: a multilevel model of memory for television content. *Commun Res* 2005;**32**(1):112–40.

18 Southwell BG, Blake SH, Torres A. Lessons on focus group methodology from a science television news project. *Tech Commun* 2005;**52**(2):187–93.

19 Pidgeon N, Kasperson RE, Slovic P. *The Social Amplification of Risk*. Cambridge, UK: Cambridge University Press; 2003.

20 Romantan, A. *A Longitudinal Model of Social Amplification of Commercial Aviation Risks: Exploring United States News Media Attention to Fatal Accidents and Media Effects on Air Travel Behavior, 1978—2001*, Dissertation. Philadelphia, PA: University of Pennsylvania; 2004.

21 Slovic P. *The Perception of Risk*. London, UK: Earthscan Publications; 2000.

22 Vasterman P, Yzermans CJ, Dirkzwager AJE. The role of the media and media hypes in the aftermath of disasters. *Epidemiol Rev* 2005;**27**:107–14.

23 Fishbein M, Ajzen I. *Belief, Attitude, Intention, and Behavior: An Introduction to Theory and Research*. Reading, MA: Addison-Wesley; 1975.

24 Ajzen I., Fishbein M. *Understanding Attitudes and Predicting Social Behavior*. Englewood Cliffs, NJ: Prentice Hall; 1980.

25 Fishbein M. The role of theory in HIV prevention. *AIDS Care* 2000;**12**:273–8.

26 Fishbein M, Yzer MC. Using theory to develop effective health behavior interventions. *Commun Theor* 2003; **13**(2):164–83.

27 Hobbs J, Kittler A, Fox S, Middleton B, Bates DW. Communicating health information to an alarmed public facing a threat such as a bioterrorist attack. *J Health Commun* 2004;**9**(1):67–75.

28 Fine A, Layton M. Lessons from the West Nile viral encephalitis outbreak in New York City, 1999: implications for bioterrorism preparedness. *Clin Infect Dis* 2001;**32**:277–82.

29 WHO Expert Consultation on Outbreak Communications. Outbreak communication: best practices for communicating with the public during an outbreak; September 2004. Available from: http://www.who.int/csr/resources/publications/WHO_CDS_2005_32/en/index.html. Accessed April 21, 2007.

30 Pennings JME, Wansink B, Meulenberg MTG. A note on modeling consumer reactions to a crisis: the case of the mad cow disease. *Int J Res Mark* 2002;**19**:91–100.

31 Yzer MC, Cappella JN, Fishbein M, Hornik R, Ahern RK. The effectiveness of gateway communications in anti-marijuana campaigns. *J Health Commun* 2003;**8**(2):129–43.

32 Southwell BG. Health message relevance and disparagement among adolescents. *Commun Res Rep* 2001; **18**(4):365–74.

33 Seeger MW. Best practices in crisis communication: an expert panel process. *J Appl Commun Res* 2006;**34**(3):232–44.

34 Hornik R. Public health education and communication as policy instruments for bringing about changes in behavior. In: Goldberg ME, Fishbein M, Middlestadt SE (eds.), *Social Marketing: Theoretical and Practical Perspectives*. Mahwah, NJ: Lawrence Erlbaum Associates; 1997:45–58.

35 Smith PK, Fox AT, Davies P, Hamidi-Manesh L. Cyberchondriacs. *Int J Adolesc Med Health* 2006;**18**(2):209–13.

Communication of information about surveillance

PART 2: Case study: a healthy response to increases in syphilis in San Francisco

Jeffrey D. Klausner & Katherine Ahrens

Background

Routine surveillance data for early syphilis in San Francisco, CA, demonstrated a sharp rise in early syphilis between 1999 and 2001, with the number of cases increasing from 44 to 185 per year. Most cases (>80%) occurred in men who had sex with men. That finding was of substantial concern to public health authorities because syphilis had become increasingly rare in the gay male community during the first two decades of the AIDS epidemic, down to only 9 cases in 1998. A resurgence in syphilis in gay men could lead to severe complications like neurosyphilis and might presage further increases in HIV incidence given the known biologic interaction between genital ulcer diseases like syphilis and HIV transmission.

Early syphilis infection can be asymptomatic but is easily diagnosed with a simple blood test and can be treated with single dose antibiotic therapy (intramuscular benzathine penicillin G). Based on disease characteristics, input from a newly developed community partners group, and the values of the San Francisco Department of Public Health ("harm reduction" and "sex positive" policies guide the response to sexually transmitted disease control), we determined what would be required in a syphilis education campaign. Because a large proportion of syphilis case patients were also coinfected with HIV (>60%) and sexual risk behavior was rapidly changing in San Francisco gay men due to altered attitudes about HIV/AIDS given the success of antiretroviral therapy, we decided it was important to partner with a professional agency with experience

in HIV/AIDS prevention in gay men. We selected a San Francisco-based social marketing firm, Better World Advertising, to create the campaign.

Healthy Penis campaign

The primary goals of the campaign were to raise the community-level awareness of the outbreak, enhance knowledge about syphilis and increase the frequency of syphilis testing in those at risk. We wanted to be innovative, build trust between the Department of Public Health and the community, and have an impact. Our budget was limited given other priorities in the response to epidemic syphilis, such as assuring adequate clinical services in already overburdened public facilities and conducting timely partner notification [1]. To further leverage resources, we collaborated with the Los Angeles Department of Health Services; this department was responding to similar increases in syphilis in their jurisdiction. In summer 2002, we launched The Healthy Penis campaign (see www.HealthyPenis.org) and continued it through 2005.

The campaign incorporated the use of humorous cartoon strips that featured a developing storyline with characters like Healthy Penis and Phil the Sore (Plate 32(2).1). In addition to messages contained within the cartoon strip, text was displayed on the bottom of the cartoon images describing modes of syphilis transmission and symptoms and noting that syphilis is treatable. Those cartoon strips were published semimonthly as full-page color advertisements in a popular gay San Francisco area newspaper. The Healthy Penis campaign was promoted through posters, billboards, palm cards, and Internet banner advertisements in neighborhoods and venues where the greatest concentration of gay or bisexual men lived and congregated. Two novel items added to the potential impact of the campaign: (1) a rubber 3-in.-high squeezie toy penis stamped on the bottom with "Get Tested for Syphilis" and a telephone number and Web site for more information and (2) 7-ft-high penis and syphilis-sore costumes worn by outreach workers at places frequented by the target population (Plate 32(2).2).

All campaign materials were developed, reviewed, and approved by focus groups of gay men, key community leaders, and health department executive staff. It was anticipated that scare tactics would be tuned out and that didactic messages could be perceived as preachy. Focus groups expressed a need for facts about syphilis and information on testing and other services—but they did not want to be judged or talked to about behavior. The community was already inundated with HIV prevention messages—the campaign would have to stand out. The approach chosen was specifically designed to be sex-positive, bold, and humorous; the controversial elements were intended to raise awareness and generate secondary waves of discussion.

Evaluation of campaign

To evaluate the effectiveness of the campaign, we supported two series of street-based surveys in campaign-targeted neighborhoods conducted by a local gay community-based organization. About 400 respondents were asked about awareness of the Healthy Penis campaign, perceived key messages of the campaign, knowledge of syphilis, and syphilis testing practices in the past 6 months.

Campaign awareness was high with more than 80% of respondents aware of the campaign [2,3]. Gay men who were aware of the Healthy Penis campaign had a greater knowledge about syphilis than those who were not aware of the campaign. There was a strong positive association between campaign awareness and recent syphilis testing—

the primary objective of the campaign. Each increase in campaign awareness level (none versus aided versus unaided) was associated with a 76–90% increase in likelihood of recent syphilis testing. In 2005, incidence of early syphilis was lower than in the previous 3 years, with sustained decreases in gay/bisexual syphilis cases accounting for the decline [4].

Lessons learned

We believe that a campaign developmental process inclusive of the values and participation of the affected community led to the high level of campaign awareness observed and the reduction in disease incidence in 2005. Participating in prominent leadership roles of the campaign, community leaders could provide insight, feedback, credibility, and balance. We also learned that partnering with another jurisdiction (Los Angeles) helped us lower start-up costs and identify cost efficiencies of scale. And most importantly, we learned that well-planned evaluations were critical in assessing the impact of a campaign; this in turn enabled us to foster support for continuing the campaign even in the face of criticism. Although health department executive staff was aware of the campaign from its inception, not all local authorities felt comfortable with every component of the campaign despite its impact. In the future, further communication with and participation of an expanded group of political and community stakeholders might be helpful. Time and logistical constraints, however, must be balanced against the need to assure complete support from all leaders.

In summary, the Healthy Penis campaign was developed in response to increases in syphilis affecting a certain subpopulation. The active participation of that subpopulation in the creation of campaign messages and materials assured its acceptance. The Healthy Penis campaign achieved its public health goals and components of the campaign were recently adopted in other health jurisdictions.

Acknowledgments

The authors thank Les Pappas from Better World Advertising, the STD Community Partners Group for Syphilis Elimination, and the San Francisco Department of Public Health and STOP AIDS Program staff who participated in the development, distribution, and the evaluation of the campaign.

References

1 Klausner JD, Kent CK, Wong W, *et al*. The public health response to epidemic syphilis, San Francisco, 1999–2004. *Sex Transm Dis* 2005;**32**(suppl 10):S11–8.

2 Montoya JA, Kent CK, Rotblatt H, *et al*. Social marketing campaign significantly associated with increases in syphilis testing among gay and bisexual men in San Francisco. *Sex Transm Dis* 2005;**32**(7):395–9.

3 Ahrens KA, Kent CK, Montoya JA, *et al*. Healthy Penis: San Francisco's social marketing campaign to increase syphilis testing among gay and bisexual men, PloS Medicine, 2006;**3**(12):e474.

4 Klausner JD, Kent CK, Kohn RP, *et al*. The changing epidemiology of syphilis and trends in sexual risk behavior, San Francisco, 1999–2005. In: *Poster, National STD Prevention Conference*, Jacksonville, FL, May 2006.

33 Evaluation of surveillance systems for early epidemic detection

James W. Buehler, Daniel M. Sosin & Richard Platt

Background

Epidemics come to the attention of public health authorities in a variety of ways. Typically, a healthcare provider notices or suspects an unusual increase in the frequency of disease and alerts public health officials. When increases in cases of disease are geographically diffuse, outbreaks may be recognized when information is funneled to central locations, such as reference laboratories or epidemiology units that receive specimens or case reports from multiple regions. In other instances, a single case report may prompt an investigation that uncovers other outbreak-associated cases.

To supplement these traditional approaches to epidemic detection, increasing attention has been focused over the past decade on alternative surveillance methods, loosely defined as "syndromic surveillance," that monitor disease syndromes or manifestations (e.g., medication purchases, work, or school absenteeism) that may be detectable before diagnoses are established [1–5]. Although some syndromic surveillance systems have used manual, paper-based data collection, automated methods for collecting electronically stored health data and for managing, analyzing, and disseminating information are favored. In the United States (US) and other countries, investments in syndromic surveillance increased substantially after 2001, when terrorist attacks led to heightened concerns about bioterrorism and syndromic surveillance was viewed as a promising strategy for early detection of bioterrorism-related epidemics. In Chapter 26, Pavlin and Mostashari provide a more detailed overview of the development and performance of syndromic surveillance systems [5]).

Despite the theoretical advantages, widespread adoption, and the increasing sophistication of epidemic models for testing syndromic surveillance methods, *practice-based* evidence regarding the utility of syndromic surveillance for early epidemic detection remains inconclusive. Given ongoing uncertainties regarding the utility of syndromic surveillance for early epidemic detection, as well as criticism from some regarding the wisdom of investing in this approach [6], evaluation of syndromic surveillance systems is warranted.

This chapter describes strategies for evaluating the utility of syndromic surveillance, with a focus on early epidemic detection, based on guidelines published by the US Centers for Disease Control and Prevention (CDC) [7,8]. The challenge of early epidemic detection can be illustrated by the following description of a hypothetical bioterrorist attack using *Francisella tularensis*, the etiologic agent of tularemia:

Release [of an aerosol] in a densely populated area would be expected to result in an abrupt onset of large numbers of cases of acute, nonspecific febrile illness beginning 3 to 5 days later (incubation range, 1–14 days), with pleuropneumonitis developing in a significant proportion of cases during the ensuing days and weeks. Public health authorities would most likely become aware of an outbreak of unusual respiratory disease in its early stages, but this could be difficult to distinguish from a natural outbreak of community-acquired infection, especially influenza or various atypical pneumonias. The abrupt onset of large numbers of acutely ill persons, the rapid progression in a relatively high proportion of cases from upper respiratory symptoms and bronchitis to life-threatening pleuropneumonitis and systemic infection affecting, among others, young, previously healthy adults and children should, however, quickly alert medical professionals and public health authorities to a critical and unexpected public health event and to bioterrorism as a possible cause [9].

Syndromic surveillance represents an effort to automate and hasten the process of epidemic recognition described in this scenario, raising the following questions:
• At what stage should syndromic surveillance provide an alert—when most patients have nonspecific prodromal illness or when more have developed severe disease?
• Which data source(s), syndrome definitions, and statistical alert criteria are most likely to assure the earliest possible event detection?
• What frequency of false alarms is acceptable to assure that the event is not missed before it would otherwise be recognized?

Together, these questions establish a fundamental dynamic in the evaluation of syndromic surveillance. Last, how should the information gathered through syndromic surveillance be used? Should epidemiologists respond to alerts in ways that maximize opportunities for early epidemic detection *and* make effective use of health department and partners (i.e., healthcare workers and laboratorians)? Ideally, syndromic surveillance should provide an alert before clinical recognition of the epidemic, enabling a more timely investigation, more rapid institution of prevention and treatment interventions, and prompter consideration of bioterrorism as a possible cause.

The purpose of evaluation

Adapting standard public health program evaluation questions [10] to syndromic surveillance, three questions must be answered: (1) what types of epidemics should be detected, (2) does the system detect such epidemics quickly, and (3) do actions triggered by system alerts represent an effective use of public health resources? The efficacy of syndromic surveillance in detection of bioterrorism-related epidemics will remain hypothetical and require simulations in the absence of an attack, whereas practice-based evaluations will necessarily focus on detecting upswings in seasonal illness or epidemics arising from natural causes or nonintentional events. The detailed steps used in an evaluation, based on CDC recommendations [7,8], are described in the sections below.

Evaluation Step A: describing the existing or proposed system

Responsibility for managing the system
Who are the parties involved in managing the system? Syndromic surveillance systems are typically managed by public health agencies. Because the development of syndromic surveillance has required the application of advanced epidemiologic, statistical, and informatics methods, university-based investigators are often involved [4]. Commercial vendors may provide software or manage systems that tap specific information sources, such as hospital or ambulance dispatch records. In the US, the military has also been substantially engaged in surveillance, reflecting its role as a major healthcare provider and insurer [11].

Data source
What are the data sources and data elements collected? Also, how might various stages of epidemic illness result in perturbations of the source data?

Legal authorities, confidentiality policies, and terms of collaboration
Under what legal authority are data collected, stored, and used? What policies are in place to protect against inappropriate or unauthorized release? Are data collection and management procedures compliant with applicable privacy or confidentiality laws? To what extent are data de-identified? Have agreements been established regarding access to additional information, including possible follow-back to patients, when investigations are warranted? When systems involve collaborations between health departments and university-based or commercial partners, how are

data-sharing arrangements defined so that health departments can execute their legal mandate to investigate suspect epidemics?

Data transmission, storage, and security
How are data transmitted, including the frequency and timing of data transmission? What procedures are used to encrypt or otherwise protect data security during transmission? How are computer systems secured to protect against unauthorized access? Are system users with different roles (e.g., staff at facilities that provide data, public health officials in local or state governments) granted different degrees of access to detailed information? How is system access governed?

Syndrome definitions
How are indicators aggregated into syndrome categories? To what extent have syndrome classification criteria been validated?

Statistical methods for aberration detection
What statistical tests are employed? Do these methods test for temporal abnormalities alone or for temporal and geospatial clustering? How are thresholds set for triggering alerts?

Display methods
How are trend results, geographic patterns, and statistical alerts displayed on Internet sites? How frequently are reports updated? To what extent does the system–Internet interface allow users to probe reported data in follow-up to an alert?

Response to alerts
What procedures or policies have been established to determine whether, when, or to what extent follow-up investigations are conducted? Are findings from one data source interpreted in concert with findings from others? How is responsibility for human oversight assigned? Who is responsible for follow-up investigations? What has been the experience with investigations triggered by alerts? To what extent have epidemics detected by other means also been recognized by the system?

Evaluation Step B: assessing the attributes and performance of the system

CDC surveillance evaluation guidelines list a series of criteria (also listed in Table 33.1) that describe desirable attributes of surveillance [7]. It is impossible for any system to fully achieve all of these attributes, since some are mutually antagonistic. For example, efforts to enhance timeliness and sensitivity of outbreak detection are likely to result in a lower predictive value of alerts [8]. However, a balance must be obtained to maximize the effectiveness of a surveillance system. For syndromic surveillance, performance attributes will likely reflect answers to the questions in Table 33.1.

The cost of conducting syndromic surveillance will be shaped by how these attributes are valued, and costs of systems may vary widely depending on the scope of data collection. Whereas a discussion of formal cost–benefit assessment [12,13] is beyond the scope of this chapter, it is useful to consider the various types of costs [7,8] and benefits that may be associated with the operation of a syndromic surveillance system. Direct costs include the salary of personnel who operate the system and expenses associated with computing resources, establishing connections to data sources, and other operational expenses. Information on direct costs may be available from budgets submitted to funding agencies. There may be costs borne voluntarily by collaborating organizations, such as hospitals or others who provide data for syndromic surveillance, or these entities may require at least partial reimbursement for their efforts in establishing links with public health agencies. When syndromic surveillance systems produce alerts, there are costs associated with follow-up efforts, both for public health agency staff and for staff at collaborating healthcare institutions, and these costs will be heightened by frequent false alarms. Some costs are more intangible, such as potential loss of credibility for public health agencies if false alarms are excessive or if the promise of syndromic surveillance is unfulfilled.

Benefits of syndromic surveillance may include the following: early indication of situations that herald epidemics, assurance that outbreaks are not occurring if rumors arise or if environmental sampling detects the presence of a suspect agent in air samples, and flexibility to monitor a spectrum of health threats beyond infectious diseases. In some situations it may be possible to estimate the savings associated with reductions in morbidity and mortality when syndromic surveillance provides an early warning.

Table 33.1 Attributes of a surveillance system.

Simplicity	To what extent is the system easy to access and use, from the perspectives of various users?
Flexibility	How readily can the system be adapted to meet changing information needs or priorities?
	To what extent can users customize system utilities to suit local information needs or display preferences?
Data quality	Is the source data of sufficient quality and consistency to assure reliable use for the intended purpose?
	Are variations in data quality apt to increase the likelihood of alerts that do not represent actual disease trends or decrease the likelihood of alerts when meaningful changes in actual trends occur?
Acceptability	From the perspective of data providers, are procedures for obtaining data nonintrusive and are the data useful for institution-specific purposes?
	For the public and policymakers, is syndromic surveillance perceived as a wise investment of public resources and a warranted exercise of governments' authority to tap health records?
Sensitivity	What percentage of epidemics or outbreaks targeted for detection are detected by the system?
	Is the cost of syndromic justified by greater sensitivity (or timeliness or predictive value) when compared to other epidemic detection methods?
Predictive value	When systems send statistical alerts, what is the likelihood that alerts represent events that public health agencies are seeking to detect?
Representativeness	To what extent is the pattern of disease detected by syndromic surveillance representative of the health of the population within a public health jurisdiction?
Timeliness	Does the syndromic surveillance system provide alerts early enough to allow timely investigations and effective public health interventions?
Stability	Does the surveillance operation assure that observed trends reflect community health and not variations in how data are collected or managed?

Examples of evaluations of syndromic surveillance

There is general concurrence that existing evaluations of syndromic surveillance are insufficient to guide decisions about its use and development [3,4,14]. Approaches are needed to delineate the *sensitivity* and *predictive value* of different outbreak detection methods, the lead time gained or lost (*timeliness*), and the impact on morbidity and mortality resulting from syndromic surveillance [8].

Evaluation studies described below are presented to exemplify two different evaluation approaches, rather than provide a review of the literature in this field. Readers seeking additional information about evaluations, practice experience, and developmental research regarding syndromic surveillance should consult the CDC Annotated Bibliography for Syndromic Surveillance [15] and the Internet site of the International Society for Disease Surveillance (http://www.syndromic.org).

Use of simulation methods in a hypothetical anthrax attack

Simulations are useful for evaluating the performance of statistical methods for detecting aberrant disease trends, particularly for outbreak scenarios that may be extremely rare. Simulations allow comparison of the timeliness of alerts from different analysis algorithms, definition of the limits of detection, and assessment of the effect on detection of variations in the epidemiologic parameters of an outbreak. A key advance in simulation methods is the use of actual electronic health data into which hypothetical outbreak cases are injected, as opposed to using entirely hypothetical data. Since these methods involve subjecting data to an analysis algorithm, a limitation is that they do not test the effect of variations in the flow of data from reporting sources to public health agencies or variations in data quality.

435

In a study by Buckeridge *et al.*, simulated cases of inhalational anthrax were superimposed on ambulatory care visit data for active duty military personnel [16]. Investigators used a statistical model to predict the timing and number of people seeking healthcare following the attack, varying the number of infected people and using different assumptions about the incubation period, the rate of disease progression, and healthcare use. The sensitivity and timeliness of a particular statistical method for detecting aberrant trends in "respiratory syndrome" visits were then assessed at different alert thresholds. In the "base case" scenario (i.e., 50,000 people infected, 11-day incubation period, 2.5-day duration of illness prodrome, 40% seeking care in prodromal stage of illness), the earliest alert was 3 days after release of an anthrax aerosol. The model allowed assessment of decrements in alert sensitivity and timeliness as the number of infected people and as the proportion seeking care in the prodromal stage were lowered.

Assessment of systems monitoring health indicators
Comparisons of health indicators captured through syndromic surveillance with more definitive measures of illness, such as medical records reviews or laboratory testing, can validate or inform refinements of syndrome classification schemes. For example, Fleischauer *et al.* assessed the validity of syndrome classifications made by emergency department staff as part of a time-limited syndromic surveillance system operated over a 23-day period around two high-profile sporting events in Phoenix, AZ [17]. During the surveillance period, triage nurses used a checklist to classify patients into one or none of 10 syndrome categories. Investigators retrospectively reviewed a sample of patient records from this interval and made syndrome classifications based on patients' descriptions of their symptoms (i.e., "chief complaints") and on diagnoses recorded by emergency department healthcare providers. Concordance between syndrome classifications made by triage staff and the investigators' retrospective reviews was deemed "fair to good." Concordance between syndrome classifications based on chief complaints and diagnoses varied by syndrome. However, because there was no outbreak during the surveillance period, there was no opportunity to assess the impact of these differences on epidemic detection.

Burgeois *et al.* evaluated syndromic surveillance of respiratory infections among children by comparing trends over an 11-year period for visits attributed to "respiratory syndrome" and trends in virus isolations from specimens collected as part of routine care during the same period [18]. The investigators observed that "respiratory syndrome" trends were closely linked to trends in respiratory syncytial virus and influenza infections, leading to the conclusion that the "respiratory syndrome" category was a reliable indicator for trends in viral respiratory infections among children.

There continue to be very few published studies demonstrating the usefulness of syndromic surveillance in public health practice. In New York City, a locality with an array of mature syndromic surveillance systems, the ability of syndromic surveillance to detect the onset of seasonal increases in influenza and viral gastroenteritis has been well documented, affording opportunities to alert the medical community and provide prevention information to the public [19]. In contrast, the ability of syndromic surveillance to detect outbreaks not associated with seasonal illness has been disappointing [20,21]. For example, during a 32-month period in 2001–2004, syndromic surveillance from emergency departments yielded nearly 100 citywide alerts and over 100 focal geographic alerts for gastrointestinal illness. Investigators were unable to relate any of the focal geographic alerts to disease outbreaks, although studies prompted by citywide alerts confirmed the occurrence of seasonal norovirus infections. In contrast, of 49 outbreaks of gastrointestinal illness investigated by the health department during the same period, none were detected by emergency department syndromic surveillance, mainly because relatively few patients sought emergency department care [21]. In one outbreak of foodborne disease, 25 ill residents of a long-term care facility were transported by ambulance to four hospitals, including two that were part of the emergency department surveillance system. Syndromic surveillance did not detect this cluster of gastrointestinal illness because patients were transported to hospitals over a 3-day period, diffusing the temporal impact on syndrome trends, and for some patients the recorded chief complaint was unrelated to gastrointestinal illness, further diminishing the capacity of the system to detect an increase in visits meeting the gastrointestinal syndrome criteria [20].

In March 2003, emergency department syndromic surveillance in New York City detected a substantial increase in "fever syndrome" in a predominantly Asian neighborhood. Concerned that this alert could represent the introduction of severe acute respiratory syndrome (SARS) into the city, health department staff conducted a field investigation and determined that the increase in cases of "fever syndrome" represented a mix of unrelated illnesses that had clustered by chance. This "false alarm" triggered an intense public health investigation, but public health authorities deemed the alert and investigation worthwhile given the threat of SARS [22]. City health officials consider the emergency department syndromic surveillance system worthwhile because of the information it provides on seasonal illness and because it enables citywide assessments of health status at times when concerns about outbreaks, such as the SARS threat, are heightened [20].

Lessons learned from a comprehensive evaluation project

The National Bioterrorism Syndromic Surveillance Demonstration Program in the US [23], funded by CDC and several state/local health departments, has been using CDC guidelines to conduct a comprehensive evaluation of syndromic surveillance in ambulatory care settings [24]. In this study, investigators are assessing the utility of syndromic surveillance for routine public health purposes. Experience to date indicates multiple challenges in designing syndromic surveillance evaluations.

The evaluation focuses on syndromic surveillance being conducted in localities in five states. Surveillance is based on diagnoses coded using the International Classification of Diseases, Clinical Modification, 9th Revision (ICD-9), and patient temperatures as recorded in electronic medical records. Syndromes are defined using CDC/US Department of Defense (DoD) criteria [25], plus an additional "influenza-like illness" syndrome. Illness events are attributed to the postal zone (i.e., zip code) where patients live. Surveillance focuses on

first visits in an episode of illness by ignoring repeat patient visits for a single syndrome category within 6 weeks; the Poisson model SaTScan method is used for detecting unusual clusters of events. Real-time notification of alerts is provided to public health agencies and staff at participating healthcare facilities are available at all times to provide clinical detail about cases that contribute to alerts.

Although this evaluation is in progress at the time of this writing (May 2007), multiple challenges have become clear as described below.

Need for standardization
The five participating health departments differed in their definition of a disease cluster or outbreak. Additionally, some health departments maintained no centralized mechanism for tracking clusters or outbreaks they identified. Among those that did, there was considerable variation in the types of events captured. Thus, the same syndromic surveillance system will have different sensitivities due to differences in disease or outbreak definitions.

Choosing syndrome definitions
The CDC/DoD syndrome definitions include a large number of diagnoses within syndrome categories to increase their sensitivity for bioterrorism events. This has two consequences. First, very common diagnoses, such as pharyngitis or cough in the respiratory illness syndrome, dominate alerts. Such alerts are often uninteresting for routine public health practice because they represent minor illness that are not a priority for intervention. Even when there is no alert, the large number of common diagnoses can mask a small but important alert that might arise if syndrome definitions were limited to less common and more severe diagnoses. Additionally, some ICD-9 codes, like 368.9 (visual disturbance unspecified) that is part of the botulism-like syndrome, are sometimes used to code diagnoses made during routine care. In one instance, an alert for "botulism-like" syndrome resulted from a family of five having visual refractions on the same day.

Determining alert notifications useful to health departments
Health departments need to make three kinds of decisions about the types of alerts they wish to receive; each requires a value judgment. First, it is necessary

to decide on alerting thresholds. These thresholds can vary for different syndromes and for different responders within a single locality. For example, frontline staff epidemiologists may review all alerts, but senior public health officials may be notified only of alerts that generate a high level of concern. Second, it is common for alerts attributable to the same illness in a community to occur on many consecutive days or for multiple geographically overlapping alerts to occur on the same day for respiratory and influenza-like illness syndromes. This happens routinely during winter respiratory illness season. These sequential temporal alerts or simultaneous geographic alerts are of little value for identifying new disease clusters; however, they can be of value for determining that there is excess disease in a locale. It is necessary to decide which health department responders should receive notice of initial alerts, and who (if anyone) should receive the additional related alerts. Finally, it is necessary to determine the time interval that may be considered a potential outbreak period. A short, intense outbreak may be best identified by a 1-day time frame, while a subacute problem with more gradual accumulation of cases, such as cases of giardiasis associated with a swimming pool, may be best identified by using a time frame of several weeks. Using longer time frames to test for aberrant trends reduces the power to find a cluster that occurs in a shorter period and also increases the number of alerts.

Choosing an alert detection algorithm
A critical issue for syndrome surveillance systems is the ability to model the natural temporal and geographical variation in the data, such as day-of-week or holiday-related variations in the use of healthcare services, effects of multiple healthcare visits by the same person during a single illness episode, and artifacts due to delayed or missing data. The types of events unrelated to disease outbreaks that can affect trends in syndromic indicators are very data-source specific. If statistical modeling is not done well, there will be many false positives and true positives will be hidden. Signal detection algorithms are evolving rapidly. Although the specific signal detection method has profound influence, the performance of algorithms across an array of conditions and circumstances is not well understood. Even modest changes in the parame-

ters of the model-adjusted SaTScan algorithm used by the Demonstration Program change the number of alerts by severalfold. Additionally, different intended uses of syndromic surveillance, for instance detecting new events versus monitoring ongoing disease occurrence, almost certainly need different signal detection strategies.

Accounting for variation in clinicians' coding practices
Variations in the way clinicians assign ICD-9 codes affects system performance in unanticipated ways. For example, at one of the five evaluation sites, surveillance generated relatively frequent alerts for the "shock/death" syndrome category. This resulted from the practice, limited to that site, of using the code 799.9 ("other ill-defined and unknown causes of morbidity and mortality") for telephone calls when the cause of the patient's problem was unclear.

Using recent history to predict illness levels
Public health officials often have a well-formed, intuitive sense of what is unusual based on many years of cumulative experience. In contrast, alert detection methods typically have access to relatively little historical data from the specific health system being evaluated. An example is the effect of the unusually early onset of the 2003–2004 influenza season in the Denver metropolitan area. The large number of early cases of influenza-like illness in November 2003, with a substantial decline by December (Figure 33.1), had an enduring effect on alerts in subsequent years and resulted in many alerts that represented "false alarms" in following "normal" Decembers. Frequent alerts generated by statistical algorithms in December 2004 and December 2005 occurred not because levels of respiratory illness were unusually high in those Decembers but because the statistical reference period, which included a large decrease from November to December 2003, was atypical. It is unclear at present how to choose the most appropriate duration of historical data to use in specific circumstances.

Identifying and accounting for changes in electronic medical records
Electronic medical record products undergo frequent modifications, which are sometimes

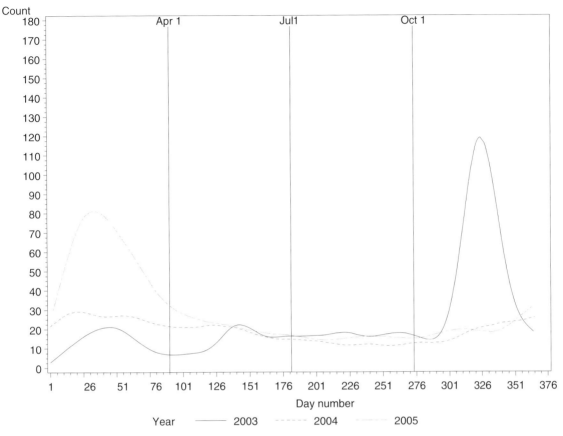

Fig 33.1 Denver metro influenza-like illness counts, 2003–2005. The sharp early peak in 2003 substantially perturbed the expected number of events in subsequent years and led to many false signals.

unapparent to users and may not be documented. These changes, for instance alterations in the way ICD-9 codes are assigned or modification of the number of diagnoses that are recorded, can have profound effects on the performance of syndromic surveillance. At the Denver site, a modification in late 2003 in the number of diagnoses captured from the electronic medical record provided an inaccurate baseline for comparison with current diagnoses. This led to an increase in alerts for influenza-like illness in October 2003 and an erroneously early "identification" of the start of the 2003–2004 influenza season (Figure 33.2).

Accommodating delayed information from clinicians
Clinicians may delay assignment of diagnoses for a day or more after seeing patients, for instance, while

they wait for laboratory information to arrive. Additionally, clinical information systems may be subject to delays in processing or transmitting information. These delays can seriously distort the performance of trend assessment algorithms, particularly if they focus on trends for specific geographic areas within a single public health region. Numerous spurious alerts have been attributed to such delays, and alerts have vanished when the missing data arrived.

Accommodating real or apparent changes
in the population under observation
Changes in the size or distribution of the population being served influence the number of expected events. Changes in postal codes cause observed counts to be higher or lower than expected based

439

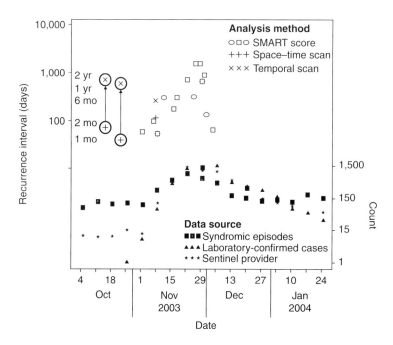

Fig 33.2 Influenza and influenza-like illness, Denver metro area 2003. Initial analyses showed two erroneous signals (shown by X) of increased activity several weeks before the outbreak was recognized by other means. The true values are shown by +. The reason for the false signals was an increase in the number of diagnoses captured from the electronic medical records. There was an increase in the number of events identified, but historical records from the same system had undercounted events. The correct analysis was published by Ritzwoller *et al.* [27].

on historical boundaries, although these population changes are not real.

Determining the size of the area in which clusters should be sought

Managers of syndromic surveillance systems that cover large geographic areas need to decide whether it is meaningful to identify alerts based on data from disparate or widespread areas and whether geographic or other boundaries should be considered. These considerations arose in separate work using data from a national telephone triage company. In principle, it may be worthwhile to identify very widespread outbreaks. In practice, using national-level data may lead to alerts that are of no interest. For example, analyses of data from this system using an algorithm that scanned for geographic clusters by randomly sampling geographic regions led to an alert from a zone centered in Honolulu, Hawaii, and extending across the Pacific Ocean to Las Vegas, Nevada. Although this is an extreme example of the way an automated statistical tool can produce illogical results, it is a reminder of the importance of informed oversight of syndromic surveillance so that nonsense calculations are recognized.

Conclusions

Syndromic surveillance is a relatively new addition to types of systems used to conduct disease surveillance. This chapter has focused on strategies for evaluating the utility of syndromic surveillance for early epidemic detection. Experience to date has been mixed, as evidenced by reports of outbreaks missed by syndromic surveillance. Given continued investments in syndromic surveillance and continued uncertainties about its value for early outbreak detection, more evaluations are needed to better define population, outbreak, and surveillance parameters associated with the sensitivity and timeliness of outbreak detection and the predictive value of system alerts. Further evaluations are also needed to assess the efficiency of different approaches to outbreak detection, taking into account not only the process of deriving initial statistical alerts, but also the process of preliminary assessments to determine whether full-scale investigations are warranted. Lastly, as the application of syndromic surveillance extends beyond epidemic detection to include monitoring the course of epidemics and other uses, new evaluation strategies will be necessary.

Acknowledgments

The authors thank Martin Kulldorff, Irene Shui, and Katherine Yih for their contributions to insights gained from the National Bioterrorism Syndromic Surveillance Demonstration Program.

References

1 Mandl KD, Overhage M, Wagner MM, *et al.* Implementing syndromic surveillance: a practical guide informed by the early experience. *J Am Med Inf Assoc* 2004;**11**:141–50.

2 Buehler JW, Berkelman RL, Hartley DM, Peters CJ. Syndromic surveillance and bioterrorism-related epidemics. *Emerg Infect Dis J* 2003;**9**:1197–204. Available from: http://www.cdc.gov/ncidod/EID/vol9no10/03-0231.htm. Accessed May 30, 2006.

3 Sosin DM. Syndromic surveillance: The case for skillful investment. *Biosecur Bioterror Biodef Strategy Pract Sci* 2003;**1**:247–53. Available from: http://www.syndromic.org/pdf/pubs/2003_BIOSECURITY-Syndromic_Investment-Sosin.pdf. Accessed May 30, 2006.

4 Bravata DM, McDonald KM, Smith WM, *et al.* Systematic review: surveillance systems for early detection of bioterrorism-related diseases. *Ann Intern Med* 2004;**140**:910–22. Available from: http://www.annals.org/cgi/reprint/140/11/910.pdf. Accessed May 30, 2006.

5 Pavlin J, Mostashari F. Implementing syndromic surveillance systems in the climate of bioterrorism. In: M'ikantha N, de Valk H, Lynfield R, Van Benden C (eds.), *Infectious Disease Surveillance*, London: Blackwell; 2007: 349–358.

6 Reingold A. If syndromic surveillance is the answer, what is the question? *Biosecur Bioterror Biodef Strategy Pract Sci* 2003;**1**(2):1–5.

7 Centers for Disease Control and Prevention. Updated guidelines for evaluating public health surveillance systems, recommendations from the Guidelines Working Group, *MMWR Morb Mortal Wkly Rep* 2001;**50**(RR-13):1–35. Available from: http://www.cdc.gov/mmwr/preview/mmwrhtml/rr5013a1.htm. Accessed May 30, 2006.

8 Centers for Disease Control and Prevention. Framework for evaluating public health surveillance systems for early detection of outbreaks, recommendations from the CDC Working Group. *MMWR Morb Mortal Wkly Rep* 2004;**53**(RR5):1–11. Available from: http://www.cdc.gov/mmwr/preview/mmwrhtml/rr5305a1.htm. Accessed May 30, 2006.

9 Dennis DT, Inglesby TV, Henderson DA, *et al.* Tularemia as a biological weapon, medical and public health management. *JAMA* 2001;**285**:2763–73. Available from: http://jama.ama-assn.org/cgi/content/full/285/21/2763. Accessed May 31, 2006.

10 Centers for Disease Control and Prevention. Framework for program evaluation in public health. *MMWR Morb Mortal Wkly Rep* 1999;**48**(RR11):1–40. Available from: http://www.cdc.gov/mmwr/preview/mmwrhtml/rr4811a1.htm. Accessed May 30, 2006.

11 Lombardo J, Burkom H, Elbert E, *et al.* A systems overview of the Electronic Surveillance System for the Early Notification of Community-Based Epidemics (ESSENCE II). *J Urban Health: Bull N Y Acad Med* 2008;**80**(suppl 1):i32–42. Available from: http://www.syndromic.org/syndromicconference/2002/Supplementpdf/Lombardo.pdf. Accessed September 15, 2006.

12 Gramlich EM. *A Guide to Benefi–Cost Analysis*, 2nd edn. Longrove, IL: Waveland Press; 1997.

13 Drummond MF, Sculpher MJ, Torrance GW, O'Brien BJ, Stoddart GL. *Methods for the Economic Evaluation of Health Care Programmes*. 2nd edn. Oxford: Oxford University Press; 2005.

14 Buehler JW. Review of the 2003 National Syndromic Surveillance Conference—lessons learned and questions to be answered. In: Syndromic Surveillance: Reports from a National Conference, 2003. *MMWR Morb Mortal Wkly Rep* 2004;**53**(suppl):12–17. Available from: http://www.cdc.gov/mmwr/PDF/wk/mm53SU01.pdf. Accessed June 5, 2006.

15 Centers for Disease Control and Prevention. Annotated Bibliography for Syndromic Surveillance. Available from: http://www.cdc.gov/epo/dphsi/syndromic/evaluation.htm. Accessed April 15, 2006.

16 Buckeridge DL, Switzer P, Owens D, Seigrist D, Pavlin J, Musen M. An evaluation model for syndromic surveillance: assessing the performance of a temporal algorithm. *MMWR Morb Mortal Wkly Rep* 2005;**54**(suppl):109–15. Available from: http://www.cdc.gov/mmwr/preview/mmwrhtml/su5401a18.htm. Accessed May 30, 2006.

17 Fleischauer AT, Silk BJ, Schumacher M, *et al.* The validity of chief complaint and discharge diagnosis in emergency department-based syndromic surveillance. *Acad Emerg Med* 2004;**11**:1262–7.

18 Burgeois FT, Olson KL, Borwnstein JS, McAdam AJ, Mandl KD. Validation of syndromic surveillance for respiratory infections. *Ann Emerg Med* 2006;**47**:265–71.

19 Heffernan R, Mostashari F, Das J, Karpati A, Kuldorff M, Weiss D. Syndromic surveillance in public health practice, New York City. *Emerg Infect Dis* 2004;**10**:858–64. Available from: http://www.cdc.gov/ncidod/EID/vol10no5/03-0646.htm. Accessed May 30, 2006.

441

20 Steiner-Sichel L, Greenko J, Heffernan R, Layton M, Weiss D. Field investigations of emergency department syndromic surveillance signals—New York City. In: Syndromic Surveillance: Reports from a National Conference, 2003. *MMWR Morb Mortal Wkly Rep* 2004;**53**(suppl):184–9. Available from: http://www.cdc.gov/mmwr/PDF/wk/mm53SU01.pdf. Accessed May 30, 2006.

21 Balter S, Weiss D, Hanson H, Reddy D, Heffernan R. Three years of emergency department gastrointestinal syndromic surveillance in New York City: what have we found? In: Syndromic Surveillance: Reports from a National Conference, 2004. *MMWR Morb Mortal Wkly Rep* 2005;**54**(suppl):175–80. Available from: http://www.cdc.gov/mmwr/pkdkf/wk/mm54su01.pdf. Accessed May 30, 2006.

22 Pérez-Peña R. System in New York For early warning of disease patterns. *New York Times* April 4, 2003: A1.

23 Platt R, Bocchino C, Caldwell B, et al.. Syndromic surveillance using minimum transfer of identifiable data: the example of the National Bioterrorism Syndromic Surveillance Demonstration Program. *J Urban Health* 2003;**80**(2, suppl 1):i25–31.

24 Yih WK, Daniel J, Heisey-Grove D, et al. Assessing the impact of syndromic surveillance systems on routine public health practice: identifying and evaluating syndromic signals [abstract]. In: *2005 Syndromic Surveillance Conference*, Seattle, WA, September 14–15, 2005. Available from: http://thci.org/_Documents/temp/evaluation%20abstract%207_19_05.doc. Accessed May 30, 2006.

25 Centers for Disease Control and Prevention. Syndrome Definitions for Diseases Associated with Critical Bioterrorism-associated Agents, October 23, 2003. Available from: http://www.bt.cdc.gov/surveillance/syndromedef/. Accessed June 5, 2006.

26 Kulldorff M. Prospective time-periodic geographical disease surveillance using a scan statistic. *J R Stat Soc A* 2001;**164**:61–72.

27 Ritzwoller DP, Kleinman K, Palen T, et al.. Comparison of syndromic surveillance and a sentinel provider system in detecting an influenza outbreak—Denver, Colorado, 2003. In: Syndromic Surveillance: Reports from a National Conference, 2004. *MMWR Morb Mortal Wkly Rep* 2005;**54**(suppl):151–6. Available from: http://www.cdc.gov/mmwr/pdf/wk/mm54su01.pdf. Accessed May 30, 2006.

Law, Ethics, Training, and Partnership in Infectious Disease Surveillance

34 Ethics and the conduct of public health surveillance

Amy L. Fairchild & Marian Moser Jones

Should data collection and analysis be viewed as research? This question has provoked debate, because research must be scrutinized by the watchful eyes of institutional review boards (IRBs) and other ethical bodies. Activities that involve data collection, such as quality assurance, program evaluation, oral history, and public health surveillance lie at the center of this controversy.

In October 2003, for example, the Office for Human Research Protection (OHRP) in the Department for Health and Human Services (HHS) addressed the issue of whether those conducting oral history studies had to subject their work to IRB review. Using the definition that research is any activity aimed at producing "generalizable knowledge," the office described oral history as falling outside the broad boundaries of research. "Oral history interviewing activities, in general, are not designed to contribute to generalizable knowledge and, therefore, do not involve research as defined by HHS regulations and do not need to be reviewed by an institutional review board," the office wrote in a memo [1].

Another attempt to draw a clear line between research and non-research-related data gathering was when the World Bank issued a report in 2002 designed to underscore the central importance of public health surveillance [2]. "Surveillance is not research," the report simply stated. "Public health surveillance is essentially descriptive in nature. It describes the occurrence of injury or disease and its determinants in the population. It also leads to public health action... If we confuse surveillance with research, we may be motivated to collect large amounts of detailed data on each case. The burden of this approach is too great for the resources available." This effort to make a sharp distinction between research and surveillance turned on economics, not ethics.

Concern for human rights accompanying the AIDS epidemic within the United States, and internationally, is what fostered recent efforts on the part of the Centers for Disease Control and Prevention (CDC) and World Health Organization (WHO) to extend to surveillance ethical considerations heretofore restricted to research [3,4]. WHO endeavors represented a response to years of experience working in different countries and settings, where ethical questions arose when implementing HIV surveillance (C. Obermeyer, personal communication, January 12, 2004). Examination of the events leading to these decisions reveals that the efforts to use a fixed and sometimes arbitrary definition of research in order to justify or reject oversight of data gathering activities can yield inconsistent results.

The debate over whether data collection is research began in the 1970s, when a federal government commission moved to establish protections for human subjects involved in research. These protections focused mainly on the principle of informed consent, which requires researchers to notify potential participants of the risks and benefits of any research before they agree to participate. In response to this set of protections for human subjects, epidemiologists and ethicists began to discuss whether the principle of informed consent extended to the use of patients' medical records and whether the insistence on individual consent would stifle epidemiological research [5–7]. In 1981, HHS regulations for the protection of human subjects explicitly exempted epidemiological research involving already existing data from informed consent requirements, provided the risk to subjects was minimal, the research did not record data in a way that was individually identifiable, and the research could not otherwise be conducted [8]. But the discussion did not extend to public health surveillance, which includes not only reporting of patients' names for conditions like tuberculosis and HIV, but also monitoring of food poisonings and blood lead levels.

The 1991 International Guidelines for Ethical Review of Epidemiological Studies issued by the Council for International Organizations of Medical Sciences (CIOMS) stated that although the vast majority of surveillance should be subject to approval by ethical review committees, "[a]n exception is justified when epidemiologists must investigate outbreaks of acute communicable diseases. Then they must proceed without delay to identify and control health risks" [9]. The CIOMS guidelines did indicate there were still areas of uncertainty, such as "when both routine surveillance of cancer and original research on cancer are conducted by professional staff of a population-based cancer registry." To resolve difficult situations, CIOMS called for the guidance of ethical review committees [9].

In this chapter, we recount the controversy that has set into bold relief the ethical challenge posed by surveillance. We argue not that we require a better definitional solution but rather a better mechanism for the ethical oversight of public health practice where it touches on issues of individual privacy. Although there have been episodes in which public health data have been inadvertently released, such as an incident in Florida in which a health department official from Pinellas County reportedly showed a list containing 4000 names of people with HIV to patrons in a Tampa gay bar or, more recently, when a laptop with medical and other records from the Veterans Administration was stolen, it is not these occasional breaches in data privacy but the routine practice of public health that requires continual ethical evaluation and guidance. This task, we argue, requires envisioning a new method for assuring accountability and responsibility, not the extension of IRB oversight.

The surveillance debate

In the early 1990s, critics charged that the CDC's blinded, or anonymous, HIV seroprevalence studies among childbearing women—which tracked the overall rates of HIV in these women but did not include identifying data on individual women's HIV status—constituted research conducted without informed consent. In response, HHS's Office for Protection from Research Risks (OPRR) began to advance the idea that all surveillance was research and might require particular kinds of review [10]. This stance alarmed the CDC as well as the Council of State and Territorial Epidemiologists (CSTE). According to the CDC, "The implications of calling public health surveillance research are broad and far reaching. . . . If all surveillance activities were research, it might mean each local health department would have to form institutional review boards (IRBs)" [11]. In the CDC's view, this decision could have dire implications: if surveillance activities were designated research, the CDC feared that "people with TB could prevent their names from being reported to the health department or refuse to provide information about their contacts," thus inhibiting disease prevention efforts. A first set of CDC recommendations drafted in 1996 made the case that public health surveillance is different from pure research because its aim is fundamentally different: Whereas "[t]he intent of research is to contribute to or generate generalizable knowledge, the intent of public health practice is to conduct programs to prevent disease and injury and improve the health of communities" [12].

The CDC is rarely involved in the use of surveillance for public health interventions like contact tracing. However practical their research might be, it remained research requiring IRB review in the minds of CDC officials. As the CDC began to work with state health departments to refine their guidelines, the profound differences in how the states and the federal government drew the boundary between research and public health surveillance became clear.

States, typically operating under statutes mandating departments of health to collect and act on individual-level morbidity data for the explicit purpose of controlling disease, tended to view most surveillance activities as public health practice. The

New York City Department of Health, for example, maintained that "we derive knowledge that may protect the particular 'victims' before us. However, it may also be that it is too late to help the particular victims, but that the activity, or the information derived from it, becomes generalizable so as to protect the general population." CSTE concurred, arguing that "we are rarely able to conduct an investigation that provides any medical benefit to those already infected" [13]. For example, in the case of foodborne outbreak investigations, the "major benefit has been to others than those we identified and obtained data and specimens from" [14].

Additionally, the nature of the entity conducting surveillance played a key role in determining whether an activity was research or practice for the states. CSTE explained that its members consistently collected data with an eye not only to the present but also to the future.

The Alaska state health department, for example, in a review of previous investigations of trichinosis outbreaks, not only developed an early diagnostic test for the disease but also identified an animal species not previously known to harbor *Trichinella*, as well as a new subspecies of the disease-causing organism: "We do not view these activities as research" when conducted by the state, a CSTE official stated in a letter to the CDC: "if conducted by an entity other than the state public health agency," however, "we would define it as research and require an outside researcher to obtain IRB approval" [14]. For many local public health officials, "If an intervention or action is delegated to the health officer by statute or regulation, such intervention is *per se ethical* and not human subjects research" [15]. CSTE broadly concurred: "What distinguishes the activities as nonresearch at the state level is that the public health authority undertakes them and the data are collected under the authority of explicit state law" [16]. By definition, then, any data collection that public health departments did was not research.

In the end, the CDC maintained that "activities can be viewed differently at federal and state levels" [13]. That is, the same initiative might be designated research at the federal level and require IRB review and yet be considered practice if performed at the state level, requiring no ethical review. But even at the federal level, some health officials have found

that they do not distinguish between research and practice consistently and that they sometimes face political pressure to define an activity as practice rather than research.*

Conclusion

The recent efforts to provide definitional solutions to the question of research and public health practice have inevitably produced results riddled with inconsistencies. It is time to resolve the matter by acknowledging the necessity of ethical review of public health surveillance activities at both state and federal levels, whether such activities fall neatly under the classification of research or practice or exist in a gray borderland.

Those involved in public health efforts appear increasingly ready to embrace ethical principles to govern the practice of public health surveillance [17]. And, indeed, there have been a number of recent efforts to develop an ethics of public health in order to help inform and guide the analysis of the issues presented in this chapter [18,19]. Public health professionals have not, however, greeted with enthusiasm proposals to establish specific mechanisms to assure ethical review [20]. Yet in the history of research ethics, it was only when forums were created to assure consideration of the rights of subjects that guiding principles were given any meaningful force. The creation of institutionally based review procedures was not without conflict, as researchers resisted the idea that their own self-review was inadequate [21]. Although the establishment of bodies responsible for the review of the ethics of surveillance need not mirror the already extant IRBs, as has been proposed by some experts on human subjects research [22], it is clear that some form of explicit, systematic, *internal* review is necessary. There is a long history of resistance on the part of state officials to the creation of federal standards, which become viewed as an intrusion upon state prerogatives. Nevertheless, we believe that there is a need for broadly acknowledged ethical norms to protect against the vagaries of state activities, whatever the law might permit.

---

* Reported to authors on condition of anonymity.

It is because individuals are compelled to participate in all surveillance efforts in the name of the common good that some form of ethical review is imperative. It might be useful to think of such review within public health agencies as analogous to the environmental impact statements that many agencies are currently required to issue.

This stance is not intended to undermine public health surveillance, which represents a vital bulwark against disease. Surveillance is an essential tool in directing interventions to protect the public. There is, after all, an ethical mandate to undertake surveillance that enhances the well-being of populations. Although reform may require changes in the legal and regulatory context within which surveillance occurs, recognizing the need to subject public health reporting to scrutiny need not challenge the constitutional foundations of state surveillance activities. Indeed, a procedure for distinguishing legal requirements from ethical necessity may well strengthen public health surveillance by providing a means to scrutinize current practice and law. Examples of such potential areas of conflict include cases where state law mandates surveillance practices that ethical bodies would prohibit, such as linkage of HIV registries with school registries. Alternatively, state law may forbid practices, such as the linkage of HIV and tuberculosis registries, which might be ethically demanded if they enhanced the capacity of a health department to fulfill its central mission.

Creating the means to conduct a full and transparent airing of the issues involved is all the more critical when important issues of privacy and the collective good are at stake, as they are in the instance of surveillance. As Gostin, Hodge, and Valdisseri have concluded, "extant state laws concerning public health information privacy are inconsistent, fragmented, and inadequate" [23]. While health departments in some states, such as Minnesota, have established clearly that the public has a right to obtain public data collected by the health department, and procedures for doing so as well as warning and consent forms when private data are obtained, "current law and policy often fail to reconcile individual privacy interests with collective public health interests in identifiable health data," according to Ackerman. "Laws often fail to narrowly define who may have access to such data

and require persons to demonstrate why they need access" [24]. Controversies continue about the circumstances under which public health officials may disclose the names of those with infectious disease, as in the instance of hepatitis outbreaks, SARS, and even HIV transmission. These circumstances include release of de-identified data to communities for purposes of their assessing for themselves the existence of a disease cluster, as has been the case in cancer, or warning the community of, say, the presence of lead paint in apartments; extending disease management practices traditional for tuberculosis to diabetes and HIV; or even the possibility of releasing public health data to law enforcement in response to a bioterrorist attack. These are just some of the examples where there exists a need to develop a means for judging the acceptability of public health means and ends [25]. In the context of public health surveillance, a review mechanism can serve as a means of avoiding inadvertent breaches in confidentiality and in preventing stigma; it can help to ensure that the public understands that surveillance will occur and what purposes it serves; and it can protect politically sensitive surveillance efforts. Indeed, it can become part of a broader call for ethical oversight of efforts to change health delivery systems or health coverage [26].

In developing the ethics of public health surveillance and envisioning a mechanism for oversight, it would be wise to recognize that simple rules will never suffice: ethical sensitivity necessitates an open discussion of how the ethical trade-offs and tensions between the claims of the individual and those of the common good can be fairly resolved. This will be especially challenging given the fact that the proposed changes are not driven by the kinds of scandal and abuse that spurred the ethical oversight of clinical research. But just as review need not be precipitated by a crisis, it need not create one.

References

1 Brainard J. Federal Agency says oral-history research is not covered by human-subject rules. *Chronicle of Higher Education* October 31, 2003;SectA:25.
2 World Bank Group's homepage on the Internet. Public health surveillance toolkit. Washington, DC: World Bank; c2003. Available from: http://survtoolkit.worldbank.org. Accessed November 12, 2003.

3 Fairchild AL, Bayer R. *Ethical Issues in Second-Generation Surveillance: Guidelines*. Geneva: World Health Organization; 2004. Available from: http://www.who.int/hiv/pub/epidemiology/sgs_ethical/en/. Accessed October 30, 2006.

4 HIV/AIDS Public Health Data Uses Project: Second pre-consultation meeting of the Centers for Disease Control, Agendas; June 16, 2003, Atlanta, GA, and September 19, 2003, New York, NY.

5 Gordis L, Gold E, Seltzer R. Privacy protection in epidemiologic and medical research: a challenge and a responsibility. *Am J Epidemiol* March 1977;**105**(3):163–8.

6 Capron AM. Protection of research subjects: do special rules apply in epidemiology? *Law Med Health Care* Fall–Winter 1991;**19**(3–4):184–90.

7 Cann CI, Rothman KJ. IRBs and epidemiologic research: how inappropriate restrictions hamper studies. *IRB* July–August 1984;**6**(4):5–7.

8 Protection of Human Subjects, 45 C.F.R. Sect. 46 (1991).

9 International Guidelines for Ethical Review of Epidemiological Studies. *Law Med Health Care* Fall–Winter 1991;**19**(3–4):247–58.

10 Evaluation of human subject protections in research conducted by the Centers for Disease Control and Prevention and the Agency for Toxic Substances and Disease Registry. Atlanta, GA: Centers for Disease Control and Prevention, Division of Human Subject Protections, Office for Protection from Research Risks; July 1995.

11 Minutes of Meeting on Protection of Human Research Subjects in Public Health. Centers for Disease Control; March 18–19, 1996.

12 Snider DE, Stroup DF. Defining research when it comes to public health. *Public Health Rep* January–February 1997;**112**(1):29–32.

13 Minutes of Meeting of CDC and the Council of State and Territorial Epidemiologists; March 4–5, 1999.

14 Middaugh J. Letter to Marjorie Speers. Atlanta, GA: Centers for Disease Control and Prevention; June 7, 1999.

15 Mojica B. Letter to Donna Knutson, Executive Director, Council for State and Territorial Epidemiologists; August 25, 1999.

16 Middaugh J. Letter to Marjorie Speers, Centers for Disease Control and Prevention; June 7, 1999. Birkhead, G. E-mail to Marjorie Speers, Centers for Disease Control and Prevention; June 1, 1999. Moore K. E-mail to Marjorie Speers; June 9, 1999. Simpson, D. E-mail to Donna B. Knutson, Council of State and Territorial Epidemiologists; July 20, 1999. Waterman S. E-mail to Fran Reid-Sanden, Centers for Disease Control and Prevention; March 3, 1999. Hoffman, R. E-mail to Guthrie Birkhead, New York State Department of Health AIDS Institute; August 26, 1999). Hoffman R. E-mail to Dixie Snider, Centers for Disease Control and Prevention; March 3, 1999.

17 American Public Health Association's Homepage on the Internet. APHA Code of Ethics. Washington, DC: American Public Health Association; 2006. Available from: www.apha.org/codeofethics/. Accessed October 30, 2006.

18 Childress JF, Faden RR, Gaare RD, Gostin LO, Kahn J, Bonni RJ. Public health ethics: mapping the terrain. *J Law Med Ethics* 2002;**30**:170–8.

19 Callahan D, Jennings B. Ethics and public health: forging a strong relationship. *Am J Pub Health* 2002;**92**:169.

20 Middaugh JP, Hodge JG, Cartter, ML. The ethics of public health surveillance [letter]. *Science* April 30, 2004;**304**(5671):681–4.

21 Rothman DJ. *Strangers at the Bedside: A History of How Law and Bioethics Transformed Medical Decision Making*. New York: Basic Books; 1991:63.

22 Levine R. Interview with Amy Fairchild; (December 2, 2002).

23 Gostin L, Hodge J, Valdisseri R. Informational privacy and the public's health: the Model State Public Health Privacy Act. *Am J Public Health* September 2001;**91**(9):1388–92.

24 Information for the Public About Public Access to MDH Data and Rights of Data Subjects. Minnesota Department of Health Data Practices Policy 607.02. St. Paul, MN: Minnesota Department of Health [updated October 28, 2005]. Acdkerman TH. In: Vanderpool HY (ed.), *The Ethics of Research Involving Human Subjects: Facing the 21st Century*. Frederick, MD: University Publications Group; 1996:83–6.

25 Fairchild AL, Gable L, Gostin LO, Bayer R, Sweeny P, Janssen P. Public goods, private data: history, ethics, and the uses of personally identifiable public health information. *Public Health Rep* 2007;**122**(Suppl 1):7–15.

26 Daniels N. Toward ethical review of health system transformations. *Am J Public Health* March 2006;**96**(3):447–51.

35 Legal considerations in surveillance, isolation, and quarantine

PART 1: Legal basis for infectious disease surveillance and control

Richard E. Hoffman & Renny Fagan

This chapter will discuss current issues related to the legal basis for communicable disease control by public health agencies in the United States (US). Topics will include discussion of disease surveillance, the role of the federal government in communicable disease surveillance, investigation of communicable diseases threatening the public health, confidentiality of surveillance reports and public health records, sharing of information from public health records, the exercise of the public health powers to control the spread of communicable diseases, and legal authority in public health emergencies. As the authors are from Colorado, the examples of state statutes and regulations are primarily from Colorado.

The US Supreme Court established the parameters of modern public health law in *Jacobson v. Massachusetts*, 197 US 11 (1905), upholding a law requiring smallpox vaccinations for all adults [1]. First, the Court found that individual liberty can be subject to the needs of the community. "There are manifold restraints to which every person is necessarily subject for the common good. On any other basis organized society could not exist with safety to its members. Safety based on the rule that each one is a law unto himself would soon be confronted with disorder and anarchy." Second, the Court confirmed that the police power of the state includes "reasonable regulations ... [to] protect the public health and the public safety." Third, courts must defer to the legislative basis for public health measures if supported by some scientific evidence. Finally, a public health measure

cannot be arbitrary nor impose an unreasonable risk of harm to an individual [1].

Because public health protection is not a specific enumerated power of the federal government in the US Constitution, state and local governments have the primary domestic responsibility for public health. While public health policy is commonly formulated as a balance of individual rights versus public good, we propose an alternate formulation of communicable disease control that balances the rights of uninfected persons with those of infected persons, with the public health agency charged with protecting both. Within this framework, the laws, regulations, and ordinances of state and local governments applicable to communicable disease control have two principal purposes: (1) preventing uninfected persons from becoming infected and (2) assuring that infected persons are diagnosed and treated in a timely manner consistent with contemporary community standards and that they are rendered noninfectious as rapidly as possible.

For decades, state legislatures have passed statutes that give state health departments and state boards of health broad, general authority pursuant to the state police power to control the spread of epidemics and communicable diseases. In those states with autonomous, independent local health agencies (e.g., New York, Pennsylvania), there are typically authorizing state statutes for local health agencies (e.g., New York City, Philadelphia) that correspond to the state agency authority. These statutes usually do not prevent the local legislative body from enacting additional public health laws or ordinances so long as they are consistent with state law. In addition to broad public health powers, most states also have enacted statutes for specific diseases, such as tuberculosis, HIV/AIDS, sexually transmitted infections, vaccine-preventable diseases and immunizations required for school entry, and bioterrorism. Disease-specific statutes may be enacted because the control of a particular disease has aroused political or legal sensitivities in certain groups (e.g., HIV/AIDS), the disease has implications beyond the normal realm of public health, (e.g., bioterrorism), or funding may be linked to specific disease control activities in a legislative bill.

Infectious disease surveillance conducted by state and local health departments

The starting point for communicable disease control is surveillance, which commonly involves mandatory, name-based reporting to public health agencies in all 50 states and US territories [2]. Reporting of personal identifying medical information by healthcare providers represents a compact of the citizens with government: in return for reporting without the consent of the individual the government must provide strong confidentiality protections. If reporting were voluntary and only with the ill person's consent, then the duty of the public health agency to prevent uninfected persons from unnecessary exposure to disease could easily be compromised.

Communicable disease surveillance systems are the means by which public health agencies detect outbreaks, monitor the course of an outbreak, and determine when the outbreak is over. Case reports trigger investigations by local or state officials. The results of such investigations may lead to several actions such as further investigations by other state or federal agencies or implementation of control measures. The specific diseases under surveillance are determined by each state and therefore, vary across the nation. In 2006, there were 61 nationally notifiable infectious diseases that are mutually agreed upon by the Council of State and Territorial Epidemiologists (CSTE) and Centers for Disease Control and Prevention (CDC) [3].

In most jurisdictions, the legislature gives statutory authority to state boards of health to adopt regulations requiring the reporting of individuals with specific diseases and conditions as determined by the board. In a minority of states, reportable conditions are determined either by the state legislature (through enactment of statutes) or by the state health commissioner. Local health agencies generally do not have explicit legal authority for establishing ongoing disease reporting within their jurisdiction, but occasionally may invoke broad public health authority to conduct limited surveillance and control activities for a disease.

The authorizing entity approves not only of placing a particular disease under surveillance, but also what persons or institutions are required to report the disease or condition and within what timeframe. In Colorado, the usual process for modifying the list of reportable infectious diseases begins with a proposal brought by staff of the state health department to the state board of health. The impetus for a proposal may come from a local situation, such as an increase in pediatric mortality related to influenza infection, or from national or international circumstances, such as the SARS epidemic in 2003. The board then follows a statutorily mandated administrative procedure that includes a public notice of the proposed changes, a public hearing with opportunity for comment by affected persons and organizations, and a regulatory analysis of the cost and impact of the proposed rule changes that is prepared by the state health department staff. Beyond the addition or deletion of diseases from the reporting requirements, the state board of health may limit reporting to specified jurisdictions within the state and for limited periods of time or limit reporting to persons with certain characteristics, such as influenza-associated pediatric mortality.

Reporting laws and regulations imply that public health agencies will receive reports filed by all physicians as discussed in Chapter 15. In practice, many physicians do not report, some of the barriers to physician reporting include not knowing what, when, and how to report. In addition, some physicians do not see the importance of reporting or think that someone else will file the report. We have found it useful to view the disease reporting statutes and regulations as a framework that promotes reporting while reassuring physicians that named reporting to the public health agency is not a breach of the confidential doctor–patient relationship. Colorado statute states that reports made in good faith "shall not constitute libel or slander or a violation of any right of privacy or privileged communication" [4], and the Health Insurance Portability and Accountability Act (HIPAA) the Privacy Rule provides that covered entities may disclose protected health information (without individual authorization) to public health authorities authorized by law to collect or receive such information for preventing or controlling disease [5]. The state and federal laws protect the reporting entity from liability and allow the public health agency access to medical information. While there are penalties for noncompliance with reporting requirements, it is rare for a physician to be sanctioned unless an outbreak occurs that could have been prevented if the case had been reported as required. To overcome underreporting by physicians, states have developed overlapping or duplicative surveillances systems, e.g., laboratory reporting, to maximize their chances of identifying all cases of a particular infectious disease.

Across the nation certain communicable diseases, such as measles, diphtheria, polio, typhoid fever, and meningococcal meningitis, have been under surveillance (i.e., mandatory reporting by name) for many decades [6]. Communicable disease surveillance, however, is not static. Case definitions may change (e.g., the case definition for AIDS has changed several times since national surveillance was begun in the early 1980s) [7]. With the emergence of many newly recognized infectious diseases since the 1980s and the heightened threat of bioterrorism within the US since 2001, the conditions under surveillance in the states have been repeatedly modified. Public health agencies are developing networks with different types of providers, such as infection control practitioners in hospitals and nursing homes and veterinarians, and are targeting physicians who normally do not report many diseases but may encounter rare and important conditions, such as dermatologists diagnosing cutaneous anthrax. Furthermore, infections by microorganisms resistant to "standard" antibiotics have increased over the past 15 years. Infections caused by drug-resistant *Streptococcus pneumoniae* (see Chapter 4), and vancomycin-resistant *Staphylococ-*

cus aureus are now included on the list of nationally notifiable infectious diseases [3], and for these infections, the laboratory, not the physician, is the primary source of the reports The diagnosis of infectious diseases and the methods of surveillance by public health entities have also evolved. The legal authority for public health surveillance must keep pace with these changes.

Probably the most significant development in communicable disease surveillance in the past 30 years has been an increasing reliance by public health agencies on laboratories to report specified findings. All states require laboratories to report certain findings in addition to required reporting by physicians and hospitals. Clinical laboratories are good reporting sources because the reports are usually confirmatory and timely. There are far fewer laboratories than physicians, and for public health agencies, this reduces the work necessary to collect reports. The strategy of requiring laboratory reporting may lead to duplicate reporting, but it also helps prevent missing a report. Laboratory methods for confirming infections, drug resistance, and epidemiologically linked cases have dramatically changed in the past 25 years through the introduction and use of polymerase chain reaction assays and pulsed-field gel electrophoresis. Reporting requirements for laboratories that list specific test findings quickly become out of date. For numerous specified microorganisms in Colorado, in lieu of repeatedly modifying a list of specific laboratory findings, the state board of health has required reporting of any positive laboratory test results [8].

The emergence of SARS in the spring of 2003, hantavirus pulmonary syndrome in 1993, and West Nile virus infection in 1999 led many states to develop and install reporting systems for theses diseases on an urgent basis. Two approaches for accomplishing this are proposing to the board of health the adoption of emergency rules that require the newly recognized disease to be reported, or alternatively, the reporting rules can be written broadly to require the reporting of any outbreak or epidemic which may be a threat to the public health whether or not it is known to be communicable. Such language permits the state and local health departments to begin surveillance immediately. With either approach, the state health department can return to the board of health to revise the reporting rules in a standard, nonemergent manner, that is, with public notice and public hearing, when more is known about the disease and how and whom should be reporting.

Along similar lines, syndromic surveillance (i.e., collecting reports of the number of persons with specified clusters of signs and symptoms seen in emergency departments or urgent care centers) and pharmacy surveillance (i.e., collecting reports on the number of particular types of medications sold, such as antidiarrheal medicines) are emerging surveillance methods [9] (also see Chapter 21). These surveillance approaches are being developed to prepare for large-scale bioterrorist attacks, but could also be applicable to influenza epidemics. In both types of surveillance, the names of ill persons are not reported to the public health agency. If the public health agency wanted to contact individuals listed in a syndromic or pharmacy surveillance system to investigate or confirm a diagnosis, the legal authority to interview the patient and access their medical information would be considerably strengthened if such authority were explicit in statute or regulation, rather than implied from broad public health powers.

An important operational change in communicable disease surveillance is the introduction and development of Internet-based reporting. Obviously, safeguards must be installed to assure that Internet-based disease reporting is secure and confidential. This is relatively straightforward, and an increasing proportion of communicable disease reports are now being transmitted to public health agencies electronically, as opposed to mailing hardcopy forms, sending faxes, or making a telephone call. Many state health departments are developing Internet-based disease reporting systems to improve timeliness. Making online entries in a database maintained by a public health agency does not automatically generate a hardcopy for reporting entities, and they cannot easily document compliance with the reporting requirements. The Colorado reporting regulations were modified, therefore, to state that when reports are made electronically using systems and protocols developed by the state health department, the reporting entity is released from liability.

When Internet-based disease reports are made to a server shared by state and local public health agencies, the state and local health agency receive the report simultaneously. This obviates legal issues of whether a particular report should go first to the local or the state health agency or both and whether and how these agencies may share disease reports. However, it requires a system that limits viewing and use of disease reports to the appropriate local jurisdictions, e.g., the county of residence.

Infectious disease surveillance conducted by the CDC

In 1961, CDC assumed responsibility at the federal level for the coordination, collection, and publication of data concerning national notifiable infectious diseases [6]. CDC exerts its leadership in multiple ways, such as training epidemiologists, laboratorians, and public health administrators; funding surveillance systems; providing reference laboratory tests; providing epidemiologic assistance in unusual outbreaks; convening expert panels; and publishing practice guidelines and standards. CDC also maintains and updates the list of nationally notifiable infectious diseases along with CSTE; operates National Notifiable Diseases Surveillance System; and reports internationally quarantinable and notifiable diseases (e.g., cholera) to the World Health Organization pursuant to international regulations.

Routine reporting of notifiable infectious diseases by states to CDC is not only voluntary, but also without names. State reporting, nonetheless, occurs reliably, and tabulations are published weekly in the *Morbidity and Mortality Weekly Reports* (see Table II in MMWR Weekly Report Current Volume at www.cdc.gov/mmwr).

CDC's legal authority to conduct communicable disease surveillance and control in the nation is limited to specific circumstances. These include preventing the introduction of diseases, both foreign and interstate, where state and municipal ordinances were deemed insufficient or state and municipal authorities refused to act, as determined by the Secretary of the US Department of Health and Human Services or his designee, the Director of CDC [10]. Surveillance in 2003 for SARS at ports of entry is an example of CDC exercising this responsibility. These legal authorities are expressed in federal regulations concerning quarantinable diseases, which are undergoing revision as of this writing [10].

Independent of state health agencies, CDC has conducted surveillance for hospital-associated infections since the early 1970s. The system is called the National Nosocomial Infections Surveillance (NNIS) system [11]. Unlike mandatory disease reporting in states, hospital participation in NNIS is voluntary. The legal basis for this activity is pursuant to CDC's responsibilities for research and investigation authorized in the Public Health Service Act. The NNIS has been granted a guarantee of confidentiality, pursuant to Section 308(d) of the Public Health Service Act, and this permits it to collect patient-specific and hospital-specific data, but neither patient-specific nor hospital-specific information is released in reports of NNIS data.

Investigation of communicable diseases by state and local health departments

Once the diagnosis of a reportable condition has been confirmed or strongly suspected, health officials attempt to identify the source of the infection and the persons who may have been exposed either to the reported person or to the same source as the reported person. This usually involves an interview with the infected person and review of pertinent medical records. The legal authority for case investigation activities may be broad (e.g., "the department has … the powers and duties … to investigate and control the causes of epidemic and communicable diseases affecting the public health … ") [12], but with the implementation of the HIPAA Privacy Rule in 2003, it is essential to rely on specific and explicit authority to access pertinent medical and laboratory records, if there is not written patient consent.

A traditional method of communicable disease investigation is to trace contacts of a contagious disease (also referred to, generally, as "case finding" [13] and with respect to sexually transmitted infections, "partner notification"). The public health official interviews the reported case to identify potential sources of infection (e.g., common sources, other persons) and to determine who was exposed to the person. Who these people are depends on the epidemiologic parameters (e.g., incubation period, period of communicability) of the disease and

how it is transmitted. The contacts may be household members, classmates in a school or child care center, sexual partners, etc.

The reported person provides contact information voluntarily in all instances; it is never coerced or ordered, and we are not aware of any statutes that explicitly mandate a reported person to disclose contacts and/or sexual partners. Therefore, to be effective public health officials must explain the rationale for their investigation as well as the service they can provide to the person by locating and notifying his or her partners. Under most circumstances, the public health official can assure the person that the information will be confidential and his or her name will not be revealed unnecessarily to contacts or sexual partners. Depending on the laws of a given jurisdiction, the collected information, however, may not remain strictly confidential within the health department if the investigation determines there has been criminal activity, e.g., bioterrorism, rape, homicide, child abuse.

Public health investigations may require additional methods besides interviewing the case and reviewing records in order to determine exposed persons. Because such investigations may involve private businesses or commercial products, such as restaurants, foods, medicines, medical devices, healthcare facilities, airline flights, cruise ships, etc., for which the investigation could result in significant liability, loss of revenues, or negative publicity, it is useful to have potential investigative procedures published, if not legally authorized in statute or regulation, in advance. This reduces resistance, advancing the investigation when public health officials are seeking to contact customers who may have been potentially exposed to an infectious agent and are rapidly dispersing. Colorado has addressed this by promulgating regulations that list investigative methods, including performing follow-up interviews with persons knowledgeable about the reported case and or relevant information about the exposure; conducting surveys of employees or clients of business associated with an outbreak; obtaining lists of passengers, transportation crews, and travelers; and entering businesses to investigate the premises [8].

Outbreak investigation is not restricted to contact tracing, product traceback, and environmental inspection. Determining the cause and risk factors for outbreaks frequently requires epidemiologists to conduct descriptive and analytic studies. These studies may require selection and enrollment of unaffected control subjects, and the results may be published in peer-reviewed journals months to years after an outbreak has ended. In recent years, CDC, CSTE, and the Department of Health and Human Services' Office for Human Research Protections have discussed whether such studies are public health practice or research. The applicable definition of "research" in federal regulation is extremely broad [14]. The distinction between practice and research is important because research protocols would be subject to federal Protection of Human Subjects regulations (45 CFR 46 available at http://ohsr.od.nih.gov) and potentially HIPAA requirements, while official state and local public health investigations (e.g., practice) are conducted pursuant to the statutes and regulations of the jurisdiction. The difference is not clear-cut, and agencies and institutions typically resolve the issue internally, sometimes on a case-by-case basis. In 2004, CSTE published a report on public health practice vs. research containing guidelines for state and local public health officials [15].

While they may exercise statutory powers to control outbreaks of disease, state and local communicable disease control units generally have little regulatory responsibility, and CDC has none, except for the limited circumstances described above. Public health outbreak investigations, however, may involve activities, operations, or products that cross political jurisdictions and/or are regulated by state or local government agencies (e.g., drinking water protection agencies, restaurant inspection agencies, healthcare facility licensing), or by federal agencies (e.g., the Food and Drug Administration, the US Department of Agriculture, the US Environmental Protection Agency, the Occupational Safety and Health Administration). Traceback of implicated products to determine how a product was produced and distributed may require another agency besides the communicable disease control unit to assume the investigatory lead. It is essential for public health agencies to coordinate investigations with regulatory agencies, but it is beyond the scope of this chapter to discuss the legal authorities of these agencies in communicable disease investigations.

Confidentiality of surveillance data and case reports held by state and local health departments

We attribute current high levels of legal protection for the confidentiality and security of public health records to the concerns raised in the 1980s about discrimination and coercion resulting from unauthorized disclosure of AIDS and HIV surveillance information. In 1987, the Colorado General Assembly passed a bill that strengthened the confidentiality protections of AIDS and HIV reports. Prior to enactment of this law, AIDS and HIV reports had been handled the same as all other communicable disease investigation reports: the reports were confidential and not subject to public records requests, but they could be subpoenaed by courts. The statute provided that AIDS and HIV public health reports were not to be made public upon subpoena, search warrant, or discovery proceedings and could not be shared with any agency or institution [16].

This degree of protection was explicitly extended to all other surveillance and investigatory records for reportable conditions in 1991 in Colorado [4], and a similar degree of confidentiality and security protection was considered the "gold standard" for all states by a collaborative workgroup that published model public health legislation in 2003 [17].

There are, however, legally permitted disclosures of records and information in public health records concerning reportable conditions. The list of permissible disclosures varies from state to state. In Colorado these include releasing records to the individual who is the subject of the record, to agencies responsible for receiving or investigating child abuse or neglect (e.g., filing a report of gonorrhea in an 8-yr-old), and in judicial proceedings when necessary to enforce public health orders or to determine whether individuals charged with sexual assault knew that they had HIV infection at the time of the assault. There is also broad discretion given to the public health agency to release information as necessary to protect the public health. This may include releasing information to other agencies, including federal regulatory agencies, which are participating in a public health investigation [4].

In a bioterrorist-caused epidemic, such as the 2001 outbreak of anthrax, both public health officials and law enforcement would conduct investigations seeking similar information about the diagnosis of infected individuals and their source of exposure. While the primary public health goal would be to prevent further cases of the disease and law enforcement's goals would be to identify arrest, and prosecute the individuals responsible for introducing the disease into the population, such events clearly call for coordination and collaboration among government agencies. Laws that explicitly permit such interagency cooperation are very helpful in a crisis.

In 2003, Colorado amended its statutes to give public health officials discretion to disclose information to law enforcement "to the extent necessary for any investigation or prosecution related to bioterrorism; except that reasonable efforts shall be made to limit disclosure of personal identifying information to the minimal amount necessary to accomplish the law enforcement purpose" [4]. The Model State Emergency Health Powers Act (MSEHPA) contains similar provisions, requiring public health and law enforcement to notify each other if they learn of a "suspicious event" and authorizing the sharing of information restricted to that "necessary for the treatment, control, investigation and prevention of a public health emergency" [17]. As of May 2006, 12 states have adopted a version of this information-sharing provision.

Because confidentiality protection and acquisition of public health information are interdependent and a breach of confidentiality in one location may threaten the collection of public health reports in all locations, we have not lightly considered requests from other government agencies to provide personal information directly to them. An alternative is for the public health agency to contact the reported cases and obtain written permission to release the information to the other agency. This approach appears reasonable when there is no extreme urgency to intervene to control an outbreak, prevent the spread of disease, and calm the public.

The police power of the state and communicable disease control measures

Governments protect the public's health through the police power authorized by the federal and state constitutions, legislatively enacted statutes, and administratively adopted regulations. Courts broadly interpret public health laws to give governments wide latitude to prevent and control communicable diseases. At the same time, the Constitution protects individual liberty from unwarranted restriction. Therefore, public health actions must be necessary, scientifically based, and reasonably related to disease control while imposing the least restrictive burden on individual liberty.

In the decades after *Jacobson v. Massachusetts*, 197 US 11 (1905), courts affirmed public health measures responding to the threat of various diseases. For example, state courts upheld the mandatory smallpox vaccination of school children [18], quarantine and treatment of venereal diseased individuals [19], closure of public theatres during the influenza pandemic of 1918–1919 [20], prohibiting a typhoid carrier from operating and serving food at her boardinghouse [21], and the isolation and quarantine of a tubercular person [22]. In these cases, the courts determined that the public health measures that restrained individual liberty were reasonably necessary to combat a communicable disease and were within the legislatively authorized discretion of the public health authority.

These principles continue to supply the legal authority for disease control measures. However, courts have applied modern procedural due process standards to long-term treatment and quarantine orders to treat multidrug-resistant tuberculosis. While recognizing the power of public health to control tuberculosis, the courts have required that the government provide a written notice detailing the grounds under which the commitment of the patient is sought, provide the right to counsel and the right to confront witnesses, prove the need for commitment by clear and convincing evidence, and provide a written transcript of the proceedings for purposes of appeal [23]. The courts also evaluated whether confinement in a hospital was the least restrictive means necessary to accomplish the public health goal. Some have argued that this heightened due process standard requires that states modernize public health laws that affect individual liberty by including extensive notice and hearing opportunities [17].

Typical control measures and enforcement through administrative procedures

The use of a particular disease control measure depends on the source of the disease or the manner in which the disease is communicated. For example, a restaurant or some other public building may be the source of a disease spread by food, air, or water. These conditions may constitute a nuisance to public health. To remedy or "abate" the nuisance, public health authorities may order the property owner, at the owner's expense, to decontaminate the premises or to destroy any materials or goods and to close the premises until this is accomplished [17].

If a particular disease spreads by person-to-person contact, public health authorities will want to separate ill or exposed individuals from the healthy population. State statutes generally authorize public health to order the isolation of individuals who have the disease and restrict or quarantine those people who have been exposed to an ill person. The order may require a person to stay at home, at a healthcare facility, or some other place [24]. Short of confinement, a person's movements may be restricted. For example, a student with measles would be prohibited from attending school or a food handler with salmonellosis or hepatitis A would be prevented from going to work until they were no longer contagious. When a virulent disease spreads easily and widely through close person-to-person contact, such as influenza, public health officials may impose measures to achieve social distancing, such as the closure of public entertainment facilities, public buildings, office buildings, schools, or other gathering places [25]. The legal authority for all of these actions may derive from a specific statute or from the general statutory authority to control disease.

Public health authorities will likely seek voluntary compliance with their directives before resorting to formal orders. By providing clear information about the disease and its treatment, how it is transmitted, the danger that a contagious person poses to others, the reason for controlling individual behavior, and how to obtain healthcare for the disease, public health officials are likely to gain voluntary cooperation. As for well, exposed persons, individuals will be more likely to comply with a voluntary quarantine order if the government supplies them and their families with necessities such as food or medicine [26].

A full discussion of the legal considerations for isolation and quarantine is contained in Chapter 35, Part 2.

Legal authority in public health emergencies

While public health officials have a great deal of legal authority to control disease, a pandemic or bioterrorist event may create a public health emergency that requires extraordinary resources and actions. Many states have general emergency disaster statutes that authorize public officials, typically the governor, to mobilize emergency preparedness forces and to issue directives necessary to combat disasters such as flooding, wildfires, blizzards, or other natural or manmade occurrences that threaten public safety or widespread destruction of property. A disaster statute may authorize the governor to activate the National Guard, impose travel restrictions, seize control of property, and order public employees or private citizens to help meet the disaster. The disaster statute may also authorize the governor to suspend the operation of any statute or regulation if strict compliance would hinder or delay any action necessary to meet the emergency [27].

Similar legal authority may be needed in a public health emergency. In 2000, Colorado enacted a statute [28] creating the Governor's Expert Emergency Epidemic Response Committee consisting of state and local public health officials, healthcare and infectious disease personnel, emergency management personnel, state veterinary and wildlife officials, and the attorney general. Upon the occurrence or imminent threat of an emergency epidemic caused by bioterrorism, pandemic influenza, or other novel and highly fatal infectious agents, the expert committee will convene to advise the governor on reasonable and appropriate measures to reduce or prevent the spread of the disease. The governor acts by declaring a disaster emergency and issuing appropriate executive order(s) that may suspend an existing statute(s). For example, if a disease can be treated or prevented by the distribution of antibiotics, the governor could order the seizure and control of supplies of the antibiotic. To distribute the antibiotic rapidly, the governor could suspend the normal pharmacy and medical practice laws to enable nonlicensed individuals to dispense the antibiotics and to do so through a general prescription issued by a public health official. An executive order may also direct conduct, such as ordering isolation or community quarantine or disposing of corpses or infectious waste. The statute confers civil and criminal immunity on any healthcare provider or public health worker who complies in good faith with the executive orders as well as members of the expert committee.

In the aftermath of September 11, 2001, CDC requested that the Center for Law and the Public's Health at Georgetown and Johns Hopkins University draft a Model State Emergency Health Powers Act (MSEHPA) in collaboration with policymakers and public health officials [15,29]. The MSEHPA and its application to quarantine law are discussed in detail in Chapter 35, Part 2.

Summary

Epidemiologists, other public health workers, and infectious disease specialists have been challenged by a long list of infectious diseases that have emerged since the time smallpox was officially declared to be eradicated from the world in December 1979 [30]. The principles that underlie communicable disease surveillance, investigation, and control are constant. However, the laws and regulations necessary to conduct infectious disease surveillance and control have been repeatedly modified in the past 20 years in response to changes in microbial threats, the manner of exposure to microbes, diagnostic methods, medical treatment, disease prevention, data collection, telecommunications, movement of populations, sensitivity of unauthorized disclosure of medical information, and cultural stigma attached to various communicable diseases. Local, state, and federal public health agencies have often met the emerging challenges by using broad, general statutes passed many years ago; in other situations, very specific laws and regulations have been passed to counter new threats and enable new responses. This chapter has presented a review of the legal issues that are integral to infectious disease control in the US in the early twent-first century.

References

1 *Jacobson v. Massachusetts*, 197 US 11 (1905). Available from: www.publichealth.net/Reader/ch7/ch7.htm. Accessed April 29, 2007.
2 Council of State and Territorial Epidemiologists. Reporting patterns for Notifiable Diseases and Conditions. Available from: www.cste.org/NNDSSHome2005.htm.
3 Centers for Disease Control and Prevention. Nationally notifiable infectious diseases, United States 2006. Available from: www.cdc.gov/epo/dhpsi/phs/infdis.htm.
4 Colorado Revised Statutes 25-1-122. Available from: www.leg.state.co.us.
5 Centers for Disease Control and Prevention. HIPAA Privacy Rule and Public Health: guidance from CDC and the US Department of Health and Human Services. *MMWR Morb Mortal Wkly Rep* 2003;52(suppl):2.
6 Centers for Disease Control and Prevention. Notifiable disease surveillance and notifiable disease statistics—United States, June 1946 and June 1996. *MMWR Morb Mortal Wkly Rep* 1996;45:530–6.
7 Centers for Disease Control and Prevention. 1993 Revised classification system for HIV infection and expanded surveillance case definition for AIDS among adolescents and adults. *MMWR Morb Mortal Wkly Rep* 1992;41(RR-17).
8 Colorado Code of Regulations 1009-1. Colorado Board of Health Rules and Regulations pertaining to epidemic and communicable disease control. Available from: www.cdphe.state.co.us.
9 Centers for Disease Control and Prevention. Syndromic surveillance: reports from a national conference, 2004. *MMWR Morb Mortal Wkly Rep* 2005;54(suppl), 27–54, 133–180.
10 42 CFR parts 70 and 71. Available from: www.cdc.gov/ncidod/dq/nprm/index.htm.
11 Centers for Disease Control and Prevention. National nosocomial infections surveillance system. Available from:www.cdc.gov/ncidod/dhqp/nnis.html.
12 Colorado Revised Statutes 25-1.5-102 (1)(a)(I). Available from: www.leg.state.co.us.
13 Last JM (ed.). *A Dictionary of Epidemiolgy*, 4th edn. New York: Oxford University Press; 2001:24.
14 46.102 CFR. Available from: www.hhs.gov/ohrp.
15 Council of State and Territorial Epidemiologists. Report on Public Health Practice vs. Research. Available from: www.cste.org.

16 Colorado Revised Statutes 25-4-1404 (1). Available from: www.leg.state.co.us.

17 Center for Law and the Public's Health at Georgetown and Johns Hopkins Universities. Available from: www.publichealthlaw.net/Resources/Modellaws.htm.

18 *Board of Trustees of Highland Park Graded Common School District v. McMurtry*, 184 SW 390 (Ky. 1916); *Vonnegut v. Baun*, 188 NE 677 (Ind. 1934); *Wright v. De Witt School District*, 385 SW2d 644 (Ark. 1965).

19 In re *Johnson*, 180 P 644 (Cal. App. 1919) and *Rock v. Carney*, 185 NW 798 (Mich. 1921).

20 *Alden v. State*, 179 P 646 (Ariz. 1919).

21 *People ex rel. Barmore v. Robertson*, 134 NE 815 (Ill. 1922).

22 In re*Halko*, 246 Cal.App.2d 553 (1966).

23 See, e.g., *Souvannarath v. Hadden*, 95 Cal.App.4th 1115 (2002); *City of Newark v. J.S.*, 652 A2d 265 (N.J.Super. 1993); *City of New York v. Antoinette R.*, 630 NYS2d 1014 (Sup.Ct. 1995); *Greene v. Edwards*, 263 SE2d 661 (Ct.App. 1980).

24 Centers for Disease Control and Prevention. Public Health Law Program. Quarantine and isolation related materials. Available from: www2a.cdc.gov/phlp/.

25 United States Department of Health and Human Services, Pandemic Influenza Plan, Part 2, Supplement 8; March 2006. Available from: www.hhs.gov/pandemicflu/plan/.

26 The SARS Commission, Second Interim Report—SARS and Public Health Legislation; April 2005:250–252. Available from: www.health.gov.on.ca/english/public/pub/ministry_reports/campbell05/campbell05.html.

27 Colorado Revised Statutes 24-32-2104(7)(a). Available from: www.leg.state.co.us.

28 Colorado Revised Statutes 24-32-2104(8) and 2111.5. Available from: www.leg.state.co.us.

29 Gostin LO, Sapsin JW, Teret SP, *et al.* The Model State Emergency Health Powers Act, planning for and response to bioterrorism and naturally occurring infectious diseases. *JAMA* 2002;**288**:622–8.

30 Centers for Disease Control and Prevention. Preventing emerging infectious diseases: a strategy for the 21st century. *MMWR Morb Mortal Wkly Rep* 1998;**47**(RR-15), 1–15.

35 Legal considerations in surveillance, isolation, and quarantine

PART 2: Legal considerations for isolation and quarantine in the United States

Frederic E. Shaw & Richard A. Goodman

All individuals found occupying the premises at ___ are hereby ORDERED to COMPLY with the following control measures required by State law NCGS § 130A-144 and all relevant provisions of 15A-NCAdmin Code § 19A.0208: REMAIN AT HOME FOR ___ (specify time, no greater than 10 days); DO NOT LEAVE YOUR HOUSE AND DO NOT HAVE ANYONE VISIT YOU AT HOME.

—Draft quarantine order from North Carolina, 2003 [1]

Since the earliest recognition that some diseases are communicable, human beings have sought to control these diseases by separating the sick from the well. Somewhere in history, quarantine and isolation (see Box 35(2).1 for definitions) became part of the law. Ancient Hebrew law mentions banishing persons afflicted with leprosy and other communicable diseases from the general population [2]. In 1347, during the Black Death (a plague epidemic that killed 25–50% of Europe's population), the Great Council of Venice established a general quarantine of 40 days on incoming ships as a way to stave off importation of the disease [3]. The word quarantine probably derives from this practice through the Italian word, *quarantina*, meaning forty, or the French word, *quarantaine*, which means a group of forty [4].

This chapter reviews the legal foundation for quarantine in the United States (US) at the federal and state levels. The chapter discusses quarantine authorities in law and in the American constitutional scheme, the characteristics of federal and state quarantine laws, and legal challenges to quarantine. Chapters on the epidemiological and public health aspects of quarantine appear elsewhere in this volume.

Quarantine law in the US

In the US, quarantine laws trace back to the earliest formations of American society. Since Colonial times, public health officials have invoked these laws to control diseases such as smallpox [5], typhoid fever, tuberculosis, scarlet fever, and poliomyelitis [6]. In the mid-twentieth century, as communicable diseases became less important as causes of premature morbidity and mortality, public health practitioners used quarantine laws less often. Since the control of poliomyelitis by vaccination in the 1950s, US officials have invoked quarantine laws mainly to detain persons with highly infectious pulmonary tuberculosis who refuse to comply with antibiotic treatment regimens, to detain persons infected with HIV who are considered dangerous to unwitting sexual partners (occasionally) [7], and for other diseases (rarely) [8].

Recently, quarantine laws took on new prominence with three historic developments: the magnified threat of bioterrorism after the attacks of September 11, 2001, and the October 2001 anthrax-laced letter mailings; the advent of severe acute respiratory syndrome (SARS) in 2003 [9]; and new global ambitions to control pandemic human influenza. At the time of this writing (fall 2006),

Box 35(2).1 Definitions.

Quarantine refers to the separation and restriction of movement of well persons who have been exposed to a communicable disease.

Isolation refers to the separation and restriction of movement of persons who are ill with a communicable disease.

Note: In this chapter, the word *quarantine* refers generically to quarantine, isolation, and all other forms of civil detention used to control the spread of communicable diseases.

avian influenza has again become a major global health concern. Although wide-scale compulsory quarantine is unlikely to play a large role in the control of an influenza pandemic in the US, voluntary quarantine might be recommended in some circumstances. Isolation of sick persons and other social distancing measures might also be used to slow spread of the virus [10].

Even as quarantine law has reawakened, it has evolved. A century ago, quarantine was sometimes used to stigmatize unpopular social groups (Figure 35 (2).1) [11,12]. Modern notions of quarantine embrace the predicament of the person whose movement is restricted and emphasize *aiding* such persons, while also protecting the larger population [13]. Some legal scholars have suggested that quarantine law in the US has not kept pace with contemporary legal doctrine in civil rights and they have recommended a series of statutory guarantees for persons placed under quarantine [14]. Some of these guarantees have been enacted into law in the states [15].

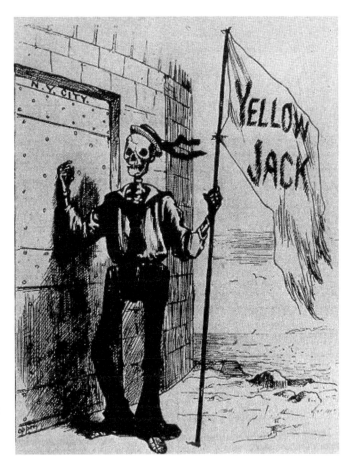

Fig 35(2).1 Death in a sailor's uniform holding the yellow quarantine flag knocking on the door of New York City during the 1878 yellow fever epidemic. (Source: Frank Leslie's Illustrated Newspaper, September 1878.)

Quarantine law in the US constitutional scheme

Under the US constitutional scheme of federalism, the federal government and the governments of the 50 states share power. Under this doctrine, the federal government's powers are limited to those expressly granted to it by the US Constitution, plus those others that are "necessary and proper for carrying into execution" the powers granted to it [16]. This means that all other governmental powers are reserved to the states, a reality that was affirmed in 1791 by the ratification of the Tenth Amendment, which states, "The powers not delegated to the United States by the Constitution, nor prohibited by it to the States, are reserved to the States respectively, or to the people." Among the reserved powers is the "police power," the inherent prerogative of the states to protect and promote the public health, safety, and welfare of their populations [17]. Most traditional public health powers, including quarantine, are part of the police powers of the states.

Federal quarantine authority

The federal government exercises responsibility for quarantine in two situations: when needed to prevent the introduction of communicable diseases from foreign countries into the US and when needed to prevent transmission from one US state or possession to another. These powers derive from the power given to Congress by the Constitution: "To regulate Commerce with foreign Nations, and among the several States, and with the Indian Tribes".

The US government has exercised quarantine power since just after the formation of the republic. Congress enacted the first quarantine statute in 1796 in response to a yellow fever epidemic [18, 19]. Congress amended the federal statute in 1878, but the legislation was extremely limited. Only in 1893 did Congress amend the federal quarantine statute to include prevention of foreign disease importation and interstate spread and to give the federal government the explicit authority to act in the event of inadequate state or local control.

Although federal quarantine authority vests in the Secretary of Health and Human Services, the Director of the Centers for Disease Control and Prevention (CDC) exercises the authority by delegation. The federal quarantine statute is very broad. It authorizes the Secretary to "make and enforce such regulations as in his judgment are necessary to prevent the introduction, transmission, or spread of communicable diseases from foreign countries into the States or possessions, or from one State or possession into any other State or possession" [20]. To carry out these duties, the statute authorizes the use of "measures, as in his judgment may be necessary." Specifically with regard to quarantine, the Secretary may prescribe regulations for the "apprehension and examination of any individual reasonably believed to be infected with a communicable disease..." [21]. Under the Code of Federal Regulations, whenever the CDC Director determines that measures taken by health authorities of any state or possession are insufficient to prevent the interstate spread of communicable diseases, the Director can "take such measures... as he/she deems reasonably necessary..." [22].

Although the CDC Director's authority to quarantine persons is broad, the authority applies only to a short list of communicable diseases that must be specified in an executive order of the President [23]. Prior to the SARS epidemic in 2003, the list consisted of just seven diseases: cholera, diphtheria, infectious tuberculosis, plague, suspected smallpox, yellow fever, and suspected viral hemorrhagic fevers. By an executive order signed on April 4, 2003, the President added SARS to the list. Two years later, the President amended the order to add "[i]nfluenza caused by novel or reemergent influenza viruses that are causing, or have the potential to cause, a pandemic" [24].

In 2005, the Department of Health and Human Services proposed the first significant change in federal quarantine regulations in 20 years. The new regulations were designed "to update and streamline practices to reflect modern quarantine practice" [19]. The proposed regulations spell out procedures for many aspects of federal quarantine for the first time. For example, they make provisions for detaining airplanes and passengers (including quarantine) and for screening passengers to control communicable diseases. As of this writing (fall 2006), the proposed regulations are still in the rulemaking process and have not yet taken effect.

State quarantine authority

Although the federal government is primarily responsible for quarantine to prevent the foreign importation and interstate spread of communicable diseases, other quarantine powers reside in the states under their police powers [25]. Each of the 50 states has a set of quarantine laws unique to itself, and the authority to revise those laws rests exclusively with the legislature of each state. Through their inherent police powers and enacted statutes, every US state has the basic authority to order quarantine when needed to control the spread of communicable diseases. However, the quarantine statutes of the states vary widely in almost every characteristic. For example, the laws vary by the level of detail provided, by the procedure for instituting or rescinding quarantine, by the types of movement restrictions that can be ordered, and by the procedures provided for individuals who wish to appeal the quarantine in court [26].

With some exceptions, the quarantine laws of the states reflect their origins—successive waves of legislation over two centuries, with each wave aimed at solving a contemporary set of medicolegal needs in the state. The resulting laws are often weakly organized, overlapping, and difficult to read and interpret [14]. Even so, antique laws are not necessarily bad laws, and many state public health attorneys view them as eminently serviceable.

One example of the variation in state quarantine laws is the authority to order group quarantine (the quarantine of groups of persons whose individual identities are not known). Group quarantine can be useful when many persons are exposed simultaneously to a communicable disease (e.g., at a gathering or event). Some states have statutes giving express authority for group quarantine, but other state statutes do not mention it [26].

Many states have "umbrella" public health statutes that give broad authority to state officials to restrict the movement of persons. For example, the California Department of Health Services has the power to "commence and maintain all proper and necessary actions and proceedings ... for any or all of the following purposes: (a) To enforce its regulations; (b) To enjoin and abate nuisances dangerous to health; (c) To compel the performance of any act specifically enjoined upon any person, officer, or board, by any law of this state relating to the public health; (d) To protect and preserve the public health" [27]. The Department also has specific quarantine authority [28]. Other states have a similar mix of laws. When public health officials need to use quarantine (including variants of quarantine such as group quarantine), they can rely on express statutory authority if it is available, or on umbrella statutes based in the police power [29].

Most states have some form of special statutory authority that is triggered by the declaration of an emergency by the governor or other official. During public health emergencies, state powers to order quarantine reach their apogee. For example, in Illinois, after declaring an emergency, the governor has broad authority to "control ingress and egress to and from a disaster area, the movement of persons within the area, and the occupancy of premises therein" [30]. States' emergency quarantine powers are further buttressed by courts' traditional deference to public health judgment and their reluctance to invalidate reasonable countermeasures taken by public health authorities [31,32]. As one court famously wrote, "It is not for the courts to determine which scientific view is correct in ruling upon whether the police power has been properly exercised. 'The judicial function is exhausted with the discovery that the relation between means and end is not wholly vain and fanciful, an illusory pretense.' (*Williams v. Mayor of Baltimore*, 289 US 36, 42)" [33].

Federal versus state quarantine authority: who is in charge?

For public health, one of the benefits of American federalism is that, in many disease control situations, the federal and state governments share legal authority; by working together, they can attain a better result than if only one level of government were able to act. But federalism also means that there is often no bright line dividing federal and state legal authority.

No doubt, however, exists about the federal government's authority to quarantine persons with certain infectious diseases arriving in the US. CDC has statutory responsibility for maintaining quarantine stations at major US ports of entry (both air and sea) and for ensuring that infectious diseases are not introduced into the country [34]. The federal government also has authority to detain persons to prevent the interstate spread of disease. Here is where the federal authority could, and in national and regional epidemics almost certainly would, overlap the authority of the states. Interpretation of the division between federal and state authorities is part of the long and evolving jurisprudence of federalism and the Commerce Clause and is beyond the scope of this chapter. However, most experts acknowledge that the power of the federal government to restrict the movement of persons is not confined to situations in which *actual* interstate disease transmission is occurring. *Potential* interstate transmission is enough to trigger federal authority, in part because Congress has the power to regulate "the channels of interstate commerce," "the instrumentalities of interstate commerce, or persons or things in interstate commerce, even though the threat may come only from intrastate activities," and "those activities having a substantial relation to interstate commerce," or "that substantially affect interstate commerce" [35]. Indeed, the relevant federal statute provides that, in such a situation, the federal government's authority extends to the "apprehension and examination of any individual reasonably believed to be infected with a communicable disease in a qualifying stage [36] and (A) to be moving or about to move from a State to another State; or (B) to be a probable source of infection to individuals who, while infected with such disease in a qualifying stage, will be moving from a State to another State" [21].

Very often, during sizeable outbreaks, concurrent legal authority for quarantine may exist and include not just the federal and state governments, but also local governments (counties, cities, interstate airport authorities). For example, if a person with a dangerous, highly transmissible disease (one of those listed in the executive order of the President) arrived at a US international airport, it is possible that the quarantine powers of the federal government, the state government, the county, and the airport authority could all apply in parallel (this would depend in part on whether the person had been officially admitted into the US, which is in the

purview of US Customs and Border Protection, an agency of the Department of Homeland Security). Working cooperatively, public health officials from the overlapping jurisdictions would choose one or more legal authorities to employ, depending on the characteristics of the disease, the characteristics of available legal authorities, the admission status of the detainee, due process requirements, available enforcement mechanisms, and other factors.

The federal government has broad quarantine authority, but it does not necessarily have broad operational capacity. In the US, the federal government has a limited role in the delivery of public health services [37]. The bulk of the public health manpower needed to operate large-scale quarantines (e.g., to coordinate and manage the restrictions, notify persons subject to quarantine, monitor compliance, provide food, medical care, and other aid, communicate with the public, enforce restrictions, and other tasks) resides in state and local agencies. Thus, in national or large regional outbreaks requiring quarantine, the role of CDC and other federal agencies would most likely be limited to strategy, coordination, and formulating recommendations. Most of the practical work of instituting and maintaining quarantine would fall on state and local health departments and other agencies [38].

Legal challenges to quarantine

Because quarantine involves the deprivation of freedom of movement, a basic liberty, it is not surprising that detainees have periodically challenged the legality of quarantine orders (detainees have also, presumably, challenged the facts on which quarantine orders have been based). These legal challenges can be grouped into three general claims: (1) the detention order is defective because it violates a statute or regulation, (2) the agency ordering the detention lacks the authority to do so, and (3) the detention infringes on the detainee's constitutional rights. The principle underlying the first claim comes from traditional precepts of the rule of law and the administrative law model—in general, where statutes or regulations provide procedures or standards for government agencies' actions, the agencies must follow them. Thus, if an agency or official issued a quarantine order but failed to obey applicable laws, procedures, or standards, the order could be invalid. In one such case in California, a person with tuberculosis quarantined in a jail cell argued that a state statute prohibited the use of such venues for quarantine detention. In deciding for the plaintiff, the California court emphasized that, when the government institutes quarantine, it must comply with its own statutes: "It is not within this court's power to release appellants from their statutory obligations . . . " [39].

It is a principle of law that no government action, including quarantine, is valid if the officer or agency taking the action is not legally authorized to do so. For example, if a plaintiff could prove that a town board of health lacked the legal authority to order quarantine of a certain type or in a certain situation, then a court could find the order invalid.

In many states, the quarantine statutes themselves provide details about how detained persons can challenge quarantine orders [40]. In some such states, the health department must either grant an administrative hearing allowing the detained person to challenge the quarantine order, or the department must go to court (often within a set time period) to obtain judicial approval for the detention.

Persons detained in quarantine have also challenged quarantine orders by asserting that it violated their individual constitutional rights. Often, these challenges have been brought through a petition for a writ of habeas corpus (Latin: "you have the body"), through which criminal or civil detainees have the constitutional right to challenge the confinement in federal or state court.

In deciding constitutional challenges to quarantine detentions, courts have examined whether the government has a legitimate basis for taking the action (i.e., whether the government can demonstrate a necessity for the detention). In the landmark 1905 US Supreme Court case, *Jacobson v. Massachusetts* (197 US 11, US Supreme Court, 1905), a compulsory vaccination case, the Court affirmed that legislatures have the right to restrict personal liberty for the good of the whole: "[T]he liberty secured by the Constitution of the United States to every person within its jurisdiction does not import an absolute right in each person to be, at all times and in all circumstances, wholly free from restraint . . . [A] community has the right to protect itself against an epidemic of disease which threatens the safety of its members." The Court also set four limits on the government's prerogative: the government's intervention must be necessary to prevent an unavoidable harm, it must bear a "real or substantial relation" to the threat, the human burden of the intervention must not be disproportionate to its expected benefits, and the measure must not pose a health risk to the subject. Although courts show great deference to public health expertise, under the principles set out in *Jacobson* and subsequent affirming cases, they have occasionally invalidated quarantine measures applied arbitrarily, capriciously, or unfairly.

Many federal and state courts have heard challenges to quarantine orders to control tuberculosis, smallpox, scarlet fever, leprosy, cholera, and plague. In one early case, *Compagnie Francaise de Navigation a Vapeur v. Louisiana State Board of Health* (186 US 380, US Supreme Court, 1902) a maritime quarantine case, the Supreme Court established that a state's exercise of quarantine was well within its police powers and did not interfere with interstate commerce.

A theme of the quarantine cases is the courts' deference to the wisdom of the legislature and the judgment of public health authorities. However, the cases also establish limits on governmental discretion, holding that government officials who wish to restrict individuals' movement must establish the necessity for doing so, must follow procedures that comport with constitutional due process, and must answer to the courts when challenged.

An illustrative case was *People ex rel. Barmore v. Robertson* [29], in which the keeper of a boarding house brought a petition for a writ of habeas corpus to seek relief from an order of isolation. Having found that the keeper was a "carrier of typhoid bacilli," the city health department had ordered her to remain confined to her house, forbade her from preparing food for anyone but her husband, and barred anyone from coming into her house (thus ending her rooming business). The court rejected the keeper's arguments that because she had never been sick with typhoid fever nor apparently transmitted it to anyone else, her liberty had been improperly restrained. In holding for the city health department, the court said, "Although courts will not pass upon the wisdom of the means adopted to

465

restrict and suppress the spread of contagious and infectious diseases, they will interfere if the regulations are arbitrary and unreasonable. A person cannot be quarantined upon mere suspicion that he may have a contagious and infectious disease, but the health authorities must have reliable information on which they have reasonable ground to believe that the public health will be endangered by permitting the person to be at large."

A great many constitutional challenges to quarantine orders have been based on violations of the right to "due process." Under the Fifth and Fourteenth Amendments, "No person shall be ... deprived of life, liberty, or property, without due process of law. ... " Under the *Jacobson* principles (discussed above), applied to quarantine "substantive due process" means that the government must show necessity for the detention. "Procedural due process" means that the government cannot order quarantine except through a procedure that is fundamentally fair.

For civil confinements, less procedural process is due than that required for a criminal detention, but it probably includes a right to notice of the confinement, a hearing before an impartial fact finder, access to legal counsel, presentation of evidence, cross-examination, a written decision, and an appeal [17]. Procedural due process is, however, a flexible concept that varies with "the interests of the individual and of society in the particular situation circumstances" [41]. One can imagine that, if the government ordered several thousand people into quarantine suddenly to stop the progression of a dangerous outbreak, it might be impossible to offer a full-scale court hearing to every person individually. Depending on the applicable law, courts could consolidate the hearings, hold hearings by telephone, or make other special arrangements to cope with the workload.

Persons under quarantine orders have also challenged the detention based on constitutional "equal protection" claims. The Equal Protection Clause of the 14th Amendment prohibits government actions that treat people differently based on classifications such as race or national origin (to name just two), unless the government has a strong justification for doing so. In the most infamous US quarantine case, *Jew Ho v. Williamson* [12], a California court struck down an order of the San Francisco Board of Health that quarantined sections of the city's Chinatown based in part on the race of the persons living within the quarantined area. The court held that the quarantine violated the Constitution's 14th Amendment guarantee of equal protection.

In the last 50 years, because quarantine has been used so rarely in the US, legal challenges have been infrequent and only a few cases have reached appellate courts. Because of the paucity of recent cases, it is difficult to predict how courts would now view challenges to quarantine, especially in the context of a large epidemic. Over the past 50 years, the civil rights era has dawned and the right to privacy (i.e., personal autonomy), which emerged in case law beginning with *Griswold v. Connecticut* (381 US 479, US Supreme Court, 1965), has become part of the constitutional landscape. Over the same period, the law of civil confinement for persons with mental disabilities or mental illness (which has been analogized to quarantine) has also expanded [14]. In addition, as mentioned above, the public health concept of quarantine has evolved to include a governmental duty to provide aid to persons confined.

Using an analogy to the law of civil commitment for mentally disabled persons [42], scholars have postulated that contemporary courts would categorize bodily restraint for communicable disease control as implicating a "fundamental right," that would trigger the highest level of judicial review, called strict scrutiny [14,17]. Under strict scrutiny, the government must show that its action is justified by a "compelling government interest"—in the case of quarantine, a crucial need for the restriction to prevent the transmission of a dangerous disease. The government would also have to show that the quarantine restrictions were "narrowly tailored" and employed the least restrictive means of confinement available. Courts might also require that persons in quarantine have a safe and healthful environment and be provided with high-priority medical care, food, and shelter [43].

Persons who challenge their quarantine detention in court carry a distinctly heavy burden. Under current constitutional doctrine, courts give general deference to government agency interpretations of law [44] and, traditionally, they give specific deference to public health officials' judgments on the need for quarantine [29,31–33]. In addition, the actual potential for governmental abuse of quarantine in the US now is likely lower than in the pre-civil rights era, especially the blatant racial/ethnic abuse "with an evil eye and an unequal hand," described in *Jew Ho v. Williamson*. Furthermore, public health officials can now apply quarantine more judiciously than in the past because of faster access to consultation with experts, better epidemiologic data [45], and an improved understanding of infectious disease transmission dynamics.

Despite these factors in their favor, public health officials can expect courts to referee petitions from detained persons impartially and to invalidate detentions that are justified inadequately or applied unfairly, ineptly, or unlawfully. Officials who plan to use quarantine laws should be prepared to make a strong case based on sound medical and epidemiologic evidence, rational and unbiased decision making, and due consideration for the good of the whole population and the welfare of the individuals confined.

Conclusions

In the US, quarantine does not exist outside the law. Thus, as the law changes, so must quarantine. The ethical concept of quarantine has certainly evolved in recent decades. As discussed above, some public health scholars believe that the law and ethics of quarantine have already adapted to consider developments in civil rights and disability law (standards for declaring quarantine, due process requirements, etc.), and that these adaptations only await recognition by the courts during future litigation. Time will prove this right or wrong.

In the present moment, however, several important questions about quarantine law await resolution. A detailed discussion of these is beyond the reach of this chapter, but some of the most salient ones are summarized as follows:

• How would a large-scale quarantine (regional or national) be enforced under existing law? Are federal and state resources sufficient to enforce a mass quarantine order? These questions are under active discussion and planning within federal and state agencies.

• What mechanisms can be used to encourage people to comply with quarantine orders? For example, what legal routes exist to compensate detainees for economic losses incurred because of compliance with quarantine orders? In a recent survey, 27% of respondents said they or a family member would be likely to lose their job or business if they stayed home for 7–10 days because of government orders during an influenza pandemic [46].

• What is the proper amount of specificity for quarantine procedures in state law? To what extent should state quarantine laws be reformed? Immediately after the September 2001 attacks and the subsequent anthrax-laced letter mailings, CDC commissioned a group of scholars to write the Draft Model State Emergency Health Powers Act [47]. The Draft Model Act was offered as a tool that states could use in reviewing their public health emergency laws. The Draft Act provides model language for state quarantine laws that is substantially more specific and detailed than many existing state laws. As of July 15, 2006, 44 states had adopted one or more statutory provisions consistent with the Draft Model Act [15]. However, some legal experts and observers have criticized the Act as a threat to civil liberties [48,49]. Others, concerned that a high level of specificity in state laws could hamper the litheness needed by state officials to respond to emergencies, or could increase the potential for litigation, have stated their preference for less specific, more flexible statutes [50].

No wide-scale intensive quarantine has been imposed in the US since the 1918 influenza pandemic. No one can foretell the future use of quarantine because no one can foretell the communicable diseases that will emerge in the future and the technological alternatives to quarantine (vaccines, prophylactic antibiotics, etc.) that will be available. Furthermore, because quarantine is, in one sense, a temporary interruption of social communities, the future of quarantine is tied to the future configuration of those communities. Whatever the future of quarantine, law will be an essential part.

References

1 Forensic Epidemiology Quarantine Task Force, Buscombe County, NC. Final Report. 2003. Available from: http://www2.cdc.gov/phlp/docs/BuncombeCounty.pdf. Accessed April 30, 2007.
2 The Holy Bible, Leviticus.

3 Gottfried RS. *The Black Death*. New York: The Free Press; 1983.

4 Clemow FG. The origin of "quarantine." *BMJ* 1929;**1**: 122–3.

5 Hopkins DR. *Princes and Peasants: Smallpox in History*. Chicago: University of Chicago Press; 1983.

6 Parmet WE. Health care and the Constitution: public health and the role of the state in the framing era. *Hastings Constitutional Law Q* 1993;**20**:267–335.

7 Hoffman RE. Quarantine in the United States in the 1990s. *Curr Issues Public Health* 1995;**1**:16–9.

8 Centers for Disease Control and Prevention. Quarantine and other measures to control an import-associated measles outbreak—Iowa, 2004. *MMWR Morb Mortal Wkly Rep* 2004;**53**:969–71.

9 Svoboda T, Henry B, Shulman L, *et al*. Public health measures to control the spread of the severe acute respiratory syndrome during the outbreak in Toronto. *N Engl J Med* 2004;**350**:2352–61.

10 Department of Health and Human Services. Community Strategy for Pandemic Influenza Mitigation [report online]. Washington: Department of Health and Human Services; 2007. Available from: http://www.pandemicflu.gov/plan/community/commitigation.html. Accessed April 30, 2007.

11 Markel H. *Quarantine! East European Jewish Immigrants and the New York City Epidemics of 1892*. Baltimore: The Johns Hopkins University Press; 1997.

12 *Jew Ho v. Williamson et al.*, 103 F 10 (Circuit Court, N.D. California, 1900).

13 Cetron M, Landwirth J. Public health and ethical considerations in planning for quarantine. *Yale J Biol Med* 2005;**78**:1–6.

14 Gostin LO, Burris S, Lazzarini Z. The law and the public's health: a study of infectious disease law in the United States. *Columbia Law J* 1999;**99**:59–128.

15 The Model State Emergency Health Powers Act: Legislative Update [report online]. Available from: http://www.publichealthlaw.net/Resources/Modellaws.htm#MSEHPA. Accessed April 30, 2007.

16 US Const. Art 1, Sect. 8.

17 Gostin LO. *Public Health Law: Power, Duty, Restraint*. Berkeley: University of California Press; 2000.

18 Goodman RA, Kocher PL, O'Brien DJ, Alexander FS. The Structure of law in public health systems and practice. In: Goodman RA *et al*. (eds.), *Law in Public Health Practice*. Oxford: Oxford University Press; 2007.

19 Department of Health and Human Services. Control of Communicable Diseases; Proposed Rule 42 CFR Parts 70 and 71. 70 *Fed Reg* 71892–948 (November 29, 2005).

20 42 USC Sect. 264(a) (2006).

21 42 USC Sect. 264(d) (2006).

22 Measures in the event of inadequate local control, 42 CFR Sect. 70.2 (2006).

23 Misrahi JJ, Foster JA, Shaw, FE, Cetron MS. HHS/CDC legal response to the SARS outbreak. *Emerg Inf Dis* 2004;**10**(2):353–55.

24 Exec. Order No. 13375, 70 *Fed Reg* 17299 (April 5, 2005), amending Exec. Order No. 13375, Sect. 1 (April 3, 2003).

25 Fried C. *Saying What the Law Is: The Constitution in the Supreme Court*. Cambridge, Mass.: Harvard University Press; 2004.

26 Shaw FE, McKie KL, Liveoak CA, Goodman RA. State Public Health Counsel Review Team. Variation in quarantine powers among the 10 most populous US states in 2004. *Am J Pub Health* 2007;**97**:S38–43.

27 California Health & Safety Code Sect. 100170 (2006).

28 California Health & Safety Code Sect. 120140, 120145, 120210 (2006).

29 *People ex. rel Barmore v. Robertson*, 302 Ill. 422 (Supreme Court of Illinois, 1922).

30 20 ILCS 3305/7 (2006).

31 Richards, EP, Rathbun, KC. Public health law. In: Wallace RB (ed.), *Public Health and Preventive Medicine*. 14th edn. Stamford: Appleton & Lange; 1998.

32 Stier DD, Nicks DM. Public health and the judiciary. In: Goodman RA, *et al*. (eds.), *Law in Public Health Practice*. Oxford: Oxford University Press; 2007.

33 *Chiropractic Assn. v. Hilleboe*, 12 NY2d 109 (Court of Appeals of New York, 1962).

34 42 USC Sect. 264–272 (2006).

35 *United States v. Lopez*, 514 US 549 (US Supreme Court, 1995).

36 "The term 'qualifying stage', with respect to a communicable disease, means that such disease is (A) in a communicable stage; or (B) in a precommunicable stage, if the disease would be likely to cause a public health emergency if transmitted to other individuals." 42 USC Sect. 264(d) (2006).

37 Institute of Medicine. *The Future of the Public's Health in the 21st Century*. Washington, DC: National Academies of Science; 2002.

38 Associated Press. Report: Don't count on federal bird flu rescue: White House says local communities must prepare for pandemic disruptions [news report online]. MSNBC Web site; May 3, 2006. Available from: http://www.msnbc.msn.com/id/12607854/. Accessed April 30, 2007.

39 *Souvannarath v. Hadden*, 95 Cal. App. 4th 1115 (Court of Appeal of California, Fifth Appellate District, 2002).

40 See Tex. Health & Safety Code Sect. 81.151–81.211 (2006).

41 *Morales v. Turman*, 562 F2d 993 (US Court of Appeals for the Fifth Circuit, 1977).

42 See, *Greene v. Edwards*, 263 SE2d 661 (Supreme Court of Appeals of West Virginia, 1980).

43 *Youngberg v. Romeo*, 457 US 307 (US Supreme Court, 1982).

44 *Chevron, U.S.A., Inc. v. NRDC*, Inc., 467 US 837 (US Supreme Court 1984).

45 CDC. PHIN: Biosense [homepage]. Available from: http://www.cdc.gov/biosense/. Accessed April 30, 2007.

46 Harvard School of Public Health. HSPH press release: In the case of an outbreak of pandemic flu, large majority of Americans willing to make major changes in their lives; Survey also finds many people would face critical work-related problems [press release online]; October 26, 2006. Available from: www.hsph.harvard .edu/press/releases/press10262006.html. Accessed April 30, 2007.

47 The Model State Emergency Health Powers Act [report online]; 2001. Available from: http://www.public healthlaw.net/MSEHPA/MSEHPA2.pdf. Accessed April 30, 2007.

48 Turley J. A prescription for disaster. *Chicago Tribune*, January 2, 2002:15.

49 Annas GJ. Bioterrorism, public health, and civil liberties. *N Engl J Med* 2002;**346**:1337–42.

50 Richards EP, Rathbun KC. Legislative alternatives to the Model State Emergency Health Powers Act (MSEHPA). LSU Program in Law, Science, and Public Health White Paper #2. Available from: http://biotech.law.lsu .edu/blaw/bt/MSEHPA_review.htm. Accessed April 30, 2007.

36 Training in applied epidemiology and infectious disease surveillance: contributions of the Epidemic Intelligence Service

Denise Koo, Douglas H. Hamilton & Stephen B. Thacker

The Centers for Disease Control and Prevention's (CDC) Epidemic Intelligence Service (EIS) (US Department of Health and Human Services) is a 2-year training and service program with a focus on applied epidemiology [1]. The EIS program emphasizes the public health practice of epidemiology and plays a critical role in developing practitioners experienced in the most current methods of public health surveillance, an area not often covered in academic training. In addition to learning about surveillance, EIS officers learn how to evaluate and contribute to actual surveillance systems, and through their training and work, they disseminate new surveillance methods across the country. The EIS program serves as an international model for training public health practitioners of epidemiology, with >30 programs around the world patterned after it [2]. This chapter describes the history of the EIS program, its contributions to surveillance and challenges encountered, and includes sample training curriculum and references for teaching tools for public health surveillance, all of which may be used to develop similar training programs in applied epidemiology and infectious disease surveillance outside of the United States (US).

Background

In 1951, the EIS program was formed at what was then the Communicable Disease Center as a combined training and service program in the public health practice of epidemiology. The program was established initially in response to concerns about the threat of biologic terrorism and the related shortage of epidemiologists who could respond to such threats [3]. The training program, which relies heavily on EIS officers' "learning while doing," was based on a concept originated by Joseph W. Mountin and implemented subsequently by Alexander Langmuir [4]. The implementation adapted a combination of the hands-on experience of the medical residency and the case-study method then used at the Johns Hopkins School of Hygiene and Public Health. After a brief foundational course in applied epidemiology, EIS officers were assigned to CDC headquarters programs, to field positions in state and local health departments, or to universities. In all of these assignments, officers conducted special studies in epidemiology, participated in disease surveillance, and were available to respond to epidemic threats, including threats of biologic or chemical terrorism.

The EIS program has flourished based on Langmuir's assumption that good things would happen if bright, motivated, and ambitious young officers are given challenging problems to solve in the real world. High expectations for performance both in the field and in the formal presentation of epidemiologic research to their peers and through publication in peer-reviewed journals further drive the successes of the program and of the individual officers. The connection of EIS officers to a formal training program even when assigned in the field domestically and internationally enhances the expectation to conduct credible science in all settings. In short, officers are required to solve problems in the field in service to a community, and they also must defend

---

Box 36.1 Epidemic Intelligence Service requirements.

• Professionals with a strong interest in applied epidemiology who meet one of the following qualifications are eligible to apply to the EIS:
• Physicians with at least 1 yr of clinical training—specialties of incoming officers have included internal medicine, pediatrics, family practice, preventive medicine, occupational medicine, surgery, and obstetrics and gynecology
• Other doctoral-degree holders (e.g., PhD or DrPH) in relevant sciences such as epidemiology, biostatistics, and biological, environmental, social behavioral, or nutrition sciences

• Dentists, physician assistants, and nurses with a Master of Public Health (MPH) or equivalent degree
• Veterinarians with an MPH or equivalent degree or relevant public health experience
• Approximately 10 international applicants are selected to enter the in-coming class each year
Note: US citizens or permanent residents with a clinical degree of eligibility must have an active US unrestricted license to practice that clinical specialty.

---

their science to their supervisors both in the field and at CDC. At the same time, public health programs at CDC and in the states benefit from the service provided by officers not only in acute situations, but also through the more in-depth investigations and evaluations required by the program.

Since 1951, over 3000 professionals have served in the EIS, including physicians, veterinarians, nurses, dentists, engineers, and persons with doctoral degrees in multiple health-related fields (e.g.,

epidemiology, anthropology, sociology, and microbiology). The fields of experience have expanded beyond the initial infectious disease focus to include environmental health, occupational health and safety, chronic disease, injury prevention, birth defects, and developmental disabilities (see Box 36.1 and www.cdc.gov/eis for eligibility criteria). A majority of EIS graduates remain employed in public health upon completion of the program (Table 36.1).

Table 36.1 Professional experience of six cohorts of Epidemic Intelligence Service officers following completion of the program.

EIS class year (no. of officers)	Additional training obtained following EIS				Initial employment following EIS										Total no. and % of EIS officers employment in in public health	
	Clinical residency		CDC Preventive Medicine Residency*		CDC		Other public health		Academic		Private practice					
	No.	%	No.	%	No.	%	No.	%	No.	%	No.	%			No.	%
1955 (36)	18	50	—	—	12	33	3	8	10	28	11	31			20	56
1965 (31)	21	68	—	—	11	35	7	23	10	32	3	10			16	52
1975 (49)	23	47	7	14	20	41	6	12	16	33	7	14			30	61
1985 (67)	3	4	18	27	32	48	24	36	8	12	3	4			59	88
1995 (75)	1	1	12	16	31	41	35	47	5	7	4	5			66	88
2004 (81)	4	5	2	2	46	57	23	28	11	14	1	1			69	85

*The Centers for Disease Control and Prevention (CDC) Preventive Medicine Residency was established in 1972.

Box 36.2 Surveillance training schedule for EIS officers, Class of 2005.

Surveillance Training for EIS Officers

EIS officers receive several surveillance lectures during the Summer Course, the initial didactic training at the beginning of their two year assignment (see below). Once officers move to their permanent assignments one of their first tasks is to conduct a formal evaluation of a surveillance system. This evaluation is then presented to their classmates and staff three months later during the first year Fall Course.

Summer Course Lectures—Learning Objectives

Surveillance Overview
- Define public health surveillance and its role in the practice of epidemiology.
- List the various uses of surveillance data.
- Give examples of several sources of data used for surveillance and discuss their applicability to the area of their EIS assignment.

Analysis & Interpretation of Surveillance Data
- List several features of surveillance data that influence data analysis
- Describe the main strategies for analysis and interpretation of data from various types of surveillance systems.
- Describe the difference in analytic approach when surveillance data are used for outbreak detection vs. other purposes.

Display & Dissemination of Surveillance
- Describe the role of clear visual representation of data in promoting accurate interpretation of surveillance findings.
- Describe how a variety of data presentation formats, including graphs, maps, and tables, may be used to support surveillance system objectives.
- Review best practices for effective graphical/tabular display of surveillance data and provide examples.

Evaluating a Surveillance System
- Describe the steps in organizing and carrying out an evaluation of a surveillance system
- Describe the major parameters that need to be assessed or measured as part of a surveillance system evaluation
- Describe how evaluation of a surveillance system for outbreak detection differs from one for individual case detection.

Case Study – Public Health Surveillance in New York City – Then and Now
- Define surveillance and identify the key features of a surveillance system
- List the types of information that should be collected on a surveillance case report form
- Describe the differences between notifiable disease surveillance and syndromic surveillance
- Summarize and interpret surveillance data

Fall Course—Learning Objectives

EISO Surveillance System Presentations
- Identify the critical elements of a surveillance system
- Describe the limitations of surveillance data
- Discuss a specific health event
- Describe a critical review of an existing or proposed surveillance system using "Guidelines for Evaluating Surveillance Systems" (MMWR 2001; 50: RR-13) in organizing your presentation.
- Write a 600 word summary of selected surveillance system including the subheadings: (1) stakeholders, (2) system description (3) evaluation design, (4) critical evidence (5) recommendations (7) lessons learned

Surveillance During a Disaster
- Describe the operation of an emergency surveillance system during a disaster response.
- Recognize the potential obstacles to establishing an emergency system.
- Define the surveillance needs during a disaster at the local, state and national levels.

Box 36.3 Recent EIS surveillance evaluations.

Emerging microbial threats: "Southern Sudan Early Warning and Response Network (EWARN)." "Active surveillance for acute respiratory illness, Sa Kaeo, Thailand."

Antimicrobial resistance: "Evaluation of the surveillance system for antimicrobial susceptibility of invasive *Streptococcus pneumoniae* in Chicago." "Methicillin resistant *Staphylococcus aureus* surveillance in North Dakota, 2000–2005."

Chronic disease: "Evaluation of a surveillance system for cancer clusters using cancer registry data."

Behavioral: "Physical inactivity surveillance in U.S. pre-school and school-age children: the National Health and Nutrition Examination Survey (NHANES)." "Evaluation of the Emergency Medical Services (EMS) suicide surveillance system of Maine." "Surveillance of methamphetamine use among sexually active female youth: the National Youth Risk Behavior Surveillance System (YRBSS)."

Occupational: "Surveillance of hospitalized injuries in Alaskan workers." "Silicosis surveillance in New Mexico." "Incidence of West Nile Virus among workers in four U.S. states in 2002."

Environmental: "Evaluation of the Kansas childhood lead poisoning prevention program." "Development of a statewide surveillance system for childhood asthma in Texas elementary schools."

Natural disasters: "A drop-in surveillance system for outbreak detection and disease reporting among Hurricane Katrina evacuees in San Antonio, Texas 2005." "Emergency department-based surveillance during hurricanes: implementation of the Early Aberration Reporting System (EARS)—Florida, 2004."

Biologic and chemical terrorism: "Evaluation of a syndromic surveillance system—Philadelphia, 2004."

International: "International cholera surveillance." "Evaluation of the TB/HIV surveillance system in Ethiopia."

Proposed systems: "Surveillance system for occupational amputation injuries in California workers: a design proposal." "Determining the prevalence of hyperbilirubinemia: feasibility of a surveillance system."

the next year, 246 cases of CSD were reported to the Connecticut Department of Health. Analysis of these surveillance data or studies derived from them enabled investigators to characterize the epidemiology of this disease among residents of Connecticut and to identify risk factors for acquisition of this disease, including exposure to kittens and the possible role of fleas in transmission [19,20].

• In September 1997, the Tennessee Department of Health was notified of an apparent cluster of encephalitis cases among children examined at a hospital in the eastern part of the state. The children were infected with the La Crosse virus, a leading cause of pediatric arboviral encephalitis in the US and endemic in the upper-Midwestern US, but an uncommon cause of encephalitis in Tennessee [21]. As part of the investigation, the EIS officer assigned to the Tennessee Department of Health

established an active surveillance system for La Crosse virus infection at a large pediatric-referral hospital in eastern Tennessee. During the next 2 years, this surveillance system confirmed that eastern Tennessee had become an endemic region for the transmission of La Crosse virus infection [22]. The health department used this information to educate area clinicians about the importance of including La Crosse virus infection in the differential diagnosis of a febrile illness presenting among children in the summer.

Cutting edge contributions to surveillance

Surveillance paradigms began shifting in the 1990s, particularly for infectious diseases, and they continue to evolve today [23]. The focus of surveillance has broadened from an emphasis primarily on diseases and outcomes to include syndromes or indicators that occur earlier in the disease process (i.e., syndromic surveillance; covered in Chapter 26) [24]. For such data, relying solely on traditional sources of collection (i.e., clinicians and laboratories) is insufficient, and practitioners have begun exploring the usefulness of such data sources as pharmacies, school or workplace absentee records, or 9-1-1 calls. Cognizant of the opportunities provided by advances in information technology, public health officials hoped to collect the majority of these data through electronic capture or transfer of existing data, and not through manual data-collection methods that remain common practice. CDC also took the lead by funding the National Electronic Disease Surveillance System ((NEDSS), www.cdc.gov) initiative. Moreover, throughout the 1990s and into the twenty-first century, the need to detect deliberately caused as well as naturally occurring illnesses remains paramount.

EIS officers have been at the forefront of these cutting edge efforts. Officers and graduates have played key roles in the development of short-term ("drop-in") surveillance systems such as surveillance systems for specific events (e.g., the 1999 World Trade Organization meeting in Seattle, the major political party conventions in 2000, and the Utah Winter Olympics in 2002) and innovative early warning systems (e.g., tracking dead birds as sentinel surveillance for West Nile virus) [25,26], in addition to the efforts to develop longer-term, automated links with the healthcare system [27–30]. Seventy-five EIS officers implemented, under direction of an EIS graduate, emergency department-based syndromic surveillance in 15 hospitals throughout New York City, and at ground zero within days of the September 11, 2001, attack on the World Trade Center (Plate 36.1)

Challenges in teaching public health surveillance

The EIS program has had a long and successful history of training EIS officers who learn while they provide service. However, the program faces challenges to maintaining its relevance and currency in a rapidly changing field. The fundamental challenge

is the tension between the pressure on the program and on EIS supervisors to provide training to the officers and the pressure on the officers to provide service. Typically, the program achieves the right balance between these forces, because EIS officers frequently do learn while performing services, especially when they have been provided with sufficient preparation and ongoing mentoring on the job. However, the applied field of public health surveillance also poses additional challenges that must be considered when teaching surveillance.

Although surveillance is a cornerstone of epidemiology and the public health approach, this is not well-understood by EIS officers at the beginning of their training. In fact, it might even be resisted by them; the need for careful critique (including review of quality, completeness, and representativeness) of a particular surveillance system and the critical role surveillance plays in the estimation of disease burden and development and evaluation of public health interventions may not be appreciated. The foundational role of surveillance warrants its inclusion early in the curriculum, but the short time frame between the end of the summer course and the fall surveillance course often does not permit actual analysis of surveillance data, making the surveillance evaluation more of a descriptive exercise. In addition, surveillance data quality is difficult to ensure, often because of the distributed nature of data collection or because the data were collected for other purposes. Appropriate interpretation and use of surveillance data, therefore, remain a critical challenge for applied epidemiologists. For some, the surveillance evaluation is simply an item to check off on the list of EIS requirements, an attitude that can be mirrored by some supervisors, who echo the officers' impatience to get out and do "real work" (e.g., an outbreak investigation or analytic epidemiology), a situation where they have more control over the data collection and quality. Not until later in their EIS experience do officers fully understand surveillance and its importance to public health practice.

The EIS program staff also face challenges of finding the appropriate timing and supply of didactic and interactive training material, lecturers, and supervisors. For example, since the early 1990s, EIS officers had often complained that the curricular material on different surveillance approaches, analyses, and evaluations were provided (if at all) during the fall course, after the EIS officers had completed their evaluations, rather than during the summer, at a time that they felt would have been more useful for preparation. The curricular plan was revised in 2004 so that these materials appeared in the summer course and included tips on how to conduct a surveillance evaluation. In addition, given the rapidly evolving nature of modern surveillance approaches with links to public health informatics, fewer experts or established scientific principles were available; where experts are available, whether epidemiologists or informaticists, they often have limited experience with teaching (and in the case of informaticists, a tendency to use jargon not easily understood by epidemiologists), and too few case examples are used to illustrate the principles. The majority of epidemiologists at CDC and from state and local health departments, for example, do not know the difference between the conceptual, logical, and physical data models crucial for building links among disparate electronic information systems, much less how to participate in building these data models. Officers sometimes resist using data standards, citing lack of responsiveness to their program needs, and too few are able to analyze data distributed in relational databases, rather than simple flat files. Yet, these are critical competencies for epidemiologists practicing in this electronic era.

Future directions

The increasing emphasis on reuse of data already captured for other purposes (e.g., National Health Information Network, www.hhs.gov, and NEDSS) presents exciting new opportunities for public health, but it also highlights challenges and gaps in the science and methods of surveillance and the training needs of epidemiologists. CDC and CSTE convened an expert panel in October 2004 to define competencies for applied epidemiologists (www.cdc.gov and www.cste.org). These competencies, finalized in mid-2006, define knowledge, skills, and abilities necessary for epidemiologists practicing in local, state, and federal public health agencies, based on current and emerging needs of applied epidemiology practice.

Surveillance was specifically identified as a competency area in the major epidemiologic domain of assessment and analysis, with 5 subcompetencies and 28 sub-subcompetencies explicitly described for mid-level epidemiologists under the surveillance heading (Box 36.4). Additionally, a subgroup of the panel paid particular attention to defining the informatics competencies needed by epidemiologists for effective engagement with such initiatives as NEDSS. CDC and CSTE anticipate that the competencies will be used as the basis of instructional competencies for the training of governmental epidemiologists, and as the framework for developing position descriptions, work expectations, and job announcements for epidemiologists practicing in public health agencies.

Teaching surveillance to EIS officers has been built on the insights of Alexander Langmuir and has evolved to reflect the expansion of the CDC mission; the training program also has adapted to changing times and incorporated the newest tools and technologies to enhance the surveillance process. The EIS program will certainly assess which of the CDC/CSTE competencies constitute an appropriate focus for a 2-year program of on-the-job learning and service in applied epidemiology. Subsequently, the training of EIS officers will be revised to ensure they have the tools and experiences to achieve competence in modern-era public health surveillance.

Select teaching tools for public health surveillance

- Key references in the literature:
  ◦ Thacker SB, Berkelman RL. Public health surveillance in the United States. *Epidemiol Rev* 1988;**10**:164–90.
  ◦ Centers for Disease Control and Prevention. Updated guidelines for evaluating public health surveillance systems: recommendations from the guidelines working group. *MMWR Morb Mortal Wkly Rep* 2001;**50**(No. RR-13).
  ◦ Dean AD, Dean JA, Burton AH, Dicker RC. Epi Info™: a general purpose microcomputer program for public health information systems. *Am J Prev Med* 1991;7:178–82.

Box 36.4 Surveillance competencies for mid-level epidemiologists.

Conduct surveillance activities

1 Design surveillance for the particular public health issue under consideration
   • Identify types of surveillance methods for specific public health problems
   • Identify information system(s) to support surveillance systems
   • Recommend types of surveillance systems for specific public health problems
   • Identify additional burden to public health system and reporting entity anticipated to result from the proposed surveillance system
2 Identify surveillance data needs
   • Create case definition(s) based on person, place, and time
   • Describe sources, quality, and limitations of surveillance data
   • Define the data elements to be collected or reported
   • Identify mechanisms to transfer data from source to public health agency
   • Define timeliness required for data collection
   • Determine frequency of reporting
   • Describe potential uses of data to inform surveillance system design
   • Define the functional requirements of the supporting information system
3 Implement new or revise existing surveillance systems
   • Define objectives and uses of surveillance system
   • Test data collection, data storage, and analytical methods
   • Create working surveillance system
   • Verify that data collection occurs according to the defined surveillance system parameters (e.g., timeliness, frequency)
   • Ensure correct classification of cases according to the case definition
   • Interview persons with illness to solicit necessary information
   • Monitor data quality
   • Create good working relationships with reporting entities
   • Provide feedback to reporting entities and other organizations or individuals who need to know about the data or system
4 Identify key findings from the surveillance system
   • Examine system's results in the context of current scientific knowledge
   • Identify implications to public health programs
   • Develop conclusions from the surveillance data
   • Communicate results to agency managers and to reporters of surveillance data
5 Conduct evaluation of surveillance systems
   • Evaluate surveillance systems using national guidance and methods (German RR and the Guidelines Working Group. Updated Guidelines for Evaluating Public Health Surveillance Systems. *MMWR* 2001;50(RR-13):1–35)
   • Propose recommendations for modifications to surveillance systems on the basis of evaluation
   • Implement changes to surveillance system on the basis of results of evaluation

---

○ Teutsch SM, Churchill RE (eds.). *Principles and Practice of Public Health Surveillance*, 2nd edn. New York: Oxford; 2000.

○ Koo D, Wharton M, Birkhead G. Case definitions for infectious conditions under public health surveillance. *MMWR Morb Mortal Wkly Rep* 1997;46(No. RR-10). Available from: http://www.cdc.gov/epo/dphsi/casedef/index.htm.

• Some online resources for teaching surveillance and epidemiology:

○ Overview of Public Health Surveillance lecture, Dr. Denise Koo:
- http://www.pitt.edu/~super1/lecture/cdc0071/index.htm (University of Pittsburgh Supercourse) or
- http://www.cdc.gov/epo/dphsi/phs/overview.htm
○ Other resources on public health surveillance: http://www.cdc.gov/epo/dphsi
○ EIS case studies: http://www.cdc.gov/eis/casestudies/casestudyex.htm
○ *Principles of Epidemiology*, 3rd edn:
- http://www.2a.cdc.gov/PHTNOnline/registration/detailpage.asp?res_id=1394

References

1 Thacker SB, Dannenberg AL, Hamilton DH. The Epidemic Intelligence Service of the Centers for Disease Control and Prevention: 50 years of training and service in applied epidemiology. *Am J Epidemiol* 2001;**154**:985–92.

2 White M, McDonnell SM, Werker D, Cardenas V, Thacker SB. The applied epidemiology and service network in the year 2000. *Am J Epidemiol* 2001;**154**:993–9.

3 Langmuir AD, Andrews JM. Biological warfare defense. 2: The Epidemic Intelligence Service of the Communicable Disease Center. *Am J Public Health* 1952;**42**:235–8.

4 Schaffner W, LaForce FM. Training field epidemiologists: Alexander D. Langmuir and the Epidemic Intelligence Service. *Am J Epidemiol* 1996;**144**:S16–22.

5 Nathanson N, Langmuir AD. The Cutter incident: poliomyelitis following formaldehyde-inactivated poliovirus vaccination in the United States during the spring of 1955. I: Background. *Am J Hyg* 1963;**78**:29–81.

6 Rosenberg MJ, Gangarosa EJ, Pollard RA, Wallace M, Brolnitsky O, Marr JS. *Shigella* surveillance in the United States, 1975. *J Infect Dis* 1977;**136**:458–60.

7 Marier R. The reporting of communicable disease. *Am J Epidemiol* 1977;**105**:587–90.

8 Kimball AM, Thacker SB, Levy ME. *Shigella* surveillance in a large metropolitan area: assessment of a passive reporting system. *Am J Public Health* 1980;**70**:164–6.

9 Schaffner W, Scott HD, Rosenstein BJ, Byrne EB. Innovative communicable disease reporting: the Rhode Island experience. *HSMHA Health Rep* 1971;**86**:431–6.

10 Thacker SB, Berkelman RL. Public health surveillance in the United States. *Epidemiol Rev* 1988;**10**:164–90.

11 Thacker SB, Berkelman RL, Stroup DF. The science of public health surveillance. *J Public Health Policy* 1989;**10**:187–203.

12 Thacker SB, Parrish RG, Trowbridge FL. A method for evaluating systems of epidemiological surveillance. *World Health Stat Q* 1988b;**41**:11–8.

13 Klaucke DN, Buehler JW, Thacker SB, Parrish RG, Trowbridge FL, Berkelman RL. Guidelines for evaluating surveillance systems: Centers for Disease Control. *MMWR Morb Mortal Wkly Rep* 1988;**37**(No. S-5):1–18.

14 Centers for Disease Control and Prevention. Updated guidelines for evaluating public health surveillance systems: recommendations from the guidelines working group. *MMWR Morb Mortal Wkly Rep* 2001;**50**(No. RR-13):1–51.

15 Dean AD, Dean JA, Burton AH, Dicker RC. Epi Info™: a general purpose microcomputer program for public health information systems. *Am J Prev Med* 1991;**7**:178–82.

16 Centers for Disease Control. National electronic telecommunications system for surveillance—United States, 1990–1991. *MMWR Morb Mortal Wkly Rep* 1991;**40**:502–3.

17 Furness BW, Beach MJ, Robert JM. Giardiasis surveillance, United States 1992–1997. *MMWR Morb Mortal Wkly Rep* 2000;**49**(No. SS-7):1–13.

18 Ghosh TS, Vogt RL. The implementation and evaluation of an active influenza surveillance system at the local level: a model for local health agencies. *Am J Public Health* (in press).

19 Hamilton DH, Zangwill KM, Hadler JL, Cartter ML. Cat-scratch disease—Connecticut, 1992–1993. *J Infect Dis* 1995;**172**:570–3.

20 Zangwill KM, Hamilton DH, Perkins BA, *et al.* Cat scratch disease in Connecticut: epidemiology, risk factors, and evaluation of a new diagnostic test. *N Engl J Med* 1993;**329**:8–13.

21 Jones TF, Craig AS, Nasci RS, *et al.* Newly recognized focus of La Crosse encephalitis in Tennessee. *Clin Infect Dis* 1999;**28**:93–7.

22 Jones TF, Erwin PC, Craig AS, *et al.* Serological survey and active surveillance for La Crosse virus infections among children in Tennessee. *Clin Infect Dis* 2000;**31**:1284–7.

23 Koo D. Leveraging syndromic surveillance. *J Public Health Manag Pract* 2005;**11**:181–3.

24 Centers for Disease Control and Prevention. Syndromic surveillance: reports from a national conference, 2003. *MMWR Morb Mortal Wkly Rep* 2006; **53**(suppl):1-268.

25 Eidson M, Komar N, Sorhage F, *et al.* Crow deaths as a sentinel surveillance system for West Nile virus in the northeastern United States, 1999. *Emerg Infect Dis* 2001;**7**:615–20.

26 Mostashari F, Kulldorff M, Hartman JJ, Miller JR, Kulasekera V. Dead bird clusters as an early warning

system for West Nile virus activity. *Emerg Infect Dis* 2003;9:641–6.

27 Effler P, Ching-Lee M, Bogard A, Ieong M, Nekomoto T, Jernigan D. Statewide system of electronic notifiable disease reporting from clinical laboratories. *JAMA* 1999;**282**:1845–50.

28 Jernigan DB. Electronic laboratory-based reporting: opportunities and challenges for surveillance. *Emerg Infect Dis* 2001;7:538.

29 Panackal AA, M'ikanatha NM, Tsui F, *et al*. Automatic electronic laboratory-based reporting of notifiable infectious diseases at a large health system [serial online]. *Emerg Infect Dis* July 2002 [last updated May 13, 2002]. Available from: http://www.cdc.gov/ncidod/EID/vol8no7/01-0493.htm. Accessed May 26, 2006.

30 Mostashari F, Fine A, Das D, Adams J, Layton M. Use of ambulance dispatch data as an early warning system for communitywide influenza-like illness, New York City. *J Urban Health* 2003;**80**(2, suppl 1):i43–9.

37 New York State International Training Program for Fogarty Fellows

Dale L. Morse, Louise-Anne McNutt & Robert A. Bednarczyk

Introduction

Surveillance is a critical element in assessing global infectious disease trends. This chapter describes the challenges and successes of providing surveillance training through the New York State (NYS) International Training Program for Fogarty Fellows to international students from Eastern Europe and Central Asia. The chapter is organized to:
• give an overview of the need for and obstacles to providing international surveillance training
• summarize the NYS program
• provide examples of surveillance methods successfully utilized by our trainees
• describe the benefits and lessons learned during training
• reflect on the importance of providing international surveillance training

Background

Challenges and barriers to implementing surveillance in target countries

The infectious disease surveillance program in the former Soviet Union was supported by the central government and managed by infectious disease surveillance systems in each of its 15 republics. When the Soviet Union dissolved in 1991 and the republics became autonomous nations, the individual infectious disease surveillance systems were suddenly required to continue their responsibilities without any central directives or resources. These systems had a talented pool of trained public health professionals, but no government funds to train new surveillance personnel, support current personnel, or maintain equipment. The social, political, and economic changes that occurred after the fall of the Soviet Union resulted in infectious disease outbreaks that could not be efficiently monitored and controlled by the resource-poor Infectious Disease Surveillance Systems (IDSS) operating in each country [1,2].

The postindependence Armenian IDSS exemplified the problems across the former Soviet Union. Measurement and reporting practices were incomplete, focusing on laboratory confirmation rather than epidemiologic investigation methods [3]. Surveillance staff were hampered by the need to perform time-consuming paper-based reporting through multiple levels of the Armenian Ministry of Health hierarchy. Diseases for which there are few potential public health or medical interventions, such as infectious mononucleosis, or diseases that are not highly pathogenic, such as scabies, were among the 64 diseases monitored in the Armenian IDSS. In preindependence Armenia, coordination between physicians in the health system and epidemiologists in the Ministry of Health allowed the Armenian IDSS to be successful, as cases of infectious disease could easily be identified, tracked, and communicated to the appropriate health officials [3]. Following the collapse of the Soviet Union, immediate financial crises resulted in reduced access to healthcare and an unraveling of the coordinated systems that previously existed. Combining this with the lack of central resource support for public health functions, it is easy to see how the public health infrastructure, including surveillance programs would suffer. This example of infectious disease surveillance in Armenia is representative of the other Soviet Republics [4,5].

The centralized nature of the surveillance systems in the former Soviet Union allowed for homogeneous surveillance methods throughout the Soviet Republics. Even when these programs were fully funded, the lack of risk factor analysis during epidemiologic investigations suggested that resources were not utilized to their full potential, and possibly missed important epidemiologic associations. The reliance on laboratory methods served the surveillance programs well in identifying infectious disease outbreaks; however, the lack of continuous improvements in laboratory facilities and technology left the newly independent republics struggling to address the health challenges of the late twentieth and early twenty-first century, including multidrug-resistant bacteria and mounting sexually transmitted disease (STD) epidemics, including human immunodeficiency virus (HIV) [3,6].

For diseases that are reported and tracked in most IDSS, such as syphilis, surveillance depends on the ability of the healthcare providers to identify and report cases of disease. When Soviet state-sponsored healthcare existed, this type of case finding was easily accomplished. However, when independence triggered a shift in healthcare delivery to the private sector in some newly independent republics, infectious disease reporting decreased, and the impoverished surveillance systems were unable to make up the difference through active case finding. Epidemics that had previously been seen in these countries, such as syphilis, peaked in the mid- to late 1990s then appeared to be under control. Although public health interventions may have effected some of the decline in new syphilis infections, lack of active case finding appears to have created detection bias, resulting in underreporting and an artificially low incidence [7]. This change in the ability to find cases appears to parallel struggles observed in the United States (US) as a result of the privatized nature of healthcare delivery [8].

NYS International Training Program

The NYS International Training Program was initially funded in late 1993 by an NIH Fogarty AIDS training grant to focus on three countries: the Czech Republic, Hungary, and Poland. By 1996, coverage was expanded to include the three Baltic States, Armenia, and Georgia with additional NIH emerging infection and tuberculosis (TB) training monies. The program was further expanded in 1998 and 1999 to Russia, Kazakhstan, Kosovo, and Mongolia (Figure 37.1). Today, the NIH Fogarty AIDS and Global infectious disease research training grants allow the program to focus on four countries: Russia, Georgia, Estonia, and Armenia.

The program goal is to train laboratory scientists, epidemiologists, and other health professionals from Eastern Europe and Central Asia to develop the public health infrastructure of the region and to specifically improve the ability of the infrastructure in these countries to respond to AIDS, its associated infections (such as TB, STDs, and hepatitis) and other emerging infections. This integrated program includes the core areas of surveillance and epidemiology as well as biomedical sciences, and the training incorporates both theoretical and applied instructional methods. The program facilitates needed research and fosters collaborative relationships between US and foreign scientific institutions.

The training objectives are as follows:
• Provide state-of-the-art postdoctoral laboratory training in the US
• Provide training in the US leading to advanced degrees in epidemiology
• Provide short-term on-site training workshops to address AIDS and its associated infections and emerging infectious diseases
• Provide advanced in-country research training on targeted projects in collaboration with US faculty
• Assist foreign institutions with the development of technical expertise to support sustainable independent research
• Train candidates to write competitive research grant proposals
• Provide training in the responsible conduct of research and the incorporation of international perspectives

Fellows are recruited with the help of alumni and in-country partners at collaborating institutions. The program is also advertised via newsletters, mailings to previous trainees and conference attendees, journal advertisements (e.g., *Georgian*

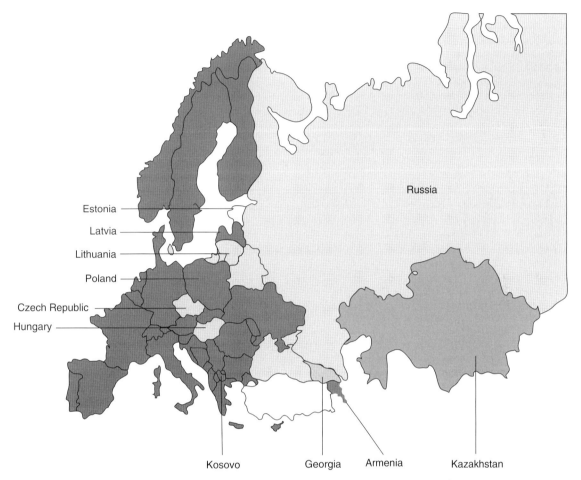

Fig 37.1 Twelve countries in Eastern/Central Europe covered by the New York State International Training Program.

Medical News), and through information provided on the New York State Department of Health's Wadsworth Center's Web site (http://www. wadsworth.org/educate/fogarty/index.htm). The target population for the program consists of physicians and other public health professionals, microbiologists, basic scientists, and other infectious disease specialists. Potential candidates must complete formal written applications and are interviewed by our in-country partners and by NYS International Training Program faculty. They are required to demonstrate academic, scientific, and English proficiency via transcripts, degrees, publications, and standardized exams (e.g., Graduate Record Examination, Test of English as

a Foreign Language). Most have MD or PhD degrees and some work experience. The long-term training is generally for 1–2 years and Fellows sign an agreement to serve an equal amount of time in their home countries; this time is sometimes supported by advanced in-country mini-research grants.

During the past 10 years, the NYS International Training Program has provided support for 67 long-term trainees, 12 of whom are still in training. Of the 55 long-term program graduates, 46 either have returned to positions in their home countries or are pursuing doctorates in the US or Canada, and 3 are US-based researchers conducting AIDS-related studies in Eastern Europe and Central Asia. The program has also provided support for short-term (<6 mo) apprenticeships at US institutions for 40 trainees.

In-country training is a cornerstone of this program: 60 short-term courses in 10 countries have been sponsored over the past 10 years. Approximately 90 US and European faculty have participated and the courses have reached more than 5300 healthcare professionals in Eastern Europe and Central Asia.

As a result of their training, program participants have made significant scientific contributions during and after their training; the impressive volume of scientific publications and presentations at national and international meetings comprises 287 publications, 149 of which list a trainee as first author. In addition, the program develops strong research partners who can successfully compete for funding. Two notable awards include the Fogarty International Research Collaboration Award (FIRCA) and the Fogarty International Center (FIC) funded Global Health Research Initiative Program for New Foreign Investigators (GRIP) Award; 11 other trainees have received funding from a variety of sources.

Provision of surveillance training

Because of its critical importance to epidemiology, surveillance training is a crucial part of the NYS International Training Program and is emphasized in coursework, internships, field projects, and laboratory fellowships as described in the sections that follow.

University at Albany SPH curriculum

The School of Public Health (SPH) is a unique partnership between the University at Albany and the New York State Department of Health (NYSDOH). The programs focus on an applied public health education in both epidemiology and laboratory sciences. A significant part of the instruction is provided by public health professionals who work full-time at the NYSDOH, but have faculty appointments at the School of Public Health. Disease surveillance, a fundamental component of public health, is integrated throughout the curriculum,

providing students an understanding of its design and use for a multitude of communicable diseases (Table 37.1).

Fundamentals of surveillance are covered in the core epidemiology courses taken by all students. This introduction provides an overview of surveillance across public health, including disease (infectious, chronic, and genetic) and exposure (behavioral and environmental) surveillance systems. The basics of person, place, and time are taught and more complex topics, such as syndromic surveillance and evaluation of surveillance systems, are introduced to prepare students for more advanced studies in topic-specific courses.

The basic infectious disease epidemiology course provides an overview of notifiable disease surveillance at the local, state, national, and international levels. Laboratory and hospital surveillance are utilized as specific examples of communicable disease surveillance systems. Zoonoses epidemiology takes students out of the classroom to learn about surveillance of nonhuman animal and vector species in addition to human surveillance. Students learn to geographically mark the location of bats, mice, and mosquitoes they collect. The course then turns to laboratory testing methods and development of geographically clustered analyses. In hospital epidemiology, students are exposed to the fundamental role surveillance plays in infection prevention and control, and the difficulties associated with monitoring healthcare-associated infections.

All epidemiology courses utilize surveillance data in the discussion of disease burden, identification of risk factors and outbreaks, and evaluation of intervention strategies. Students who expand their epidemiology coursework to include chronic and environmental disease learn about exposures and large registries, such as cancer registries. In addition to coursework, all epidemiology degree students are required to complete either a 240-hour field placement and thesis (MS degree) or 960 hours of internship with a paper (MPH degree). Whenever possible, fellows are encouraged to complete these capstone experiences in their home countries. The projects often include analysis and evaluation of surveillance data at the local, state, or national level. These projects are often planned in collaboration with mentors from home country institutions and occasionally with nongovernment

Table 37.1 Surveillance topics covered in epidemiology courses.

Course	Topics covered in class
Epidemiologic methods	• Introduction to public health surveillance, including the rationale for surveillance, types of surveillance systems, and evaluation of surveillance systems. • Review of current surveillance systems in the US and NYS
Infectious disease epidemiology	• Overview of infectious disease surveillance at the local, state, national, and international levels. • Review of laboratory, epidemiology, and healthcare surveillance systems • Case examples of how surveillance is used for multiple communicable diseases. • Detailed evaluation of surveillance systems
Hospital epidemiology	• Surveillance methods used in healthcare settings, including discussion of the fundamental role surveillance plays in infection prevention and control. • Surveillance of occupational exposures including risk reduction and assessment of interventions for occupational exposures. • Discussion of the various surveillance strategies utilized to monitoring trends, identify risk factors, evaluate intervention strategies, identify outbreaks, and evaluate patient safety and/or quality improvement initiatives. Use of case definitions, standard terminology, and their implications for inter and intra-facility comparisons.
HIV/AIDS epidemiology	• Types of surveillance systems including electronic surveillance, syndromic surveillance, and behavioral surveillance. • Methods of data quality assessment for surveillance systems • Data/registry maintenance including confidentiality protections • Surveillance issues arising in less developed areas, during war and conflict, and in a natural disaster setting • Ethics, privacy, and human rights vs. public health needs • Review of NYS regulations and HIV/AIDS surveillance activities comparison to US and other states
Zoonoses epidemiology	• Comparison of epidemiologic and laboratory-based surveillance methods for zoonotic diseases vs. nonzoonotic diseases, and for surveillance in humans, nonhuman animals, and vector species. • Learn statistical and geographical clustering methods for assessing surveillance data and determining clusters of interest in time and space.
Cancer epidemiology	• Overview of the extent and nature of cancer problems in the US and internationally • Familiarity with the different types of cancer registries and their roles in etiologic studies and cancer surveillance. • Medical record review (i.e., abstracting information that is reported to a central cancer registry) • Results of cancer surveillance (i.e., responding to citizen concerns) including issues involved in conducting cancer cluster investigations.
Reproductive epidemiology	• Overview birth defects surveillance and registries • Discuss specific issues with vital statistics data in Infant mortality surveillance systems
Diabetes epidemiology	• Introduction to the course includes a brief historical summary/overview of diabetes surveillance • Epidemiological methods for diabetes surveillance
Occupational and environmental epidemiology	• Discussion of environmental public health tracking and the conceptual difference it has with infectious disease surveillance • Review of occupational injury surveillance systems with a discussion of the conceptual difference between surveillance and epidemiological studies • The use of outcome registries (e.g., cancer registries) in combination with exposure registries to monitor for occupational and environmentally related diseases • Review federal and state surveillance databases and registries

organizations (e.g., John Snow, Inc., Civilian Research Defense Foundation) and other partners (e.g., Centers for Disease Control and Prevention, World Health Organization). Through these extensive applied experiences, fellows become familiar with the strengths and limitations of surveillance data from a combined practical and academic perspective. Thus, as a result of these experiences, students have a solid foundation to participate in surveillance activities once they return to their home countries.

The program places a high priority on providing instruction on the responsible conduct of research including the protection of human subjects. Fellows receive formal training in research and public health ethics as part of the Albany SPH curriculum and most complete research ethics education required for researchers by their affiliated institutions. This training is crucial since human subjects training certificates and Institutional Review Board approval are required for most of the fellow's research projects.

Research and use of infectious disease surveillance

A major goal of the program is to assist fellows in the development of the public health research infrastructure in Eastern Europe and Central Asia. Fellows are encouraged to identify projects of interest in their home countries during their education in the US, and then work with US and home country mentors to develop these projects. The field work is often conducted with funding in their home country during the summer after the first year and the data used to complete their thesis during the second year of study.

Combining surveillance education with knowledge of their home countries' public health infrastructure, many fellows have identified important infectious disease surveillance projects that may define their careers. Surveillance is instrumental in identifying disease incidence and prevalence in rapidly changing environments. These projects include basic serosurveillance studies, evaluation of surveillance systems for specific diseases, and development of new surveillance methods. The following examples provide some perspective on the significance of projects that fellows have conducted.

Surveillance case histories of international fellows

Serosurveillance studies in blood donors, Dr Maia Butsashvili, Georgia

To obtain an estimate of the prevalence of hepatitis B (HBV), hepatitis C (HCV), syphilis, and HIV in the population, Dr Butsashvili conducted a serosurveillance study of Georgian blood donors in 1998. Blood donors were primarily from low-income, low-risk groups, although individuals with high-risk behaviors also gave blood for pay. The study identified three HIV-infected individuals, an indicator of the beginning of the HIV epidemic in Georgia. In addition, the HCV level (7%) was higher than neighboring countries with the exception of some regions in Russia and served as a sentinel warning of the potential for an HIV epidemic. Similar to the Russian experience, HCV was particularly common in men (8.6%), signifying the transmission of HCV among injection drug users, of whom about half were already infected with HCV. Findings from this study were presented at the 10th International Symposium on Viral Hepatitis and Liver Disease, published in the *European Journal of Epidemiology* [9] and used to obtain a subsequent 3-year Biotechnology Engagement Program grant. A recent graduate, Dr Nino Badridze, is now planning a follow-up study to better evaluate the risk factors among blood donors to improve understanding of how the HCV and HIV epidemics are spreading throughout the country.

Evaluation of hepatitis C surveillance, Dr Jacek Mazurek, Poland

In the 1990s, Poland expanded its infectious disease surveillance system to include hepatitis C virus. Dr Mazurek decided to assess this addition to the list of notifiable diseases and was assisted by mentors from the Albany SPH, CDC, and his home institution. He based his evaluation on discussions with public health staff and physicians, and a thorough review of surveillance records [10]. To estimate the proportion of acute cases among the total reported, he conducted a study in the Warsaw district to validate case reports. A total of 1661 hepatitis C cases were studied nationally. Hepatitis C surveillance was timely and acceptable to the user, but did not provide a number of information elements required to differentiate acute from chronic cases of infection. Of the 268 case reports available in the Warsaw district, only 15 (5.6%) met the acute HCV case definition. Dr Mazurek concluded that the current HCV surveillance system in Poland could provide neither useful incidence estimates nor information regarding risk factors for acute infection. While it initially appeared logical to simply add HCV to the existing hepatitis collection forms, it may be necessary to develop a new form to include specific items to identify acute HCV infections, including questions to identify HCV transmission routes. These same issues are being addressed in US HCV surveillance systems.

Surveillance of HIV, HBV, and HCV IDUs, Dr Anneli Uuskula, Estonia

Estonia has been hit hard by the HIV epidemic and currently has the highest incidence of HIV per capita in the European region. The epidemic centers around the injection-drug using (IDU) population. Dr Uuskala wanted to develop a simple, valid method for monitoring this epidemic, but lacked resources. She hypothesized that testing syringes returned to needle-exchange programs may meet the surveillance needs of public health. Testing IDUs and their returned needles/syringes showed that the syringes could be utilized to assess the HIV prevalence among IDUs who use the programs [11]. Interestingly, HCV rates were underestimated based on syringe results, suggesting that trends in HCV can be monitored, but prevalence estimates would not be accurate.

Analysis of tuberculosis surveillance, Drs Judit Messer and Akos Somoskovi, Hungary

Two laboratory fellows worked under the direction of New York State Wadsworth Center and home country mentors to undertake analysis of the first year of data reported from Hungary's revised National Tuberculosis Surveillance System. Major findings of this published study showed that only 40% of tuberculosis (TB) cases were bacteriologically confirmed and only 68% of those were tested for susceptibility [12]. Drug resistance was detected in 10.7 and 23.5% of those previously untreated and treated, respectively. Publication of these findings led to government recommendations to increase bacteriologic and susceptibility testing. Unfortunately, despite some progress, the level of testing can still be improved.

Surveillance of tickborne encephalitis, Pawel Stefanoff, Poland

During his fellowship, Dr Stefanoff conducted a summer field placement in his home country and completed his thesis on the evaluation of tickborne encephalitis (TBE) case classification in Poland. He was able to summarize surveillance findings using standardized case definitions on 607 cases over 4 years. Major findings included the need for a uniform and valid case definition for European countries. These results were presented at the 2004 CDC International Conference on Emerging Infectious Diseases and published in the *Eurosurveillance Journal* [13]. In an accompanying editorial, two editors commented on two important questions raised by the paper: the lack of a generally accepted case definition and the quality of national surveillance of TBE cases. Thus, Stefanoff's surveillance evaluation has the potential to influence future public health policy in Poland and Europe.

Obstacles to conducting surveillance in Eastern Europe and Central Asia

A survey of these and other graduating fellows identified a number of obstacles in conducting surveillance that remain to be overcome:
• Lack of standardized case definitions
• Disappearance of traditional surveillance systems
• Reliance on handwritten records
• Absence of computerized data
• Severe restrictions in access to medical records
• Lack of governmental resources
• Limited collection of risk factor data
• Absence of monitoring and evaluation processes
• Reluctance of public health officials to use surveillance data for decision making

For Fogarty Fellows, these obstacles were overcome with careful planning, close collaboration between US and home country mentors, funding to support field work and data collection, and the hard work of our fellows and supervising faculty.

Advance preparations often included study briefings with government and institutional officials during our annual visits and submission of detailed proposals for IRB approval. Projects were sometimes supplemented with grant funds from other agencies.

Conclusions

Although it has been relatively easy to provide academic training on various surveillance methods, we have found it more challenging to apply this knowledge directly to projects within the fellows' home countries. The disintegration of the former Soviet Union with elimination of its centralized data structure and lack of resources to establish effective replacement systems with adequate demographic, epidemiologic, risk factor, and evaluation components has provided significant deterrents to progress. Despite these challenges, substantial progress has been made as demonstrated by the case histories presented here and scientific presentations and publications of our fellows. The most successful projects have received the support of in-country institutions and mentors, and collaboration with external partners (e.g., WHO, CDC, the World Bank, other international agencies, and private foundations) that have provided expertise and financial support to allow our fellows to conduct surveillance within their own countries.

The surveillance training provided through this program has been successfully used by our fellows not only to analyze data, but to evaluate old and develop new surveillance systems. The key advantage of this program has been to equip trainees with a strong scientific foundation to conduct these analyses and evaluations. The training has resulted in not only peer-reviewed publications, but more importantly, improvements in public health practice. Without this type of focused attention, the critical review of existing surveillance programs might not occur in the day-to-day practice of public health. These lessons have not been lost on the participating US faculty who have also benefited immensely from the emphasis on high level academic and applied surveillance training.

While our program is a relatively small one, it has been multiplied by surveillance training efforts provided via NIH Fogarty [14] and CDC [15] funded training programs in a number of countries. Such training is a critical element for the development and implementation of surveillance programs to address the myriad of emerging and chronic health issues throughout the world.

Acknowledgments

We acknowledge the contributions of SPH faculty and NIH Fogarty trainees who provided valuable insight on their surveillance training activities. We would particularly like to thank Maia Butsashvili, Jacek Mazurek, Anneli Uuskula, Judit Mester, Akos Somoskov, and Pawel Stefanoff whose hard work made the case history section possible.

References

1 McNabb SJN, Chorba TL, Cherniack MG. Public health concerns in the countries of Central and Eastern Europe and the New Independent States. *Curr Issues Pub Health* 1995;**1**:136–45.

2 Vitek CR, Bogatyreva EY, Wharton M. Diphtheria surveillance and control in the Former Soviet Union and the Newly Independent States. *JID* 2000;**181**: S23–6.

3 Wuhib T, Chorba TL, Davidiants V, MacKenzie WR, McNabb SJN. Assessment of the infectious diseases surveillance system of the Republic of Armenia: an example of surveillance in the Republics of the former Soviet Union. *BMC Public Health* 2002;**2**(3):1–8. Available from: http://www.biomedcentral.com/1471-2458/2/3. Accessed March 9, 2006.

4 Farmer RG, Goodman RA, Baldwin RJ. Health care and public health in the Former Soviet Union, 1992: Ukraine—a case study. *Ann Intern Med* 1993;**119**: 324–8.

5 Vlassov V. Is there epidemiology in Russia? *J Epidemiol Community Health* 2000;**54**:740–4.

6 MacLehose L, McKee M, Weinberg J. Responding to the challenge of communicable disease in Europe [review]. *Science* 2002;**15**;295:2047–50.

7 Riedner G, Denhe KL, Gromyko A. Recent declines in reported syphilis rates in eastern Europe and central Asia: are the epidemics over? *Sex Transm Inf* 2000;**76**:363–5.

8 Golden MR, Hogben M, Handsfield HH, St. Lawrence JS, Potterat JJ, Holmes KK. Partner notification for HIV and STD in the United States: low coverage for gonorrhea, chlamydial infection and HIV. *Sex Tranm Dis* 2003;**30**(6):490–6.

9 Butsashvili M, Tsertsvadze T, McNutt LA, Kamkamidze G, Gretadze R, Badridze N. Prevalance of hepatitis B, hepatitis C, syphilis and HIV in Georgian blood donors. *Eur J Epidemiol* 2001;**17**:693–5.

10 Mazurek J, Hutin Y, McNutt LA, Morse DL. Evaluation of hepatitis C surveillance in Poland in 1998. *Epidemiol Infect* 2002;**129**:119–25.

11 Uuskula A, Heimer R, DeHovitz J, Fischer K, McNutt LA. Surveillance of HIV, hepatitis B virus and hepatitis C virus in Estonian injection drug-using population: sensitivity and specificity of testing syringes for public health surveillance. *J Infect Dis* 2006;**193**: 455–7.

12 Mester J, Vadasz I, Pataki G, *et al*. Analysis of tuberculosis surveillance in Hungary in 2000. *Int J Tuberc Lung Dis* 2000;**6**:966–73.

13 Stefanoff P, Eidson M, Morse DL, Zeilinski A. Evaluation of tickborne encephalitis case classifications in Poland. *Eurosurveillance* 2005;**10**:1–3.

14 Research Training Grants. Retrieved June 8, 2006 from NIH Fogarty International Center's Web site: http://www.fic.nih.gov/funding/training-grants.htm. Accessed June 8, 2006.

15 White M, McDonnell SM, Werker D, Cardenas V, Thacker SB. The applied epidemiology and service network in the year 2000. *Am J Epidemiol* 2001;**154**:993–9.

38 Public–private partnerships in infectious disease surveillance

Andrew Friede

Introduction

The objectives of this chapter are to:
1 Illuminate the roles that public and private sectors play in infectious disease surveillance;
2 Explore the role of public–private partnerships; and
3 Review policy alternatives that might promote more fruitful working relationships between government and private organizations.

This chapter is distinct from the others in this book in that it addresses the business/organizational context of infectious disease surveillance. The focus is on the United States (US) but other countries are discussed, including those with fewer resources. Because this chapter uses terms that are often poorly understood, it begins with definitions of (1) types of organizations and (2) government procurement mechanisms.

Types of organizations and procurement mechanisms

Types of organizations

The business terms for the three fundamental types of organizations in US law (and very many countries) are (1) government (also called public), (2) nonprofit (also called not-for-profit), and (3) for-profit. Nonprofit and for-profit organizations may be owned and operated by individuals or be organized as corporations. Corporations have different rights and responsibilities than individuals, including having no right to vote and—depending on the subtype—various degrees of limited liability (pierced by froud). In many minds, the word "corporation" signifies for-profit [1]—this is, however, a misconception.

• *Government organizations* may be federal, state, or local (regional, county, city, or parish). They typically also include public universities, which may be organized as wholly owned "government nonprofits." Government organizations may be organized as corporations and their operations are subject to public oversight. In many circumstances, they provide services to other organizations via government procurement mechanisms described below, or by forming separate nonprofit corporations (e.g., Amtrak, the US Postal Service). Multinational organizations, for example, the United Nations (UN) and its affiliates, are best viewed as governmental organizations, even though some (such as the World Bank) are highly focused on generating a surplus that is used to further the mission.

• *Nonprofit organizations* are private concerns organized for charitable, educational, or humanitarian purposes. Their income minus expenses is termed surplus (or loss) and they must either use it internally or distribute it for the above purposes. Typically, a Board of Directors oversees nonprofit organizations. Nonprofits include some universities. Other nonprofits include foundations, religious and charitable institutions, and many large professional services organizations. Although they are all private, confusion arises because they are obligated by tax law to provide a "public service" in exchange for be-

490

ing tax-exempt (www.irs.gov). In common parlance, one often sees the phrase "private and nonprofit" as if they were mutually exclusive; however, all nonprofit organizations are private. Outside the US, the term *nongovernmental organization (NGO)*—despite suggesting a broader meaning—is widely used to refer to nonprofits only. Notwithstanding all these distinctions, nonprofits can own for-profits.

• *For-profit organizations* generate a surplus that is called "profit." In return for paying taxes, their owners may retain this profit. Individuals or other entities may own them. An individual or a board, which serves a proxy for other owners, may govern a for-profit organization. Finally, for-profits can own nonprofits, provided that the governance is wholly separate.

How the US government procures goods and services

Procurement types often control the role that organizations can play in possible partnerships. Hence, to elucidate the description of public–private partnerships, it is necessary to clarify how the government procures goods, such as a computer, and services, such as maintenance for that computer. The government typically uses grants, cooperative agreements, and contracts for procurement; all three mechanisms are competitive unless the government decides that only one organization is qualified. Second, in all cases the government pays "overhead," which is typically 25–75% of the procurement cost. Interestingly, nonprofits and governmental organizations often have a higher overhead than for-profits: in the case of educational institutions, overhead is often two to three times greater than the average for private corporations. Overhead is paid explicitly or as part of a fixed price, and covers costs that are part of running the organization that cannot reliably be allocated to a specific good or service (e.g., rent, fringe benefits, salaries of administrative and executive personnel, shared equipment). Certain business costs are excluded from overhead, such as entertainment and lobbying expenses. Finally, there are often direct costs attributable to specific activities, which are treated separately (e.g., travel, equipment, consultants).

The mechanisms for procurement by the government vary in the degree to which the government can demand specific performance.

• Grants are awarded for work whose outcome is typically a process (e.g., research in computer science, teaching), rather than for a specific deliverable (a computer program).
• Contracts demand very specific performance.
• Cooperative agreements are in between grants and contracts, with the government and the grantee working closely together on performance objectives and the work itself.

Only contracts allow the government to pay more than the cost of the service or product (including overhead); this extra amount is called a "fee." Accumulated fees are called "profit" by for-profits and "surplus" by nonprofits, but the cost to the procuring agency is identical. It is important to emphasize that many contracts are awarded to government and nonprofit organizations, which then take a fee. It is the procurement mechanism—not the class of awardee—that determines if a fee can be awarded. The fee can be fixed; or it can depend wholly or in part on performance. Officials sometimes think they can save money by using a nonprofit in the mistaken belief that the nonprofit cannot make a fee. There is also the widespread belief that nonprofits have lower overhead, because "they don't have to make a profit." In fact, nonprofits strive to make surplus that they can reinvest or distribute as part of their public mission. On the obverse, for-profit firms may elect to do grants or cooperative agreements to gain experience, make a contribution to society, or for intellectual interest. In any case, fees are wholly disconnected from overhead in cost proposals (except in fixed price contracts, which are rare in federal public health contracts, although more common in state and local contracts).

Finally, nonprofit firms often have a different relationship with government outside the procurement process per se. For example, government committees and advisory groups are typically open to nonprofit firms, but closed to for-profits. Homologously, government officials are often allowed to serve on the boards or advisory committees of nonprofits but are barred from serving on advisory boards of for-profits, to avoid real or perceived conflicts of interest. Taken together, these factors allow nonprofit firms to work closely with government officials, exchange information, and influence policy.

In summary, it is widely believed that organizations of different types have wholly different motivations and operating characteristics. This would suggest that they would have very different roles in infectious disease surveillance. In fact, these types of organizations are less different than commonly believed; and for practical purposes, their structure has a constrained influence on how they behave and what roles they might play in partnerships. Rather, many of those roles have been determined by history and custom rather than a strategic evaluation of best practices. The next section clarifies the different roles organizations play in infectious disease surveillance.

The history of infectious disease surveillance business practices

The current role of government

How did infectious disease surveillance become a largely governmental function? Is it a historical accident or a result of a carefully designed policy? Should that policy be revisited? Consider a counter example. The government's role in pharmaceutical product development is largely restricted to carrying out and promoting research, regulation, and monitoring. This is the accepted business model, which arose because drugs have had a commercial value since antiquity. In fact, drugs have only been regulated by the government since the 1960s, instigated by a crisis of congenital malformations due to thalidomide. Given the potential dangers of modern drugs and their costs, including costs to the government, regulation was overdue.

Few policy analysts have ever seriously considered suggesting a larger role for the government in drug development, notwithstanding the commonly held beliefs that pharmaceutical firms make excess profits by selling products that may have dangerous side effects or uncertain utility. Instead of government control, market forces decide the importance of many pharmaceutically related issues, with regulation and obligatory information provision acting as gatekeepers and safety nets.

By contrast, historically, infectious disease surveillance arose from government needs and oversight. In the US, infectious disease surveillance began with post-World War II malaria surveillance in the southeastern US, leading to the founding of the US Centers for Disease Control and Prevention (CDC) in Atlanta. Today, current infectious disease surveillance is almost wholly a governmental function, although there has not been a substantive public debate on whether this is always the best approach.

Public–private partnerships in infectious disease surveillance

While initially it may seem as if there is no business case for infectious disease surveillance, this same argument was originally made for formerly inherently governmental functions, such as mail delivery in the US and medical care in the United Kingdom (UK). Moreover, there are major businesses that sell health information to pharmaceutical and device firms, insurance companies, and indeed, the government. It seems reasonable to assume that there would be a similar market for infectious disease surveillance data.

Is it accurate to say that infectious disease surveillance is solely a governmental function? A large number of infectious disease surveillance programs in the US depend on the private sector. For example, private hospitals send a large amount of data (e.g., electronic laboratory reports) to state and local health departments, and to CDC, at a cost to themselves. Except for data provided by the Department of Defense, the Department of Veteran's Affairs, state public health laboratories, and epidemiology programs, virtually all infectious disease surveillance data in the US originates in the private sector; a *de facto* public–private partnership lies at the heart of this type of infectious disease surveillance.

The private sector's role in these systems is not restricted to providing data. CDC contracts the private sector for operational components of national surveillance programs, including components of the Vaccine Adverse Event Reporting System, BioSense, and the national mortality system. In addition, CDC's Base System version of the National Electronic Disease Surveillance System (NEDSS) and NEDSS compatible systems in many state and local health departments have been developed in part by private firms, typically on contract.

The US government, through agencies like the US Agency for International Development (USAID), CDC, and the US Department of Agriculture, funds the private sector, often US and non-US universities, to build and run disease surveillances systems in other countries for tuberculosis, HIV/AIDS, malaria, and other conditions. Many of these systems have been built with grants and cooperative agreements that have been won by private firms. Again, a de facto public–private partnership underlies these programs.

Roles in partnerships

Is contract work a partnership? Are grants and cooperative agreements partnerships? Some would say not; but that would be a constrained view. What is a partnership? Literally, everyone has a part: everyone brings something to the table, and derives some benefit. Collegial working relationships and shared values are a requirement. Many types of organizations contribute to these associations, and derive some benefit; sometimes the benefit flows to citizens, beneficiaries of a foundation, or investors who have put their private funds at risk. The government gains work and the private firms gain experience, exposure, and have a chance to contribute their expertise for public good.

On the obverse, private sector foundations with a public health focus (e.g., Gates, Ford, Rockefeller, Robert Wood Johnson, Clinton Foundations) are funding disease surveillance programs that are being carried out by public and/or private agencies in parts of the world with few resources. "Business as usual" in infectious disease surveillance is changing right before our eyes.

Examples of current public–private partnerships

Vaccine adverse events reporting system (VAERS)

VAERS (described in detail in Chapter 18, Part 2) is a joint CDC/Food and Drug Administration (FDA) surveillance system that collects and analyzes reports of side effects associated with immunizations. Nurses call reporters to collect more detailed data and investigate unusual events. Data are analyzed for patterns and new syndromes. VAERS data have been used to investigate vaccine safety concerns such as intussusception reported in association with early rotavirus vaccines [2] (a relationship was indeed found, and the vaccine was withdrawn from the market), and autism putatively associated with DPT vaccine [3] (no association was found).

In what sense is VAERS a pubic–private partnership? For over a decade, for-profit firms have operated components of VAERS. The government (CDC/FDA) sets programmatic objectives, determines deliverables, and provides technical oversight, while the process of collecting the data, working with data providers, and providing clinical support to healthcare facilities is contracted. Contractor staff greatly outnumber the government staff. Over the years, there has been variability in each of these roles, but there has always been a substantive scientific contribution from the contractor.

BioSense

Initially created in response to the September 11, 2001, bioterrorism attacks, BioSense is a CDC initiative to collect real-time (or close to real-time) clinical data on cases of putative bioterrorism [4]. BioSense contracts with hundreds of hospitals around the country to build information systems which link these hospitals to the CDC. A variety of for-profit businesses have been involved in all phases of this work. For-profits have participated in the delicate negotiations with the nonprofit and government healthcare institutions that contribute data, and have collaborated in the implementation of complex information systems. This has become a public–private partnership in the fullest sense, with active participation from hundreds of organizations of many types.

Autonomous detection systems

In 2004, the US Postal Service instituted an airborne anthrax surveillance program that grew to include 283 mail-handling facilities. It is based on an Autonomous Detection Systems, i.e., an automated air-sampling and testing machine that uses real-time polymerase chain reaction testing. The equipment was developed by for-profit firms under contract; CDC has provided technical assistance and guidance on response protocols; local public authorities are alerted if there are positives [5]. This is a complex public–private partnership. The Postal Service is actually a government corporation that is part of the Executive Branch (it is operated by its Postmaster General/CEO as a business with a break-even mandate). Installing the hardware and establishing clear communication channels and associated action plans requires close coordination between the Postal Service, local public health authorities, CDC, and the manufacturers of the system. Partnership members bring a range of capabilities, including requirements analysis; scientific, public health, and logistical expertise; and funds. In 2005, the San Francisco Department of Public Health conducted an exercise that included the Postal Service, the San Francisco Mail Processing and Distribution Center, and local emergency responders [6].

Drug and vaccine development

The development and promotion of new drugs and vaccines depends heavily on infectious disease surveillance for understanding the distribution and determinants of infectious diseases, case finding, and evaluation of efficacy and cost–benefit. Although for-profit pharmaceutical firms are often most identified with these projects, they could not do their work without the active participation of researchers in government and nonprofit universities (supported by public and private funds), and the many contract research organizations (mostly for-profit) that work with healthcare providers in government and nonprofit healthcare facilities.

For drugs and vaccines that have a limited commercial market (e.g., drugs for HIV infection and prevention in high-risk populations), government and foundations play an essential funding role. Government and foundations are also active in research involving these drugs and vaccines. There are studies and new promotion programs in countries with limited resources, especially for diseases that are prevalent in those areas (e.g., tuberculosis, malaria) or for which new vaccines hold special promise (e.g., childhood diseases caused by pneumococcus or *Haemophilus influenzae*). Each of these projects has a cadre

of partners from government including UN agencies; nonprofits (foundations, nonprofit services firms); and for-profit services and research firms (www.vaccinealliance.org).

International disease detection and prevention

USAID and its counterparts in other countries (e.g., the UK Department for International Development), and foundations (Gates, The Global Fund) and World Health Organization (WHO) agencies, operate many projects in developing countries that are devoted to monitoring and preventing infectious diseases. There is a special focus on HIV/AIDS, tuberculosis, and malaria. These programs typically involve public–private partnerships between government experts in their home countries and in offices abroad, host government experts, universities in developed and developing countries, local religious and community-based organizations, and nonprofit and for-profit firms. Two projects that have been in operation for over two decades and that operate as public–private partnerships include the Demographic Health Surveys [7] (http://www.measuredhs.com/aboutdhs/whoweare.cfm) and the Health Policy Initiative [8] (http://www.policyproject.com/). These projects cover the waterfront of infectious disease surveillance (especially for HIV/AIDS and malaria), including data collection and analysis, development of prevention strategies, and policy formulation [9].

Policy alternatives

Current policy

Since the dawn of the 21st century, a number of macro factors—bioterrorism, emerging infectious diseases, and globalism—have combined to radically heighten public health's profile in the US and other countries. It has been widely thought that a better-funded public sector would assume more responsibility for protecting Americans by implementing surveillance programs like BioSense (enhanced surveillance of clinical syndromes associated with agents of bioterrorism), BioWatch (sampling for airborne agents of bioterrorism), and BioShield (vaccines and medications), and by implementing more vigorous, worldwide surveillance for emerging and re-emerging infectious diseases (influenza, malaria, tuberculosis) (see Chapter 1). The private sector has been seen as an implementer of infectious disease surveillance systems that have been conceptualized and designed by the government; or, in the case of foundations, as a co-funder. As the above examples make clear, it is more accurate to say that each type of organization can at times play one or more roles in research, funding, and oversight.

In particular, it has been assumed that there is no natural commercial market for these services, because the benefit would be perceived to redound to groups, not the individual; or the benefit/cost ratio would not appeal to the individual. However, this assumption has not been tested. It is possible that individuals or smaller communities would like their air sampled, would pay to detect patterns of disease that could represent bioterrorism or influenza or an unreliably pure water supply. Various payers might well buy an improved anthrax vaccine, just as the military likely will, perhaps at subsidized costs. In the crisis atmosphere following 9/11, it was reasonable to act urgently. The crisis has now evolved into a chronic concern that may last decades: it may be time to explore policy alternatives.

The large governmental role in public health activities, and infectious disease surveillance in particular, stands in contrast to the overwhelming role of the private sector in clinical medicine in the US. This role has been widely accepted for many years, and is now taken for granted, although it was not always self-evident [10]. Moreover, the dominant role of the private sector in medicine is far from being generally accepted in many developed countries (e.g., Canada, Sweden). In the US, despite the enviable economies that a larger governmental role in medicine is thought to bring to some countries (especially in reimbursement), Americans have decided to pay for the perception of flexibility and innovation associated with our system. Would Americans pay for infectious disease surveillance if they had a choice?

Some social critics think that the private sector should operate under more special constraints in medicine and in public health, as contrasted with the operation of other parts of our economy (such as housing or transportation), even though they may touch on similarly vital needs. Indeed, in 1977 the WHO declared that "Health for All" is a right; no UN agency has a policy of, say, "housing for all," nor even "food for all" or "clothing for all" or "education for all." Put another way, the value of health has often been considered "priceless"; the concern is that individuals will not pay for public health services because the benefits accrue to groups. But given the emergence of markets for health information, is it time to consider making (or allowing) a market for infectious disease surveillance information?

In summary, we have:

- the dominance of the private sector in clinical care (with some calls for changing the balance);
- an apparent monopoly of the government sector in public health (with few critics of the *status quo*), although the role of pubic-private partnerships is in fact large and growing, especially as foundations grow;
- the elevation of health—private and public—to a special status; and
- the emergence of new health information markets.

The time seems ripe to reexamine some of the basic "business as usual" *modus operandi*, and review the relative role of the private sector in public health. Put another way, the "public" in public health need not mean that government goes it alone.

A new paradigm?

Since the 1970s, there has been a worldwide movement toward privatizing functions that were previously considered "inherently governmental." Should infectious disease surveillance be more fully privatized, too? Certainly some privatization experiments have gone awry. Similarly, the privatization and sometimes-simultaneous deregulation of some industries (airlines, telecommunications, utilities, prisons, public hospitals) have led to massive market and business disruptions, although actual service interruptions have been remarkably rare. China has a mixed model system, with the state owning many for-profits; this model bears close watching.

No discussion of privatization—and indeed, modern business—is complete without touching on the potential for criminal behavior. In the US, recent cases of corporate theft, securities fraud, and violation of privacy laws have led to numerous indictments but surprisingly few criminal convictions. New laws and regulations such as the Sarbanes–Oxley Act [11] have been designed to improve oversight and due diligence in this new world, largely by forcing executives to be personally responsible for audits. The business community has largely embraced these regulations as a way to strengthen their own internal processes and promote transparency.

There is a natural and real concern that if infectious disease surveillance were to be wholly or partly privatized, public agencies could be denied access to the data (or be forced to pay high prices). First, those data are in fact very difficult to access now and are frequently unavailable for research or program purposes. In the case of true emergencies, there are ample public health laws that would require firms to turn over data, just as healthcare providers are required to report notifiable disease data now without being reimbursed. Second, it should be recognized that public agencies are currently paying for infectious disease surveillance data; those costs are buried in government programs and grants; and frequently borne by providers as unfunded and unaccounted for mandates.

Finally, privatizing infectious disease surveillance data may make it *more available* if there were vast markets for it; the emergence of "prediction markets" (essentially, betting pools for measurable events) may create such a new market (and new hitherto untapped sources) for surveillance data. There would be an important societal advantage: there would be hundreds or thousands of analysts around the world pooling their collective data and analytical wisdom to help predict epidemics of, say, SARS or highly pathogenic avian influenza [12,13].

Summary and conclusions

There are policy choices that could promote public–private partnerships in infectious disease surveillance:

• The substantial and multifaceted roles the private sector already plays in infectious disease surveillance, especially with respect to data provision and management (and sometimes, funding) should be acknowledged, and form part of the policy debate.

• The private sector may be able to add value to infectious disease surveillance process, as opposed to government working alone. There is no reason to invoke an "all or none" approach; partnerships of several types are working now; it would seem reasonable to consider more mixed models.

• There may also be a role for new quasi-governmental agencies that operate in a business model similar to the US Post Office, General Services Administration, and Amtrak.

• Different degrees of decrementing regulation should be explored, especially for what economists call "natural monopolies" (e.g., utilities, toll-ways). Many of these processes might evolve during transitions, especially as new technology and market forces dissolve monopolies. This has occurred to some degree in communications (satellite replacing cable) and new energy sources (solar and tide).

• The capacity to enforce business regulations to minimize the risk of abuse or outright fraud should be considered when exploring private public partnerships.

• There may be untapped markets for infectious disease surveillance data (pharmaceutical and device firms, insurance firms, healthcare providers, prediction markets) which could provide important revenue streams to support a more robust system, to carry out research, and to support surveillance for new, rare, and emerging conditions, as well as to improve the process overall.

• There is no reason to do a "big bang" and there is every reason to explore different models, especially for different diseases. As an example, models that work for salmonellosis may not work for malaria.

• Infectious disease surveillance may be in a position to lead the way for more robust partnerships in the surveillance of noninfectious diseases.

Acknowledgments

We gratefully acknowledge Dr James W. Buehler, Emory University, for his thoughtful suggestions regarding private–public partnerships. We also thank

Martin I. Meltzer, Centers for Disease Control and Prevention for his insightful comments.

References

1 Micklethwait J, Wooldridge A. *The Company: A Short History of a Revolutionary Idea*. Modern Library Chronicles; 2003.

2 Murphy T, Gargiullo P, Massoudi MS, *et al.* Intussusception among infants given an oral rotavirus vaccine. *N Engl J Med* 2001;**344**(8):564–72.

3 Jick H, Kaye JA. Autism and DPT vaccination in the United Kingdom. *N Engl J Med* 2004;**350**(26): 2722–3.

4 Centers for Disease Control and Prevention. PHIN: BioSense. Available from: http://www.cdc.gov/phin/component-initiatives/biosense/ index.html. Accessed December 22, 2006.

5 Meehan PJ, Rosenstein NE, Gillen M, *et al.* Responding to detection of aerosolized *Bacillus anthracis* by autonomous detection systems in the workplace. *MMWR Recomm Rep* 2004;**53**(RR-7):1–12.

6 Department of Public Health, City and County of San Francisco. Bioterrorism and Infectious Disease Emergency Programs and Activities. Available from http://www.sfcdcp.org/index.cfm?id=65. Accessed December 22, 2006.

7 Demographic Heath Surveys. Available from: http://www.measuredhs.com/aboutsurveys/dhs/start.cfm. Accessed December 22, 2006.

8 Policy Project. Available from: http://www.policyproject.com/. Accessed December 30, 2006.

9 Kirungi WL, Musinguzi J, Madraa E, *et al.* Trends in antenatal HIV prevalence in urban Uganda associated with uptake of preventive sexual behaviour. *Sex Transm Infect* April 2006;**82**(suppl 1):i36–41.

10 Starr P. *The Social Transformation of American Medicine*. New York: Basic Books; 1983.

11 Sarbanes-Oxley SEC Rules & Regulations. Available from: http://www.sarbanes-oxley.com/section.php?level=1&pub_id=SEC-Rules. Accessed December 22, 2006.

12 Polgreen PM, Nelson FD, Neumann GR. Use of prediction markets to forecast infectious disease activity. *Clin Infect Dis* 2007;**44**:272–9.

13 Surowiecki J. *The Wisdom of Crowds: Why the Many Are Smarter Than the Few and How Collective Wisdom Shapes Business, Economies, Societies and Nations*. New York: Little, Brown; 2004.

Conclusions

39

Lessons learned from smallpox eradication and severe acute respiratory syndrome outbreak

PART 1: The use of surveillance in the eradication of smallpox and poliomyelitis

D.A. Henderson

Introduction

The surveillance-containment program in smallpox eradication was, ultimately, the essential factor in its success. The data generated through surveillance provided critical information as to where the disease was present and how extensive it was; it provided information as to the characteristics of cases by age, sex, and vaccination status; and it served to chart progress in controlling the disease. The data were invaluable in providing ongoing quality control and in guiding program management. Strategic decisions were made on the basis of this information as, for example, the decision to focus on primary vaccination at the expense of revaccination efforts; the development of special strategies to reach resistant, high-risk groups; and special programs to control endemic foci of smallpox in urban settings during the seasonal low in incidence. Most important was the revelation that smallpox spread less readily and rapidly than the conventional medical texts suggested and that fairly simple containment vaccination strategies could stop transmission more readily than had been anticipated.

It is difficult to understand how this or any other disease control program could be effectively executed without recognizing the obvious—that the ongoing collection of morbidity and mortality data regarding the disease in question is the ultimate indicator of progress and that the currency of those data is a critical guide to policy decisions and program management. However, from the inception of the program, it proved difficult for national leaders and, indeed, some international staff to com-

prehend this and to give this activity the priority it required [1,2]. As a measurement of progress in vaccine programs, most were accustomed to relying on reports of vaccinations performed. They resisted assigning personnel to surveillance and containment activities when, as they saw it, those persons could be more usefully engaged in performing vaccinations.

Development of the surveillance concept

Disease surveillance, as we conceive it today, is a surprisingly recent component of disease control programs. Credit for the development of this concept goes to Dr Alexander Langmuir who became Chief of the US Communicable Disease Center's (CDC's) Epidemiology Branch in 1949. Until then, the term "surveillance" had been applied to a continuing watchfulness of contacts of cases of serious communicable diseases, such as plague and yellow fever, so as to detect the earliest signs of development of the disease [3]. In 1950, he broadened the use of the term to apply it to a systematic program of data collection in watchfulness for the occurrence and spread of a disease. Malaria in the southern US was the disease to which surveillance was first applied but this was soon followed by programs for poliomyelitis, hepatitis, influenza, and others [4]. The intrinsic features of a disease surveillance program as he defined them were "the continued watchfulness over the distribution and trends of incidence through the systematic collection, consolidation and evaluation of morbidity and mortality reports and other relevant data. Intrinsic in the concept is the regular dissemination of the basic data and interpretations to all who have contributed and to all others who need to know" [3,5]. Implicit in this was the expectation that having in hand the accumulating surveillance data and its interpretation, authorities with responsibilities for disease control would be motivated and guided in taking appropriate action. For smallpox eradication, surveillance was a critical factor that was stimulated and directed by those responsible for instituting control measures, and thus surveillance and containment came together as a single operational entity.

The concept of surveillance was deemed to be of sufficient international importance, yet so little recognized, that Langmuir was asked to serve as principal consultant for a special technical program and discussion at the Twenty-First World Health Assembly (May 1968) on the "National and Global Surveillance of Communicable Diseases" [5].

Surveillance in the smallpox program

Having myself served as Chief of the CDC Surveillance Section from 1961 to 1965, it was only natural, in 1967, as the new World Health Organization (WHO) Director of Smallpox Eradication, to stress surveillance and containment as key components of global smallpox eradication. Indeed, the importance of surveillance to smallpox eradication was implicit in the object of the program itself—"zero" human smallpox cases [6]. A decision that the objective had been achieved implied a sufficiently sensitive surveillance system to discover cases if they were present.

Fortunately, surveillance for smallpox infection is easier than for most other communicable diseases. Because chronic carriers are unknown and there is no known natural reservoir [6–8], the presence of smallpox infection in an area can be detected and its prevalence measured by the number of human cases. Detection and diagnosis of such cases is reasonably straightforward. A distinctive rash is produced which is wholly characteristic in the great majority of cases. While smallpox infection without rash is known to occur, such persons do not

further transmit infection and thus their detection is of no practical epidemiological importance [8,9].

At the inception of the intensified global smallpox eradication program in 1967, it was believed that for surveillance-containment activities to be effective, it would first be necessary to reduce smallpox incidence to less than 5 cases per 100,000 population [10]. It was expected that systematic vaccination programs designed to reach 80% of the population would achieve a reduction in incidence to this level. While such vaccination programs were in progress, sufficient time would be provided for surveillance systems to develop. Surprising, however, was the discovery in Nigeria during the first year of the program that an extensive area could become smallpox-free even when half or less of the population bore scars of primary vaccination [11]. This observation was soon confirmed in other countries of western Africa [12–14], India, Brazil, and Indonesia. Accordingly, the strategy of the program was altered to place more stress on the development of surveillance-containment activities, if necessary, at the expense of mass vaccination.

The epidemiology of smallpox facilitated the success of the surveillance-containment approach. Since the patient does not transmit virus until rash first develops, early isolation of obviously infected individuals is effective in reducing spread [1]. For contacts, a highly effective and stable vaccine is available which offers virtually complete protection even when given 3–4 days after exposure to the index patient. Since an incubation period of 2 weeks intervenes between generations of cases and since the patient does not usually infect more than two to five additional persons, prompt intervention through patient isolation and vaccination of actual or potential contacts is most efficient in rapidly stopping transmission. Finally, identification of the source of infection of each case is relatively easy since transmission almost always requires face-to-face contact between a patient with rash and susceptible contacts. The chain of disease transmission can thus be readily identified and previously unknown outbreaks detected.

At the beginning of the global program, smallpox surveillance in the endemic areas was vestigial to nonexistent. Schemes employed in implementing surveillance varied from country to country according to differences in health structures and their sophistication. Thus, emphasis in this chapter is given to the more generally used approaches.

Status of routine case detection and reporting—1967

The International Health Regulations required that all countries notify WHO promptly of all cases of smallpox. In 1967, 44 of 129 member countries of WHO reported 131,418 cases of smallpox. Reporting was recognized to be incomplete but how serious the problem was became apparent early in the global program through two studies. Jacobus Keja, the WHO Senior Smallpox Advisor in the WHO Southeast Asia Regional Office, working in Indonesia in 1968, reasoned that the prevalence of facial scars among infants would provide a basis for the approximation of true smallpox incidence during the preceding year [15]. A cluster sample survey in Java, which involved the examination of 56,000 children, provided data. That year, 10,010 cases were reported to Javanese provincial authorities. Based on the survey, this represented less than 1% of the total of estimated cases in Indonesia [7]. Foster found the situation in Nigeria to be not dissimilar [16]. Using a similar approach but a larger sample and a more precise method of estimation, he calculated that about 1–3% of cases in rural areas and 8% of cases in urban areas were being reported. Based on subsequent experiences in the program, the efficiency of reporting systems in Indonesia and Nigeria was then probably better than the average among endemic countries.

Reports of smallpox cases which came to notice and which were reflected in the official disease notifications were found to be primarily those that had been seen in government hospitals or health centers. In most countries, reporting systems asked that government health establishments provide monthly reports of numbers of cases of 20–50 or more diseases. Follow-up to assure that reports were consistently submitted was usually lacking; rarely were the data employed in guiding program operations; and almost never was there a mechanism to obtain reports from nongovernment health facilities. Cases that were discovered during field investigation of an outbreak were usually not enumerated in the official data.

These observations were consistent with the observations of the 1964 WHO Expert Committee on Smallpox Eradication, which stated bluntly: "the reporting of smallpox, as of any other communicable disease, is frequently unreliable and the data available to the Committee are not accurate" [17].

Actions taken to improve case detection and reporting

Primary surveillance system

A first step in improvement of the surveillance system was to increase progressively the completeness and regularity of reporting from all fixed medical units such as hospitals, health centers, and dispensaries. While for many, the image of the developing countries was that of a vast, medically uncharted wilderness, there was, in all countries, a surprising number of medical units scattered throughout the countryside which provided some form of medical care to patients, including those ill with smallpox. Although only a portion of all smallpox cases were seen by such units, it was thought, and so it proved, that this basic reporting network would provide valuable information as to the general prevalence of the disease in different areas, as well as the distribution of cases by age and sex. Based on such data, resources both for outbreak control and systematic vaccination would be able to be more effectively deployed.

The usual procedure for developing the system was to first prepare a list of all fixed medical units and to coerce, persuade, and cajole each unit to submit each week a report indicating numbers of cases of smallpox seen that week and a limited amount of data regarding each case—name, age, sex, village, date of onset of rash, and whether or not previously vaccinated. If no cases were seen, a "nil" report was requested. The concept that a report should be submitted even when no cases were seen (so-called negative reporting) proved a far more difficult principle to establish than that of reporting known cases (Figure 39(1).1). However, it was soon obvious that the most ineffective health units were the ones that often failed to report but, at the same time, the ones that most frequently had cases.

Development of a reasonably effective primary surveillance system usually took between 18 and

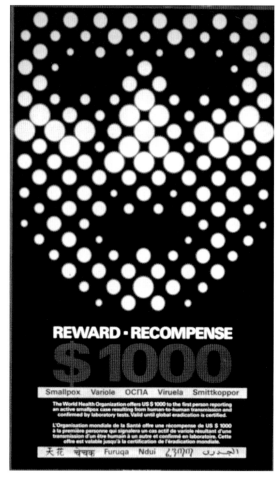

Fig 39(1).1 During smallpox eradication campaigns, public health officials vaccinated in a concentric ring around an outbreak but this required prompt reporting of all smallpox cases. Cash bounties were paid to people who reported smallpox cases.

24 months. Experience showed that development was best achieved by establishing for each administrative unit of perhaps 2–5 million persons a surveillance team of perhaps two to four persons with transport. Each team, in addition to its other duties in outbreak containment, visited each reporting unit regularly to explain and discuss the program, to distribute forms (and often vaccine), and to check on those who were delinquent in reporting. Regularly distributed nationally produced surveillance reports helped to motivate these units. However, the best stimulus for reporting seemed to be the knowl-

edge that a surveillance team for outbreak investigation and control would visit promptly if cases were reported. This simple indication that the routine weekly reports were a cause for public health action accomplished more than what a multitude of government directives could have done.

Many examples could be cited to illustrate the usefulness of the surveillance data. They served to guide the timing of vaccination campaigns within the country—the most heavily afflicted areas being scheduled first. They revealed that most of the cases during the summer low in seasonal incidence occurred in urban areas—a cause for intensified surveillance and containment in that period. In Afghanistan, costly and time-consuming plans developed especially to vaccinate women in purdah were abandoned when detailed follow-up of case reports revealed that almost 90% of all cases were in children and only rarely were women afflicted [1]. Emphasis on priorities for vaccination also changed. Medical teaching indicated that revaccination every 5–10 years was necessary. However, revaccination of adults had seldom been practiced in the endemic countries, yet cases among adults were rare. Presumably, this reflected the occurrence of subclinical infections that served to reinforce vaccination immunity [9]. Accordingly, emphasis in the vaccination campaign was shifted to primary vaccination with a considerable gain in efficiency.

Secondary surveillance systems

In addition to the primary network for routine case notification, supplementary systems, known as secondary surveillance systems, were developed. For improvement in the completeness of reporting, the surveillance teams which investigated reports of cases were the most critical. During the early stages of the systems, teams frequently discovered 20–50 cases for every case officially reported [18]. As time progressed, these ratios steadily decreased but, even in the best programs, the teams consistently discovered at least two additional cases for every case reported.

Assistance in reporting was actively solicited from various other groups such as agricultural extension workers, block development officers, railway workers, police, security forces, and others. Although such groups were sometimes of assistance in winning the confidence of villagers when vaccination was conducted, none contributed substantively to the reporting of cases.

The most widely used of the secondary surveillance systems and most effective for the time expended was querying teachers and schoolchildren about suspect cases [19]. Smallpox with its characteristic rash was remarkably well known to villagers. A brief visit to a school permitted a surveillance team to inquire about possible cases of smallpox in villages located over a wide area. The use of large colored pictures of smallpox encased in plastic (WHO Recognition Card) and small postcard-sized pictures of smallpox proved invaluable. The children proved to be a mine of information regarding illnesses in their villages. After a few visits of the surveillance teams, teachers undertook the questioning themselves and often to better advantage.

Almost as useful as the schools was a similar type of query at markets [19,20]. Within a few hours a surveillance agent with a picture and sometimes a megaphone could obtain information about possible smallpox cases in rural villages within at least a 10-km radius of the market. The efficiency of this approach was improved by a practical training program for the market searches on how to approach the people (a neutral opening gambit on weather or crops), when (usually toward the end of the market day), where (tea shops were useful), etc. Monitoring the work of surveillance agents in markets was facilitated in India by the development of a "Market Survey Book." The agent asked each person queried which village he was from and noted this on a list in a book, a new village being added to the list each time a new one was named. At the end of a day, scrutiny of the book indicated the geographical area covered by the market search and by the number of "x's" after each village, how many people from that village had been queried.

Systematic house-by-house search, the ultimate in the development of secondary surveillance systems, matured in India beginning in 1973 [2] and, soon after, was used widely in Pakistan and Bangladesh. The accelerated disappearance of smallpox in Asia was closely linked with this development [21–25]. In concept, the plan was simple. Once every 4–8 weeks, many health staff in each administrative area devoted a week to a planned village-by-village (later, house-by-house) search for smallpox. Where health staff were as plentiful as they were in some countries of southern Asia and, at the same time, underutilized, such a scheme was surprisingly feasible. The requisite planning, organization, training, and motivation to ensure that each worker knew specifically what to do, where and when, was a formidable task but proved more soluble than was initially thought.

In order to ascertain the completeness of the search activities, independent teams, staffed by district and higher level officials, assessed a 5–10% sample of villages. The results were compiled monthly, distributed to, and discussed with supervisors and corrective and disciplinary measures decided. Assessed coverage rose to the level of 80% and later to more than 90%.

As smallpox incidence fell and it became increasingly important to quickly detect cases, the periodic special searches were supplemented by specially organized searches in problem areas such as the slum areas of cities. The interest of the public in the reporting of cases and the motivation of health workers in their discovery were further increased by the offer of a reward initially of Rs. 50 (about US$6.00) to the person who reported a case and a similar sum to the health worker who received the report. The reward was widely advertised by radio and loudspeakers in markets; by house visits of search workers; and by stenciled announcements on house walls. Posters were also sometimes employed but their "half-life" on most walls was so brief and the costs of their production so great that other methods of advertising were preferred.

Dissemination of information within countries

A national weekly (or sometimes fortnightly or monthly) surveillance report was of great help in encouraging prompt notifications. National surveillance reports varied in character but, as a minimum, each contained data regarding cases reported weekly from each reporting unit plus interpretative comment. Each included, variably, epidemiological reports, schedules for search weeks, procedures for submitting specimens, information regarding other programs, etc. They were usually mimeographed and distributed promptly so as to contain the latest data and were sent to a large number of people directly and indirectly associated with the program. In most cases, preparation required only a few hours' work each week by the program director or an epidemiologist and the assistance of a part-time clerk for stenciling, addressing, and mailing.

A difficult problem in some countries, especially at national and state/provincial levels, were existing organizational systems in which all data were dealt with by a statistical unit usually working without effective contact with any other part of the health structure. Rarely did any of the national statistical units consider it their responsibility to assure that reports were received from all reporting units. Many refused to accept reports of cases discovered by surveillance teams on the grounds that cases could only be submitted by permanent government medical units. Almost never did the statistical units query "unusual" reports such as the report perhaps of hundreds of cases of smallpox in 1 week from an area that had reported no cases whatsoever for a year or more. In many countries, available data at higher administrative levels were frequently misleading. Often it was found, for example, that 100 cases of smallpox registered by units at a subdistrict level diminished to 70 cases in reports from the district level, to 40 cases at provincial levels, and to 25 cases officially registered nationally. Sometimes this occurred because of deliberate suppression of case reports, but more frequently, the problem was cumbersome and inept data-handling systems. By insisting that program officers responsible for smallpox activities assume primary responsibility for smallpox case reporting and by helping them to see the use for and importance of the data, most of the difficulties were able to be resolved.

International data collection and dissemination

Although the national reporting of cases of smallpox at the inception of the program was recognized to be woefully deficient, it was considered important nevertheless to try to improve the regularity and rapidity of reporting at all levels of the system while endeavoring at the same time to improve the system so as to obtain the "best available data," however incomplete, regarding smallpox cases worldwide. These data were sometimes referred to by the ironic acronym BAD to emphasize their tentative nature.

When the eradication program began, two systems for data recording were in place at WHO Headquarters. The International Sanitary Regulations explicitly called for prompt and regular telegraphic reports to WHO of smallpox cases from all member countries. The Quarantine unit which dealt with the International Sanitary Regulations published these data in the *Weekly Epidemiological Record*. A second set of data was published annually by the WHO Statistics Division, an entirely separate group, employing summary information which originated from special statistical units within the national governments.

The Statistics Division received and faithfully published in the *World Health Statistics Annual*, data based on the summaries provided each year by national governments. With no technical officer knowledgeable of the global smallpox situation to query strange or unusual reports, numerous anomalies appeared in the *World Health Statistics Annual*. Each year, a number of reports of smallpox cases were received from countries thought to be smallpox-free. After 1967, such reports were queried and most turned out to be simple clerical errors. As an example, the 1967 *World Health Statistics Annual* [26] shows for Columbia seven deaths due to smallpox but no cases; for Sao Tome and Principe, one smallpox death but no cases. Neither country experienced smallpox that year. Conversely, there were several endemic countries that reported having no cases whatsoever in 1967.

In brief, smallpox data that were available to and published by WHO through the 1960s bear only a vague resemblance to the smallpox situation as it actually was. The underlying deficiency at WHO was little different than the problems in each of the countries. There was no single responsible and knowledgeable public health official or unit that was actively using the data and doing all possible to assure that it was of the best possible quality. After 1967, the Smallpox Eradication Unit took full responsibility for monitoring and harmonizing the data system and obtaining uniformity of reports on smallpox from all of the countries.

The problem of official suppression of reports of smallpox cases was found to pertain to comparatively few countries. These were reasonably readily identified through an unofficial smallpox information network of university scientists, embassies, and a variety of national and international contacts. Most governments responsible for case suppression quickly reversed their policies when approached diplomatically with a full explanation of the need for reporting and the fact that suppression on their part was harmful to the program's credibility and was damaging to the reputation of their own health services.

Of special value was an international surveillance report that was distributed regularly to national and international staff concerned with smallpox and which included information regarding the current status and trends of smallpox incidence, interpretative summaries, and information regarding program developments. This was achieved by modifying the traditional format of the *WHO Weekly Epidemiological Record* to permit such reports to be included as a regular feature. The first report appeared on May 30, 1968, and subsequent reports appeared at intervals of 2–4 weeks thereafter. Report number 120 was published on September 16, 1975, and distributed to the *Weekly Record's* 5000 subscribers while an additional 2900 reprints of the Smallpox Surveillance portion were distributed to national and international field staff throughout the world.

Polio surveillance—a next step

Clearly, the most powerful and effective tool in smallpox eradication was that of surveillance. In essence, it represented, organically, the brain and the nervous system in a management process. Its importance was described and documented in many publications and discussed in scientific meetings. Thus, it was only logical that with the launch of the next major eradication program—that for poliomyelitis—surveillance should again play an important role. This it did in the Americas but extending surveillance to most other parts of the world proved to be far more difficult than any had imagined.

Problems of polio diagnosis

The opening phase of the global poliomyelitis program began in the Americas in 1985 with a commitment by its Directing Council to eradicate polio by 1990 [27]. Surveillance was accorded a high priority, its principles of operation deriving from those of smallpox eradication. However, it was recognized that the program of surveillance and containment would have to be adapted to the clinical and epidemiological realities of poliomyelitis. Weekly reports of cases of acute flaccid paralysis were called for, to be provided by health units throughout each of the countries. However, diagnoses were far more difficult, and containment, such as was possible in smallpox, was impossible given the fact that only about 1 in 200 poliovirus infections resulted in paralysis [28].

Certainty of diagnosis was clearly a major problem from the inception of the program and has continued to be so ever since. Initially, a suspected case was defined as "acute onset of paralysis in a person less than 15 years of age for any reason other than severe trauma, or paralytic illness in a person of any age in whom polio is suspected" [29]. The case was considered to be "confirmed" if a wild poliovirus was isolated from the stool; or if there was epidemiological linkage to a confirmed case; or if there was residual paralysis 60 days after onset; or if there was either death or lack of a follow-up of a case. As is apparent, the definition deliberately biased the system toward sensitivity over specificity.

At the beginning, it was believed that the finding of a case of acute flaccid paralysis, not due to trauma, and which persisted for 60 days or longer, was all but pathognomonic of poliomyelitis. If this were so, laboratory confirmation would seldom be required. However, it was soon discovered that there were a surprising number of cases in polio-free areas of acute flaccid paralysis in which poliovirus could not be recovered from patients nor their contacts. Examination by neurologists and pediatricians found the cases to be indistinguishable from polio. Various nonpolio causes were thought to have been responsible, including Guillain–Barré syndrome, acute transverse myelitis and traumatic neuritis. Eventually, it was determined that these cases occurred at the rate of approximately 1 per 100,000 children under the age of 15 years.

Greater diagnostic certainty was needed in order to prioritize vaccination programs and program operations and so it was decided that greater efforts would be made to obtain stool specimens from patients within 14 days after onset of illness and to transport these, under refrigeration, to designated polio virus diagnostic laboratories. Thus, a network of laboratories had to be established. It was decided eventually that only those cases from whom poliovirus was isolated would be categorized as "confirmed." Cases from whom no virus could be isolated but who had clinically compatible residual paralysis at 60 days, or who were lost to follow-up or had died were placed in the category of "polio compatible" [30].

Establishing the laboratories proved to be far more difficult and time-consuming than had been anticipated. The selected diagnostic laboratories were few in number but they were among the most experienced laboratories in Latin America in tissue culture diagnosis. Nevertheless, despite use of standardized protocols and the provision by Pan American Health Organization of supplies and reagents, more than 2 years were to elapse before results from each of them could be fully relied upon.

Needless to say, the "confirmed cases" were those upon which most attention was focused; at the same time, all were conscious of the fact that there was a not inconsequential number of patients in the "compatible" category from whom virus might have been recovered if patients had been seen more promptly after onset; or if the stool specimens had been transported under better conditions of refrigeration; or if the laboratory itself were functioning more adequately. Clearly, it was critical to minimize the number in the uncertain "compatible" category in order to understand and to be able to follow polio epidemiologically. This was accomplished with ever more rigorous supervision of programs in Latin America to assure that reported cases were investigated rapidly, that proper specimens were obtained and transported, and that laboratories were regularly tested for quality control. As reporting improved, program staff became more confident that they could delineate the remaining endemic areas and take active measures to stop transmission. Of special help was the discovery that by genomic sequencing of the viruses, specific lineages of each strain could be identified as well as the likely epidemiological linkages between cases and outbreaks in different parts of Latin America [31].

Special contributions of the surveillance program in the Americas

Soon after the program began, outbreaks of type 3 polio were discovered in Brazil and later in Mexico. Brazilian investigators found that most of those with polio had been fully vaccinated and thus they suspected possible deficiencies in the vaccine. Special studies were undertaken and this proved to be the case. It was found that by doubling the concentration of the type 3 component of the vaccine, three times as many children had a satisfactory serological response [29]. With the reformulated vaccine, type 3 polio rapidly disappeared.

As polio incidence declined, it became apparent that sustained transmission of the disease, as with smallpox, was occurring in crowded, lower socioeconomic populations. Accordingly, areas at special risk were delineated based on the occurrence of the most recent cases, information on vaccination coverage, population density, and size of migrant populations. These areas encompassed approximately 10% of the Latin American population. In these areas, special house-to-house programs were mounted to vaccinate all children less than 5 years of age [32]. These were termed "Mopup" campaigns. Polio rapidly disappeared from the Americas; the last documented case occurred in October 1991.

The international surveillance program for poliomyelitis

It was clear from the experience in the Americas that reasonably sophisticated health structures and adequate transportation and communication infrastructures were requisite to a successful eradication program. To endeavor to repeat the experience of the Americas in areas of Asia and Africa where medical care facilities were more limited and experienced health personnel much fewer in number was recognized to be a formidable undertaking, undoubtedly requiring significant adaptations of strategy and considerable financial resources. However, without evaluation or further study nor a written plan, the 1988 World Health Assembly voted to embark on a global polio eradication initiative [33].

The strategies and methodology for the eradication effort in the Americas were adopted essentially without modification albeit with one important exception. For more than a decade, little attention was paid to fostering the development of polio surveillance in most developing countries, even in countries as populous as India [34] and other countries of south Asia. Not until the late 1990s did the global magnitude of the polio problem begin to be defined. However, even as recently as 2006, the actual status of the program was blurred. WHO officials remained constantly optimistic and each year they proclaimed that transmission would be interrupted 18 months hence. The year 2000 goal progressively retreated to 2009. At the end of 2006, WHO stated that there were only four endemic countries (India, Afghanistan, Pakistan, and Nigeria) and, on average, only about 20–25 cases per week. However, there were four other countries where endemic cases had been reported regularly for nearly 2 years (Angola, Democratic Republic of Congo, Yemen, and Ethiopia) but were not considered by WHO to be "endemic," because, at one time, they appeared to have interrupted transmission. These countries were still trying to contain outbreaks that ensued after an importation. In July 2006, one country (Namibia) reported more than 150 cases of severe clinical polio following an importation from Angola. However, since less than 25 cases had been confirmed by virus isolation, the official number that WHO recorded was far lower than the probable number. Moreover, reports from a number of African countries, primarily those geographically proximate to heavily endemic Nigeria, showed exceptionally high rates of cases of acute flaccid paralysis which were identified as "compatible but not confirmed" as polio. What with limited resources for early case detection and investigation, difficulties in transporting properly cooled specimens and laboratories with difficulties in sustaining high qualities of performance, it is likely that, under better circumstances, a substantial number of wild poliovirus would have been isolated. Only then would the cases be registered on the official list of "confirmed" cases. Of even greater concern is the question of how many cases may be occurring in the extensive areas of the Democratic Republic of the Congo, Angola, and southern Sudan where surveillance, at best, is possible only in a comparatively few cities and towns under government control.

Conclusion

An eradication program necessitates a demanding and well-managed surveillance program, a fact that had been apparent during the smallpox eradication campaign and was even more apparent in the original polio eradication program in the Americas. A comparable polio surveillance program on an international scale was greatly delayed in its development. Although many efforts have been made in recent years to rectify serious deficiencies, there is still a great deal of work yet to be done. Meanwhile, encouraging progress is being made in a number of countries to develop additional surveillance programs which could provide an important foundation for effective control of other diseases.

Note: Much of the material in this chapter is drawn from a more comprehensive paper on the surveillance of smallpox which was published in the *International Journal of Epidemiology* in 1976 [35]. An even more complete treatment of the subject with many specific details pertaining to key national programs appears in the book, *Smallpox and Its Eradication* [1].

References

1 Fenner F, Henderson DA, Arita I, Jezek Z, Ladnyi ID. *Smallpox and Its Eradication*. Geneva: World Health Organization; 1988.
2 Bhattacharya S. *Expunging Variola: The Control and Eradication of Smallpox in India 1947–1977*. New Delhi: Orient Longman Private Limited; 2006.
3 Langmuir AD. Evolution of the concept of surveillance in the United States. *Proc R Soc Med* 1971;**64**:681–4.
4 Langmuir AD. The surveillance of communicable diseases of national importance. *N Engl J Med* 1963;**268**:182–92.
5 World Health Organization. Report of the technical discussions at the Twenty-First World Health Assembly. Geneva: World Health Organization; 1968.

6 Henderson DA. Current status of smallpox in the world. *J Commun Dis* 1975;**7**:165.

7 World Health Organization. Expert Committee on Smallpox Eradication; 1972. Second report. WHO technical report series, No. 493.

8 Sarkar JK, Mitra AC, Mukherjee MK, De SK. Virus excretion in smallpox. 2: Excretion in the throat of household contacts. *Bull World Health Organ* 1973;**48**:523–7.

9 Heiner GG, Fatima N, Daniel RW, Cole JL, Anthony RL, McCrumb FR. A study of inapparent infection in smallpox. *Am J Epidemiol* 1971;**94**:252–68.

10 World Health Organization. *Handbook for Smallpox Eradication in Endemic Areas*. Geneva: World Health Organization; 1967.

11 Foege WH, Millar JD, Lane JM. Selective epidemiologic control in smallpox eradication. *Am J Epidemiol* 1971;**94**:311–5.

12 Foege WH, Millar JD, Henderson DA. Smallpox eradication in West and Central Africa. *Bull World Health Organ* 1975;**52**:209–22.

13 Hopkins DR, Lane JM, Cummings ED, Thornton JN, Millar JD. Smallpox in Sierra Leone: the 1968–1969 eradication program. *Am J Trop Med Hyg* 1971;**20**:697–704.

14 Imperato PJ, Sow O, Benitieni F. The persistence of smallpox in remote unvaccinated villages during eradication programme activities. *Acta Tropica* 1973;**30**:261–8.

15 Keja J. *Report on a Visit to the Smallpox Program*. Indonesia: World Health Organization; 1968.

16 Foster SO. *Persistence of Facial Scars of Smallpox in West African Populations*. Geneva: World Health Organization; 1972.

17 World Health Organization. Expert Committee on Smallpox; 1964. First report. WHO technical report series, No. 283.

18 de Quadros CA, Morris L, Azeredo EA, Arnt NT, Tigre CH. Epidemiology of variola minor in Brazil based on a study of 33 outbreaks. *Bull World Health Organ* 1972;**46**:165–71.

19 De Quadros CA, Weithaler KL, Siemon J. Active search operations for smallpox-an Ethiopian experience. *Int J Epidemiol* 1973;**2**:237–40.

20 Sharma MID, Foege WH, Grassett NC. National smallpox eradication programme in India—progress, problems and prospects. *J Commun Dis* 1974;**6**:160–70.

21 Sharma MID, Grassett NC. History of achievement of smallpox "Target Zero" in India. *J Commun Dis* 1975;**7**:171–82.

22 Jha SP, Achari AG. Smallpox eradication programme in Bihar. *J Commun Dis* 1975;**7**:183–7.

23 Srivastave GP, Agarwal RS. Intensive campaign against smallpox in Uttar Pradesh. *J Commun Dis* 1975;**7**:188–94.

24 Basu Mallick KC, Mukerjee RN. Progress of national smallpox eradication programmed in West Bengal until the smallpox "Target Zero" was reached. *J Commun Dis* 1975;**7**:195–8.

25 Singh M. Intensified campaign against smallpox in the Eastern States of India. *J Commun Dis* 1975;**7**:198–202.

26 World Health Organization. *World Health Statistics Annual (1967)*. Geneva: World Health Organization; 1970.

27 Pan American Health Organization. Director announces campaign to eradicate poliomyelitis from the Americas by 1990. *Bull Pan Am Health Organ* 1985;**19**:213–5.

28 Sutter RW, Kew OM, Cochi SL. Poliovirus vaccine-live. In: Plotkin SA, Orenstein WA (eds.), *Vaccines*. Philadelphia: Saunders; 2004:651–705.

29 de Quadros CA, Andrus JK, Olive JM, Macedo CG, Henderson DA. Polio eradication from the Western Hemisphere. *Annu Rev Public Health* 1992;**13**:239–52.

30 Pan American Health Organization. *Polio Eradication Field Guide*, 2nd edn. Washington, DC: Pan American Health Organization; 1988.

31 Kew OM, Nathanson N. Molecular epidemiology of viruses. *Semin Virol* 1995;**6**:357–8.

32 Pan American Health Organization. Operation Mopup. *Expanded Programme on Immunization Newsletter* 1989:3–6.

33 World Health Organization. *Global Eradication of Poliomyelitis by the Year 2000*. Geneva: World Health Organization; 1988.

34 Sathyamala C, Mittal O, Dasgupta R, Priya R. Polio eradication initiative in India: deconstructing the global polio eradication initiative. *Int J Health Serv* 2005;**35**:361–83.

35 Henderson DA. Surveillance of smallpox. *Int J Epidemiol* 1976;**5**:19–28.

Lessons learned from smallpox eradication and severe acute respiratory syndrome outbreak

PART 2: SARS surveillance in Hong Kong and the United States during the 2003 outbreak

Lauren J. Stockman, Thomas Tsang & Umesh D. Parashar

Introduction

The outbreak of severe acute respiratory syndrome (SARS) in late 2002 and early 2003 represents an important and historic example of global, epidemic disease surveillance. The emergence of SARS challenged the global public health community to confront a novel epidemic that spread rapidly from its origins in southern China until it had reached more than 25 other countries within a matter of months [1]. The disease had profound economic and social repercussions in affected regions [1,2]. With its cause initially unknown, anxiety was felt worldwide and the SARS outbreak posed several unique challenges to public health practice and infectious disease surveillance.

Overall the global epidemic of 2003 produced 8098 probable cases of SARS with 774 deaths reported in 29 countries [3]. Some areas were severely affected; in Hong Kong, there were 1755 SARS cases, including 300 deaths within 5 months. In contrast, low incidence areas such as the United States (US) were largely spared and mainly dealt with imported SARS cases. Despite the variation in case number, the efforts to detect, respond to, and prevent SARS spread were immense and required rapid, coordinated response of multiple governments, agencies, and professions. These aspects of SARS surveillance provide us with an opportunity to consider responses that may be effective for future outbreaks of new or emerging pathogens.

In this chapter, we describe the SARS outbreak in Hong Kong and in the US. We compare the surveillance systems implemented in each locality, highlight some of the key challenges, and outline some of the key lessons learned from measures implemented during and after the emergency response; the goal of this assessment is to improve surveillance for future outbreaks of SARS or other global infectious disease threats.

In the winter of 2002, an outbreak of atypical pneumonia (later identified as SARS) characterized by fever, cough, and dyspnea that could rapidly progress to respiratory distress and death was first noted in Guangdong Province, China [4]. A novel coronavirus, called SARS-associated coronavirus (SARS-CoV) was later identified as the etiologic agent of SARS [5–7]. A notable feature of SARS-CoV was its ability to spread efficiently from infected persons to their close contacts, mainly through respiratory droplets. In February 2003, a physician from Guangdong Province who had himself become infected while treating SARS patients traveled to attend a social gathering in Hong Kong. He stayed at a Hong Kong hotel (Hotel M) for one night while he was ill with SARS symptoms and is believed to have infected at least 12 other guests at the hotel [8]. Some of these infected guests subsequently traveled to other countries and seeded large outbreaks in Hong Kong, Vietnam, Singapore, and Canada (Figure 39(2).1). It was this dramatic chain of transmission that first led to the recognition of

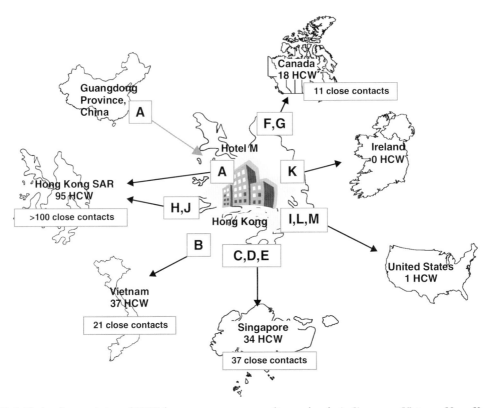

Fig 39(2).1 Chain of transmission of SARS from guests at Hotel M, Hong Kong, March 2003. A = Index guest at Hotel M the night of February 21, 2003. B through M = Guests who reported staying at Hotel M when other persons staying in the hotel were symptomatic. Arrows indicate travel of guests who were ill or subsequently became ill, seeding outbreaks in Singapore, Vietnam, Hong Kong SAR, and Canada. HCW = suspect cases in healthcare workers. Close contacts = a person having cared for, lived with, or had direct contact with respiratory secretions of bodily fluids of a person with SARS. (Adapted from Ref. [8].)

SARS by the global community and prompted the World Health Organization (WHO) to issue an historic alert calling for immediate global efforts to contain the outbreak [9].

Several measures were used to control the global SARS outbreak [10]. Nearly all countries implemented fundamental measures for early identification of SARS cases and prompt implementation of appropriate infection control measures and monitoring of contacts of SARS cases. Countries that were severely affected by the SARS outbreak, such as Hong Kong, used additional measures such as quarantine of close contacts of SARS patients, enhanced overall infection control measures in healthcare facilities, as well as social distancing measures such as suspension of schools and border health measures. Through these measures, the SARS outbreak was effectively contained within 4 months of its global spread. Control of the SARS outbreak was facilitated by the facts that SARS transmission generally required close contact with infected persons, the virus was only moderately infectious [11–13], patients were not infectious prior to symptom onset, and patients were less infectious in early stages of illness than during the second week of illness, allowing additional time to implement containment measures before peak infectiousness [14].

Unique aspects of SARS

- The agent of disease was novel.
- Modes of transmission and effective preventative measures were not initially known.
- WHO issued a rare global alert in response to the spread of SARS to several countries in a short period of time.
- SARS invoked international fear and anxiety.
- Healthcare workers were among the most affected.
- Surveillance for SARS required the integration of international organizations.

SARS surveillance in Hong Kong and the US

Hong Kong

In response to an announcement on February 10, 2003, by the Health Department of Guangdong Province, China, about an outbreak of 300 cases of atypical pneumonia, Hong Kong initiated a surveillance system for severe community-acquired pneumonia. The case definition was community-acquired pneumonia that required intubation or admission to intensive care unit. All public and private hospitals were required to report patients who had illnesses fulfilling the severe community-acquired pneumonia case definition to the Department of Health. Each patient underwent laboratory investigation for a defined panel of respiratory pathogens and their contacts were traced and placed under medical surveillance. During February, surveillance detected 39 cases, a few of whom later turned out to have SARS. In addition, the Department of Health monitored the number of hospital discharges due to pneumonia on a weekly basis.

When an outbreak at Prince of Wales Hospital was identified in early March, a case definition was developed based on epidemiological, clinical, and radiological features of atypical pneumonia seen at the hospital. Active surveillance was initiated and all hospitals were required to submit daily reports including zero reporting (reports of no cases) to the Department of Health and the Hospital Authority, which managed all public hospitals in Hong Kong.

In mid-March, WHO published its case definition for SARS. This definition proved difficult to apply in Hong Kong because it included residence in or travel to a SARS-affected area as one of the epidemiologic criteria, and by definition all patients in Hong Kong met the criteria. By the third week of March, a revised case definition was developed by Hong Kong health authorities and cases were categorized into probable, suspected, under observation, and noncases. Persons meeting the various case classifications elicited a different set of public health measures. Toward the end of March, SARS was made a statutorily notifiable disease in Hong Kong. In early April, diagnostic tests for SARS-CoV gradually became available and polymerase chain reaction and serologic testing for SARS-CoV emerged as the gold standard. SARS-CoV testing was performed at three centers in Hong Kong: the Department of Health Public Health Laboratory Center and laboratories at two local medical universities.

On March 31, 2003, the Department of Health required persons meeting the WHO definition for close contacts of SARS cases to visit one of four designated medical centers daily for 10 days after last contact with a SARS case. Starting April 10, 2003, household contacts of SARS cases were put under compulsory home quarantine for 10 days. Quarantine was supervised by teams of visiting nurses who monitored each household and enforced by police who made spot compliance checks. To prevent the spread of SARS through international travel, household contacts of SARS patients who were being monitored and under quarantine were not allowed to leave Hong Kong during their quarantine period. This was further enforced by the Department of Health which required all departing, arriving, and transit passengers at airport, seaport, and land border control points to undergo thermal screening (a practice used to measure body temperature by either full-body scan or skin) and to complete health declaration forms.

The US

On March 17, 2003, the US Centers for Disease Control and Prevention (CDC) developed an initial

SARS case definition based on the WHO definition and launched national surveillance. The surveillance system was based on detection and passive reporting from clinicians rather than active surveillance to identify potential SARS cases. State and local health authorities received reports from clinicians and reported to CDC all respiratory illnesses that met the WHO case definition for SARS or were considered under investigation for SARS for other reasons. The case definition included clinical and epidemiologic criteria and the latter were based on links to either another SARS patient or travel to a SARS-affected area. SARS-affected areas that constituted an epidemiologic link changed throughout the outbreak, requiring continual modification of the case definition (Table 39(2).1). In general, cases classified as "suspect" presented with moderate respiratory illness of unknown etiology and, within 10 days prior to symptom onset, had close contact with a person suspected to have SARS or recent history of travel to areas reporting cases of SARS. Cases were classified as "probable" if they met the definition of

suspect case with the addition of radiographic evidence of pneumonia, respiratory distress syndrome, or autopsy findings of respiratory distress syndrome without an identifiable cause. At the end of April, the case definition was changed to incorporate criteria for laboratory-confirmed illness.

Clinical specimens, including acute- and convalescent-phase serum, stool, and nasopharyngeal or oropharyngeal swabs were sought from all case patients. Serum specimens were tested for SARS-CoV antibodies and stool and respiratory specimens were tested for SARS-CoV by reverse-transcriptase polymerase chain reaction. Diagnostic testing was initially centralized at CDC, but was later expanded to public health laboratories in various states after reagents were distributed more widely. Diagnostic testing for a wide array of bacterial and viral pathogens was also ordered at the discretion of the physician.

For surveillance among travelers, domestic ports of entry were staffed with surveillance officers who distributed information on SARS symptoms

Table 39(2).1 Changes to the US SARS case definition.

Date	Change to CDC case definition used in the US
March 17, 2003	Initial case definition for SARS is developed based on WHO definition *All* cases classified as suspect cases • Clinical criteria: Respiratory illness of unknown etiology with onset since February 1, 2003, including temperature >38°C and findings of respiratory illness • Epidemiologic link criteria: Travel within 10 days of symptom onset to area with documented or suspected community transmission of SARS, *or* Close contact within 10 days of symptom onset with either a person with respiratory illness who had traveled to SARS area or a person suspected to have SARS [8]
March 28, 2003	• Hong Kong Special Administrative Region and Guangdong Province, China; Hanoi, Vietnam, and Singapore are defined as areas with documented or suspected community transmission of SARS [15]
April 29, 2003	• CDC adopts WHO definition and now includes suspect and probable classifications • Clinical criteria are revised to reflect the possible spectrum of respiratory illness associated with SARS-CoV • Criteria for laboratory-confirmed illness are added after SARS-CoV is identified as the etiologic agent of SARS. Requirement for convalescent-phase serum is >21 days • Mainland China, Taiwan, and Toronto are added to the list of areas with documented or suspected community transmission of SARS [16]
July 18, 2003	• Requirement for convalescent-phase serum is revised to >28 days after symptom onset based on data that some persons with SARS-CoV infection might not mount a detectable antibody response until >28 days after illness onset [17]

to passengers arriving from SARS-affected areas. Thermal scanning to screen incoming passengers for SARS was not used. Contact investigations of household contacts, healthcare workers, and airline contacts were initiated by state and local health authorities. Apart from healthcare workers who had a high-risk exposure (e.g., intubating a SARS patient), quarantine of asymptomatic contacts of SARS patients was not routinely performed in the US.

Descriptions of SARS outbreaks in Hong Kong and the US during 2003

Hong Kong

The index patient of the Hong Kong SARS outbreak was admitted to Prince of Wales Hospital on March 4, 2003, due to respiratory symptoms. This patient was infected during the outbreak at Hotel M that was initiated by a visiting professor from Guangdong Province (Figure 39(2).1). Transmission among hospital staff and visitors, as well as secondary transmission among household members, resulted in over 250 SARS cases. In 3 weeks time, the epidemic had spread to other hospitals in Hong Kong and to a limited extent in the community, amounting to a case count of 624. In late March,

there was a large community outbreak of 329 cases at Amoy Gardens, a densely populated residential housing estate. Environmental transmission, mediated via a contaminated sewer system and high concentrations of viral aerosols in estate buildings, was believed to have played a significant part in the genesis of this outbreak [18–20]. By the time the SARS outbreak in Hong Kong was contained in early June, 1755 SARS cases, including 300 deaths, were reported (Figure 39(2).2). Although the initial identification of SARS cases was based on clinical and epidemiologic criteria only, approximately 80% of the 1755 cases were confirmed by laboratory testing to be infected with SARS-CoV. Hong Kong health authorities also monitored close contacts and household contacts of SARS patients. Thirty-nine close contacts out of approximately 15,800 attendances monitored at designated medical centers and 34 of 1262 quarantined household contacts developed SARS.

The US

The initial cases of SARS in the US were also among guests who were infected at Hotel M in Hong Kong in early March 2003. From March 17 to July 20, 2003, CDC received reports from

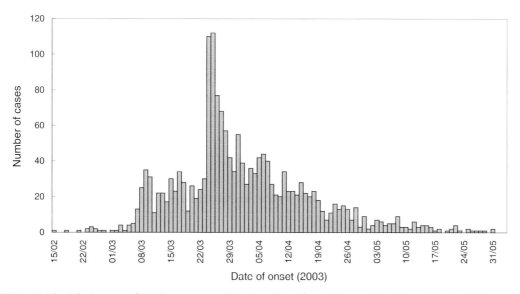

Fig 39(2).2 Epidemiologic curve of SARS cases reported in Hong Kong from February 15, 2003 to May 31, 2003.

41 states and Puerto Rico of 1460 respiratory illnesses under evaluation for SARS [21]. Of these, 326 met the case definition for suspect SARS and 72 met the definition for probable SARS. In contrast to the situation in Hong Kong, a very small proportion of these reported patients were confirmed by laboratory testing to be infected with SARS-CoV. Of 398 patients meeting the definitions for suspect and probable SARS, 8 (2%) were confirmed to be infected with SARS-CoV, 206 (52%) were confirmed to be negative, and the status of 184 (46%) patients could not be determined because convalescent-phase serum was not available (Figure 39(2).3). All 8 patients with SARS-CoV infection were initially classified as probable SARS; no deaths were reported among these patients. Investigations among healthcare workers caring for these 8 patients and household members of the patients failed to identify evidence of secondary transmission except in one possible instance [22–24].

Challenges in SARS surveillance

Nonspecific and evolving case definition

Prompt detection of SARS cases followed by rapid implementation of infection control measures was the fundamental strategy for control of SARS. However, two features of SARS-CoV disease posed challenges for case surveillance. First, the early signs and symptoms were not specific enough to reliably distinguish SARS-CoV disease from other common respiratory illnesses. Second, existing laboratory diagnostic tests were not adequately sensitive early in the course of illness to exclude a diagnosis of SARS. The initial WHO case definition was broad and described a nonspecific, influenza-like illness with epidemiologic linkages of contact with other SARS patients or travel to SARS-affected areas. This broad and sensitive case definition allowed for early identification of all possible SARS cases. However, the definition lacked a high specificity and this meant that many patients with nonspecific respiratory illnesses were mislabeled as SARS, thereby generating considerable anxiety among patients and consuming substantial healthcare and public health resources for response. The absence of a laboratory test to rule out SARS during early illness meant that decisions on patient management and public health measures had to be based on consideration of the nonspecific clinical and epidemiologic criteria alone. Even in countries that were severely affected by the outbreak such as Hong Kong, approximately two-thirds of initial SARS notifications

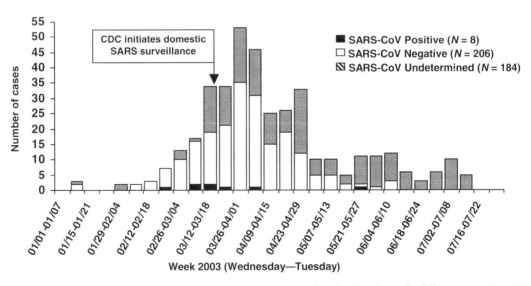

Fig 39(2).3 Epidemiologic curve of the number of US SARS cases reported to the CDC by week of illness onset ($N = 398$), January 8, 2003 to July 15, 2003. (From Ref. [21].)

Challenges to SARS surveillance

- Early signs of SARS were not specific. Symptoms appeared similar to common respiratory illnesses.
- Laboratory diagnostic tests were not sensitive early in the course of illness.
- Transmission dynamics were not completely understood.
- The need for healthcare and public health resources to identify and monitor people in quarantine or isolation was substantial.
- The case definition was reliant on exposure within or travel to SARS-affected areas.
- Awareness of SARS activity by all who applied the case definition in surveillance efforts was necessary.
- Contacts needed to be monitored for development of disease across international boundaries.
- Policies of management of contacts and mandate of quarantine varied between countries.

turned out not to be true SARS-CoV cases on subsequent investigation. In countries such as the US that were not severely affected, less than 1% of all SARS notifications were confirmed to be true SARS-CoV cases.

Modifications to the clinical and epidemiologic criteria in the case definition were necessary as more was learned about the clinical features of SARS, as diagnostic tests became available, and as the epidemic spread to involve additional countries. Changing case definitions were a potential source of confusion for reporting doctors and public health authorities, and sometimes required user interpretation (e.g., radiological features in chest X-rays). Furthermore, each change in the case definition required coordination at both the global and national levels, notification at all levels in the clinical and public health systems, and modifications to reporting forms and databases.

Screening for SARS among travelers

Travel across international borders, especially air travel, played a key role in rapid global spread of the SARS outbreak. Therefore, many countries and WHO issued advisories against travel to SARS-affected areas and extensive efforts were made to identify potential SARS cases among travelers. A variety of approaches were used to inform and screen entering and exiting travelers, including signs, videos, public address announcements, health alert notices that asked passengers to see a physician if they began to have any symptoms related to SARS, screening questionnaires to assess symptoms and possible exposure, visual inspection to detect symptoms, and thermal scanning. These methods required substantial resources (e.g., the US deployed more than 50 CDC staff to various ports of entry to distribute health alert notices to incoming passengers), and in many instance no predefined mechanisms for effective implementation existed.

Contact tracing and monitoring

Rapid identification, evaluation, and monitoring of contacts of SARS patients were important for identifying potential prospective SARS cases and for containing further transmission. Contact tracing, however, was particularly challenging as the dynamics of transmission of SARS were not completely understood. It was clear early in the outbreak that healthcare workers and household contacts of SARS patients were at risk of infection. Monitoring these groups alone for the full range of incubation of 10 days required substantial effort. However, the duration and intensity of exposure required for transmission was not completely understood and it was not clear if individuals exposed to SARS patients in other settings with less intense exposure (e.g., airplanes, schools, or offices) were also at risk. In addition, it was not known in the early stages of the outbreak if patients were infectious prior to the onset of clinical disease and at what phase of their illness they were most infectious. The lack of knowledge on these key epidemiological parameters created substantial challenges in deciding the optimal strategy for contact tracing and management.

Contact tracing and monitoring across international borders posed special challenges. Information on potential contacts of SARS patients that traveled had to be rapidly communicated to public health authorities in destination countries, requiring substantial coordination and effort. In some instances, because policies regarding management of contacts of SARS patients varied between countries (e.g., the US did not impose mandatory quarantine for close contacts unlike most other countries), there was confusion and disagreement between health authorities in different countries on appropriate strategies for management of contacts. Many legal and ethical issues had to be addressed as in most countries large-scale quarantine of this magnitude had not been imposed in decades and public health laws required modification. Notification of passengers that may have been exposed to SARS patients during air travel was sometimes difficult because contact information was not rapidly available in an electronic format from airline manifests.

Data management

Collecting clinical and epidemiological information from case patients and contacts and real-time analysis of the data to monitor trends in the epidemic was critical to the effective response to SARS but proved to be a challenge in all countries. In Hong Kong, during the first 3 weeks of the SARS outbreak, the Department of Health received notifications of SARS cases from hospitals via fax and e-mail. Each SARS report was followed up and a standardized questionnaire was administered to collect data. Case data was entered into static electronic databases for epidemiological analysis and daily situation updates. The escalating outbreak soon overwhelmed this system of data management. The information systems managing patient clinical data, epidemiological data, and laboratory data operated on different platforms and direct electronic data transfer and automatic linkage of records across the different systems could not be achieved. Instead, databases and spreadsheets of SARS cases kept by the Department of Health and the Hospital Authority were exchanged at periodic intervals. This led to considerable confusion in differentiating new cases from old cases, eliminating double entries, reconciling conflicting data, updating case status, and incorporating laboratory results. Data input was also problematic as the system relied considerably on paper forms (e.g., patient hospital records, epidemiological questionnaires, laboratory results) and the questionnaires were revised numerous times. Finally, there was no automated system to support contact tracing and quarantine of the large number of contacts involved.

Similar challenges were encountered in the US. US physicians were asked to report suspect and probable SARS cases to their local and state health departments. State health departments then reported these data on paper-based forms to CDC; there the information was entered into a centralized database. As updated information (e.g., new clinical or radiographic data, laboratory results) on each case became available, it was reported again through a similar paper-based mechanism and each entry was manually updated. The results of laboratory testing at CDC were entered into a different database. Although the centralized database at CDC could be used to link results of specimen testing with the clinical and epidemiological information, the real-time analysis capabilities were limited because reporting to the CDC was paper-based and data were entered manually.

Communications

In Hong Kong, many communication challenges were identified during the SARS epidemic. Some private doctors expressed concern that due to inadequacies of information systems and the sheer volume of work, they did not receive feedback concerning the progress and outcome of SARS case patients that they reported. In some instances, data ownership and sharing issues, especially when cross-disciplinary stakeholders were involved, created obstacles in compiling integrated databases and putting the surveillance data to full use.

In the US, similar challenges in communicating surveillance information were encountered. Because of the paper-based reporting mechanisms, obtaining information on cases reported to CDC and feedback of results of laboratory testing at CDC was arduous and time-consuming. In addition, there was considerable media interest in progression of the SARS epidemic and it was a challenge to provide accurate reports on the numbers of suspect and probable SARS cases on Web sites of the state health departments and CDC.

Lessons learned and measures to improve future surveillance efforts

Case-based surveillance

For diseases such as SARS for which early identification of cases is needed for containment of transmission, developing case definitions based on clinical and epidemiological features alone requires a suitable balance of sensitivity and specificity. At the operational level, the problem of low specificity arising from a broad case definition can be partially mitigated by stratification of cases into categories according to the likelihood of being true cases (e.g., confirmed, probable, suspect, under observation) and implementing different levels of public health action for cases in each category, as was done in Hong Kong. Since missing even a single case of SARS can have tremendous implications in terms of propagating the outbreak, aggressive public health action should be implemented for each potential case. As more is learned about the clinical and epidemiological features of the disease, case definitions

must be continually refined. The formation of an expert panel consisting of clinicians and public health experts that had experience with SARS helped to reduce interobserver variation in interpreting clinical and radiological features and improved the specificity of diagnosis; such a strategy should be considered for future epidemics. When diagnostic tests for SARS first became available, compatibility of test results and quality assurance across different laboratories were important issues to address. To the extent possible, standardized protocols for testing and interpretation of test results should be developed. Verification of test results by another laboratory or a designated reference laboratory is another useful safeguard, especially in the early stages of an outbreak.

Screening for SARS in travelers

Although SARS was contained largely by aggressive use of traditional public health interventions, the effectiveness of entry and exit screening and other

What was needed	Action taken or solution proposed

• A constant exchange and update of information	• Case counts and information were disseminated via:
	   - Daily press conferences
	   - Daily postings on the Internet
	   - Relayed to WHO via e-mail
	• A command post was established to provide data to media through one official source

• Consistent case counts between local, national, and international health agencies	• Health agencies communicated more frequently and sought confirmation before posting counts • Clearer and more consistent case definitions evolved
• A rapid and accessible system to receive case data	• Initially, existing information systems were adopted or modified for SARS • A Web-based, real-time system for collecting case records was developed
• A timely and complete manifest of airlines which carried a potential SARS case	• Public health agencies worked closely with the airline industry • Standardized forms and secure data systems have been developed to collect passenger contact information
• Test results that were compatible across different and international laboratories	• Protocols for testing and interpretation were standardized • Test results were verified by a reference laboratory

measures to detect SARS among travelers remains uncertain. Reviews of these measures, such as the distribution of health alert notices to passengers departing flights from SARS-affected areas, thermal screening of incoming travelers, and quarantine of incoming travelers, was conducted [10,25]. The data suggest that measures to enhance surveillance for SARS among travelers required considerable resources to implement and the effectiveness of these measures requires further evaluation. In addition to determining which measures are most effective, efforts should also focus on determining the most resource-efficient ways to implement these measures.

Contact tracing and monitoring

During the height of the SARS outbreak in Hong Kong, nurses, auxiliary medical personnel, and even police officers were recruited to conduct telephone interviews with contacts of SARS cases to monitor their health. In addition, administrative and executive personnel provided the much needed back-end logistics support for the execution of quarantine. A predetermined manpower mobilization and training plan at different stages of an outbreak was vital for effective implementation of contact tracing and monitoring. The number of individuals needed to employ a monitoring and quarantine program, with or without activity restriction, highlights the need to build up surge capacity for future outbreaks of SARS or other diseases for which such a response would be needed.

Several countries, including the US, have implemented changes that will allow passenger contact information to be more easily accessed by public health authorities in a timely manner and have also identified mechanisms to rapidly contact and notify passengers. The CDC has developed a passenger locator form to collect contact information from passengers in a machine-readable format. In the event of an international disease outbreak, this locator form has been made available to the airlines and can be used if a request is initiated by CDC. Since the SARS outbreak, a software application called eManifest has been developed by the CDC for internal use to securely import, sort, and assign passenger-locating information to jurisdictions in order to facilitate timely identification of

exposed persons. These data can be securely transmitted to state and territorial health departments for notification of potentially exposed passengers [26].

Data management

In Hong Kong, three information systems were developed to improve reporting of information on SARS cases and their contacts and to identify common exposures among patients. The urgency of the situation did not allow time to build entirely new systems de novo. Instead, existing information systems were adopted, modified, and connected to produce the desired functions. In early April 2003, a real-time electronic platform for SARS reporting (E-SARS) was set up linking public hospitals and the Department of Health. E-SARS is a Web-based, online clinical record system capturing patient data entered at all public hospitals. It contained a limited set of data for each SARS patient, such as demographics, hospital admission details, basic symptoms, laboratory test results, and probable source of infection. Because of its online nature, registered users could access and update case records on a common, single platform at any time and in real time. E-SARS thus eliminated the problems associated with managing a large number of different static databases operated by different groups. It was particularly useful for monitoring changing case status of patients with suspected SARS. The second application was a contact-tracing system relating data on SARS case patients and their contacts. It included cluster analysis functions for the construction of cluster trees from SARS case patients with known probable exposures. The third system was derived from a criminal tracking system known as MIIDSS used by the police. This system was capable of standardizing names of local buildings and street addresses, displaying alerts on geographical clusters and common exposures among cases. Together, these systems vastly improved the speed and efficiency of gathering, management, and analysis of data on SARS patients and their contacts.

In the US, a Web-based case reporting system that allows transmission of data from state health departments to CDC was developed to eliminate the many problems of using a paper-based reporting system. This system allows direct entry of patient information on a Web-based interface through a secure log-in system and also allows the upload of information from existing databases at state health departments that wish to maintain their own database. This electronic reporting system allows for frequent updates of data as additional clinical, epidemiological, and laboratory data become available. It also allows linkage with laboratory results of testing of specimens centrally at CDC and transmission of the information back to state health departments (Figure 39(2).4). To facilitate identification and monitoring of contacts of SARS patients, a software platform that contains relational databases has been developed and disseminated to various jurisdictions.

Communications

At a national level, it was paramount to maintain good communications with all parties involved in the SARS surveillance and response. Communication channels needed to be rapid and flexible enough to accommodate the highly dynamic situation (e.g., changing case definitions, laboratory test requirements). Similar coordination was required at

the international level to facilitate communications across countries, to monitor global progression of the epidemic, and to disseminate new data as they become available.

In Hong Kong, case counts and related information on SARS were disseminated via daily press conferences, posted daily on the Internet, and relayed to the WHO via e-mail. To facilitate daily update of case counts and communication of surveillance data, the Department of Health set up a designated command post staffed with doctors and personnel experienced with database management. This command post acted as a central data repository and became the sole official source providing SARS statistics to the media enquiries, thereby reducing the chance that inconsistent or conflicting data would be disseminated. At the height of the SARS outbreak, more than 100 manned hotlines were set up addressing public enquiries on SARS. However, the utility of hotline as a case surveillance tool was limited. Learning from the SARS experience, the Department of Health developed an electronic Web-based case reporting system covering all notifiable infectious diseases (including SARS) that could be used by all registered doctors.

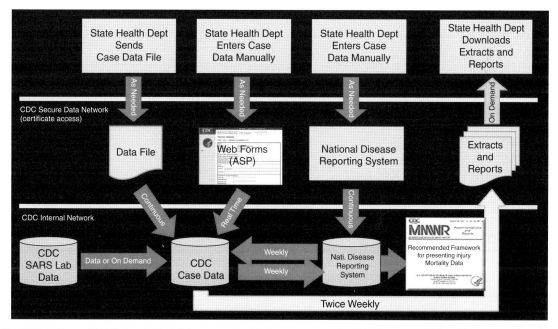

Fig 39(2).4 Flow of SARS data in the US from state health departments to the CDC by means of data files, Internet-based forms, and a national disease reporting system.

In the US, rapidly evolving information on the outbreak, including changes in the case definition, was disseminated to state and local health departments through an electronic network of public health professionals, through CDC's Health Alert Network and though CDC's Web site. Telephone hotlines were also set up at CDC and staffed by epidemiologists who could verify that local health authorities reported case patients using the most current case definition. Case-reporting activity by state was posted on the CDC Web site and case counts were sent to WHO by e-mail.

Conclusions

Containing the 2003 SARS outbreak required a rapid, intense, and coordinated global public health response. Surveillance for early detection of SARS cases and for management of their close contacts was a key component of this response. Although the SARS outbreaks in Hong Kong and the US differed considerably in scope, many of the challenges in implementing effective surveillance and lessons learned were similar. Immediate establishment of a working case definition is crucial, even in situations with a new illness like SARS for which key clinical and epidemiological information is lacking, and this definition will likely require modification as more information becomes available. Monitoring of illness among travelers and contacts of SARS cases required considerable resources, and efforts are needed to determine the most effective and practical implementation strategies for use in similar outbreaks in the future. Collection of real-time data on SARS cases and their contacts that could be rapidly analyzed to provide information to guide the public health response was a major challenge. Global coordination of these efforts was further complicated by differences in technological capability and resources across countries. Effective communication strategies are vital to rapidly disseminate new findings and strategies. Many of these lessons were utilized by countries around the world to enhance preparedness for effective surveillance and response to a possible resurgence of SARS or other diseases. These preparedness measures will also improve the capacity of the global healthcare and public health community to respond to other emergencies such as a possible pandemic of influenza.

References

1 Knobler S, Mahmoud A, Lemon S, Mack A, Sivitz L, Oberholtzer K (eds.). *Workshop Summary in Learning from SARS: Preparing for the Next Disease Outbreak.* Washington: National Academies Press; 2004. Available from: http://www.iom.edu/CMS/3783/3924/18086.aspx. Accessed November 6, 2006.

2 World Travel and Tourism Council. The impact of travel and tourism on jobs and the economy, China and China Hong Kong SAR, 2003. Available from: http://www.wttc.org/publications/pdf/China-Hong%20Kong.pdf. Accessed November 6, 2006.

3 World Health Organization. Cumulative number of reported probable cases of severe acute respiratory syndrome (SARS) 2003. Available from: http://www.who.int/csr/sars/country/table2004_04_21/en/index.html. Accessed November 6, 2006.

4 Breiman RF, Evans MR, Preiser W, *et al.* Role of China in the quest to define and control severe acute respiratory syndrome. *Emerg Infect Dis* September 2003;**9**(9):1037–41.

5 Peiris JS, Lai ST, Poon LL, *et al.* Coronavirus as a possible cause of severe acute respiratory syndrome. *Lancet* April 2003;**361**(9366):1319–25.

6 Ksiazek TG, Erdman D, Goldsmith CS, *et al.* A novel coronavirus associated with severe acute respiratory syndrome. *N Engl J Med* May 2003;**348**(20):1953–66.

7 World Health Organization. A multicentre collaboration to investigate the cause of severe acute respiratory syndrome. *Lancet* May 2003;**361**(9370):1730–3.

8 Update: outbreak of severe acute respiratory syndrome—worldwide, 2003. *MMWR Morb Mortal Wkly Rep* March 2003;**52**(12):241–6, 248.

9 World Health Organization. World Health Organization issues emergency travel advisory; March 15, 2003. Available from: http://www.who.int/csr/sars/archive/2003_03_15/en. Accessed July 3, 2006.

10 Bell DM. Public health interventions and SARS spread, 2003. *Emerg Infect Dis* November 2004;**10**(11):1900–6.

11 Lipsitch M, Cohen T, Cooper B, *et al.* Transmission dynamics and control of severe acute respiratory syndrome. *Science* June 2003;**300**(5627):1966–70.

12 Dye C, Gay N. Epidemiology: modeling the SARS epidemic. *Science* June 2003;**300**(5627):1884–5.

13 Riley S, Fraser C, Donnelly CA, *et al.* Transmission dynamics of the etiological agent of SARS in Hong Kong: impact of public health interventions. *Science* June 2003;**300**(5627):1961–6.

14 Peiris JS, Chu CM, Cheng VC, *et al.* Clinical progression and viral load in a community outbreak of coronavirus-associated SARS pneumonia: a prospective study. *Lancet* May 2003;**361**(9371):1767–72.

15 Outbreak of severe acute respiratory syndrome—worldwide, 2003. *MMWR Morb Mortal Wkly Rep* March 2003;**52**(11):226–8.

16 Updated interim surveillance case definition for severe acute respiratory syndrome (SARS)—United States, April 29, 2003. *MMWR Morb Mortal Wkly Rep* May 2003;**52**(17):391–3.

17 Update: severe acute respiratory syndrome—worldwide and United States. *MMWR Morb Mortal Wkly Rep* July 2003;**52**(28):664–5.

18 World Health Organization. Environmental Health Teams Reports on Amoy Gardens. Available from: http://www.info.gov.hk/info/sars/who-amoye.pdf. Accessed July 3, 2006.

19 McKinney KR, Gong YY, Lewis TG. Environmental transmission of SARS at Amoy Gardens. *J Environ Health* May 2006;**68**(9):26–30.

20 Yu IT, Li Y, Wong TW, *et al.* Evidence of airborne transmission of the severe acute respiratory syndrome virus. *N Engl J Med* April 2004;**350**(17):1731–9.

21 Schrag SJ, Brooks JT, Van Beneden C, *et al.* SARS surveillance during emergency public health response, United States, March–July 2003. *Emerg Infect Dis* February 2004;**10**(2):185–94.

22 Park BJ, Peck AJ, Kuehnert MJ, *et al.* Lack of SARS transmission among healthcare workers, United States. *Emerg Infect Dis* February 2004;**10**(2):244–8.

23 Peck AJ, Newbern EC, Feikin DR, *et al.* Lack of SARS transmission and US SARS case-patient. *Emerg Infect Dis* February 2004;**10**(2):217–24.

24 Isakbaeva ET, Khetsuriani N, Beard RS, *et al.* SARS-associated coronavirus transmission, United States. *Emerg Infect Dis* February 2004;**10**(2):225–31.

25 Bell DM. Non-pharmaceutical interventions for pandemic influenza, international measures. *Emerg Infect Dis* January 2006;**12**(1):81–7.

26 Exposure to mumps during air travel—United States, April 2006. *MMWR Morb Mortal Wkly Rep* April 2006;**55**(14):401–2.

40 Future directions in infectious disease surveillance

Ruth Lynfield, Nkuchia M. M'ikanatha, Chris A. Van Beneden & Henriette de Valk

Infectious diseases will continue to plague, challenge, and inspire us to improve and protect the public's health. Surveillance, the instrument of detection, is truly the cornerstone for the prevention and control of infectious diseases. This book has attempted to describe practical approaches toward conducting surveillance for a number of different infectious diseases using classical and innovative methods. Our aim was to provide a framework of possibilities for the reader to review and apply to his or her situation. We also attempted to warn the reader of potential stumbling blocks to implementation and maintenance of effective surveillance for various pathogens.

The specific applications of an infectious disease surveillance program will depend upon local needs, priorities, and resources. Just as infectious diseases evolve, so too will surveillance programs. However, some common lessons emerge. Successful surveillance depends upon the cooperation and collaboration of many individuals across many disciplines including professionals in clinical medicine, infection control, microbiology, veterinary medicine, agriculture, entomology, law, public safety, communication, and health economics. These partnerships will help identify obstacles and explore tools already available. It is invaluable to utilize experiences and lessons learned by other public health professionals. Also, to maintain advancements in the fields of infectious disease surveillance and epidemiology, collaborations with academic researchers are important. More than in any other field of science or medicine, public health profession-

als must know how to work with local, regional, and central governments in order to effectively carry out activities. We have also learned from smallpox and severe acute respiratory syndrome (SARS) that infectious diseases do not recognize borders and collaboration of public health entities across geographic boundaries can be key to the success of an infectious disease program.

Political unrest continues to result in the formation of refugee populations, with amplification of poverty and disease. In addition, natural disasters such as the tsunami of 2005 have afflicted various parts of the globe, resulting in displaced populations and public health challenges. Geographic areas with limited abilities to provide basic sanitation needs, including clean water, are common. Unfortunately, lack of sanitation, overcrowding, and poverty are unlikely to disappear in the near future, maintaining the stage for large outbreaks of disease. Global cooperation, resources, and innovative thinking in multiple disciplines will be needed to tackle associated population health issues. Infectious disease surveillance will be an important tool to measure the impact of interventions.

There already has been great progress made in international partnerships. For example, the revised International Health Regulations describe a framework for international collaboration for surveillance, provide a means for Member States to build public health capacity by sharing expertise and experience, and in some cases, facilitate training opportunities. It is hoped that the international community will continue to assist resource-limited countries in developing and maintaining core public health capacities for surveillance and outbreak response.

Large outbreaks also occur in industrialized countries. Increases in food production through industrialized agriculture occurring in a small number of big producers can result in large, multistate outbreaks of foodborne disease. Advances in molecular epidemiology can allow the detection of widespread and diffuse outbreaks and provide the momentum for safer agriculture and handling of food. Nevertheless, the continued globalization of food supply and distribution is likely to be matched with more and larger foodborne outbreaks, requiring an ongoing role for surveillance and control. Similarly, international travel provides opportunities for acquisition and transmission of infectious diseases as evidenced by SARS and predicted for avian influenza. The speed at which diseases are spread globally is matched by the need for more rapid, effective tools for integrating surveillance data from multiple countries.

Adverse consequences of advances in medical technology result in additional populations at risk for infectious disease through the increased use of invasive procedures, immunosuppression resulting from therapeutic agents for transplant or treatment of malignancies, a growing population with co-morbidities, and an increased number of elderly. Progress in xenotransplantation introduces unique zoonotic challenges, and engineered bioterrorism remains a global concern. A major tangible issue is the rapid pace at which antimicrobial resistance is increasing, resulting in a significant impairment of our current and future ability to treat infections. At-risk populations for these public health threats include those residing in the community in addition to those in acute-care, long-term-care, or other facilities. Surveillance systems will need to advance in scope and flexibility to effectively encompass and serve all of these populations.

The future will likely bring technological advances in information systems and in other tools that ease the collection and analysis of data. It should be remembered that interpretation of surveillance data and application into public health practice requires a deep understanding of local behaviors, practices, customs, and traditions; the success of interventions to prevent and control disease depends upon the relevance and acceptability of these measures at a local level. Public health is a cooperative venture and the involvement of stakeholders is a critical component of success. This includes the education of many groups, such as the general public, clinicians, and government officials. The investment into establishing a mutual and clear understanding of the issues and the solutions will yield long-standing dividends.

Finally, because surveillance is a rapidly developing field, we would like to emphasize that regular assessment is important to ensure that surveillance systems function optimally and that data are used effectively. The efficiency of the system should be reviewed, taking into account the accuracy of the system, potential obstacles encountered by participants, and the costs and resources required. Public health resources are always finite and in many cases very limited. Responsible use of these resources to identify areas for intervention, identify types of control measures, and monitor the impact of these control measures is an important role for public health professionals. Infectious disease surveillance should be utilized to provide data for decision making. We hope that the future will bring innovations that simultaneously produce an increase in data quality, a decrease in system resources, and applications that advance health locally and globally.

Index